Current Advances in Breast Cancer Research

Current Advances in Breast Cancer Research

Edited by **Sandra Lekin**

hayle medical

New York

Published by Hayle Medical,
30 West, 37th Street, Suite 612,
New York, NY 10018, USA
www.haylemedical.com

Current Advances in Breast Cancer Research
Edited by Sandra Lekin

International Standard Book Number: 978-1-63241-098-6 (Hardback)

Printed in China.

Contents

Preface

Scientists all over the world are researching the causes of breast cancer. In the past few years, it has become pretty apparent that breast cancer encompasses a number of molecularly separate tumors emerging from the epithelial cells of the breast. There is a vital need to comprehend these separate subtypes and build up modified diagnostic procedures and treatments suitable to each. This book considers breast cancer from a lot of original standpoints. New developments in the essential biology of breast cancer are discussed jointly with high throughput approaches to molecular profiling. Modern techniques for analysis and imaging are presented along with evolving perspectives on breast cancer treatment. This book includes contributions from prominent experts in their fields and will be beneficial for readers interested in learning more about breast cancer.

Significant researches are present in this book. Intensive efforts have been employed by authors to make this book an outstanding discourse. This book contains the enlightening chapters which have been written on the basis of significant researches done by the experts.

Finally, I would also like to thank all the members involved in this book for being a team and meeting all the deadlines for the submission of their respective works. I would also like to thank my friends and family for being supportive in my efforts.

Editor

Part 1

Biology

1

Progestogens and Breast Cancer Risk – In Vitro Investigations with Human Benign and Malignant Epithelial Breast Cells

Alfred O. Mueck, Harald Seeger and Hans Neubauer
University Women's Hospital, Tübingen, Germany

1. Introduction

Two recent studies, the Women's Health Initiative (WHI) and the Million Women Study (MWS), have above all raised concerns over the relationship between progestogens and increased risk of breast cancer in the climacteric and postmenopause (Million Women Study collaborators, 2003; Writing Group, 2002). The Women's Health Initiative study was terminated early after five years, due to an increased incidence of breast cancer in the group treated with combined estrogen and progestogen therapy (EPT). The MWS concluded that breast cancer risk was increased two-fold in current users of combined HRT compared to a factor of 1.3 for estrogen-only therapy.

A crucial role of progestogens in increasing breast cancer risk was supported by the WHI estrogen mono-arm showing no increase but rather a reduction of breast cancer risk, which was significant for patients with more than 80% adherence to study medication (The Women's Health Initiative Steering Committee, 2004).

However, in the French E3N-EPIC trial of over 80 000 postmenopausal women it was reported that hormone therapy containing the progestin medroxyprogesterone acetate or norethisterone was associated with a significant increase in risk of breast cancer, whereas hormone therapy including progesterone and certain other progestins did not induce an increased risk (Fournier et al., 2008).

By stimulating the production of survival factors, estradiol (E2) and other steroid hormones may influence cell proliferation. These survival factors include growth factors and cytokines. Epithelial and stromal cell-derived growth factors are understood to be significant in the regulation of breast epithelial cells directly via autocrine, paracrine, juxtacrine or intracrine pathways. Further responses stimulated by growth factors may activate signalling pathways which support the growth of cancer cells (Dickson & Lippman, 1995).

Progestogens are conventionally thought to act via the activation of the intracellularly-located progesterone receptors (PR), PR-A and PR-B. Several *in vitro* studies indicate that progestogens may exert an antiproliferative effect by activation of these receptors in human breast cancer cells (Cappellatti et al. 1995; Krämer et al., 2006; Schoonen et al., 1995). These data are in contrast to the above mentioned clinical data. Other data suggested a proliferative effect of synthetic progestogens (Catherino et al., 1995; Franke & Vermes, 2003). Thus the mechanisms by which progestogens act on human breast cells remain unclear.

Recent experimental data revealed that in addition to the intracellular-located receptors, progesterone receptor membrane component-1 (PGRMC1) is associated with a membrane-associated progesterone receptor activity (Cahill, 2007). PGRMC1 was originally cloned from the endoplasmatic reticulum from porcine hepatocytes (Meyer et al., 1996). It contains several predicted motifs for protein interactions, and overlapping sites for phosphorylation, whose phosphorylation status might correlate with its localisation in the cell (Ahmed et al., 2010, Cahill, 2007; Munton et al. 2007). PGRMC1 has been detected in several cancers and cancer cell lines e.g. breast cancer (Neubauer et al., 2008, 2009). It is overexpressed in lung cancer and colon cancer (Cahill, 2007).

There is a long-standing link between PGRMC1 and progesterone signaling. However, because bacterially expressed PGRMC1 does not bind to progesterone (Min et al., 2005), and since the majority of PGRMC1 is not localized to the plasma membrane (Crudden et al., 2005; Nolte et al., 2000; Peluso et al., 2008) it is now tentatively assumed that PGRMC1 does not bind P4 by itself (Cahill, 2007), but requires an unknown protein that is associated only in partially purified PGRMC1 preparations (Peluso et al., 2008). PGRMC1-associated progesterone binding is functionally important in cancer cells because progesterone inhibits apoptosis in granulosa cells, and this anti-apoptotic activity requires PGRMC1 (Peluso et al., 2008a, 2008b). However, it is unclear how PGRMC1 transduces anti-apoptotic signaling by progesterone. Expression of PGRMC1 has been identified in several subcellular compartments including cell membrane, cytoplasm, endoplasmatic reticulum and nucleus (reviewed in Cahill, 2007). Swiatek-De Lange et al. (2007) reported that PGRMC1 localizes to the plasma membrane and microsomal fraction of retinal cells.

In the following our investigations on the effect of progesterone and various synthetic progestins on the proliferation of human benign and malignant breast epithelial cells with and without expressing PGRMC1 are summarized.

2. Normal breast epithelial cells

MCF10A, a human, non-tumorigenic, estrogen and progesterone receptor-negative breast epithelial cell line was used for these experiments (Catherino et al., 1995, Soule et la., 1990). Progesterone (P4), chlormadinone acetate (CMA), norethisterone (NET), medroxyprogesterone acetate (MPA), gestodene (GSD), 3-ketodesogestrel (KDG) and dienogest (DNG) were tested at the concentration range of 10^{-9} to 10^{-6} M. For stimulation of the MCF-10A cells a mixture of growth factors was used. As outcome proliferation and apoptosis were measured and the ratio of apoptosis to proliferation was compared. Proliferation is quantified by measuring light emitted during the bioluminescence reaction of luciferene in the presence of ATP and luciferase. Apoptosis was measured by the Cell Death Assay, which is based on the quantitative sandwich-enzyme-immunoassay principle using mouse monoclonal antibodies directed against DNA and histones. Photometric enzyme immunoassay quantitatively determines cytoplasmic histone-associated DNA fragments after induced cell death.

The combination of the stroma-derived growth factors epithelial growth factor (EGF),basic-fibroblastic growth factor (FGF) and insulin-like growth factor-I (IGF-I) alone confirmed a proliferative response compared to the assay medium-only control. These growth factors were chosen, since they have been shown to be most effective in terms of breast epithelial cell proliferation (Dickson & Lippman, 1995).

In combination with growth factors, the ratio was reduced significantly compared to the growth factor alone by MPA and CMA (i.e., favouring an additional proliferative effect). MPA produced a four-fold reduction in the ratio in comparison to growth factors alone at 10^{-7} M and 10^{-6} M ($p<0.05$), CMA had a significant effect at 10^{-6} M only, reducing the ratio 3-fold. P4, NET, LNG, DNG, GSD and KDG had no significant effect on the growth factor-induced stimulation of MCF10A (Table 1).

	Normal cells
	Growth factors
Progesterone	Ø
Medroxyprogesterone acetate	--
Chlormadinone acetate	--
Norethisterone	Ø
Levonorgestrel	Ø
3-Keto-desogestrel	Ø
Gestodene	Ø
Dienogest	Ø

Table 1. Effect of various progestins on the ratio of apoptosis to proliferation in normal breast epithelial cells in the presence of stroma-derived growth factors as stimulans. (+ = increase; - = decrease of the ratio; Ø = no effect as compared to the stimulans alone)

3. Cancerous breast epithelial cells

HCC1500, a human estrogen and progesterone receptor-positive primary breast cancer cell line was used (Gazdar et al., 1998). For stimulation of the cells estradiol alone, a growth factor mixture alone as well as a combination of both was used.

The combination of the growth factors EGF, FGF and IGF-I alone confirmed a proliferative response compared to the assay medium-only control. MPA in combination with growth factors caused a significant increase in the ratio of apoptosis to proliferation at both concentrations compared to growth factors alone ($p<0.05$), the greatest effect being at 10^{-7} M, with a doubling of this ratio, i.e., an inhibitory effect. CMA also caused a significant increase in this ratio, with the greatest effect seen at 10^{-6} M, yielding over a 2-fold ratio increase. Conversely, NET, LNG, and DNG at both concentrations and GSD and KDG at 10^{-6} M led to a significant reduction in the ratio of apoptosis to proliferation, enhancing the initial proliferative effect induced by the growth factors. P4 had no significant effect at either concentration.

The results of the combination of the steroids and E2 on the estrogen-receptor positive (ER+) HCC1500 cells showed that the progestins CMA, MPA, NET, LNG, DNG, GSD and P4 significantly increased the ratio of apoptosis to proliferation towards an anti-proliferative

effect to varying degrees compared to E2 alone, with MPA having the greatest effect, followed by NET. KDG had no significant effect at either concentration. No progestin used was able to further enhance the stimulatory effect of E2 on HCC1500 cells, and all but KDG actually inhibited this effect.
The results of combining the steroids with the combination of growth factors (EGF, FGF and IGF-I) and E2 on HCC1500 cells revealed that MPA, GSD, CMA and NET all increased the ratio favouring an anti-proliferative effect compared to the proliferative effect of growth factors and E2 alone. P4, LNG, DNG and KDG had no significant effect at either concentration.

Progestin	**Cancerous cells**		
	Growth factors	Estradiol	Growth factors + Estradiol
Progesterone	+	+	+
Medroxyprogesterone acetate	++	++	++
Chlormadinone acetate	++	++	++
Norethisterone	--	++	++
Levonorgestrel	--	++	++
3-Keto-desogestrel	--	Ø	++
Gestodene	-	++	++
Dienogest	--	+	Ø

Table 2. Effect of various progestins on the ratio of apoptosis to proliferation in cancerous breast epithelial cells in the presence of stroma-derived growth factors, estradiol or a combination of both as stimulans. (+ = increase; - = decrease of the ratio; Ø = no effect as compared to the stimulans alone)

In summary these results indicate that progestins are different in their ability to induce proliferation or inhibit the growth of benign or malignant human breast epithelial cells dependently or independently of the effects of stromal growth factors and E2. Thus on the basis of experimental data the choice of progestin for hormone therapy may be important in terms of influencing a possible breast cancer risk.
A further important result from our experimental research seems to be the fact that the influence of the progestins can differ largely between normal and cancerous breast epithelial cells. This would have clinical relevance for the use of HRT after breast cancer, which is of course contraindicated in routine therapy. But as even in the normal population women express malignant cells, shown by post mortem analyses (Black & Welch, 1993), different, may be contrary progestins effects in benign or malignant cells may have relevance for the primary breast cancer risk of postmenopausal women treated with HRT. Therefore this field should be further investigated.

4. Cancerous breast epithelial cells cells overexpressing PGRMC1

Since the results of the WHI mono arm were published, indicating a negative effect of progestins on breast cancer risk, the molecular pathway responsible for this effect and the many questions on the extrapolation of the WHI results to all synthetic progestins and to natural progesterone remain unknown. We have published for the first time results suggesting that signaling of synthetic progestins via PGRMC1 could be one explanation (Neubauer et al., 2009).

For the experiments two synthetic progestins have been chosen that are widely used in hormone therapy, i.e. MPA and NET, as well as a new synthetic progestin, i.e. DRSP, which might differ in its behaviour to MPA and NET because of a different chemical structure. In addition progesterone and progesterone-3-(O-carboxymethyl) oxime: BSA-fluorescein-isothio cyanate conjugate (P4:BSA-FITC) was tested.

4.1 Transfection of MCF-7 cells

MCF-7 cells were stably transfected with expression vector pcDNA3.1 containing hemeagglutinin-tagged (3HA) PGRMC1 using lipofectamine™ 2000, in accordance with the manufacture's recommendation. A total of $5x10^5$ cells were transfected and plated with RPMI-medium for 24h. Then medium was changed to RPMI complete medium containing 100µg/ml hygromycin B. Cells were cultured for 2 weeks for selection of stable integration events. Transfection rates were measured by cotransfection of a GFP expressing plasmid and immune fluorescence analysis. After 2 weeks single colonies had formed and limiting dilutions were performed three times to select for colonies grown from a single cell.

Stable transfection was verified by PCR using chromosomal DNA and primers spanning intron 1 to distinguish integrated PGRMC1 cDNA from the chromosomal sequence. The sequences of the primers were 5′- CTGCTGCATGAGATTTTCACG-3′ hybridizing to nucleotides 71 to 91 of PGRMC1 open reading frame and 5′-GCATAGTCCGGGACGTCATA-3′ hybridizing to the sequence coding for the HA tag. PCR products were sequenced.

4.2 Effect of synthetic progestins alone

Dose-dependent effects on cell proliferation of P4, P4:BSA-FITC, MPA, NET or DRSP were determined using MTT assay (Fig. 3). Between 10^{-9}M to 10^{-5}M P4 did not increase proliferation of either MCF-7 or MCF-7/PGRMC1-3HA cells (WT-12). However, proliferation of WT-12 cells was significantly increased when treated with P4:BSA-FITC or the synthetic progestogens: for P4:BSA-FITC at concentrations from 10^{-7} M to 10^{-5}M with a maximal effect at 10^{-6}M, for NET reaching its maximal effect compared to untreated control at 10^{-7}M, for MPA at concentrations higher than 10^{-6}M, and for DRSP at concentrations higher than 10^{-7}M. The effect of NET was significantly different to that one of DRSP at the concentrations of 10^{-9} and 10^{-8} M and to the effect of MPA at the concentrations of 10^{-9}, 10^{-8} and 10^{-7} M. DRPS showed a significant stronger effect as compared to MPA at the concentration of 10^{-7} M. No effects were observed in MCF-7 cells within the investigated concentration ranges for all the progestogens used in this experiment.

For further kinetic experiments 10^{-6}M was chosen for all progestogens. In comparison to all other synthetic progestins tested NET significantly increased proliferation almost to maximum even at 10^{-9}M, the lowest concentration that we tested. Taken together, the results strongly suggested that some synthetic progestins elicit a PGRMC1-dependent proliferative response.

To determine time-dependent proliferative effects of progestogens a kinetic analysis over 6 days was performed (Fig. 4). MCF-7 and WT-12 cells were incubated with P4, P4-BSA-FITC, DRSP, MPA and NET at 10^{-6}M and proliferation was determined by MTT assay. The results indicate that P4:BSA-FITC, DRSP, MPA and NET increased proliferation in WT-12 cells by approximately 3.5 to 4 fold on day 6 which is highly significant compared to the simultaneously cultured untreated control cells. No effects on proliferation were observed for P4, DRSP, MPA and NET in MCF-7 cells. Only the membrane-impermeable P4-BSA-FITC caused a marginal increase of proliferation in the parental MCF-7 cells by approximately 1.5 fold compared to the control cells.

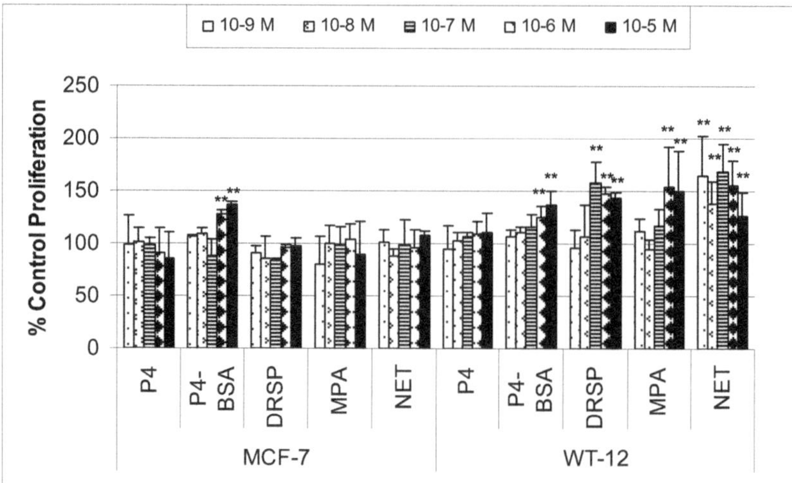

Fig. 3. Titration of progesterone and synthetic progestins. MCF-7 and MCF-7/PGRMC1-3HA (WT-12) cells were incubated with either progesterone (P4), P4:BSA-FITC, DRSP, MPA, and NET from 10^{-5}M to 10^{-9}M in tenfold dilution steps. Cell proliferation was measured after 4 days. Data were normalized to unstimulated controls. (means ± SD; ** p< 0.01 vs. controls)

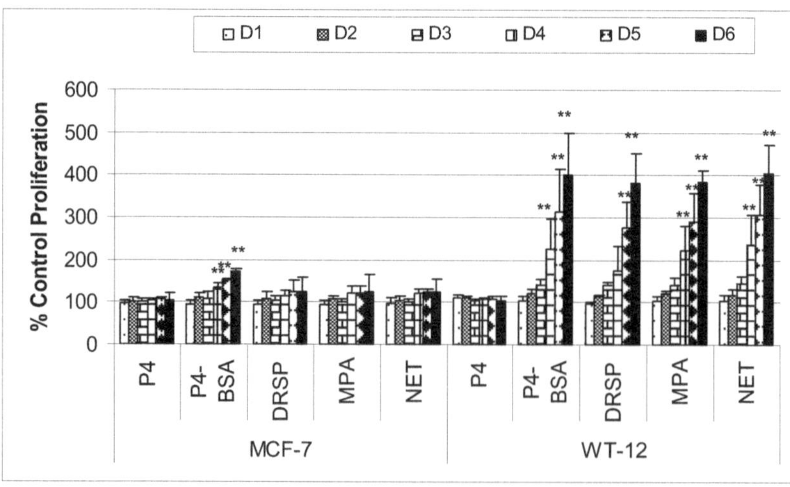

Fig. 4. Kinetic analysis of proliferation. MCF-7 and MCF-7/PGRMC1-3HA (WT-12) cells were incubated with either progesterone (P4), P4:BSA-FITC, DRSP, MPA, and NET at 10^{-6}M. Cell proliferation was measured daily for 6 days (D1–D6). Data were normalized to unstimulated controls. (means ± SD; * p< 0.05; ** p< 0.01 vs. controls)

4.3 Combination of progestogens with estradiol in PGRMC1 overexpressing cells

In our further investigations we showed that estradiol in a dosage that increased cell numbers of MCF-7 cells was able to induce an effect in WT-12 cells that doubed the effect in MCF-7 cells (Neubauer et al, 2010). The concentration of 10^{-10} M was chosen, because it is equally to in vivo serum concentrations achieved with transdermal or low orally estradiol application. The concentration of 10^{-12} M was chosen in order to imitate very low serum estradiol concentrations that were not able to induce a measurable breast cancer risk. The E2 effect could be blocked by the addition of the potent estrogen receptor antagonist fulvestrant indicating that the intracellular estrogen receptor-alpha is involved. However, since the proliferation was twice as high as in MCF-7 cells, in the presence of PGRMC1 a mechanistic interaction between the estrogen receptor-alpha and PGRMC1 signaling systems seems to be highly possible. The mechanism(s) of interaction is currently unknown. Of special significance are our findings in terms of adding progesterone or medroxyprogesterone acetate to estradiol. When PGRMC1 is overexpressed the E2-induced effect is more pronounced, but P4 still displayed a neutral effect. However, the addition of MPA triggered a strong proliferative signal in the presence of this E2 concentration (Fig. 5). The effect of other synthetic progestogens in combination with E2 on the proliferation of MCF-7 cells overexpressing PGRMC1 is currently under investigation.

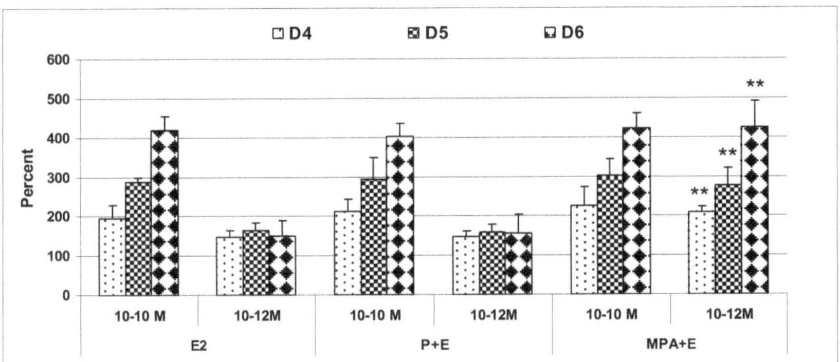

Fig. 5. MCF-7/PGRMC1-3HA (WT-12) cells were incubated with estradiol (E2, 10^{-10} M or 10^{-12} M) alone and in combination with either progesterone (P, 10^{-6} M) or medroxyprogesterone acetate (MPA, 10^{-6} M). Cell proliferation was measured after 4, 5 and 6 days. Data were normalized to unstimulated controls. (Means ±SD; ** $p< 0.01$ vs. E2)

5. Discussion

The proliferation of normal and malignant cells is under the control of both estrogen and growth factors. In normal epithelial cells, estrogen-receptor expressing cells represent only a minority of the total cells and do not proliferate (Ali & Coombes, 2002). Current opinion is that estrogens act proliferatively in a paracrine fashion by inducing the production of stromal-derived growth factors and cytokines or their receptors via the activation of epithelial or stromal estrogen receptors. Growth factors may play an important role in the promotion of receptor-positive breast cancer by cross-talk with the steroid-receptor and are mainly responsible for the progression of estrogen-receptor negative breast cancer. Among the growth factors which are important for cell growth are the epidermal growth factor (EGF) family, insulin-like growth factors I and II (IGF-I and IGF-II), fibroblast growth factors (FGFs), transforming growth factor-α (TGF-α) and platelet-derived growth factors (PDGFs).

It is important to differentiate between normal and malignant estrogen-receptor positive breast cells. Therefore, for the first time, we have investigated the effect of eight different progestogens on the proliferation of benign and malignant breast epithelial cells in the presence of growth factors and/or estradiol.

Our results indicate that MPA may enhance the mitotic rate of normal epithelial breast cells in the presence of growth factors and thus may increase the probability of faults in DNA-replication when used in long-term. Indeed, the results of WHI indicate that patients who were not using hormones prior to the start of the study had no increased hazard ratio for breast cancer whereas subjects with prior hormone use for up to five, five to ten and more than 10 years showed an increasing risk (Writing Group, 2002). These data suggest that long-term use of MPA may increase breast cancer risk by enhancing the mitotic rate of normal epithelial cells.

We could further demonstrate that progesterone had a neutral effect on growth-factor stimulated healthy breast epithelial cells. In the case of cancerous breast cells, other groups have published supporting results, where E2-induced stimulation of MCF-7 cells has been shown to be inhibited by progesterone (Cappellatti et al., 1995; Mueck et al., 2004; Schoonen et al., 1995; Seeger et al., 2003). Up to now, there is a paucity of data available regarding the effects of CMA and LNG on the proliferation of normal and malignant epithelial breast cells. There are also conflicting epidemiological data concerning these progestogens (Ebeling et al., 1991; Nischan et al., 1984; Persson et al., 1996). DNG has been shown to elicit potent anti-tumour activity against hormone-dependent cancer types in an animal model and has exhibited slight concentration-dependent inhibitory effects in combination with E2, in agreement with our results (Katsuki et al., 1997). GSD and KDG have been shown to be able to inhibit cell proliferation of a specific sub-clone of MCF-7 in the presence of E2 (Schoonen et al., 1995). Our results support the inhibitory effects of both GSD and KDG in combination with E2, however, we found both exhibited a proliferative effect on HCC1500 cells with growth factors alone.

By comparing the cell death to proliferation ratio results of growth factors alone, E2 alone and combination of growth factor and E2 on HCC1500 cells, we also found that the single proliferative effects of growth factors or E2 alone are magnified when in combination with each other, which, however, was not always statistically significant. The mechanism of the stimulatory effect of MPA (and of CMA) on MCF10A cells is currently unknown, as this cell line is both estrogen and progesterone receptor negative. The effects of the steroids on HCC1500 cells appear to be receptor-dependent, since the time course clearly shows a long-term effect rather than a rapid non-genomic action.

For the first time we could present data suggesting that signaling of synthetic progestins via PGRMC1 could be one explanation for the clinically observed possible induction of breast cancer risk by progestins. We have chosen two synthetic progestins that are widely used in hormone therapy, i.e. MPA and NET, as well as a new synthetic progestin, i.e. DRSP, which might differ in its behaviour to MPA and NET, because of a different chemical structure.

The synthetic progestins MPA, NET and DRSP significantly induced a relatively large proliferative effect in MCF-7 cells that overexpress PGRMC1. For P4, however, no such effect was found. Since progesterone and the synthetic progestins used in HT are able to activate PR-A/-B and PGRMC1 simultaneously, our data suggest that *in vivo* the balance of the expression levels of both receptors might influence whether epithelial cells proliferate or not in the presence of progestogens. Therefore, it may be instructive to determine the expression ratio of PGRMC1 and PR-A/-B before HT.

Interestingly, P4:BSA-FITC is able to induce a marginal proliferative signal in MCF-7 cells (Fig. 3). P4:BSA-FITC is thought to be unable to cross the plasma membrane and can therefore only bind to membrane associated progesterone receptors. MCF-7 cells express endogenous PGRMC1 at very low amounts (data not shown), which may transduce the weak proliferative signal since the classical PR-A/-B response is not triggered. The synthetic progestins and P4 bind to all progesterone receptors expressed by MCF-7 cells. Binding to PR-A/-B might transduce an antiproliferative signal, countermanding the proliferative signal induced by low levels of PGRMC1. In contrast, in WT-12 cells the exogenously expressed PGRMC1 might overrule the antiproliferative effect of PR-A/-B. In several human ovarian surface epithelial cell lines, P4 inhibits their proliferation (Syed et al., 2001). Because these cells express the PR-A/-B it has been assumed that P4's actions are mediated via these receptors. However, P4 exhibits antimitotic action only at micromolar doses, which have been used in these experiments (Syed et al., 2001). Given that the dissociation constant for the PR-A/-B is 1–5 nm (Stouffer, 2003) and for PGRMC1 is in the 0.20–0.3 μm range (Meyer et al., 1996), which is well within the levels of P4 in serum and in follicular fluid (Stouffer, 2003), in MCF-7 cells the classical PR-A/-B receptors are perhaps activated preferentially by gestagens inducing an anti proliferative signal. This concept is supported by a previous observation that at micromolar doses P4 inhibits granulosa cell and spontaneously immortalized granulosa cell (SIGC) mitosis (Fujii et al., 1983).

Interestingly, NET exerts its activity on proliferation already at the lowest concentration tested (10^{-9} M, Fig. 4) whereas DRSP and MPA increase proliferation only at higher concentrations (10^{-7} M and 10^{-6} M). This suggests that NET binds PGRMC1 with the highest affinity, followed by DRSP and MPA. Compared to PR-A/-B this is different since the latter binds MPA better than NET (Kuhl, 1998). These results indicate that HT including NET might result in an increased risk for breast cancer development. Indeed, some studies in which norethisterone- or levonorgestrel-derived progestogens were continuously administered a significantly higher risk for breast cancer was observed than for continuously administered progesterone-derived progestogens (Lyytinen et al., 2009; Magnusson et al., 1999). In one study the use of norethisterone acetate was accompanied with a higher risk after 5 years of use (2.03, 1.88-2.18) than that of medroxyprogesterone acetate (1.64, 1.49-1.79) (Lyytinen et al., 2009). It is known that NET can be converted in vivo into ethinylestradiol (Kuhnz et al., 1997). In as far this conversion may influence the observed NET effect is currently unknown and is under investigation.

Despite their widespread use, *in vitro* models have certain limitations: the choice of culture conditions can unintentionally affect the experimental outcome, and cultured cells are adapted to grow *in vitro*; the changes which have allowed this ability may not occur *in vivo*. Limitations of this *in vitro* study might be the high concentrations needed for an effective antiproliferative effect. The clinically relevant blood concentrations for the progestogens most commonly used for HRT, MPA and NET, are in the range of $4x10^{-9}$M to 10^{-8}M for MPA (Svensson et al., 1994) and around 10^{-8}M for NET (Stanczyk et al., 1978). However, higher concentrations may be required *in vitro* in short-time tests in which the reaction threshold can only be achieved with supraphysiological dosages. Higher concentrations may also be reached *in vivo* in the vessel wall or organs compared to the concentrations usually measured in the blood.

A further limitation of our work is the short incubation period of the cells with the substrates under investigation, in comparison to the longer time period for which hormone therapy is usually prescribed. That duration of therapy may indeed be an important factor for breast cancer risk is emphasized by the results of WHI, where breast cancer risk was significantly higher compared to placebo only in women given combined HRT for 10 years or more, but not in those treated only for the duration of the study period, i.e. 5.2 years (Writing Group, 2002). In vitro experiments can support, but not replace clinical trials, and therefore, further clinical studies are needed to determine which progestogens, if any, have the lowest breast cancer risk.

6. Conclusion

Experimental data with the comparison of various synthetic progestins in the same in vitro model present rather high evidence that there may be differences between the various progestins regarding breast cancer risk. Especially of concern may be to differentiate between primary and secondary risk i.e. between benign and malignant breast epithelial cells. This differentiation seems to be especially important for the progestin MPA. Since even in 'clinically healthy' women malignant cells can be detected (Nielsen et al., 1987), this experimental finding may have relevance and should be further investigated.

The effect of progestins on breast cancer tumorigenesis may depend on the specific progestin used for hormone therapy and the expression of PGRMC1, PR-A and PR-B in the target tissue. However, in terms of the clinical situation it remains unknown how uniformly PGRMC1 is expressed in the normal breast epithelial cells between patients. Thus screening, which might be based on determining the expression ratio of PGRMC1 and PR in cells from nipple aspirate fluid (NAF), might be of interest to identify women who show an increased expression of PGRMC1 and who might thus be susceptible for breast cancer development under HT (Sauter et al., 1997). The data presented here are of dramatic importance in terms of progesterone and breast cancer risk in HT clinical studies so far (Writing Group for the Women's Health Initiative Investigators, 2002; The Women's Health Initiative Steering Committee, 2004). The epidemiological studies and especially the WHI trial, so far the only prospective placebo-controlled interventional study, demonstrate an increased risk under combined estrogen/progestin therapy, but they have the limitations that they up to now can not discriminate between the various progestins mostly due to too small or not comparable patient numbers in the subgroups with the various progestins. However, there is evidence that the natural progesterone, possibly also the transdermal usage of synthetic progestins, may avoid an increased risk, but this must be proven in further clinical trials.

7. References

Ahmed IS, Rohe HJ, Twist KE & Craven RJ. (2010) Pgrmc1 (progesterone receptor membrane component 1) associates with EGFR and regulates erlotinib sensitivity. *Biological Chemistry*, 285, pp. 24775-82

Ali S & Coombes RC. (2002). Endocrine-responsive breast cancer and strategies for combating resistance. *Nature Reviews Cancer*, 2, pp. 101-15

Black WC & Welch HG. (1993). Advances in diagnostic imaging and overestimations of disease prevalence and the benefits of therapy. *New England Journal of Medicine*, 328, pp. 1237-1243

Cahill MA. (2007). Progesterone receptor membrane component 1: an integrative review. *Journal of Steroid Biochemistry and Molecular Biology*, 105, pp. 16-36

Cappelletti V, Miodini P Fioravanti L & DiFronzo G. (1995). Effect of progestin treatment on estradiol- and growth factor-stimulated breast cancer cell lines. *Anticancer Research*, 15, pp. 2551-2556

Catherino WH, Jeng MH & Jordan VC. (1995) Norgestrel and gestodene stimulate breast cancer cell growth through an oestrogen receptor mediated mechanism. *British Journal of Cancer*, 67, pp. 945-952

Crudden G, Loesel R & Craven RJ. (2005). Overexpression of the cytochrome p450 activator hpr6 (heme-1 domain protein/human progesterone receptor) in tumors. *Tumour Biology*, 26, pp. 142–146

Dickson RB & Lippman ME. (1995). Growth factors in breast cancer. *Endocrine Reviews*, 16, pp. 559-89

Ebeling K, Ray R, Nischan P, Thomas DB. Kunde D & Stalsberg H. (1991). Combined oral contraceptives containing chlormadinone acetate and breast cancer: results of a case-control study. *British Journal of Cancer*, 63, pp. 804-08

Fournier A, Berrino F & Clavel-Chapelon F. (2008). Unequal risks for breast cancer associated with different hormone replacement therapies: results from the E3N cohort study. *Breast Cancer Research Treatment*, 107, pp. 103-111

Franke HR & Vermes I. (2003). Differential effects of progestogens on breast cancer cell lines. *Maturitas*, 46, Suppl1, pp. S55-S58

Fujii T, Hoover DJ & Channing CP. (1983). Changes in inhibin activity, and progesterone, oestrogen and androstenedione concentrations, in rat follicular fluid throughout the oestrous cycle. *Journal of Reproduction and Fertility*, 69, pp. 307-314.

Gazdar AF, Kurvari V, Virmani A, Gollahon L, Sakaguchi M, Westerfield M, Kodagoda D, Stasny V, Cunningham HT, Wistuba II, Tomlinson G, Tonk V, Ashfaq R, Leitch AM, Minna JD & Shay JW. (1998). Characterization of paired tumor and non-tumor cell lines established from patients with breast cancer. *International Journal of Cancer*, 78, pp. 766-774

Katsuki Y, Shibutani Y, Aoki D & Nozawa S. (1997). Dienogest, a novel synthetic steroid, overcomes hormone-dependent cancer in a different manner than progestins. *Cancer*, 79, pp. 169-76

Krämer EA, Seeger H, Krämer B, Wallwiener D & Mueck AO. (2006). The effect of progesterone, testosterone and synthetic progestogens on growth factor- and estradiol-treated human cancerous and benign breast cells. *European Journal of Obstetrics, Gynecology and Reproduction*, 27, pp. 139-141

Kuhl H. (1998). Pharmakologie von Sexualsteroiden. *Gynäkologe*, 31, pp. 832-847

Kuhnz W, Heuner A, Hümpel M, Seifert W & Michaelis K. (1997). In vivo conversion of norethisterone and norethisterone acetate to ethinyl etradiol in postmenopausal women. *Contraception*, 56, pp. 379-85

Lyytinen H, Pukkala E & Ylikorkala O. (2009). Breast cancer risk in postmenopausal women using estradiol-progestogen therapy. *Obstetrics and Gynecology*, 113, pp. 65-73

Magnusson C, Baron JA, Correia N, Bergstrom R, Adami H-O & Persson I. (1999). Breast-cancer risk following long-term oestrogen- and oestrogen-progestin-replacement therapy. *International Journal of Cancer*, 81, pp. 339-344

Meyer C, Schmid R, Scriba PC & Wehling M. (1996) Purification and partial sequencing of high-affinity progesterone-binding site(s) from porcine liver membranes. *European Journal of Biochemistry*, 239, pp. 726-733

Million Women Study Collaborators. (2003). Breast Cancer and hormone replacement therapy in the Million Women Study. *Lancet*, 362, pp. 419-427

Min L, Strushkevich NV, Harnastai IN, Iwamoto H, Gilep AA, Takemori H, Usanov SA, Nonaka Y, Hori H, Vinson GP & Okamoto M (2005). Molecular identification of adrenal inner zone antigen as a hemebinding protein. *Febs J*, 272, pp. 5832–5843

Mueck AO, Seeger H & Wallwiener D. (2004). Comparison of the proliferative effects of estradiol and conjugated equine estrogens on human breast cancer cells and impact of continuous combined progestogen addition. *Climacteric*, 6, pp. 221-27

Munton RP, Tweedie-Cullen R, Livingstone-Zatchej M, Weinandy F, Waidelich M, Longo D, Gehrig P, Potthast F, Rutishauser D, Gerrits B, Panse C, Schlapbach R & Mansuy IM. (2007). Qualitative and quantitative analyses of protein phosphorylation in naive and stimulated mouse synaptosomal preparations. *Molecular and Cellular Proteomics*, 6, pp. 283-293

Neubauer H, Adam G, Seeger H, Mueck AO, Solomayer E, Wallwiener D, Cahill MA & Fehm T. (2009). Membrane-initiated effects of progesterone on proliferation and activation of VEGF in breast cancer cells. *Climacteric*, 3, pp. 230-239

Neubauer H, Clare SE, Wozny W, Schwall GP, Poznanović S, Stegmann W, Vogel U, Sotlar K, Wallwiener D, Kurek R, Fehm T & Cahill MA. (2008). Breast cancer proteomics reveals correlation between estrogen receptor status and differential phosphorylation of PGRMC1. *Breast Cancer Research*, 10, R85

Neubauer H, Yang Y, Seeger H, Fehm T, Cahill MA, Tong X, Ruan X & Mueck AO. (2010). The presence of a membrane-bound progesterone receptor sensitizes the estradiol-induced effect on the proliferation of human breast cancer cells. *Menopause,8,845-50*

Nielsen M, Thomsen JL, Primdahl S, Dyreborg U & Andersen JA. (1987). Breast cancer and atypia among young and middle-aged women: a study of 110 medico-legal autopsies. *Br J Cancer*,56, pp.814–819

Nischan P & Ebeling K. (1984). Oral contraceptives containing chlormadinone acetate and cancer incidence at selected sites in the German Democratic Republic—a correlation analysis. *International Journal of Cancer*, 34, pp. 671-74

Nolte I, Jeckel D, Wieland FT & Sohn K. (2000). Localization and topology of ratp28, a member of a novel family of putative steroid-binding proteins. *Biochimica and Biophysica Acta*, 1543, pp. 123–130

Peluso JJ, Liu X, Saunders MM, Claffey KP & Phoenix K. (2008a). Regulation of ovarian cancer cell viability and sensitivity to cisplatin by progesterone receptor membrane component-1. *Journal of Clinical and Endocrinololgical Metabolism*, 93, pp. 1592–1599

Peluso JJ, Pappalardo A, Losel R & Wehling M. (2006). Progesterone membrane receptor component 1 expression in the immature rat ovary and its role in mediating progesterone's antiapoptotic action. *Endocrinology*, 147, pp. 3133–3140

Peluso JJ, Romak J & Liu X. (2008b). Progesterone receptor membrane component-1 (PGRMC1) is the mediator of progesterone's antiapoptotic action in spontaneously immortalized granulosa cells as revealed by PGRMC1 small interfering ribonucleic acid treatment and functional analysis of PGRMC1 mutations. *Endocrinology*, 149, pp. 534–543

Persson I, Yuan J, Bergkvist L & Schairer C. (1996). Cancer incidence and mortality in women receiving estrogen and estrogen-progestin replacement therapy - long-term follow-up of a Swedish cohort. *International Journal of Cancer*, 67, pp. 327-32

Pirnia F, Pawlak M, Thallinger GG, Gierke B, Templin MF, Kappeler A, Betticher DC, Gloor B & Borner MM. (2009) Novel functional profiling approach combining reverse phase protein microarrays and human 3-D ex vivo tissue cultures: expression of apoptosis-related proteins in human colon cancer. *Proteomics*, 9, pp. 3535-3548

Sauter ER, Ross E, Daly M, Klein-Szanto A, Engstrom PF, Sorling A, Malick J & Ehya H. (1997). Nipple aspirate fluid: a promising non-invasive method to identify cellular markers of breast cancer risk. *British Journal of Cancer*, 76, pp. 494-501

Schoonen WGEJ, Joosten JWH & Kloosterboer HJ. (1995). Effects of two classes of progestins, Pregnane and 19-nortestosterone derivatives, on cell growth of human breast tumor cells: 1. MCF-7 cell lines. *Journal of Steroid Biochemistry and Molecular Biology*, 55, pp. 423-437

Seeger H, Wallwiener D & Mueck AO. (2003). The effect of progesterone and synthetic progestins on serum- and estradiol-stimulated proliferation of human breast cancer cells. *Hormone and Metabolic Research*, 35, pp. 76-80

Soule HD, Maloney TM, Wolman SR, Peterson WD, Brenz R, McGrath CM, Russo J, Pauley RJ, Jones RF & Brooks, SC. (1990) Isolation and characterization of a spontaneously immortalized human breast epithelial cell line, MCF-10. *Cancer Research*, 50, pp. 6075-6086.

Stanczyk FZ, Brenner PF, Mishell DR, Ortiz A, Gentzschein EKE & GoebelsmannU. (1978). A radioimmunoassay for norethindrone (NET): measurement of serum net concentrations following ingestion of NET-containing oral contraceptive steroids. *Contraception*, 18, pp. 615-33

Stouffer RL. (2003). Progesterone as a mediator of gonadotrophin action in the corpus luteum: beyond steroidogenesis. *Human Reproduction Update*, 9, pp. 99–117

Svensson LO, Johnson SH & Olsson SE. (1994) Plasma concentrations of medroxyprogesterone acetate, estradiol and estrone following oral administration of Klimaxil, Trisequence/Provera, and Divina, A randomised, single-blind, triple cross-over bioavailability study in menopausal women. *Maturitas*, 18, pp. 229-38

Swiatek-De Lange M, Stampfl A, Hauck SM, Zischka H, Gloeckner CJ, Deeg CA & Ueffing M. (2007). Membrane-Initiated Effects of Progesterone on Calcium Dependent Signaling and Activation of VEGF Gene Expression in Retinal Glial Cells. *Glia*, 55, pp. 1061–1073

Syed V, Ulinski G, Mok SC, Yiu GK & Ho SM. (2001) Expression of gonadotropin receptor and growth responses to key reproductive hormones in normal and malignant human ovarian surface epithelial cells. *Cancer Research*, 61, pp. 6768–6776

The Women's Health Initiative Steering Committee. (2004). Effects of conjugated equine estrogen in postmenopausal women with hysterectomy. *JAMA*, 291, pp. 1701-1712

Writing Group for the Women's Health Initiative Investigators. (2002). Risks and benefits of estrogen plus progestin in healthy postmenopausal women. *JAMA*, 288, pp.321-333

2

Parathyroid Hormone Related Protein: A Marker of Breast Tumor Progression and Outcome

Zhor Bouizar
U676 INSERM, Hôpital Robert Debré AP-HP, Paris
Université Paris Diderot, Paris
France

1. Introduction

1.1 Breast cancer

Breast cancer is the second leading cause of death among women. According to the American Medical Association and American Cancer Society, it is the most common disease of women, although it usually does not affect them until they reach their '20s. Every year millions of women are diagnosed with this disease and screening for breast cancer is now widespread, particularly among older women. Breast cancer is the most common form of cancer in women accounting for 1 in 4 of female cancers and is the leading cause of death among gynecological cancers in developed countries. Almost 10% of women in France will develop breast cancer and 75% of newly detected cases are women over 50 years. This number is constantly increasing. (The Lancet, Volume 374, Issue 9701, Page 1567, 7 November 2009 (Breast cancer in developing countries).

1.2 Background

Breast tissue is an exocrine gland of ectodermal origin. Each breast is composed of 10-20 glandular lobes, each of which is divided into lobules and acini. The acini are grouped densely around an alveolar duct (lactiferous duct 3rd order). Several alveolar ducts come together to form a lobular channel (channel 2nd order) which drains a lobule. Several lobular channels unite to form a milk duct that drains all the lobules within the glandular lobe. Each lobe acts as an independent gland with its own excretory duct (lactiferous duct). These lactiferous ducts converge toward the nipple. The mammary gland can be affected by various lesions. The more benign, include pseudo-tumoral lesions, benign epithelial tumors, fibro-epithelial and cystic fibrosis. These are also called benign breast disease. Malignant epithelial lesions may be non-invasive (lobular carcinoma *in situ* and ductal carcinoma) or infiltrating (invasive lobular carcinoma and infiltrating ductal carcinomas). Infiltrating ductal cancers are the most common, accounting for 84% of breast cancers, while infiltrating lobular cancers account for only 4% of breast tumors and non-invasive forms for 1-3%.
Breast cancer cells often metastasize to bone where they produce large amounts of parathyroid hormone-related protein (PTHrP). We have investigated the possible roles of PTHrP in breast cancer bone metastases.

1.3 Parathyroid hormone-related protein (PTHrP) gene

The sequence of parathyroid hormone-related peptide (PTHrP) is very similar to that of the N-terminal portion of parathyroid hormone (PTH). The PTHrP gene is complex and can generate at least three mature peptides by alternative splicing. PTHrP acts via a receptor that it shares with PTH and also via specific receptors. Physiologically, PTHrP is produced locally in many normal tissues where it has autocrine/paracrine functions, particularly during embryonic development, growth regulation and the differentiation of many cell types. PTHrP has an endocrine action on bone and kidney.

1.3.1 Gene structure

The PTHrP gene is located on the short arm of chromosome 12 in a position homologous to the PTH gene on chromosome 11 in humans (Naylor et al. 1983; Mangin et al. 1988; Suva et al., 1989) (*Figure 1*). Both chromosomes carry more genes belonging to the same family such as the A and B isoforms of lactate dehydrogenase (LDH), Sox 5 and 6 and forms H and K of the ras gene (Yang and Stewart, 1996). The chromosomal location and structural homology of the two genes suggest that they were produced by duplication of a common ancestral chromosome. But the PTHrP gene is much more complex than the PTH gene (Philbrick et al., 1996) *(Figure 1).*

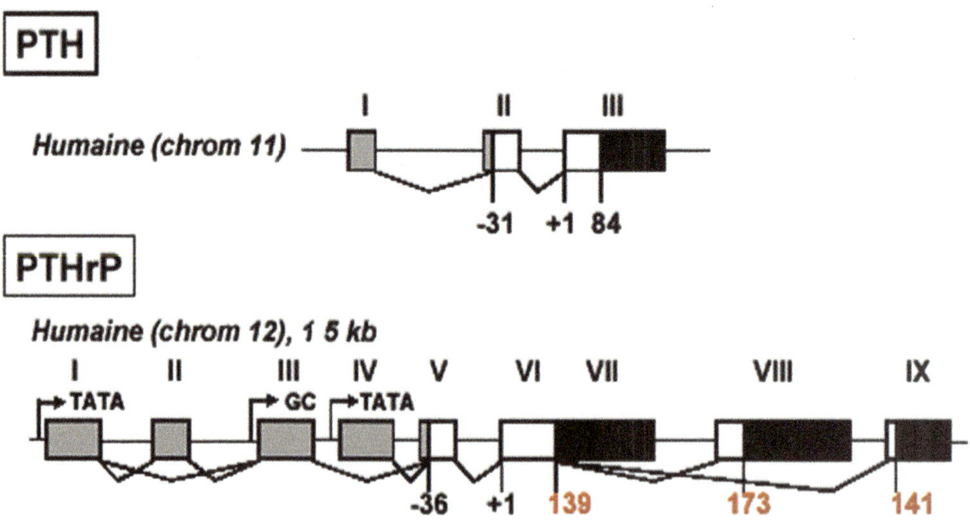

Fig. 1. *Structure and organization of the Human PTH and PTHr P genes*: Organization of the PTH (chromosome 11 in humans) and PTHrP (chromosome 12 in humans) genes and phylogenetic variations. Exons are in Roman numerals. The coding regions are shown as white rectangles, untranslated 5′ regions are in gray, untranslated 3' regions are in black, and introns are shown by solid lines. The promoter sequences are indicated by black arrows. The alternative splicings that generate the isoforms of PTHrP in each species are represented by the broken lines in each sequence.

The 15 kb-long human PTHrP gene is a complex transcriptional unit composed of nine exons and 15 different transcripts can be generated by alternative splicing of the 5′ and 3′ exons (Broadus and Stewart, 1994; Gillespie and Martin, 1994). Transcription may be initiated at any of the three promoters, P1, P2 and P3. P1 and P3 are canonical TATA promoters (Mangin et al., 1990; Campos et al., 1992; Suva et al., 1989) and initiate transcription at exons 1 and 4 respectively, while P2 is a GC-rich promoter that initiates transcription upstream of exon IC (Vasavada et al., 1993). Evaluation of PTHrP alternative promoter usage by qualitative (Southby et al., 1995 and 1996) and quantitative reverse transcription RT-PCR (Bouizar et al., 1999; Richard et al., 2003) revealed high concentrations of P3-initiated transcripts in most tumors, including breast cancers (Bouizar et al., 1999) and many tumor cell lines (Cataisson et al., 2003). The amino acid sequences encoded by only two of the 9 exons in the human gene are present in all transcripts. One is exon 5, which encodes the prepro-sequence and the other is exon 6, which encodes the common sequence of 139 amino acids. Polymerase II will transcribe exon 7 if the splice donor site located at the end of exon 6 is skipped; this exon encodes the stop codon and the 3' untranslated region of the 139 residue isoform. The splicing of exon 6 to exon 8 provides a transcript encoding the 173-residue isoform, while splicing exon 6 to exon 9 produces a transcript encoding the 141-residue isoform. *(Figue 1)*

2. PTHrP and mammary gland physiopathology

Recent studies using targeted overexpression or disruption of the PTHrP gene have demonstrated that the peptide regulates the development of the cartilaginous growth plate, the skin, teeth and mammary glands (Broadus et al 1994, Karaplis et al 1994, .Philbrick et al 1998,Wysolmerski et al 1998)

2.1 PTHrP and mammary development

Overexpression and underexpression of PTHrP disrupt the process of branching morphogenesis by which the mammary gland develops (Broadus et al 1994, Wysolmerski,et al 1994,). Wysolmerski and colleagues demonstrated that amino-terminal PTHrP is required for the development of the mammary epithelial duct system in mice. PTHrP gene expression is limited to the mammary epithelium during embryonic mammary development, while expression of the PTH/PTHrP receptor gene is restricted to the mesenchyme. In addition, mammary stromal cells in culture bind aminoterminal PTHrP and respond with an increase in intracellular cAMP (Dunbar et al 1998). This suggests that PTHrP acts as an epithelial message that must be received by mammary mesenchyme before it can support branching growth. Collagen II-PTHrP (rescued) /PTHrP knockout mice that have no PTHrP in any tissue except the cartilage lack even a vestige of mammary epithelial ducts. PTHrP-knockout mouse embryos exhibit a primary failure of branching morphogenesis during embryonic mammary gland development. Deletion of the PTH/PTHrP receptor recapitulates the failure of mammary development seen in the PTHrP knockout embryos. Transgene-mediated reintroduction of PTHrP into the mammary epithelial cells of PTHrP-knockout animals reversed the failure of embryonic mammary development and allowed the development of a complete mammary duct system within the mammary fat pad. Embryonic mammary glands are formed in two steps; the mammary bud is formed first, followed by branching morphogenesis to form the immature ductal tree (Sakakura et al 1987). The mammary buds are formed appropriately in PTHrP-knockout embryos but they fail to undergo the initial round of branching growth that leads to a typical immature ductal tree. The mammary epithelial structure fails to elongate and/or penetrate into the developing fat pad in the absence of PTHrP. Instead, the mammary bud remains in the upper dermis surrounded by dense fibro-connective tissue. The mammary epithelial cells have degenerated in newborn PTHrP-knockout mice, the nipple sheath has not formed, and all traces of the mammary epithelial duct system has disappeared, explaining the lack of mammary structures in the mature rescued PTHrP-knockout mice (Dunbar et al 1998).

2.2 PTHrP gene expression, puberty and early pregnancy

The mammary glands of newborn mice undergo little development until the onset of puberty at 3-4 weeks of age (Sakakura et al 1991). The hormonal changes that occur at this time influence the distal ends of the mammary ducts to form specialized structures called terminal end buds, where there is active cell proliferation and differentiation during ductal growth and morphogenesis (Daniel et al 1988). By the time mice are 8-10 weeks old, the epithelial duct system has grown to the borders of the mammary fat pad and the terminal buds disappear, leaving the typical branched duct system found in the adult virgin gland. Pregnancy triggers another round of epithelial proliferation that leads to the production of terminal ducts and lobular-alveolar structures.

PTHrP may also play a role in the epithelial/mesenchymal interactions that govern these later rounds of ductal morphogenesis. PTHrP was first found in the mature mammary gland during late pregnancy and lactation (Budayr et al 1987, Thiede et al 1988). More recently, Dunbar and colleagues found mRNAs encoding PTHrP in the mammary epithelium and PTH/PTHrP receptor mRNAs in the stroma during puberty and early-to-mid pregnancy. Furthermore, both genes are most actively expressed in those regions of the mammary gland that are proliferating and undergoing ductal morphogenesis, the terminal end buds. Overproduction of PTHrP in the mammary myoepithelial cells of transgenic mice results in abnormal mammary duct development during puberty and early pregnancy (Wysolmerski,et al 1994). PTHrP overproduction during puberty severely impairs both the overall rate of ductal proliferation and the pattern of side branching. In addition, PTHrP overproduction during early pregnancy impairs terminal duct development. These effects appear to be mediated by amino-terminal PTHrP acting through the PTH/PTHrP receptor.

2.3 PTHrP and lactation

Parathyroid hormone-related protein does not only influence the development of breast tissue. Human and bovine milk contain high concentrations of PTHrP (Thiede et al 1988,): a thousand times higher than the concentration in the blood plasma. The glandular epithelial and myoepithelial cells of the lactating breast produce large amounts of parathyroid hormone-related protein. Most of it is secreted into the milk although small quantities are released into the blood (Khosla et 1990). It has therefore been proposed that PTHrP may enhance blood flow to the mammary gland during lactation (Davicco et al 1993). Suckling stimulates PTHrP gene expression in the mammary gland and prolactin has been reported to increase synthesis of the peptide. This led to the idea that the protein may be the long-postulated signal that adapts maternal calcium metabolism to the stress of lactation.

While an infusion of PTHrP can increase mammary blood flow in goats (Posser et al 1994) and sheep (Rodda et al 1988), this does not appear to alter milk production or enhance the calcium content of the milk. Moreover, there is no evidence that the plasma concentration of

PTHrP induced by lactation can mobilize calcium from bone or enhance its renal reabsorption. However, there is evidence that PTHrP is involved in calcium transfer. Barlet et al showed that PTHrP increases the $P0_4$, Ca_{2+}, and Mg_{2+} content of breast milk (Barlet et al 1990). Parathyroid hormone-related protein has been detected in the serum of nursing mothers (Grill et al 1991, Sowers et al 1996). But there is no conclusive evidence that it is the long-sought lactation signal. Yet mammary parathyroid hormone-related protein probably has systemic effects, because its concentrations are high in the serum of women with rare syndromes of hypercalcemia associated with lactation and massive mammary hypertrophy (Lepre et al 1993). PTHrP increases the cAMP in myoepithelial cells and decreases the intracellular calcium induced by oxytocin in these cells (Ferrari,et al 1993, Seitz et al 1993).

3. PTHrP and breast cancer

Several studies have reported finding PTHrP in primary tumors. Ikeda and coworkers identified PTHrP transcripts in two breast tumors by Northern blotting in patients with hypercalcemia (Ikeda et al.,1988). Many subsequent immunohistochemical studies with polyclonal antibodies have revealed a significant percentage of cells staining positive for PTHrP: 60% of 102 primary tumors (Southby et al. 1990), 69% of 81 breast carcinomas (Liapis et al., 1993) and up to 72% of 367 primary tumors (Henderson et al., 2001, Henderson et al., 2006). Other more recent studies using monoclonal antibodies detected positive signals in 100% of invasive carcinomas tested (Iezzoni et al. 1998; Surowiak et al., 2003) .Similarly, both PTHrP and its receptor PTH1-R have been detected in breast cancers (Carron et al., 1997, Downey et al., 1997, Iezzoni et al. 1998; Linforth et al. 2002). There is now considerable evidence that PTHrP influences the growth and differentiation of mammary tissue, both *in vitro* and *in vivo* (Wysolmerski,et al 1995, Ferrari, et al 1992, Birch,et al 1995, Lupareilo et al 1997, Cataisson et al 2000). PTHrP is secreted by epithelial cells in the breast (Sebag et al 1994) and that both normal myoepithelial and tumoral epithelial mammary cells (Seitz et al 1993) secrete PTHrP in vitro (Birch,et al 1995 Luparello et al 1997,Cataisson et al 2000). Analyses of human breast cancer cell lines and immunological and in situ hybridization studies of human tumors indicate that neoplasic epithelial cells express both PTHrP and the PTH/PTHrP receptor (Birch,et al 1995,Iezzoni et al 1998, Cataison et al, 2000). In contrast, antibody labeling of human breast cancer tumors suggests that stromal fibroblasts surrounding the tumor produce significant amounts of immunoreactive PTHrP (Iezzoni et al 1998, Cros et al 2002).

3.1 Parathyroid hormone in invasive breast cancer

3.1.1 Role of PTHrP in the development of bone metastases

Parathyroid hormone-related protein (PTHrP) is a PTH-like calcitropic hormone, a growth factor and regulator of development (Murray et al., 2005). Tumor-derived PTHrP appears to be a crucial component of a chain of signalling events among cells of the bone microenvironment that facilitates both the destruction of bone and the growth of tumor cells (Guise et al., 1996; Thomas et al., 1999, Kozlow& Guise 2005). Many clinical studies have examined the impact of PTHrP on metastatic primary tumors. PTHrP has been detected by immunocytochemistry and *in situ* hybridization in 92% of bone metastases, but in only 17% of non-bone (soft tissue) metastases (Vargas et al., 1992). Others have found that 83% of patients who developed bone metastases had PTHrP in the primary tumor (Kohno et al.,

1994). A retrospective RT-PCR study showed increased transcripts of PTHrP in the primary tumors of patients who subsequently developed bone metastases (Bouizar et al., 1993). The results of an extension of this study to a larger cohort suggested that transcripts encoding the 139-residue isoform were overexpressed in tumors that had metastasized to bone (Bouizar et al. 1999; Guise et al. 2002).

PTHrP produced by breast cancer cells may facilitate the development of skeletal metastases by enhancing the survival of tumor cells in bone, or by promoting the invasion of bone by tumor cells (Bundred et al., 1992). Tumor cells tha have become established in bone produce factors that change normal bone remodeling, such as parathyroid hormone-related protein (PTHrP). Bone metastases of breast cancers are predominantly osteolytic and cause skeletal lesions leading to fractures, intractable bone pain, nerve compression, and hypercalcemia (Arguello et al 1988, Bouizar et al, 1993, 1999).

In vitro studies identified PTHrP in primary cultures of mammary tumors and in breast cancer cell lines, although the amount varied from one line to another (Birch et al. 1995; Guise et al. 1996; Cataisson et al., 2000, Saito et al., 2005). Breast cancer cells frequently spread to bone, where they form osteolytic metastases. Coleman and Rubens found that 69% of patients who died from breast cancer had bone metastases (Coleman and Rubens, 1987). And PTHrP has a major role in the development of such metastases. It is not only linked to the development of bone metastases; it concentration is also increased when breast tumor cells metastasize to bone (Bundred et al. 1992) Metastasis is a complex process involving a cascade of relatively well known cellular events . Many factors (Guise et al., 1996 and 2002), including PTHrP, can facilitate metastasis to bone (Vargas et al. 1992; , Guise et al., 2002, Bouizar et al., 1993 and 1999, Cataisson et al , 2000) *(Figure 4)* .These factors promote the differentiation and activation of osteoclasts, and hence bone resorption. There is considerable evidence that PTHrP promotes metastases to bone (Guise et al 1996, 2002). Studies on Animal models that mimic metastatic bone disease have helped identify the mechanisms responsible for osteolytic metastasis. A popular one is athymic mice injected with human breast carcinoma cells (Arguello et al. 1988; Guise and Mundy, 1998; Peyruchaud et al., 2001). Another uses the injection of MCF-7 mammary carcinoma cells transfected to overexpress PTHrP into the hearts of immunodeficient mice (Thomas et al., 1999). Clinical and experimental evidence indicates that it is important in malignancy; it mediates bone destruction during osteolytic metastasis. Neutralizing antibodies against PTHrP inhibit both the development and the progression of bone metastasis by cells of the human breast cancer cell line MDA-MB-231 in mice (Burtis et al 1990, 1992). The PTHrP produced by breast cancer cells may enable them to grow and invade bone by stimulating osteoclastic activity and bone resorption (Kozlow& Guise 2005).

3.1.2 Malignant humoral hypercalcemia and PTHrP

Parathyroid hormone-related protein (PTHrP) was initially identified because of its involvement in hypercalcemia associated with malignancy Bundred et al 1992. PTHrP is produced and secreted by tumors whose targets are primarily bone and kidney. It has thus been considered to be primarily a deleterious protein responsible for humoral hypercalcemia of malignancy (HHM). This metabolic phenomenon is mediated by the paraneoplastic secretion of PTHrP.The amino-terminal peptide of PTHrP induces hypercalcemia of magliancy, osteoclast-mediated resorption, elevated nephrogenous cAMP, and phosphate excretion. The plasma concentration of PTHrP may be useful for predicting the occurrence of bone metastasis in breast cancer patients. Immunochemical studies have detected the peptide in 60% of normocalcemic women with a primary breast cancer (Southby et al., 1990). Brunded et al (1992) used this methodology to show that patients who went on to develop bone metastases were more likely to have marked staining. Most (65%) of the hypercalcemic patients with breast cancers metastasizing to bone had elevated plasma PTHrP concentrations (Pvveli et al 1991). PTHrP mRNA was detected by *in situ* hybridization more frequently in bone metastases than in non-bone metastases (Vargas et al 1992). Our semi-quantitative RT-PCR studies, which are considerably more accurate than immunochemistry, showed that PTHrP mRNA was present in 82% of primary breast cancers (Bouizar et al 1993). We also found PTHrP mRNA in significantly more (97%) patients with primary breast cancer who subsequently developed bone metastases than those who remained free of metastases or developed metastases in soft tissues (Bouizar et al 1993, 1999). Patients with cancer often have severe hypercalcemia (Strewler, 2000). This is and synonymous with a poor prognosis since their median survival time is estimated to be about six weeks (Strewler, 2000; Solimando, 2001). Moreover, the PTHrP concentration is elevated in the serum of 80% of the patients who develop cancer, particularly those with solid tumors (Rankin et al. 1997).

4. PTHrP in different breast cell models

Cultured 8701-BC cells express the genes encoding PTHrP and its receptor and release immunoreactive PTHrP (iPTHrP) fragments into the extracellular medium (Luparello et al 1999) PTHrP 1-34, 67–86 and, to a minor extent, 107–139 have also been described as anti-mitogenic but invasion-promoting for the same cell line (Luparello et al 1999).
Studies with transfected MCF-7 cells have shown that the overproduction of PTHrP is associated with increased mitogenesis via the intracrine pathway. Adding PTHrP 1-34 to cultures of MCF-7 cells stimulated increases in cAMP and cell proliferation , (Falzon et al 2000), but its effects on the PLC signaling arm were not evaluated. Walker carcinoma cells are derived from mammary glands, and are used in animal models of HHM. N-terminal PTHrP and PTH act exclusively through the PLC signal pathway in these cells, and these peptides stimulate these cells to proliferate *in vitro* (Benitez-Verguizas et al 1994).
Endogenous PTHrP appears to stimulate a variety of carcinoma cell lines to proliferate (Martin et al 1997). This may be due to tumor-specific responses to the dysregulated production of PTHrP by these cancerous cells, or a reflection of the tissue-specific growth effects of the peptide. PTHrP gene expression, PTH/PTHrP receptor signaling and PTHrP-induced mitogenesis was investigated in three SV-40 large T immortalized human mammary epithelial cell lines with different degrees of tumorigenicity (Cataissionet al 2000). The S1T3 and S2T2 cell lines were established by immortalizing primary cultures of normal human breast epithelial cells from two individuals with SV40-T Ag. *(Table 1)*Like breast epithelial cells in primary culture, the S1T3 cells did not grow in soft agar and did not form tumors in nude mice. In contrast, S2T2 cells, which also did not grow in soft agar, produced slow growing tumors (<8 mm in diameter 8 to 10 weeks after inoculation) in nude mice. The NS2T2A1 cell line was derived from an S2T2 tumor that had been grown in nude mice, re-established in vitro and then repassaged in nude mice(Berthon et al 1992 , Cataisson et al 2000). The NS2T2A1 line produced colonies in soft agar and tumors that grew rapidly in nude mice. All the cell lines stained for *pan-cytokeratin and cytokeratin 18,* confirming their epithelial nature. S2T2 and NS2T2A1 cells exhibit specific chromosomal markers resembling

those of human breast cancer (Berthon et al., 1992). Cells were cultured in Dulbecco's modified Eagle's and Ham's F12 medium (DMEM/F12, 1/1, v/v) with reduced calcium, 10 mM HEPES, 2 mM glutamine, 10 mg/ml insulin, 5mM cortisol, 2 ng/ml epidermal growth factor, 50 IU/ml penicillin, 50 mg/ ml streptomycin and 5% Chelex-treated horse serum. MDA-MB-231 breast cells lines derived from pleural effusions (Cailleau et al., 1974) were used as positive control of PTHrP gene expression, were cultured in RPMI medium supplemented with 10% fetal calf serum.

	NS2T2A1 Invasive Cell line	S2T2 Tumoregenic Cell line	S1T3 Nontumorogenic Cell Line
Soft agar colonies formation	+++	-	-
Nude mouse Tumors	100%, 3 Weeks	30% , 3 Months	0%
Estrogen Receptor Status	-	-	-
Bone Mestastasis Production	+++	-	-

Table 1. Tumorigenicity, phenotype and caryotype of human mammary epithelial cell line immortalised with SV40 T antigen. (+++) strongly stained by anti–cytoketin 18 and anti-Pan-cytokeratin antibodies , 100 % of positively staining epithelial breast cancer cells (from, Berthon et al1992; Cataisson et al 2000).

The most tumorigenic NS2T2A1 cells contained the most PTHrP mRNA, produced aggressive tumors (Cataisson et al., 2000) and gave rise to bone metastases in mice. PTH/PTHrP receptor1 (PTHrP-R1) mRNA and proteins were detected in all three cell lines. Treatment with hPTHrP (1-34) and hPTH (1-34) increased intracellular cAMP, but not free Ca2+ in the non-tumorigenic S1T3 cells. They increased both cAMP and free Ca2+ levels in the moderately tumorigenic S2T2 cells, but only increased free Ca2 in the highly tumorigenic NS2T2A1 cells. Cataisson et al., 2000, studied the mitogenic effect of PTHrP (1-34) and the signaling pathways coupled to this effect in these three immortalized mammary epithelial cell lines. The tumorigenic NS2T2A1 cells had the highest concentration of PTHrP mRNA and protein. PTHrP 1-34 stimulated NS2T2A1 cells to proliferate, acting via its receptor and the R-PTH1 activation pathway of PLC. The PTHrP-R1 receptor antagonist (Asn^{10} , Leu^{11} , D Trp^{12}) PTHrP (7-34) or anti-PTHrP antibodies dose-dependently reduced [^{3}H] thymidine incorporation into the highly tumorigenic cells but did not affect the other lines. This finding that a PTHrP-R1 receptor antagonist reduced cell proliferation suggests that PTHrP signaling mediated by the phospholipase C pathway stimulated the proliferation of these highly tumorigenic NS2T2A1 cells. PTHrP also causes 8701-BC breast tumor cells to be more invasive while inhibiting tumor growth (Luparello, et al., 1995). The heterogeneity of clones within a tumor may condition the effect of PTHrP on proliferation by giving responding differently to exogenous PTHrP (Luparello, et al., 1997). Another study by Luparello et al. found that PTHrP (38-94) only inhibited the proliferation of several breast cancer cell lines in vitro and tumor growth in vivo (Luparello et al., 2001). By evaluating PTHrP protein and mRNA expression in the SV40 immortalized human mammary epithelial cell lines, we found that PTHrP protein and mRNA expression levels of the various lines are associated with tumorigenicity. The highly tumorigenic NS2T2A1 and tumorigenic S2T2 cells expressed significantly greater amounts of PTHrP protein and mRNA than the nontumorigenic S1T3 cells. (Cataisson et al 2000).

5. Regulation of PTHrP gene expression in breast cancer cell lines

PTHrP seems to influence the malignant progression of breast cancer. About 60% of primary breast neoplasms contain PTHrP immunoreactivity, as do more than 90% of metastatic foci in bone (Southby et al 1990, Downey et al 1997,). And patients with primary breast cancer who later develop bone metastases have elevated plasma PTHrP mRNA concentrations (Bouizar et al 1993, 1999). The presence of PTHrP immunoreactivity in many breast cancers has led to the suggestion that the peptide has an autocrine effect on tumor growth (Iezzoni et al 1997). And Downey et al found that 100% of the invasive breast carcinomas surveyed had PTHrP immunoreactivity and 96% were labeled with anti-PTH/PTHrP receptor antibodies (Downey et al 1997). Significantly more cells in breast cancer tumors and metastases that are rich in PTH/PTHrP receptor mRNA and protein are labeled with antibodies to the proliferation marker Ki-67, suggesting that this receptor is associated with the increased proliferation of these tumors (Downey et al 1997). We found high concentrations of PTHrP mRNA in primary breast cancers of 110 patients who later develop bone metastases (Bouizar et al 1993, 1999). It is therefore very likely that the peptide influences aspects of the disease that precede metastasis to bone.

5.1 Splicing patterns of PTHrP mRNAs

The complexity of the PTHrP gene suggests that regulation is transcriptional and post-transcriptional, which provides considerable opportunity for dysregulation in neoplastic diseases. We investigated the mechanisms underlying the synthesis of PTHrP in the three SV-40 large T immortalized human mammary epithelial cell lines (S1T3, S2T2 and NS2T2A1) with differing tumorigenicities in order to identify the splicing patterns of their PTHrP mRNAs. The PTHrP gene has three distinct promoters, P1, P2 and P3. The TATA-containing promoter, P3, lies in an intron 35 bp upstream to exon 4 [-4 94 to -486 bp, and the transcription start site is -464 relative to the ATG translation start site in exon 5]. The second TATA promoter, P1, lies 25 bp 5′ to exon 1 and ~2.7 kb upstream of P1[-3250 to -3242 and the transcription start site is -3221]. P2 is a GC-rich regulatory region located upstream of exon 3 and the transcription initiation site is 11 bp upstream of the exon 3 splice acceptor site [-726]. Initial studies of the PTHrP promoters suggested tissue-specific promoter usage. P1 was used infrequently, generally in cell lines and tumors of squamous cell origin.

5.2 Splicing patterns of PTHrP mRNAs in breast tumors

We studied 74 primary breast cancer samples by semiquantitative RT-PCR. P2- and P3-derived transcripts were much more abundant than those derived from P1. And P3-derived transcripts were more abundant in samples from patients who later developed bone metastases. The amounts of P2-derived transcripts are significantly higher in samples from patients with mixed metastasis (bone and extra-bone metastasis) than in samples of non-metastatic tumors (Bouizar et al 1999). However, almost all breast tumors that contained P2-initiated transcripts also lacked estrogen receptors and P3 transcripts were the most abundant in breast tumors that metastasized to bone (Bouizar et al., 1999). The concentration of the 1-139 isoform was significantly elevated in primary tumors from breast cancer patients who later developed bone metastases (Bouizar et al 1999), transcripts of the 1-139 isoform derived from the P2 and P3 promoters were more abundant in tumors that ultimately metastasized, and P3 transcripts were the most abundant in tumors that metastasized to bone (Bouizar et al 1999). We found a positive correlation between PTHrP-amplified cDNA and histological node involvement (Bouizar et al 1993). Levels of PTHrP 139 cDNA were increased in the breast tumors of patients with many invaded lymph nodes (Bouizar et al 1999). This suggests that the production of PTHrP 139 is directly or indirectly linked to the ability of malignant breast cancer cells to spread through the lymph system.
Various studies have reported that the incidence of bone metastases is correlated with the histologic grade in breast cancers, and 65% of breast cancers with bone metastases were SBR GRII, while only 30% were GRIII (Coleman et al 1987, Diel et al 1992). We found more 139 PTHrP cDNA in the tumors with SBR GRIl than in those with SBR GR I or III. Thus, the PTHrP 139 isoform is the most abundant in breast cancers (Bouizar et al 1993, Bouizar et al 1999) and its presence is linked to a poor prognosis and the development of bone metastases. This isoform could be a useful prognostic marker in breast cancers. The same trend was observed for P2-initiated transcripts, but the values between groups were not statistically different. The activities of the P2 and P3 promoters were significantly correlated. The upstream TATA box promoter (P1) was rarely used. Therefore, the PTHrP gene seems to use mainly its downstream TATA (P3) and mid-region GC-rich (P2) promoters in breast cancers, especially in those that developed metastases (Bouizar et al 1999) *(Figure2,3)*. The tumorigenic NS2T2A1 cells contained increased levels of the transcripts that encode for the 1–139 isoform and showed that the P3 promoter was most active in lines produced high levels of PTHrP mRNA (Cataisson et al, 2003) *(Figure 2,3)*.
GC-rich *cis* regulatory regions do not appear to be limited to a particular class of genes. They have been located in housekeeping genes and those encoding viruses, receptors, ion-channels, cytokines, structural proteins, and DNA-binding proteins. They are frequently located in the 5′ region of genes lacking typical TATA- or CCAAT-consensus elements. The 5' untranslated region of the PTHrP gene contains a 'CpG island' upstream of exon 1C (Vasavada et al, 1993). P2-initiated transcripts only in the S2T2 and NS2T2A1 neoplasic cells and not in the non-tumoral S1T3 cells. The isolated promoter 1 construct (P1) produced very little reporter gene activity in any of the cell lines, and it is not clear whether this result reflected the low endogenous activity of this promoter or whether it lacks appropriate activating sequences. Both the full length (FL) and the promoter 2 (P2) constructs, which has a minimal (30 bases) sequence upstream of the transcription initiation site, produced relatively high reporter gene activities in all three lines. Even the S1T3 line, which contained very few endogenous P2-derived transcripts, produced substantial P2-driven luciferase activity. This finding limits the utility of larger PTHrP P2 containing reporter constructs

with these specific lines. In contrast, reporter gene activity from an isolated promoter 3 construct that contained 140 bp of upstream sequence (P3-BH) reflected endogenous P3 activity because luciferase activity gradually increased in the S2T2 and NS2T2A1 cells. While P2 appears to be active in a wide variety of cell lines and tumors quantitative studies will be needed to determine the contribution of this promoter to PTHrP gene expression in breast cancer cells *(Figure 4)*

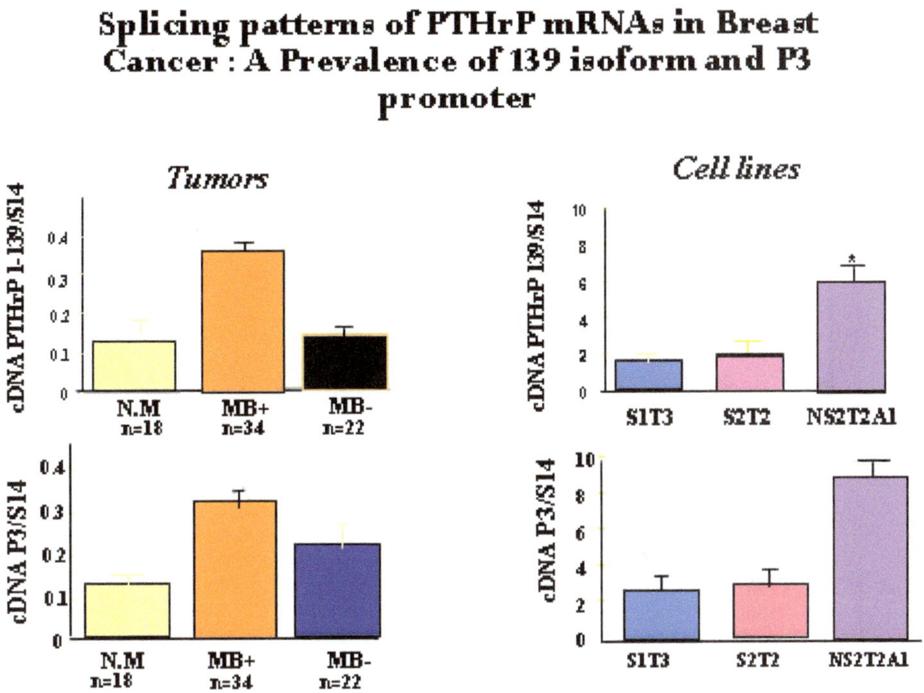

RT-PCR of the PTHrP isoforms 1-139 and 1-141/ S14 according to the development of metastases.
S14: internal control gene S14 (human small ribosomal protein 14)
n : number of patients
Tumors from patients without metastases (No Metastasis) (NM)
Tumors from patients that formed Bone Metastases (BM+)
Tumors from patients developing soft tissue metastases (BM-)

Fig. 2. Prevalence of PTHrP 139 and the P3 (TATA) promoter in invasive breast cancer and invasive breast cancer cell line (NS2T2A1)(Bouizar et al, 1999, Cataisson et al 2003).

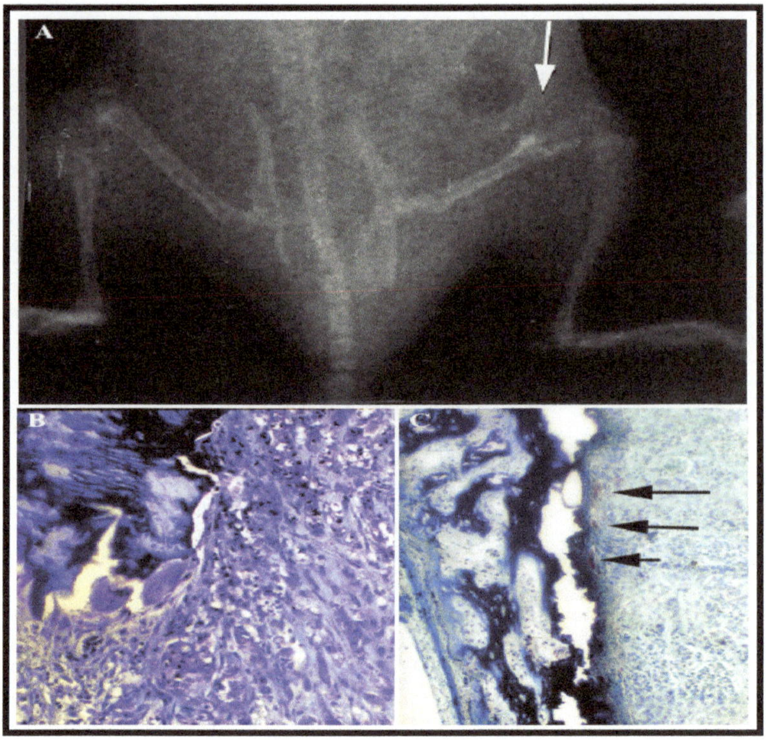

(A) Radiograph of bone metastases (white arrows) induced by injecting NS2T2A1 cells intracardially into athymic mice. (B) Histological image showing invasion of the bone marrow by the tumor mass. (C) osteoclasts stained for alkaline phosphatase (black arrows). (Bouizar et al., unpublished data).

Fig. 3. The invasive nature of NS2T2A1 cells.

6. The P3 (TATA) promoter in PTHrP transcription

The way PTHrP gene expression differs among tumors appears to result from altered transcription (Gillespie and Martin, 1994).The P3 promoter contains a series of transcription factor binding sites located ~ 50 bp upstream and downstream of the TATA box. The Ets, SMAD, and Sp1 binding sites and a CRE-like site may be involved in the control of PTHrP gene expression in some cancer cell lines (Cataisson et al., 2003; Lindemann et al., 2001; Karperien et al., 1997; Chilco et al., 1998). Also, bone osteoclasts may mediate the release of TGF-β from the bone matrix in order to stimulate PTHrP gene expression in breast cancer cells (Yin et al., 1999, Guise et al., 2002). A recent study of PTHrP promoter activity in MDA MB-231 breast cancer cells indicated that the P3 promoter is activated by TGF-β, and requires the synergistic interaction of SMADs, components of the TGF-β signaling pathway, and Ets factors (Lindemann et al., 2001).

6.1 Transcription factors that regulate the P3 promoter

We have established immortalized human mammary epithelial cell lines whose differing tumorigenicities are correlated with their PTHrP gene expression (Cataisson et al., 2000).

The Ets binding site of the PTHrP P3 promoter and the amount of Ets1 were crucial for PTHrP production by the most tumorigenic NS2T2A1 cells (Cataisson et al., 2003). However the precise mechanisms by which Ets1 activates PTHrP gene expression during tumor progression in breast cancer are unknown. We have also shown that the transcription factor Ets1 and its DNA binding site (EBS) are major determinants in the activation of PTHrP transcription in tumorigenic NS2T2A1 cells. These cells also contain higher concentrations of Ets1 protein (and mRNA) than S2T2 and S1T3 cells (Cataisson et al., 2003), which again suggests that this factor is responsible for the increased activity of the EBS-dependent PTHrP reporter gene. However, since not enough Ets1 was produced to activate PTHrP reporter gene expression in S2T2 and S1T3 cells, there are probably other transcription factors and/or coactivators contributing to the regulation of PTHrP gene expression in the fully tumorigenic cells (Cataisson et al., 2003).
Ets factors typically have a conserved winged helix-turn-helix DNA-binding domain (Wasylyk et al., 1993) that recognizes the core motif 5'GGA(A/T)3' whose flanking nucleotides determine specificity (Wasylyk et al., 1993 and (Sementchenko and Watson, 2000). Ets1 is overproduced in a variety of malignant tumors, including mammary carcinomas and tumorigenic cell lines (Delannoy-Courdent et al., 1996 and Cataisson et al., 2003). Like other regulators, the Ets proteins regulates transcription by interacting with other nuclear factors such as NFκB (Bassuk et al., 1997), AP-1 (Bassuk and Leiden, 1995), Pax (Fitzsimmons et al., 1996), (Dittmer et al., 1997 and Gitlin et al., 1993), Sp1 (Dittmer et al., 1997 and Block et al., 1996), CREB (cyclic AMP response element binding protein) (Wardle et al., 2002), CBP (Foulds et al., 2004 and Wang et al., 2004), and STAT factors (signal transducers and activators of transcription) (Aittomaki et al., 2000 and Rameil et al., 2000). CREB and Ets may cooperate to recruit CBP. We know that the P3 promoter in lung squamous carcinoma cell lines is sensitive to cAMP stimulation (Chilco et al., 1998) and there is a CRE-like site in the non-coding portion of the exon 4, 56bp downstream the TATA box. We investigated the relationship between the binding of Ets1 to the EBS site and the concentration of CBP and P3 promoter function in our three tumorigenic cell lines and whether the transcription factor CREB helps control of the PTHrP P3 promoter. The transcription factor CREB and its coactivator, CBP, were first identified as mediators of cAMP/PKA signaling (Gonzalez et al., 1989; Arias et al., 1994 and Chrivia et al., 1993). It is now clear that the coactivator CBP and the related protein p300 activate specific genes and recruit other coactivators to transcription initiation complexes. They interact with several transcription factors to form multimolecular complexes that regulate the transcription of eukaryotic genes (Janknecht and Hunter, 1996 and Goodman and Smolik, 2000). Ets1 recruits CBP and p300 during the activation of the human stromelysin promoter, while the histone acetyl transferase (HAT) activity of the proteins is required for effective transactivation of this gene (Jayaraman et al., 1999). Thus, the recruitment of CBP/p300 by DNA-bound transcription factors like Ets1 could facilitate the formation of pre-initiation complexes at promoters like P3. We used gel retardation assays with competition studies and supershift assays with specific anti-Ets1 antibodies to show that Etsl interacts with its DNA binding site (EBS) on the PTHrP P3 promoter. We found that extracts of tumorigenic cell lines contained more Ets1-DNA-binding complexes than pre-tumorigenic and non-tumorigenic cells, which correlated with their Ets1 contents (Cataisson et al., 2003). Western blot analyses showed that there were higher basal concentrations of CBP/P300 in invasive tumorigenic NS2T2A1cells than in the pre-tumoral S2T2and non-tumoral and S1T3 cells. The transfection of Ets1 and CBP/p300 expression vectors enhanced Ets1-activated P3

reporter gene activity. This cooperation was specific to tumorigenic NS2T2A1 cells. These cells not only have high concentrations of CBP/p300 and Ets1 cooperate in PTHrP P3 reporter gene transactivation, but this action is strictly dependent on the integrity of the EBS, indicating that CBP is directly recruited by Ets1. The involvement of CBP in basal and Ets1-induced P3 promoter. Our results are in agreement with previous findings showing that 12S-E1A represses PTHrP gene expression in murine keratinocytes and in human squamous carcinoma cell lines. Foley et al., 1999, Jayaraman et al., (1999) found that Ets1 recruited CBP and p300 during the transcriptional activation of the human stromelysin promoter and their HAT activity was required for effective transactivation. It is generally believed that the interaction of transcription factors with CBP/p300 localizes the coactivators to specific DNA regions, resulting in site-specific histone acetylation, chromatin remodeling and the activation of specific genes. Thus, the recruitment of CBP/p300 by DNA-bound transcription factors could facilitate the formation of pre-initiation complexes at relevant promoters (Oikawa and Yamada, 2003).

6.2 Crosstalk between transcription factors

Crosstalk between transcription factors is a commonly recognized mode of gene regulation. A STAT DNA binding site called GAS in the PTHrP P3 promoter (Richard et al., 2005) overlaps the EBS site. STAT proteins are latent cytoplasmic factors that can be activated by tyrosine phosphorylation by members of the Janus tyrosine kinase (JAK) family in response to a variety of cytokines and growth factors (Wang et al., 2005). STAT3 and STAT5 are constitutively activated in several cancers, including breast cancer, and during cell growth and transformation (Garcia et al., 2001). We found only phosphorylated STAT3 in our three cell lines and no evidence that it interacted with the EBS/GAS or was involved in the expression of the PTHrP gene. However, it is always possible that bone-derived cytokines disrupt the JAK-STAT pathway during bone invasion and influence PTHrP gene transcription.

NS2T2A1 cells should also possess additional factors required for the Ets1-mediated activation of PTHrP reporter genes (Cataisson et al., 2003). There are other regulatory sites on the P3 promoter in addition to EBS/GAS; they are SMAD, AP1, AP2 and SP1. We found binding activities for the Ap1, Ap2 and Sp1 consensus sequences in nuclear extracts of NS2T2A1 cells (data not shown), suggesting that the cognate transcription factors may participate in PTHrP-P3 promoter activity. Further studies with P3 promoter sequences, specific mutations used for EMSA and transfection experiments are required to understand how other transcription factors participate in PTHrP P3 promoter activity in tumorigenic cells.

6.3 CREB transcription factor

We also found that the transcription factor CREB was present in the cells of all three lines and that the p-CREB/CREB ratio increased with their tumorigenicity. Electrophoretic mobility shift assay (EMSA) or gel shift assay is one of the most powerful methods for studying protein-DNA interactions. Typically, ^{32}P-labeled DNA probes containing the sequence bound by the protein of interest are used in EMSA (Lance et al, 2007). However, using an electrophoresis mobility shift assay indicated that CREB was not bound to CRE-like sequences (Hamzaoui et al, 2007). This suggests no binding or a low affinity interaction, possibly due to the presence of T instead of G in the CRE-like sequence (data not shown). Nevertheless mutations in the CRE-like site abrogated activation by Ets1 as well as cooperativity between Ets1 and CBP, indicating that sequences downstream of the EBS recruit factors and coactivators that help stabilize the EBS-Ets1 complex. The CRE-like region is followed by an AP2 site. So, member of the b-ZIP family of transcription factor may form heterodimers at this composite site, recruit CBP and take part in EBS functioning. The enhancement of P3 promoter activity by CREB or constitutively active CREB overproduction, independently of the integrity of EBS and/or CRE-like sequences, may also indicate that CREB promotes DNA-binding-independent transcriptional activation, as it does in other models (Giebler et al., 2000). CREB may thus tether CBP to an as-yet-unidentified transcription factor/regulatory site on the P3 promoter. We are now working to determine how CREB acts on the P3 promoter and its relationship with the tumorigenic potential of breast cancer cell lines.

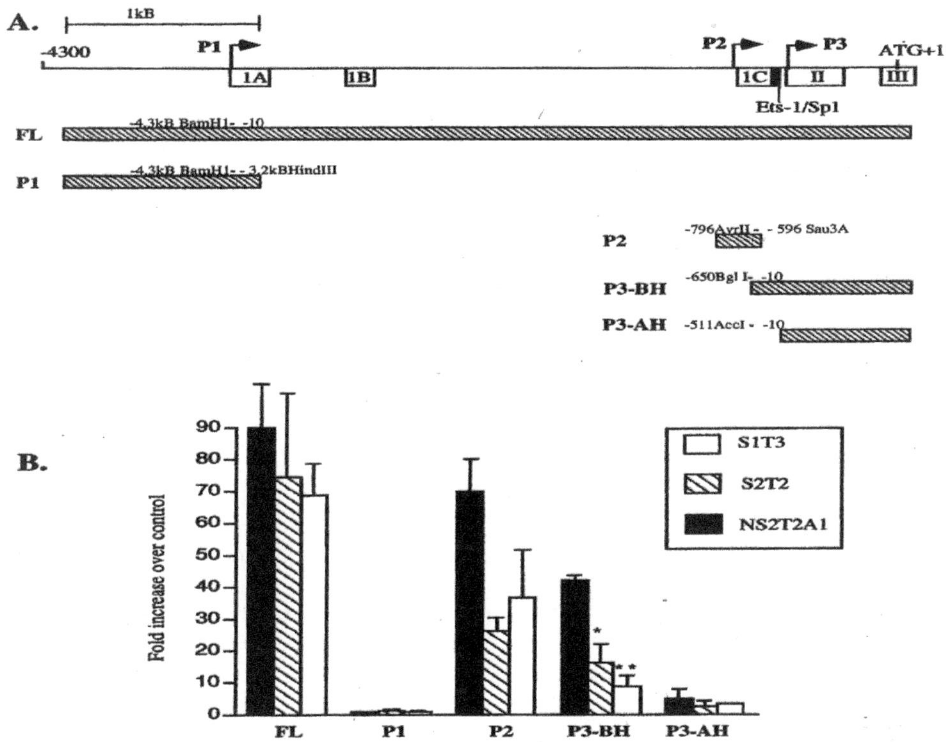

Fig. 4. Expression of reporter genes driven by 5′PTHrP sequences in S1T3, S2T2 and NS2T2A1 cells. Panel A: a schematic representation of the 5′- flanking region of the human PTHrP gene and the 5′PTHrP-Luc constructs used in the analysis: exons are indicated by boxes, promoters by arrows and the shaded region represents the region of the EBS-1 and Sp1trascription factors sites. The construct represented as FL (full length) contains 4.3 kb of upstream sequence and all three promoters. P1 contains the P1 promoter in isolation and P2 contains the P2 promoter and minimal (30 bases) sequence upstream of the transcription initiation site. P3-BH contains 140 bp upstream of the P3 TATA including the Ets-1/Sp1 site and the downstream non-translated exon II. P3-AH contains only 15 bp of upstream sequence, thus eliminating the Ets-1/Sp1 site, but contains downstream sequences. Panel B: Substantial P2-driven luciferase activity and relatively high level of the reporter gene

activity in the NS2T2A1 line *V/S* S1T2 and S1T3 lines .The bar graph depicts reporter gene activity normalized to the activity of a promoter less luciferase vector pGL-2. Bars represent the average of three samples and error bars indicate SEM. If an error bar is not present it indicates the error was not of sufficient magnitude to be illustrated on the graph. Every construct was transfected into each of the three lines in three separate experiments and similar results were obtained. * represents PB/0.05 NS2T2A1 vs S2T2; ** represents PB/0.01NS2T2A1 vs S1T3.(Cataisson et al 2003).

In conclusion, we have clearly established the importance of cooperation between Ets1 and CBP at the EBS regulatory sequence of the P3 promoter. We have proposed that there is cross-talk between Ets1 and transcription factors (like CREB) that have affinity to and share a linkage with coactivators such as CBP. (Son et al 2010), reported that metastatic MDA-MB-231 breast cancer cells contained more CREB than did non-metastatic MCF-7 cells. They used wild-type CREB and a dominant-negative form (K-CREB) to show that CREB signaling positively regulated the proliferation, migration, and invasion of MDA-MB-231 cells. K-CREB also prevented MDA-MB-231 cell-induced osteolytic lesions in a mouse model of cancer metastasis. Lastly, CREB signaling regulated the expressions of the PTHrP, MMPs, and OPG genes, which are all closely involved in cancer metastasis and bone destruction. Thus CREB is overproduced in developing breast cancer cells and this CREB upregulation is important for many steps in the metastasis of breast cancers to bone, along with the stimulation of PTHrP gene expression. These findings open up new horizons in the study of the modulation of the PTHrP promoter activity and its impact on the devastating results of PTHrP overexpression (invasion, metastasis, HHM, etc.). They may even reveal new targets forbreast c ancer therapy.

7. References

Aittomaki, S. Aittomaki, M. Pesu, B. Groner, O.A. Janne, J.J. Palvimo and Silvennoinen,o. (2000). Cooperation among Stat1, glucocorticoid receptor, and PU.1 in transcriptional activation of the high-affinity Fc gamma receptor I in monocytes, *J. Immunol.* 164 (2000), pp. 5689–5697.

Arias J, Alberts AS, Brindle P, Claret FX, Smeal T, Karin M, Feramisco J, Montminy M. (1994) Activation of cAMP and mitogen responsive genes relies on a common nuclear factor, Nature 370 (1994), pp. 226–229Bassuk and Leiden, 1995 A.G. Bassuk and J.M. Leiden, A direct physical association between ETS and AP-1 transcription factors in normal human T cells, *Immunity*,3 ,(1995), pp.223–237

Arguello, F. Baggs, R. B. and Frantz, C. N. (1988). A murine model of experimentalmetastasis to bone and bone marrow. *Cancer Res*, 48, (1988), pp. 6878–6881

Barlet,W. Davicco, M.J. Coxam,V. (1990). Synthetic parathyroid hormone-related peptide (1-34) fragment stimulates placental calcium transfer in ewes *J. Endocrinol*, 127,(1990), pp.33-37.

Birch, M. A. Carron, J. A. Scott, M. Fraser, W. D.and Gallagher, J. A. (1995). Parathyroid hormone (PTH)/PTH-related protein (PTHrP) receptor expression and mitogenic responses in human breast cancer celi lunes. *Br J Cancer*, 72,(1995), pp.90-95.

Bassuk AG, Leiden JM. (1995). A direct physical association between ETS and AP-1 transcription factors in normal human T cells, *Immunity*, 3 ,(1995), pp. 223–237

Bassuk AG, Anandappa RT, Leiden JM.(1997). Physical interactions between Ets and NF-kappaB/NFAT proteins play an important role in their cooperative activation of the human immunodeficiency virus enhancer in T cells, J Virol, 71, (1997), pp. 3563–3573.

Benitez-Verguizas, J. and Esbrit, P. (1994). Proliferative effect of parathyroid hormone-related protein on the hypercalcemic Walker 256 carcinoma celi une. *Biochem Biophys Res Commun,* 198, (1994),pp.1281-1289.

Berthon, P. Goubin ,G. Dutrillaux ,B. Degeorges, A. Faille, A, Gespach, C. and Calvo, F.(1992). Single-steep transformation of human breast epithelial cells by SV40 large T oncogene. *Int J Cancer, 52, (1992), pp.92-97.*

Bouizar, Z. Spyratos, F. Deytieux, S. de Vernejoul, MC. Jullienne, A. (1993). Polymerase chain reaction analysis of parathyroid hormone-related protein gene expression in breast cancer patients and occurrence of bone metastases. *Cancer Res,* 53(21), (1993), pp.5076-8.

Bouizar, Z. Spyratos, F. and De Vernejoul, M.C.(1999).The parathyroid hormonerelatedprotein (PTHrP) gene: Use of downstream TATA promotor and PTHrP1-139 coding pathways in primary breast cancers vary with the occurrence of bone metastasis. *J Bone Miner Res,* 14, (1999), pp.406–414.

Broadus, AE, Stewart, AF. (1994). Parathyroid hormone-related protein structure, processing and physiological actions. *The Parathyroids, Raven Press ed., New York,* pp. 259-294.

Brundred,NJ.Walker,RA.Ratciiffe,WA.Warwick,J.Morrison,JM.Ratcliffe,JG.(1992).Parathyroi d hormone related protein and skeietai morbidity in breast cancer. *Eur J Cancer,* 28, (1992),pp.690-692.

Budayr, A. A. Halbran, B. P. King, J. C. Diep, D. Nissenson, R. A.and Strewler, G. J.(1989). High levels of a parathyroid hormone-like protein in milk. *Proc Natl Acad Sci U S A* ,86,(1989), pp.183-185.

Burtis, W. J. Bady, T. F. Orloff, J. J. Ersbak, J. B. Warrell, R. P. Olson, B. R. Wu, T. L.Mitnick, M. E. Broadus, A. E. and Stewart, A. F.(1990). Immunochemical characterization of circulating parathyroid hormone-related protein in patients with humoral hypercalcemia of cancer. *N Engl J Med,* 322, (1990),pp.1106–1112..

Burtis, W. J. Fodero, J. P. Gaich, G. Debeyssey, M. and Stewart, A. F.(1992). Preliminary characterization of circulating amino- and carboxy-terminal fragments of parathyroid hormone-related peptide in humoral hypercalcemia of malignancy. *JClinEndocrinolMetab,*75,(1992),pp.1110–1114.

Campos, R.V. Wang, C. and Drucker, D.J. (1992). Regulation of parathyroid hormone-related peptide (PTHrP) gene transcription: cell- and tissue-specific promoter utilization mediated by multiple positive and negative cis-acting DNA elements, *Mol. Endocrinol,* 6, (1992), pp. 1642–1652

Cataisson, C. Lieberherr ,M. Cotton, J. Calvo, F. Cros, M. de Vernejoul, MC. Foley, J. and Bouizar, Z. (2000). Parathyroid hormone-related peptide stimulates proliferation of highly tumorigenic human SV40-immortalized breast epithelial cells. *J Bone Miner Res,* 15 (2000), pp.2129-2139.

Cataisson, C. Gordon, J.Roussière, M. Abdalkhani, A. Lindemann, R. Dittmer, J. Foley, J,·and Bouizar, Z. (2003) . Ets-1 Activates Parathyroid Hormone-Related Protein Gene Expression In Tumorigenic Breast Epithelial Cells. Molecular and Cellular *Endocrinology,* 204,(2003),pp.155-168

Chilco, P.J. Leopold,V.and Zajac, J.D.(1998).Differential regulation of the parathyroid hormone-related protein gene P1 and P3 promoters by cAMP, Mol. Cell *Endocrinol,* 138, (1998), pp. 173–184

Chrivia, J.C. Chrivia, R.P. Kwok, N. Lamb, M. Hagiwara, M.R. Montminy,M. and Goodman, R.H. (1993). Phosphorylated CREB binds specifically to the nuclear protein CBP.*Nature* 365 , (1993),pp. 855–859

Coleman, RE. Rubens, RD. (1987). The clinical course of bone metastases from breast cancer. *Br J Cancer,* 55, (1987), pp.61-66.

Cros, M. Cataisson, C. Mee Cho, Y. Berthois ,Y.Bernard-Poenaru, O. Denne, M. Graulet ,AM. deVernejoul, MC. and Bouizar, Z.(2002). Constitutive production of Parathyroi-Hormone Related Protein (PTHrP) by fibroblasts derivated from normal and pathological human tumorigenic breast cancer. *Oncol.Res/Anti-Cancer Drug Design, 13*,(2002), pp.137-146.

Daniel, CW.Silberstein, GB. (1987). Postnatal development of the rodent mammary gland. The mammary Gland Development, Regulation and Fonction. *(MC Neville, CW Daniel, pp. 3-36. New York: Plenum Press.*

Davicco, MJ. Rouffet, J. Durand, D. (1993). Parathyroid hormone-related peptide my increase manimary blood fow.*J Bone Min Res* , 8, (1993), pp. 1519-1524.

Downey. S.E. Hoyland,J. Freemont, A.J. Knox, F. Walls, J. and Bundred, N. J. (1997). Expression of the receptor for parathyroid hormone-related protein in normal and malignant breast tissue. *J Pathol,* 183,(1997),pp. 212-217.

Delannoy-Courdent A, W. Fauquette, X.F. Dong-Le Bourhis, B. Boilly, B. Vandenbunder and X. Desbiens (1996). Expression of c-ets-1 and uPA genes is associated with mammary epithelial cell tubulogenesis or neoplastic scattering, *Int J Dev Biol* 40, (1996), pp.1097–1108.

Diel, IJ. Kaufmann, M. Goerne,r R. Costa, SD. Bastert ,DG. (1992). Detection of tumor celis in bone marrow of patients with primary breast cancer: A pronostic factor for distant metastasis. *J Clin Oncol,* 10, (1992), pp.1534-1539.

Dittmer, J. Dittmer, C.A. Pise-Masison, K.E. Clemens, K.S. Choi, and Brady, J.N.(1997). Interaction of human T-cell lymphotropic virus type I Tax, Ets1, and Sp1 in transactivation of the PTHrP P2 promoter. *J Biol Chem,* 272, (1997), pp. 4953–4958.

Dunbar, M. E. Young, P. Zhang, J. P. Mc Caughern, C. J. Lanske, B. Orloff, J. J. Karaplis, A. C., Cunha, G. and Wysolmerski, J. J. (1998). Stromal ceils are critical targets in the regulation of mammary ductal morphogenesis by parathyroid hormone-related protein. *Dey Biol* , 203, (1998), pp.75-89.

Ferrari, S. L. Rizzoli, R. Chaponnier, C.Gabbiani, G. and Bonjour, J. P. (1993). Parathyroid honnone-related protein increases cAMP production in mammary epithelial cells. *Am J Physiol* , E47(1993), pp. 1-5.

Fitzsimmons, D. Fitzsimmons, W. Hodsdon, W. Wheat, S.M. Maira, B. Wasylyk and Hagman, J. (1996). Pax-5 (BSAP) recruits Ets proto-oncogene family proteins to form functional ternary complexes on a B-cell-specific promoter, *Genes Dev.* 10, (1996), pp. 2198–2211

Foley,J. Wysolmerski, C. Missero, C.S. and Philbrick, W.M. (1999) Regulation of parathyroid hormone-related protein gene expression in murine keratinocytes by E1A isoforms: a role for basal promoter and Ets-1 site. *Mol Cell Endocrinol,* 156, (1999), pp. 13–23.

Foulds, C.E. Foulds, M.L. Nelson, A.G. and Blaszczak, B.J.(2004). Graves, Ras/mitogen-activated protein kinase signaling activates Ets-1 and Ets-2 by CBP/p300 recruitment. *Mol Cell Biol,* 24,(2004), pp. 10954–10964

Garcia, T.L. Bowman, G. Niu, H. Yu, S. Minton, C.A. Muro-Cacho, C.E. Cox, R. Falcone, R. Fairclough, S. Parsons, A. Laudano, A. Gazit, A. Levitzki, A. K. and Jove, R. . (2001). Constitutive activation of Stat3 by the Src and JAK tyrosine kinases participates in growth regulation of human breast carcinoma cells, *Oncogene,* 20, (2001), pp. 2499-2513.

Giebler, H.A. Lemasson, I. and Nyborg, J.K. (2000). p53 recruitment of CREB binding protein mediated through phosphorylated CREB: a novel pathway of tumor suppressor regulation, *Mol Cell Biol,* 20, (2000),pp. 4849–4858.

Gillespie, M.T. and Martin, T.J. (1994). The parathyroid hormone-related protein gene and its expression. *Mol. Cell Endocrinol.* 100, (1994),pp. 143–147.

Gitlin, S.D. J. Dittmer, R.C.and Brady, J.N. (1993). Transcriptional activation of the human T-lymphotropic virus type I long terminal repeat by functional interaction of Tax1 and Ets1. *J Virol,* 67, (1993), pp. 7307–7316.

Gonzalez, G.A. andMontminy, M.R.(1989). Cyclic AMP stimulates somatostatin gene transcription by phosphorylation of CREB at serine 133. *Cell,* 59, (1989), pp. 675-680.

Goodman, RH and Smolik, S. (2000). CBP/p300 in cell growth, transformation, and development. Genes Dev,14, (2000),pp. 1553–1577.

Grill, V. Ho, P.Body, J. J. Johanson, N. Lee, S. C. Kukreja, S. C. Moseley, J. M. and Martin, T. J. (1991). Parathyroid hormone-related protein: elevated levels in both humoral hypercalcemia of malignancy and hypercalcemia complicating metastatic breast cancer. *J Clin Endocrinol Metab* ,73, (1991), pp.1309-1315

GuiseTA J.J. Yin S.D. Taylor Y. Kumagai M. Dallas, B.F. Boyce, T. and Mundy, G.R. (1996). Evidence for a causal role of parathyroid hormone-related protein in the pathogenesis of human breast cancer-mediated osteolysis. J Clin Invest, 98, (1996),pp. 1544–1549.

Guise,TA. J.J. Yin, R.J. Thomas, M. Dallas, Y. C. and Gillespie, M.T. (2002). Parathyroid hormone-related protein (PTHrP)-(1-139) isoform is efficiently secreted in vitro and enhances breast cancer metastasis to bone in vivo. Bone ,30, (2002), pp. 670–676.

Hamzaoui, H. Rizk-Rabin, M. Gordon, J. Offutt, C. Bertherat, J. and Bouizar, Z. (2007), PTHrP P3 promoter activity in breast cancer cell lines: Role of Ets1 and CBP (CREB binding protein*). Mol and Cell Endocrinol,268, (*2007), pp.75-84

Iezzoni, J. C. Bruns, M. E. Frierson, H. F. Scott, M. G. Pence, R. A. Deftos, L. J. and Bruns, D.E. (1998). Coexpression of parathyroid hormone-related protein arid its receptor in breast carcinoma:a potential autocrine effector system. *Mod Pathol,*11, (1998),pp. 265-270.

Janknecht, R. J. and Hunter, T. (1996). Transcription. A growing coactivator network. Nature, 383, (1996), pp. 22–23.

Jayaraman, G. R. Srinivas, C. Duggan, E. Ferreira, S. Swaminathan, K. Somasundaram, J.

Williams, C. Hauser, M. Kurkinen, R. Dhar, S. Weitzman, G. B. and Thimmapaya, B.(1999). p300/cAMP-responsive element-binding protein interactions with ets-1 and ets-2 in the transcriptional activation of the human stromelysin promoter. *J Biol Chem,* 274, (1999), pp. 17342–17352.

Ikeda, K. Mangin, M. Dreyer, B.E. Webb, A.C. Posillico, J.T. Stewart, A.F. Bander, N.H.b Weir, E.C. Insogna, K.L. and Broadus, A.E. (1988). Identification of transcripts encoding a parathyroid hormone-like peptide in messenger RNAs from a variety of human and animal tumors associated with humoral hypercalcemia of malignancy. *J Clin Invest,*81, (1988), pp. 2010-2014.

Karaplis, AC. Luz, A. Glowacki,J. Bronson, RT. Tybulewicz, VL. Kronenberg, HM. Mulligan, R.(1994). Lethal skeletal dyspiasia from targeted disruption of the parathyroid hormone-related peptide gene. *Genes Dey,* 8, (1994), pp.277-289.

Karperien, M. Karperien, H. Farih-Sips, C.W. Lowik, S.W. de Laat, J. B. and Defize, L.H. (1997). Expression of the parathyroid hormone-related peptide gene in retinoic acid-induced differentiation: involvement of ETS and Sp1. *Mol. Endocrinol.* 11, (1997),pp. 1435–1448.

Khosla, S, Johanson, KL. Ory ,SJ.(1990). Parathyroid hormone-related peptide in lactation and umbilical cord blood . *Myo Clin Proc* ,65, (1990),pp.1408-1412.

Kozlow, W. and Guise, T.A. (2005). Breast cancer metastasis to bone: mechanisms of osteolysis and implications for therapy. *J Mammary Gland Biol Neoplasia* ,10, (2005),pp. 169-180.

Lance, M. H and Fried, M.G.(2007). Electrophoretic Mobility Shift Assay (EMSA) for Detecting Protein-Nucleic Acid Interactions. *Nat Protoc,* 2, (2007), pp.1849–1861.

Lee, K. Deeds, J.Segre, G. V. (1995b). Expression of parathyroid hormorie-reiated peptide and its receptor messenger ribonucieic acids during fetal deveiopment of rats. *Endocrinoiogy* ,136, (1995b), pp.453-463.

Liapis, H. Crouch, E.C. Grosso, L.E. Kitazawa, S. and Wick, M.R. (1993). Expression of parathyroidlike protein in normal, proliferative, and neoplastic human breast tissues. *Am J Pathol* ,143, (2001), pp.1169-1178.

Lindemann, R.K. Ballschmieter, P. Nordheim, and Dittmer,J.(2001). Transforming growth factor beta regulates parathyroid hormone-related protein expression in MDA-MB-231 breast cancer cells through a novel Smad/Ets synergism. *J Biol Chem,* 276 , (2001), pp. 46661–46670

Linforth, R., Anderson, N., Hoey, R., Nolan, T., Downey, S., Brady, G., Ashcroft, L. and Bundred, N. (2002). Coexpression of parathyroid hormone related protein and its receptor in early breast cancer predicts poor patient survival. *Clin Cancer Res* ,8, (2002), pp. 3172-3177.

Lepre, F. Grill, V. Ho, P. W. and Martin, T. J. (1993). Hypercalcemia in pregnancy and lactation associated with parathyroid hormone-related protein. *N Engl J Med,* 328, (1993), pp. 666-667.

Mangin, M. K. Ikeda, B.E. and Broadus, A.E. (1990). Identification of an up-stream promoter of the human parathyroid hormone-related peptide gene . *Mol Endocrinol,* 4, (1990),pp. 851–858.

Martin, T.J. Moseley, J.M. and Williams, E.D. (1997). Parathyroid hormone-related protein:hormone and cytokine. *J Endocrinol,* 154, (1997), pp.S23-S37.

Murray, T.M. Rao, L.G. Divieti, P. and Bringhurst, F.R. (2005). Parathyroid hormone secretion and action: evidence for discrete receptors for the carboxyl-terminal region and related biological actions of carboxyl- terminal ligands. *Endocr Rev*,26, (2005), pp. 78–113.

Oikawa, T. and Yamada, T. (2003). Molecular biology of the Ets family of transcription factors. *Gene* , 303, (2003), pp. 11–34. |

Philbrick, W.M.Wysolmerski, J.J. Galbraith, S. Holt, E. Orloff, J.J. Yang, K.H. Vasavada, ,R.C. Weir, E.C. Broadus, A.E. and Stewart, A.F. (1996). Defining the roles of parathyroid hormone-related protein in normal physiology. *Physiol Rev* ,76, (1996), pp. 127-173.

Philbrick, W.M.Dreyer, B.E. Nakchbandi, l.A. Karaplis, A.C. (1998). Parathyroid hormone-related protein is required for tooth eruption. *Proc Nati Acad Sci US A*, 95, (1998), pp. 11846-11851.

Peyruchaud, O. Winding, B. Pecheur, I.b Serre, C.M. Delmas, P. and Clezardin, P. (2001). Early detection of bone metastases in a murine model using fluorescent human breast cancer cells: application to the use of the bisphosphonate zoledronic acid in the treatment of osteolytic lesions. *J Bone Miner Res* ,16, (2001), pp.2027-2034.

Pvveli, G. J. Southby, J. Danks, J. A. Stiliweil, R. G. Hayman, J. A. Henderson, M. A. and Martin, T. J. (1991). Localization of parathyroid hormone-reiated protein in breast cancer tmeastases: increased incidence in bone compared with other sites. *Cancer Res,* 51, (1991), pp. 3059-3061.

Rankin, W. Grill, V. and Martin, T.J. (1997). Parathyroid hormone-related protein and hypercalcemia. *Cancer,* 80, (1997), pp.1564-1571.

Rameil, P. Lecine, J. Ghysdael, F. Gouilleux, B. Imbert, J. (2000). IL-2 and long-term T cell activation induce physical and functional interaction between STAT5 and ETS transcription factors in human T cells. *Oncogene,* 19 , (2000), pp. 2086–2097.

Richard,V. A. Luchin, R.M. Brena, C. P. and Rosol, T.J. (2003). Quantitative evaluation of alternative promoter usage and 3' splice variants for parathyroid hormone-related protein by real-time reverse transcription-PCR. *Clin Chem,*49 , (2003), pp. 1398–1402.

Rodda, C.P. Kubota, M.J. Heath, A. Ebeling, P. R. Moseley, J. M. Care, A. D. Caple I. W. and Martin T. J. (1988). Evidence for a novel parathyroid hormone-r.elated protein in fetal lamb parathyroid glands and sheep placenta: comparisons with a similar protein implicated in humoral hypercalcaemia of malignancy. *J Endocrinol* , 117, (1988), pp. 261-271

Sementchenko ,V.I. and Watson, D.K. (2000). Ets target genes: past, present and future. Oncogene ,19, (2000), pp. 6533–6548.

Sakakura, T. (1991). aspects of stroma-parenchyma relations in mammary gland differentiation.int.Rev. *Cytology,* 125, (1991), pp 165-199.

Sakakura, T. (1987). Mammary ebryogenesis. *In the mammary Gland: development, Regulation and fonction.* (ed MC Neville, CW Daniel, pp. 37-36.), New York: Plenum Press.

Sebag, M. Henderson, J. E. Goltzman,D. and Kremer, R. (1994). Regulation of parathyroid hormone-. reiated peptide production in normal human mammary epithelial ceils in vitro. *Am J Physiol ,(1994), pp.* C723-730.

Solimando, D.A. (2001). Overview of hypercalcemia of malignancy. *Am J Health Syst Pharm* ,58 Suppl 3, (2001), pp. S4-7.

Son J,-Ho J Lee, Ha-Neui Kim, Hyunil Haand Zang Hee Lee (2010). cAMP-response-element-binding protein positively regulates breast cancer metastasis and subsequent bone destruction . *Biochem and Biophysical Rese Comm,* 398, (2010), pp. 2309-2314.

Surowiak, P. Dziegiel, P. Matkowski, R. Sopel, M. Wojnar, A. Kornafel, J. and Zabel, M. (2003). Prognostic value of immunocytochemical determination of parathyroid hormone-related peptide expression in cells of mammary ductal carcinoma. *Analysis of 7 years of the disease course.* Virchows Arch 442, (2003), pp. 245-251.

Southby, J. O'Keeffe, L.M. Martin, . T.J. and. Gillespie, M.T. (1995). Alternative promoter usage and mRNA splicing pathways for parathyroid hormone-related protein in normal tissues and tumours. *Br J Cancer,* 72, (1995), pp. 702–707.

Southby,J. Murphy, L.M. Martin, T.J. and Gillespie, M.T. (1996). Cell-specific and regulator-induced promoter usage and messenger ribonucleic acid splicing for parathyroid hormone-related protein. *Endocrinology* ,137, (1996), pp. 1349–1357.

Strewler, G.J. (2000). The parathyroid hormone-related protein. *Endocrinol Metab Clin North Am* ,29, (2000), pp. 629-645.

Suva., L.J. Suva, K.A. Mather, Gillespie, M.T. Webb, G.C. Ng, K.W. Winslow, G.A. Wood, W.I. Martin T.J. and Hudson, P.J. (1989). Structure of the 5′ flanking region of the gene encoding human parathyroid-hormone-related protein (PTHrP). *Gene, 77,* (1989), pp. 95–105.

Sowers, M. F. Hollis, B. W. Shapiro, B. Randolph, J. Janney, C. A. Zhang, D. Schork, A. Crutchfield, M. Stanczyk, F. and Russell, A. M. (1996). Elevated parathyroid hormone-related peptide associated with lactation and bone density loss. *Lama,* 276, (1996), pp. 549-554.

Thiede, M. A. and Rodan, G. A. (1988). Expression of a calcium-mobilizing parathyroid hormone-like peptide in lactating mammary tissue. *Science,* 242, (1988), pp. 278-280.

Thomas, R.J. Guise, T.A. Yin, J.J. Elliott, J. Horwood, N.J. Martin T.J. and. Gillespie, M.T (1999). Breast cancer cells interact with osteoblasts to support osteoclast formation. *Endocrinology* ,140, (1999), pp. 4451–4458.

Vargas,S. Gillespie, M.T. Poweli, G.J. Southby, J. Danks, J.A. Moseley, J.M. Martin, T.J. (1992). Localization of parathyroid hormone-related protein mRNA expression in breast cancer and metastatic lesions by in situ hybridization. *J Bone Miner Res,* 7, (1992), pp. 971-979.

Vasavada, R.C. Wysolmerski, J.J. Broadus, A.E. and. Philbrick, W.M. (1993). Identification and characterization of a GC-rich promoter of the human parathyroid hormone-related peptide gene . *Mol Endocrinol,* 7, (1993), pp. 273–282

Wang, H. R. Fang, J.Y. Cho, T.A. and Oettgen, P. (2004). Positive and negative modulation of the transcriptional activity of the ETS factor ESE-1 through interaction with p300, CREB-binding protein, and Ku 70/86. J Biol Chem, 279, (2004), pp. 25241–25250.

Wardle,F.C. Wardle, D.H. and Sive, H.L. (2002). Cement gland-specific activation of the Xag1 promoter is regulated by co-operation of putative Ets and ATF/CREB transcription factors. *Development,* 129, (2002), pp. 4387–4397.

Wasylyk, S.L. and Giovane, A. (1993). The Ets family of transcription factors. *Eur J* Biochem, 11, (1993), pp. 7–18.

Wojcik, S. F. Capen, C. C. and Rosol, T. J. (1999). Expression of PTHrP and the PTH/PTHrP receptor in purified alveolar epithelial cells, myoepithelial cells, and stromal fibroblasts derived from the lactating rat mammary gland. *Exp Cell Res,* 248, (1999), pp. 415-422.

Wysolmerski, J. J. Broadus, A. E. Zhou, J. Fuchs, E. Milstone, L. M. and Philbrick, W. M. (1994). Overexpression of parathyroid hormone-related protei in the skin of transgenic mice interferes with hair follicle development. *Proc Nati Acad Sci U S A,* 91, (1994), pp. 1133-1137.

Wysolmerski, J.J. Stewart, A.F, (1998).The physiology of parathyroid hormone-related protein: an emerging role as a developmental factor. *Annu Rev Physiol* ,60,(1998), 431-460.

Yin, J.J. Selander, K. Chirgwin,J.M. Dallas, M. Grubbs, B.G. Wieser, R. Massague, J. Mundy G.R. and. Guise, T.A.(1999). TGF-beta signaling blockade inhibits PTHrP secretion by breast cancer cells and bone metastases development. *J Clin Inves*t, 103, (1999), pp. 197–206.

3

The Electronics of HER2/neu Positive Breast Cancer Cells

Jan Baumann, Christopher Karch,
Antonis Kourtidis and Douglas S. Conklin
University at Albany, State University of New York
USA

1. Introduction

Approximately 20 to 30 % of all breast cancer cases are classified as HER2/neu-positive (McCann et al. 1991). The overexpression the HER2 receptor tyrosine kinase is most commonly caused by a gene amplification and is associated with aggressive tumor behavior (Hynes & Stern 1994). Patients with HER2/neu overexpressing tumors have a significantly shorter time to relapse as well as a reduced overall survival rate compared to patients with normal HER2/neu expression levels (Berchuck et al. 1990; Slamon et al. 1989; Slamon et al. 1987). The oncogenic properties of HER2/neu were first discovered in rat neuroblastoma ("neu") as a tumor antigen related to epidermal growth-factor receptor (EGFR) (Schechter et al. 1984). The human homologue to *neu* was mapped to chromosome 17q21 and, because of its similarity to the human EGF receptor, named human EGF receptor 2 (HER2) (Coussens et al. 1985; King et al. 1985). Two more members of the HER family, namely HER3 and HER4, were subsequently identified (Kraus et al. 1989; Plowman et al. 1993). In this review we will discuss the altered metabolism and potential downstream effects found in breast cancer cells with increased HER2/neu expression.

1.1 The HER family of receptor tyrosine kinases

The HER family of receptors are found in a variety of tissues and interact with several EGF-like ligands (Harris et al. 2003). HER2 plays an important role in human development, it has been detected in the nervous system, bone, muscle, skin, heart, lungs and intestinal epithelium (Coussens et al. 1985; Quirke et al. 1989). Deletion of HER2 in mice leads to embryonic lethality (Meyer & Birchmeier 1995). Upon ligand binding, the receptors either homo- or heterodimerize and transphosphorylate each other. This initiates downstream signaling cascades through a variety of adaptor proteins and second messengers resulting in cell cycle progression, proliferation and survival (Bazley & Gullick 2005; Alroy & Yarden 1997). Even though HER2 does not bind any ligand by itself, it has been reported to display low affinity interactions with many, if not all, ligands in any given receptor heterodimer (Tzahar & Yarden 1998). It has been suggested that HER2 is the preferred dimerization partner for all the ligand-binding members of the HER family and that HER2 heterodimers are more active than their homodimeric counterparts (Yarden 2001), which might be due to enhanced recycling of HER2 receptor heterodimers to the cell surface (Lenferink et al. 1998).

This indicates that a disregulation of HER2 levels will lead to increased receptor dimerization and thus increased signaling.
The expression levels of HER2 in malignant cells can be increased up to 100-fold compared to normal cells, resulting in as many as two million HER2 molecules per cell (Park et al. 2006; Liu et al. 1992; Venter et al. 1987). This overexpression is most commonly caused by an amplification of the HER2 gene, which leads to increased transcription and protein synthesis. Experiments utilizing fluorescence *in situ* hybridization suggest that only about 3 % of HER2 overexpressing breast cancers do not carry a corresponding gene amplification (Pauletti et al. 1996). The majority of HER2 overexpressing breast cancer cells have been shown to have 25-100 copies of the HER2 gene (Kallioniemi et al. 1992). This gene amplification and overexpression of the HER2 protein identifies a subset of the breast cancer disease which is found independent of disease stage. In fact, gene expression studies show that HER2 overexpressing tumors display a characteristic molecular pattern that is maintained as the cancer progresses, indicating that HER2 amplification is an early event in carcinogenesis (Weigelt et al. 2005; Perou et al. 2000). HER2 overexpression is found in almost half of all ductal carcinoma *in situ* (DCIS) that show no evidence of invasion but does not occur in benign breast disease (Allred et al. 1992; Park et al. 2006; Liu et al. 1992).

1.2 Treatment of HER2/neu-positive breast cancer

These advances in basic breast cancer research lead to the development of the first truly targeted cancer therapy agent, the humanized monoclonal antibody trastuzumab (Herceptin®, Genentech) (Carter et al. 1992). Herceptin was FDA approved in 1998 for the treatment of advanced metastatic breast cancer (Hortobagyi 2001). Possible mechanisms of action and the safety profile of trastuzumab are reviewed in Hudis et al. (2007). After initial success of using Herceptin in the clinic (Vogel et al. 2002), more and more reports about tumors developing Herceptin resistance were published (recently reviewed in Mukohara 2011). Truncated HER2 receptors (p95HER2) lacking the extracellular domain, which is targeted by Herceptin, were identified in human breast tumors (Molina et al. 2002). This prompted the development of new, second generation targeted therapies like tyrosine kinase inhibitors, HSP90 inhibitors, inhibitors of PI3 kinase, new anti-HER2 antibodies as well as HER2-based vaccination strategies. These novel anti-HER2 strategies are reviewed in Mukohara (2011).
Even though it has been almost 25 years since the discovery of HER2 as an identifier of a unique subset of breast cancers, we still have not conquered the disease with therapies directed against HER2. The ability of HER2 driven breast tumors to consistently develop resistance against therapies targeting HER2 underlines the importance of further research in this area. The underlying genetics associated with HER2 overexpression seem to be responsible for a more complex picture that is only hinted at by HER2 diagnostics.

2. The genetics of HER2/*neu*-positive breast cancer

Several studies in the past decade show that HER2 protein overexpression or gene amplification is not the only alteration in the breast cancer subtype denoted HER2 positive. Transcriptional profiling (meta-) analyses have demonstrated that a number of genes are commonly overexpressed along with HER2. At the beginning of this century, a specific gene expression signature was reported for HER2/neu-positive tumors and cell lines using DNA microarrays as well as comparative genomic hybridization techniques (Pollack et al. 1999; Perou et al. 2000). Co-amplification of individual genes was reported as early as 1993 (Keith et al. 1993). A microarray based screen (probes for 217 ESTs on chromosome 17) by Kauraniemi et al. (2001) using 14 breast cancer cell lines identified seven transcripts as the minimal region of co-amplification with HER2.

In a more extensive study, Bertucci et al. (2004) used a microarray platform with ~9000 cDNA probes. The analysis of 213 different tumor samples as well as 16 breast cancer cell lines yielded a characteristic gene expression signature of 37 differentially expressed genes for HER2/neu-positive tumors/cell lines. According to this "HER2-Signature", 29 genes were up- and 8 downregulated. Using this expression signature the group was able to predict the HER2 status of tumors with remarkable accuracy compared to the classical histologic classification methods (92.2% accurate compared to 85.9% for FISH and IHC). Seven of those 29 upregulated genes are located on chromosome 17q12, close enough to the HER2 gene locus to be candidates for co-amplification. Indeed, of these seven genes four were also part of the minimal region of co-amplification identified by Kauraniemi et al. (2001). The most striking targets in this "HER2 gene expression signature", apart from HER2, are the peroxisome proliferator receptor binding protein (PBP) and NR1D1, a nuclear receptor for heme and regulator of adipogenesis as well as circadian rhythm. NR1D1 is also known as Rev-erb-alpha. Later studies confirmed the overexpression and co-amplification of these genes in HER2/neu-positive breast cancer (Arriola et al. 2008; Chin et al. 2006).

Recently, an extensive RNAi-based screen by Kourtidis et al. (2010) evaluated 141 genes that were previously reported to be overexpressed in HER2/neu-positive breast cancers. Kourtidis et al. used shRNA constructs derived from a genome-wide shRNA library to transfect the well established HER2/neu-positive breast cancer cell line model BT474 and subsequently monitored changes in cell proliferation. The shRNA targets that resulted in the highest decrease of cell proliferation were confirmed by a second round of transfections. The most significant reduction in proliferation occurred after knockdown of HER2, indicating that the experimental approach was valid. Interestingly, knockdown of NR1D1 and PBP resulted in the third and fourth most significant reduction of cell proliferation which was found to be due to decreased viability. To confirm these results, SKBR3 and MDA-MB-361, both HER2/neu-positive cell lines, were transfected with the same constructs, resulting in a severe decrease of viability compared to control. Knockdown of these two targets in cell lines that do not carry the HER2 amplicon (breast cancer MCF7, MDA-MB-453, MDA-MB-468, normal human mammary epithelial cells - HMEC - and human kidney HEK293 cells) was without effect.

NR1D1 was first identified as an orphan nuclear receptor in 1989 (Miyajima et al. 1989). Since then it has been discovered that NR1D1 is a constitutive transcriptional repressor (Harding & M A Lazar 1995) and a nuclear receptor for heme, the binding of which actually enhances repression (Yin et al. 2007; Raghuram et al. 2007). NR1D1 is also an important regulator of the circadian rhythm. Circadian oscillations in gene expression are based on a 24 hour time frame and are present throughout the animal kingdom (Panda et al. 2002). They allow the organism to anticipate changes in metabolic activity and food availability. The master clock is located in the suprachiasmatic nuclus (SCN) of the hypothalamus which is responsive to light. This master clock synchronizes peripheral clocks that have an important role in organ homeostasis. The circadian regulation allows for metabolic enzymes to be expressed at the appropriate times to avoid, for example, the simultaneous expression of glycolytic and gluconeogenic enzymes (Duez & Staels 2009). Disruptions of circadian cycles have been linked to various diseases such as mental illness, metabolic syndrome and cancer (Gachon et al. 2004). The cycle of a peripheral clock starts when the two positive regulators BMAL1 and CLOCK heterodimerize and initiate transcription of their target genes. Among those targets are also negative regulators of BMAL1 and CLOCK transcription like NR1D1, which binds to their respective promoters and, by recruiting NCoR and HDAC3, represses transcription of BMAL1 and CLOCK (Yin and Lazar 2005). This creates a negative feedback loop resulting in oscillating levels of circadian rhythm regulatory proteins. NR1D1 also binds to its own promoter, thus repressing NR1D1 transcription once a critical protein concentration is reached (Adelmant et al. 1996). NR1D1 levels are high in metabolically active tissues including adipose tissue and liver (Lazar et al. 1989). NR1D1 is required for adipocyte differentiation (Wang & Lazar 2008) and its overexpression enhances adipogenesis in 3T3-L1 adipocytes (Fontaine et al. 2003). This is particularly intriguing as Kourtidis et al. observed significant differences in the amount of stored neutral fats in HER2 overexpressing breast cancer cells compared to other breast cancer cells with normal HER2 expression levels as well as human mammary epithelial cells. HER2 overexpressors consistently showed higher fat content than other breast cancer cells.

The peroxisome proliferator receptor-gamma binding protein (PBP) is a nuclear receptor co-activator also called mediator complex subunit 1 (MED1). Other names include CRSP1, RB18A, TRIP2, CRSP200, DRIP205, DRIP230, TRAP220 and MGC71488. Throughout this text we will refer to it as PBP. PBP was first identified through a yeast-2-hybrid screen using PPARγ as bait. It was capable of enhancing PPARγ dependent transcription (Zhu et al. 1997). Subsequently, PBP has been shown to be a critical component of the mediator complex, which is required for polymerase II mediated transcription (Kornberg 2005; Malik & Roeder 2005). Apart from binding to PPARγ, PBP also interacts with various other nuclear receptors like PPARα, TRβ, VDR, ERα, RARα, RXR and GR and is strongly expressed in the developing mouse embryo, suggesting an important role in cellular proliferation and differentiation (Viswakarma et al. 2010; Zhu et al. 1997). Indeed, a complete knockout of PBP in mice leads to embryonic lethality on day 11.5 (Zhu et al. 2000). In a carcinogenesis study using diethylnitrosamine followed by phenobarbital promotion, PBP null liver cells fail to undergo proliferation. All tumors that arise in mice carrying a conditional liver PBP knockout develop from cells that have retained PBP expression. This indicates that PBP is required for the development of hepatocellular carcinoma in mice (Matsumoto et al. 2010). Moreover, it has been shown that PBP is required for mammary gland development (Yuzhi Jia et al. 2005).

The PPARs belong to the superfamily of nuclear receptors and typically regulate the transcription of genes associated with lipid metabolism (Desvergne & Wahli 1999). In fact, PPARγ is required for adipocyte differentiation and NR1D1 is a transcriptional target of PPARγ (Tontonoz et al. 1994; Fontaine et al. 2003). Indeed, Kourtidis et al. showed that knockdown of PBP results in decreased mRNA levels of NR1D1. Co-transfection of BT474 cells with shRNAs targeting PBP and NR1D1 does not result in increased cell death, indicating that these two regulators work synergistically. Treatment of cells with a PPARγ antagonist results in reduced message levels of NR1D1 and induces apoptosis in BT474 cells. The survival advantage caused by PBP and NR1D1 overexpression is independent of HER2 overexpression as HER2 message levels do not change after NR1D1 knockdown. Instead, NR1D1 and PBP indirectly induce a lipogenic phenotype which results in increased fat

synthesis and storage. Disruption of this synthetic pathway results in HER2/neu-positive breast cancer cell apoptosis but does not affect HER2 negative cells.
PPARγ, PBP and NR1D1 are responsible for a markedly altered physiology in cells carrying the HER2 amplicon. These new co-amplified and overexpressed transcriptional regulators cooperatively change the metabolism of HER2/neu-positive breast cancer cells by inducing a unique, Warburg-like metabolism that is primed towards fat production. The next section will discuss this metabolism in detail.

3. The altered metabolism of HER2/neu-positive breast cancer

NR1D1, PBP and PPARγ are required for adipogenesis and many of their transcriptional targets are related to lipid metabolism. Their unregulated overexpression in HER2/neu-positive breast cancer causes a unique metabolic phenotype that relies on aerobic glycolysis and fatty acid synthesis for energy production and survival.
Kourtidis et al. show that the amount of stored neutral fats is about 20-fold higher compared to human mammary epithelial cells and about 10-fold higher compared to HER2 negative breast cancer lines. Knockdown of PBP and NR1D1 results in a significant decrease of fat stores and overexpression of NR1D1 in immortalized, non-tumorigenic, MCF10A cells increases their fat content by about 4-fold compared to vector control. Further studies using fructose and galactose as alternative fuel sources indicate that it is not the amount of fat stores but the requirement for active fatty acid synthesis that is important for the survival of HER2/neu-positive breast cancer cells. While PBP and NR1D1 knockdown decreases fat stores and viability, similar decreases in fat stores through cell growth in fructose or galactose containing media did not alter viability in these cells.
Investigation of transcript levels of potential downstream targets of PBP and NR1D1 revealed significant changes in ATP-citrate lyase (ACLY), acetyl-CoA carboxylase α (ACACA), fatty acid synthase (FASN) and fatty acid desaturase 2 (FADS2) mRNA levels after knockdown of either PBP or NR1D1. Indeed, shRNA mediated knockdown of ACLY, ACACA and FASN resulted in decreased viability in HER2/neu-positive breast cancer cells.
Other studies have already shown a tight link between FASN and HER2. Overexpression of FASN in immortalized, non-tumorigenic HBL100 and MCF10A cells induces oncogenic properties and results in upregulation and activation of HER1 and HER2 (Vazquez-Martin et al. 2008). There is evidence that HER2 posphorylates FASN, which results in increased enzymatic activity. Blocking FASN phosphorylation and enzymatic activity by either lapatinib (HER2 specific tyrosine kinase inhibitor) or C75 (FASN inhibitor) suppressed invasion of SKBR3 and BT474 cells (Jin et al. 2010).
In order to sustain this lipogenic phenotype, the cells are in constant demand of cofactors that are essential for glycolysis and fatty acid synthesis. Nicotinamide adenine dinucleotide (NAD^+) is required to take up electrons from glucose and coenzyme A is required to transfer carbons from glucose to fatty acids. Once NAD^+ is reduced to NADH the electrons need to be shuttled to NADPH so that they can be used in fatty acid synthesis. Two cytoplasmic enzymes are required for the formation of cytoplasmic NADPH. Malate dehydrogenase (MDH1) produces malate from oxaloacetate using NADH as a cofactor, whereas malic enzyme (ME1) cleaves malate to pyruvate and CO_2 while reducing $NADP^+$ to NADPH. ME1 is the primary producer of cytoplasmic NADPH which can then be used for fatty acid synthesis. Knockdown of MDH1 and ME1 with shRNAs significantly reduced mRNA levels and cell viability in BT474 cells (Kourtidis et al. 2010). This represents a new physiological

alteration that is transcriptionally independent from the NR1D1 and PBP axis since knockdown of PBP does not change mRNA levels of MDH1 or ME1. The importance of fatty acid synthesis in this type of cancer is underscored by the finding that FASN inhibition reverses Herceptin resistance in SKBR3 cells (Vazquez-Martin et al. 2007).

To date, there is not much known about the contribution of coenzyme A (CoA) metabolism to this lipogenic phenotype. One study reported that a PPARα agonist regulates CoA levels through the induction of pantothenate kinase 1α (PanK1alpha), which catalyzes the rate-limting step in CoA biosynthesis (Ramaswamy et al. 2004). The agonist used in this study is actually a pan-PPAR agonist (Krey et al. 1997), so there is a plausible connection between PPAR action and coenzyme A. Interestingly, overexpression of NR1D1 in MCF10A cells results in a 50% decrease of pantothenate levels compared to vector control, indicating increased substrate flux through pantothenate kinase (Baumann et al, unpublished data). Further studies are under way in our lab to determine how PBP and NR1D1 influence the metabolism of coenzyme A and vice versa.

The amount of palmitate produced by HER2/neu-positive breast cancer cells would normally result in cytotoxicity and apoptosis but the overexpression of PBP and NR1D1 allows for the neutralization of these toxic products by generating neutral triglycerides in a PPARγ dependent fashion. This system is operating close to the limit, as addition of free palmitic acid results in ROS mediated cell death of HER2/neu-positive but not HER2 negative breast cancer cells (Kourtidis et al. 2009). Metabolomic analysis of NR1D1 overexpressing MCF10A cells shows a drastically altered metabolite profile (Baumann et al, unpublished data). Levels of pathway intermediates in glycolysis and TCA are decreased, whereas lipids and lipid progenitor molecules are markedly increased. Overall energy levels seem to decrease with NR1D1 overexpression as nucleotide triphosphate levels are low. Nucleotide precursors from the pentose phosphate shunt are increased, while NADPH levels are low. These data indicate that NR1D1 overexpression results in increased metabolic flux through glycolysis and the pentose phosphate shunt towards nucleotide precursors and lipids. Of course this type of metabolism has to be balanced by appropriate anaplerotic reactions or the flux towards fatty acids would quickly deplete the TCA cycle of oxaloacetate, the "acceptor"-molecule for acetyl-CoA generated from pyruvate. Many cancer cells in culture have been shown to utilize glutaminolysis to achieve this goal (Weinberg & Chandel 2009). While BT474 cells also require glutamine in the culture medium, metabolomic analysis shows an unusual accumulation of glutamine in the cells, indicating that uptake rates far surpass any flux through glutamine consuming pathways (Kourtidis and Conklin, unpublished data). It is possible that glutamine is used to take up or excrete other compounds through sym- or anti-port transporters, respectively. The exact nature of the anaplerotic and glutamine utilization pathways in HER2 positive breast cancer are currently under investigation in our lab.

The synergistic action of HER2, PBP and NR1D1 allows cells carrying the HER2 amplicon to maintain a high flux rate through glycolysis and accumulate building blocks to sustain a high rate of cell proliferation. This might explain why therapies that target only HER2 are initially effective and result in the development of resistance. NR1D1 and PBP might be sufficient to drive the oncogenic metabolism once it is established. This is evidenced by the reversal of Herceptin resistance by FASN inhibition.

This metabolic phenotype is reminiscent of Warburg's original observation of aerobic glycolysis in cancer cells (Warburg 1956), except that the electrons do not end up in lactate. Metabolomic analysis indicates that overexpression of NR1D1 in MCF10A cells reduces lactate levels by approximately 56 % (Baumann et al, unpublished data). The end result for the cancer cells are the same, if not more beneficial in the case of the "Warburg-like" metabolism we observed in HER2/neu-positive breast cancer cells. In the canonical Warburg effect lactate serves as an electron sink and as a means to regenerate NAD^+, which allows for continued flux through glycolysis, but lactate is then excreted from the cells as a waste product. HER2/neu-positive breast cancer cells use fatty acids as an electron sink to regenerate electron acceptors while simultaneously generating building blocks needed for cell proliferation.

Considering the movement of electrons in these cells provides a valuable frame of reference for understanding the metabolism of HER2/neu-positive breast cancer. All living organisms rely on the oxidation of energy rich compounds like glucose to fuel cellular processes like growth and proliferation. This is achieved by directing electrons from glucose through various steps toward a terminal electron acceptor, often oxygen, to create water. During this process the potential energy of these electrons can be used to fuel endergonic reactions. The carbon backbone of glucose is terminally oxidized to CO_2 and excreted. Plants use water, CO_2 and energy to produce glucose, completing the cycle. Of course this is an oversimplified version of the real picture but it helps to illustrate a point. The problem for any metabolizing cell can be described as one of electrons and their corresponding energy levels, the nature of the compound they are part of in any system at any given time is only important in terms of its reactivity and potential inhibitory effects on enzymes. In a complex organism each cell takes up electrons at a high energy level which need to be shuttled towards stable, lower energy compounds for the cell to be able to utilize their potential energy. In a homeostatic, non-proliferative setting, when oxygen can function as the terminal electron acceptor, this process is highly regulated and very efficient. One mole of glucose generates 36 moles of ATP, 6 moles of CO_2 and 6 moles of H_2O. All electrons are bound in stable non-reactive products that can freely diffuse out of the cell. In anaerobic conditions, for example in muscle tissue, the terminal electron acceptor can be pyruvate, which generates lactate. Lactate is then excreted from the cell and further metabolized in other organs. In a proliferative setting a growth signal will instruct certain cells to deposit electrons in an intermediate stable acceptor like fatty acids and other compounds needed to create a new cell. This is again a tightly controlled and highly efficient process that will eventually return to oxygen reduction once the growth signal is removed.

In a situation where uncontrolled proliferation takes place because of chromosomal aberrations the cell needs to substantially increase its uptake of high energy electrons in the form of glucose. Most of them will end up in new cellular matter, which leaves little energy to be used by the cell for other processes. This creates a disconnection between electron uptake, energy usage and deposition of electrons in stable end products. One round of glycolysis will generate 4 electrons, 2 molecules of ATP and 2 molecules of pyruvate per molecule of glucose. The deposition of the electrons into pyruvate will generate a stable end product that can be excreted but leaves no carbons to accumulate new biomass for proliferation. Increasing the flux through glycolysis will yield an increase in usable energy and carbons that can be used by the cell but it also requires fast regeneration of electron acceptors. The best solution for this problem is to uncouple the terminal electron acceptor from the primary anabolic pathways that need to be carried out in a regulated concerted way. Increased flux through glycolysis to increase energy uptake is only feasible if electron acceptors can be regenerated quickly and if end products can be excreted or shuttled into other pathways to avoid negative feedback through product inhibition. The accumulation of one or more metabolites in cancer cells might simply be a result of an energetic necessity: the transfer of electrons into stable intermediates that have only a minor inhibiting effect on their corresponding biosynthetic pathways. HER2/neu-positive breast cancer cells produce lots of fatty acids because their genetic program enables them to further shuttle the toxic fatty acids towards non-toxic, basically inert, triacylglycerides that are then stored in the cell. Palmitic acid, which has a strong inhibitory effect on acetyl-CoA carboxylase α (ACACA), the rate-limiting step of fatty acid synthesis, never accumulate in these cells. The terminal electron acceptor in these cells is, for all practical purposes, acetyl-CoA.

The stoichiometry of these processes does not come out even and it does not have to. Stoichiometry only works if we look at a well-defined chemical reaction with a starting point and an end point, which is not necessary if we consider metabolic flux as an ongoing process. If one particular product cannot be formed any more, the preceding substrate will accumulate and be diverted into other metabolic pathways. Depending on all the different reactions going on in the cell that require either energy or carbons, any excess electrons can just flow towards other lower energy states in compounds that can serve as a substitute for oxygen, for example, pyruvate. Despite the fact that in HER2/neu-positive breast cancer cells the majority of electrons are deposited in triglycerides, these cells still produce lactate. Lactate can be excreted from the cells and will then feed into the Cori Cycle, which will result in glucose production in the liver and subsequent glucose export into the bloodstream. This type of metabolism is hardly efficient in terms of energy usage but it is very resilient and robust and allows for consistent production of energy and cellular matter. This is reflected in the slow growth rate of HER2/neu-positive cancer cell lines *in vitro*. The HER2/neu-positive cell line BT474 has a doubling time of approximately 100 hours whereas the HER2 negative line MCF7 takes about 29 hours for a population doubling. This seems counter-intuitive considering that HER2/neu-positive breast cancer has a worse prognosis and decreased survival time, but it is intriguing to speculate that in the complex environment of a human body growth rate might be less important than robust survival and growth in all conditions.

The accumulation of fat in HER2/neu-positive breast cancer cells raises other issues relating to the microenvironment, tumor growth and metastasis. By storing triglycerides these cancer cells store a vast amount of energy that is at the cells disposal if the environment of the cell changes. It is possible that these energy stores provide an advantage in case the cell enters a quiescent state or metastasizes to a new site as it will be less dependent on external energy sources if changes in metabolic regulation occur that allows the cells to switch to beta-oxidation for energy production. Tumors that produce a lot of lactate and excrete it into the tumor microenvironment will have a severe impact on the physiology of the surrounding cells. Excess lactate accumulation acidifies the tumor microenvironment and results in NF-κB and Hif1α activation which in turn results in angiogenesis and inflammation (reviewed in Allen & Jones 2011). This is likely to coincide with an increased influx of immune cells that will result in tumoricidal activity until the tumor is able to evade the immune response. In the case of HER2/neu-positive cells the efflux of lactate is decreased resulting in a less acidic tumor microenvironment, which might promote tumor immune evasion.

4. A potential role for metabolism in the epigenetics of Her2/neu-positive breast cancer

Epigenetic dysregulation is a well accepted contributing factor to tumorigenesis (Esteller 2007). Many of the cofactors that are required for the establishment of epigenetic marks are intermediates in the cellular metabolism. These include S-adenosylmethionine (SAM), NAD^+, and acetyl-CoA. Changes in the concentrations as well as in the intracellular spatial distributions of these molecules can have a profound impact on the epigenetic status of the cells. Alterations in how these molecules interact with each other can also influence the epigenetic modifications. By taking what has been learned about changes in cancer metabolism we can generate new ideas that will lead to a better understanding of how the flux of electrons in HER2/neu-positive breast cancer ultimately affects its epigenome and thus gene expression (Figure 1). More on the basics of epigenetics and cancer can be found in many recent reviews (Portela & Esteller 2010; Jovanovic et al. 2010; Sharma et al. 2010).

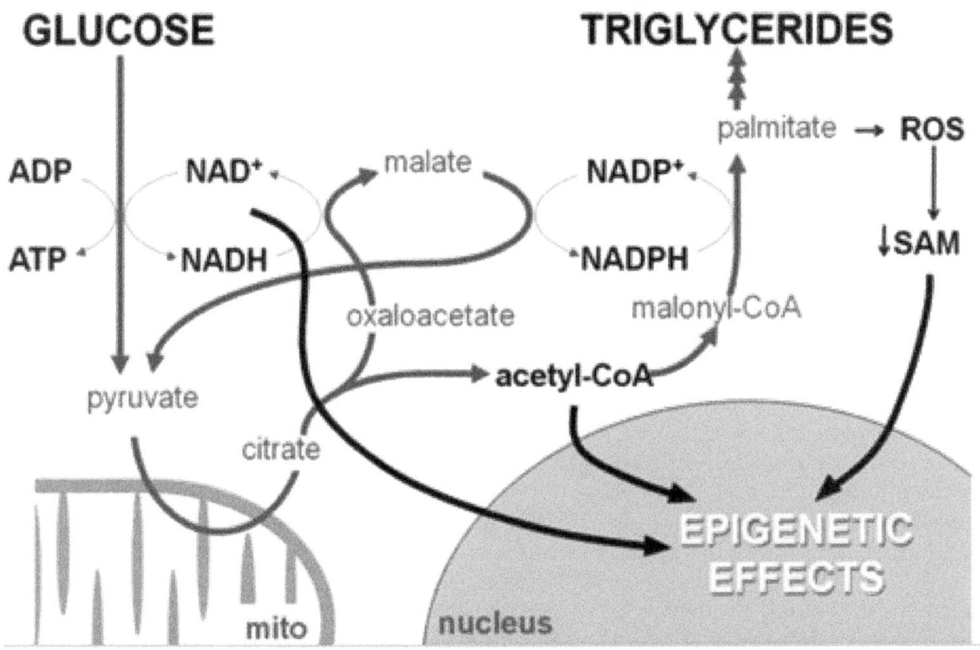

Fig. 1. The altered metabolism of HER-2/neu-positive breast cancer cells allows electrons from glucose to be deposited in triglycerides. Changes in levels of cofactors required for or affected by this process may have effects on epigenetic regulation. See text for details.

4.1 Methylation

Breast cancer, like all human cancers, is known to have differences in DNA methylation patterns (Esteller 2007; Ruike et al. 2010). During the development of the disease there is a global decrease in DNA methylation, also known as hypomethylation. However, concurrently there is an increase in CpG island (CGI) methylation at the promoters of tumor suppressor genes. Generally, genes important in apoptosis, metastasis, cell cycle regulation, angiogenesis and genes that encode non-coding RNAs (ncRNAs) are differentially methylated in breast cancer (Jovanovic et al. 2010). This improper methylation pattern begins in the primary tumor and increases upon metastasis, leading to alterations in gene expression (Feng et al. 2010). This change occurs in concert with an alteration in histone methylation, leading to a decrease in the expression of tumor suppressor genes in breast cancer (Sharma et al. 2010). It appears that histone methylation levels are decreased in HER2/neu-positive breast cancer compared to other subclasses of breast cancer and may play a role in the poor prognosis of HER2/neu-positive tumors (Elsheikh et al. 2009).

Alterations to one-carbon metabolism, specifically the methionine cycle, play a major role in all methylation reactions that occur in epigenetics. During the methionine cycle, dietary methionine is converted into SAM. SAM is then used as the methyl donor in various reactions inside the cell leaving S-adenosylhomocysteine (SAH) as a byproduct, which can be reconverted to methionine in a folate (vitamin B-12) dependent reaction (Mato et al. 1997). Dietary reductions in folate have been linked to hypomethylation of both DNA and histones in liver diseases, the neurological development of embryos, as well as the development of both liver and colorectal cancer (Mato and Lu 2007; Greene, Stanier, and Copp 2009; Pogribny et al. 2004; van Engeland et al. 2003; Davis and Uthus 2003). Experimental evidence suggests that the tumor suppressor gene p53 is hypomethylated in mice with a folate deficiency, which results in decreased protein function as well as in an increased mutation rate (Kim et al. 1997; Liu et al. 2008). Work examining the direct role of SAM on the growth of cancer cells has also shown changes in methylation patterns. In rat models of hepatocarcinogenesis and in human prostate cancer xenografts, SAM treatment slows the growth of tumors and prevents new tumor growth (Pascale et al. 2002; Shukeir et al. 2006). It is believed that this effect occurs through increased methylation at the promoters of the protooncogenes, c-myc, c-Ha-ras, and c-K-ras (Simile et al. 1994). Taken together, these results from nutritional studies and from SAM treatment studies support the hypothesis that the availability of SAM can affect the epigenetic modifications of cancer cells.

Methylation is also directly correlated with the redox potential inside the cell. Normal cells maintain a reducing environment inside the cytosol, whereas cancer cells develop a pro-oxidant cytosolic environment (Cerutti 1985). Most of the intracellular reduction potential is due to the production of glutathione (GSH) which functions as the main cellular redox buffer. The ratio of GSH to its reduced form, glutathione disulfide (GSSG), is an important indicator of the intracellular redox state. In non-pathological states, GSSG levels approach almost zero (Schafer & Buettner 2001). Results from our lab indicate that there are alterations in the redox state in a HER2/neu-positive cell line compared to a normal breast epithelial line (Kourtidis & Conklin, unpublished data). Enzymes that contain redox sensitive amino acids such as cysteine are at particular risk of losing their catalytic activity in this environment. In fact many of the enzymes important in epigenetics are altered by the pro-oxidant state of the cancer cell (Hitchler & Domann 2009).

The decreased levels of GSH found in many cancer cells can alter epigenetic patterns by affecting SAM levels. After SAM has donated its methyl group, SAH is converted into homocysteine. Homocysteine can then reenter the methionine cycle, or, as has been shown in a in a pro-oxidant environment, be shuttled into GSH synthesis (Mosharov et al. 2000). As homocysteine is shuttled away from the methionine cycle less SAM is generated, which results in a reduced supply of methyl donors for DNA methyltransferases (DNMTs) and histone methyltransferases (HMTs). This finding is confirmed when GSH is chemically depleted (Lertratanangkoon et al. 1997). This scenario is further exacerbated because the enzymes in the methionine cycle are redox sensitive and inactivated by oxidation (Hitchler & Domann 2009). DNMT and HMT also have conserved catalytic cysteine residues present in their active sites (Chen et al. 1991; Zhang et al. 2003). Oxidation of these residues impairs the function of the both the DNMT as well as the HMT, which will also influence epigenetic methylation patterns (Hitchler & Domann 2009). Taken together, all of these factors illustrate how the altered metabolism in HER2/neu-positive breast cancer cells can influence epigenetic modifications of both DNA and histones and thus influence gene expression.

4.2 Acetylation

The importance of histone modifying enzymes like histone deacetylases (HDACs) in cancer is also becoming clearer (Jovanovic et al. 2010). Breast cancer is no different. As with histone methylation, there is a global decrease in acetylation in HER2/neu-positive breast cancer in comparison with other classes of breast cancer (Elsheikh et al. 2009). It is believed that the hypermethylated CGI of tumor suppressor promoters attract HDACs either directly, or indirectly through methyl binding proteins (MBPs) increasing the repressed state of these genes (Dalvai & Bystricky 2010). Very little is known about HDAC expression in HER2/neu-positive breast cancer, despite the fact that HDAC 1 and 3 are overexpressed in most breast cancers and the expression levels of HDACs 2,4,6 decrease as the cancer develops (Dalvai & Bystricky 2010). The significance of these changes of acetylation has not yet been established, but it is intriguing to speculate that the altered metabolism in HER2/neu-positive breast cancer cells changes the availability of important co-factors that are required for histone acetylation and deacetylation.

The cofactor NAD^+ and its reduced counterpart NADH play a major role in the movement of electrons in cells. The overall cellular ratio of NAD^+/NADH effects the overall cellular redox environment, and alters the activity of various NAD^+ dependent enzymes. When cells use aerobic glycolysis as their main energy generation pathway, there is an overall decrease in the NAD^+/NADH ratio (Vander Heiden et al. 2009). We have noted that this phenomenon occurs in comparing NAD^+/NADH ratios of HER2/neu overexpressing breast cancer cell lines to normal breast epithelial cells lines (Kourtidis & Conklin, unpublished data).

Examining the effect of the decreased NAD^+/NADH ratio in relation to cancer cells is in its infancy, however, its role in lifespan extension has been studied for many years in organisms from yeast to human (Imai et al. 2000; Anderson et al. 2003; Guarente 2005). Caloric restriction, specifically a glucose reduction, leads to an increase in life span in yeast and mammals (Guarente 2005). The extension in longevity occurs because of the increase in ratio of NAD^+/NADH (Zhang & Kraus 2010). This shift is thought to inhibit the function of the sirtuins, a NAD^+ dependent class of HDAC, leading to a decrease in their functional ability to deacetylate histones, as well as other protein targets such as transcription factors (Imai et al. 2000; Zhang & Kraus 2010). These two facts together potentially allow for some of the aberrant gene expression that occurs in HER2/neu-positive breast cancer cells displaying a Warburg-like physiology.

Work in our lab has shown that the nuclear receptor NR1D1 plays a role in the proliferation and lipid production in HER2/neu-positive breast cancer cells (Kourtidis et al. 2010). NR1D1, which is overexpressed in HER2/neu breast cancer, functions as a transciptional repressor by recruiting HDAC3 to its target genes. Recent Chip-seq data from liver cells echoes this concept indicating that NR1D1 binds genes important in lipid synthesis and other metabolic pathways leading to a recruitment of HDAC3 (Feng et al. 2011). The exact effects of NR1D1 mediated transcriptional repression are likely to be tissue specific since gene expression data from HER2/neu-positive breast cancer cells shows NR1D1 dependent upregulation of lipid synthesis genes. The mechanism of this phenomenon is likely to be indirect. These findings could indicate that the overall decrease in histone acetylation in breast cancer may be caused by overexpression of NR1D1 and widespread HDAC3 recruitment.

However, some genes like HER2/neu itself display increased acetylation which results in upregulated gene expression (Mishra et al. 2001). This leads to the conclusion that while there is a global decrease in histone acetylation, differential acetylation occurs in breast cancer cells compared to normal breast cells. The Warburg-like metabolism of HER2/neu-positive breast cancer cells is likely to alter the availability and consumption of acetyl-CoA as a cofactor for acetylation and thus may influence acetylation patterns. There is not just a global decrease in histone acetylation, but also an alteration of histone modifications that lead to the expression of genes necessary for the survival and proliferation of the HER2/neu-positive breast cancer. The availability of acetyl-CoA can also have implications for other proteins that are acetylated, for example p53. The differential acetylation of transcription factors is another mechanism apart from histone acetylation, which illustrates how acetylation patterns can alter gene expression.

5. Conclusion

In HER2/neu-positive breast cancer, several genes are frequently co-amplified along with HER2. Recent evidence has shown that the co-amplified genes, NR1D1 and PBP, are required for HER2/neu-positive breast cancer cell survival. NR1D1 and PBP are important regulators of adipogenesis and their overexpression, functionally associated with PPARγ, induces a Warburg-like metabolism that uniquely primes these cells for fat production and fat storage. HER2/neu-positive breast cancer cells store significantly more fats compared to HER2 negative breast cancer cells and normal human mammary epithelial cells. Since it is the synthetic process that is required for cell survival and not the amount of stored fats, disruption of fat synthesis induces apoptosis, whereas a similar decrease in fat stores through growth on alternative carbon sources does not. NR1D1 and PBP do not act through HER2 as knockdown of NR1D1 does not change HER2 transcript levels. HER2/neu-positive breast cancer cells are dependent on this type of metabolism as disruption of other pathways required for continued fatty acid synthesis results in apoptosis. This altered metabolism allows HER2/neu-positive breast cancer cells to shuttle electrons from glucose to neutral fat stores. The constant production of fatty acids allows the regeneration of NAD^+, which in turn enables the cells to maintain a high flux rate through glycolysis. By storing those fatty acids in lipid droplets the cell avoids palmitate-induced cytotoxicity as well as feed-back inhibition of fatty acid synthase.

The accumulation of fatty acids might confer an advantage to HER2/neu-positive cells in a state of quiescence or during metastasis, however, these possibilities warrant further investigation. It is however possible that cancer cells in general might just accumulate those metabolic intermediates that their genetic program allows them to synthesize as a means of regenerating NAD^+ for continued energy production. For example, glioma cells have been reported to frequently express isocitrate dehydrogenase (IDH) mutations which result in the production of 2-hydroxy-glutarate from 2-oxo-glutarate. It is possible that this mutation poses an advantage simply because it enables the cells to use 2-hydroxy-glutarate as an electron sink, since the reaction consumes NADH, providing another parallel example of a potential Warburg-like physiology.

6. References

Adelmant, G., Bègue, A., Stéhelin, D. & Laudet, V. (1996) A functional Rev-erb alpha responsive element located in the human Rev-erb alpha promoter mediates a repressing activity. *Proceedings of the National Academy of Sciences of the United States of America*, 93 (8), p.pp.3553-8.

Allen, M. & Louise Jones, J. (2011) Jekyll and Hyde: the role of the microenvironment on the progression of cancer. *The Journal of Pathology*, 223 (2), p.pp.162-176.

Allred, D.C., Clark, G.M., Molina, R., Tandon, A.K., Schnitt, S.J., Gilchrist, K.W., Osborne, C.K., Tormey, D.C. & McGuire, W.L. (1992) Overexpression of HER-2/neu and its relationship with other prognostic factors change during the progression of in situ to invasive breast cancer. *Human Pathology*, 23 (9), p.pp.974-9.

Alroy, I. & Yarden, Y. (1997) The ErbB signaling network in embryogenesis and oncogenesis: signal diversification through combinatorial ligand-receptor interactions. *FEBS letters*, 410 (1), p.pp.83-6.

Anderson, R.M., Bitterman, K.J., Wood, J.G., Medvedik, O. & Sinclair, D.A. (2003) Nicotinamide and PNC1 govern lifespan extension by calorie restriction in Saccharomyces cerevisiae. *Nature*, 423 (6936), p.pp.181-5.

Arriola, E., Marchio, C., Tan, D.S.P., Drury, S.C., Lambros, M.B., Natrajan, R., Rodriguez-Pinilla, S.M., Mackay, A., Tamber, N., Fenwick, K., Jones, C., Dowsett, M., Ashworth, A. & Reis-Filho, J.S. (2008) Genomic analysis of the HER2/TOP2A amplicon in breast cancer and breast cancer cell lines. *Laboratory Investigation; a journal of technical methods and pathology*, 88 (5), p.pp.491-503.

Bazley, L. a & Gullick, W J (2005) The epidermal growth factor receptor family. *Endocrine-related Cancer*, 12 Suppl 1, p.pp.S17-27.

Berchuck, A., Kamel, A., Whitaker, R., Kerns, B., Olt, G., Kinney, R., Soper, J.T., Dodge, R., Clarke-Pearson, D.L. & Marks, P. (1990) Overexpression of HER-2/neu is associated with poor survival in advanced epithelial ovarian cancer. *Cancer Research*, 50 (13), p.pp.4087-91.

Bertucci, F., Borie, N., Ginestier, C., Groulet, A., Charafe-Jauffret, E., Adélaïde, J., Geneix, J., Bachelart, L., Finetti, P., Koki, A., Hermitte, F., Hassoun, J., Debono, S., Viens, P., Fert, V., Jacquemier, J. & Birnbaum, D. (2004) Identification and validation of an ERBB2 gene expression signature in breast cancers. *Oncogene*, 23 (14), p.pp.2564-75.

Carter, P., Presta, L., Gorman, C.M., Ridgway, J.B., Henner, D., Wong, W.L., Rowland, A.M., Kotts, C., Carver, M.E. & Shepard, H.M. (1992) Humanization of an anti-p185HER2 antibody for human cancer therapy. *Proceedings of the National Academy of Sciences of the United States of America*, 89 (10), p.pp.4285-9.

Cerutti, P.A. (1985) Prooxidant states and tumor promotion. *Science*, 227 (4685), p.pp.375-81.

Chen, L., MacMillan, A.M., Chang, W., Ezaz-Nikpay, K., Lane, W.S. & Verdine, G.L. (1991) Direct identification of the active-site nucleophile in a DNA (cytosine-5)-methyltransferase. *Biochemistry*, 30 (46), p.pp.11018–11025.

Chin, K., DeVries, S., Fridlyand, J., Spellman, P.T., Roydasgupta, R., Kuo, W.-L., Lapuk, A., Neve, R.M., Qian, Z., Ryder, T., Chen, F., Feiler, H., Tokuyasu, T., Kingsley, C., Dairkee, S., Meng, Z., Chew, K., Pinkel, Daniel, Jain, A., Ljung, Britt Marie, Esserman, L., Albertson, D.G., Waldman, Frederic M & Gray, Joe W (2006) Genomic and transcriptional aberrations linked to breast cancer pathophysiologies. *Cancer Cell*, 10 (6), p.pp.529-41.

Coussens, L., Yang-Feng, T.L., Liao, Y.C., Chen, E., Gray, a, McGrath, J., Seeburg, P.H., Libermann, T. a, Schlessinger, J. & Francke, U. (1985) Tyrosine kinase receptor with extensive homology to EGF receptor shares chromosomal location with neu oncogene. *Science*, 230 (4730), p.pp.1132-9.

Dalvai, M. & Bystricky, K. (2010) The role of histone modifications and variants in regulating gene expression in breast cancer. *Journal of Mammary Gland Biology and Neoplasia*, 15 (1), p.pp.19-33.

Davis, C.D. & Uthus, E.O. (2003) Cancer-Dietary Folate and Selenium Affect Dimethylhydrazine-Induced Aberrant Crypt Formation, Global DNA Methylation and One-Carbon Metabolism. *Journal of Nutrition*, 1 (June), p.pp.2907-2914.

Desvergne, B. & Wahli, W. (1999) Peroxisome proliferator-activated receptors: nuclear control of metabolism. *Endocrine Reviews*, 20 (5), p.pp.649-88.

Duez, H. & Staels, B. (2009) Rev-erb-alpha: an integrator of circadian rhythms and metabolism. *Journal of Applied Physiology* , 107 (6), p.pp.1972-80.

Elsheikh, S.E., Green, A.R., Rakha, E. a, Powe, D.G., Ahmed, R. a, Collins, H.M., Soria, D., Garibaldi, J.M., Paish, C.E., Ammar, A. a, Grainge, M.J., Ball, G.R., Abdelghany, M.K., Martinez-Pomares, L., Heery, D.M. & Ellis, I.O. (2009) Global histone modifications in breast cancer correlate with tumor phenotypes, prognostic factors, and patient outcome. *Cancer Research*, 69 (9), p.pp.3802-9.

Engeland, M. van, Weijenberg, M.P., Roemen, G.M.J.M., Brink, M., Bruine, A.P. de, Goldbohm, R.A., Brandt, P.A. van den, Baylin, S.B., Goeij, A.F.P.M. de & Herman, J.G. (2003) Effects of dietary folate and alcohol intake on promoter methylation in sporadic colorectal cancer: the Netherlands cohort study on diet and cancer. *Cancer Research*, 63 (12), p.p.3133.

Esteller, M. (2007) Cancer epigenomics: DNA methylomes and histone-modification maps. *Nature Reviews. Genetics*, 8 (4), p.pp.286-98.

Feng, D., Liu, T., Sun, Z., Bugge, A., Mullican, S.E., Alenghat, T., Liu, X.S. & Lazar, Mitch A. (2011) A Circadian Rhythm Orchestrated by Histone Deacetylase 3 Controls Hepatic Lipid Metabolism. *Science*, 331 (6022), p.pp.1315-1319.

Feng, W., Orlandi, R., Zhao, N., Carcangiu, M.L., Tagliabue, E., Xu, Jia, Bast, R.C. & Yu, Y. (2010) Tumor suppressor genes are frequently methylated in lymph node metastases of breast cancers. *BMC Cancer*, 10, p.p.378.

Fontaine, C., Dubois, G., Duguay, Y., Helledie, T., Vu-Dac, N., Gervois, P., Soncin, F., Mandrup, S., Fruchart, J.-charles, Fruchart-Najib, J. & Staels, B. (2003) The orphan nuclear receptor Rev-Erbalpha is a peroxisome proliferator-activated receptor (PPAR) gamma target gene and promotes PPARgamma-induced adipocyte differentiation. *The Journal of Biological Chemistry*, 278 (39), p.pp.37672-80.

Gachon, F., Nagoshi, E., Brown, S.A., Ripperger, J. & Schibler, U. (2004) The mammalian circadian timing system: from gene expression to physiology. *Chromosoma*, 113 (3), p.pp.103-12.

Greene, N.D.E., Stanier, P. & Copp, A.J. (2009) Genetics of human neural tube defects. *Human Molecular Genetics*, 18 (R2), p.pp.R113-29.

Guarente, L. (2005) Calorie restriction and SIR2 genes--towards a mechanism. *Mechanisms of Ageing and Development*, 126 (9), p.pp.923-8.

Harding, H.P. & Lazar, M A (1995) The monomer-binding orphan receptor Rev-Erb represses transcription as a dimer on a novel direct repeat. *Molecular and Cellular Biology*, 15 (9), p.pp.4791-802.

Harris, R.C., Chung, E. & Coffey, R.J. (2003) EGF receptor ligands. *Experimental Cell Research*, 284 (1), p.pp.2-13.

Hitchler, M.J. & Domann, F.E. (2009) Metabolic defects provide a spark for the epigenetic switch in cancer. *Free Radical Biology & Medicine*, 47 (2), p.pp.115-27.

Hortobagyi, G N (2001) Overview of treatment results with trastuzumab (Herceptin) in metastatic breast cancer. *Seminars in Oncology*, 28 (6 Suppl 18), p.pp.43-7.

Hudis, C.A. (2007) Trastuzumab--mechanism of action and use in clinical practice. *The New England Journal Of Medicine*, 357 (1), p.pp.39-51.

Hynes, N.E. & Stern, D.F. (1994) The biology of erbB-2/neu/HER-2 and its role in cancer. *Biochimica et Biophysica Acta*, 1198 (2-3), p.pp.165-84.

Imai, S.-ichiro, Armstrong, C.M., Kaeberlein, M. & Guarente, L. (2000) Transcriptional silencing and longevity protein Sir2 is an NAD-dependent histone deacetylase. *Nature*, 403 (6771), p.pp.795-800.

Jia, Yuzhi, Qi, Chao, Zhang, Z., Zhu, Y.T., Rao, S.M. & Zhu, Y.-J. (2005) Peroxisome proliferator-activated receptor-binding protein null mutation results in defective mammary gland development. *The Journal of Biological Chemistry*, 280 (11), p.pp.10766-73.

Jin, Q., Yuan, L.X., Boulbes, D., Baek, J.M., Wang, Y.N., Gomez-Cabello, D., Hawke, D.H., Yeung, S.C., Lee, M.H., Hortobagyi, Gabriel N, Hung, M.C. & Esteva, F.J. (2010) Fatty acid synthase phosphorylation: a novel therapeutic target in HER2-overexpressing breast cancer cells. *Breast Cancer Research*, 12 (6), p.p.R96.

Jovanovic, J., Rønneberg, J.A., Tost, J. & Kristensen, V. (2010) The epigenetics of breast cancer. *Molecular Oncology*, 4 (3), p.pp.242-54.

Kallioniemi, O.P., Kallioniemi, A., Kurisu, W., Thor, A., Chen, L.C., Smith, H.S., Waldman, F M, Pinkel, D & Gray, J W (1992) ERBB2 amplification in breast cancer analyzed by fluorescence in situ hybridization. *Proceedings of the National Academy of Sciences of the United States of America*, 89 (12), p.pp.5321-5.

Kauraniemi, P., Bärlund, M., Monni, O. & Kallioniemi, A. (2001) New amplified and highly expressed genes discovered in the ERBB2 amplicon in breast cancer by cDNA microarrays. *Cancer Research*, 61 (22), p.pp.8235-40.

Keith, W.N., Douglas, F., Wishart, G.C., McCallum, H.M., George, W.D., Kaye, S.B. & Brown, R. (1993) Co-amplification of erbB2, topoisomerase II alpha and retinoic acid receptor alpha genes in breast cancer and allelic loss at topoisomerase I on chromosome 20. *European Journal of Cancer*, 29A (10), p.pp.1469-75.

Kim, Y.-I., Pogribny, I.P., Basnakian, A.G., Miller, J.W., Selhub, J., James, S.J. & Mason, J.B. (1997) Folate deficiency in rats induces DNA strand breaks and hypomethylation within the p53 tumor suppressor gene. *The American Journal of Clinical Nutrition*, 65 (1), p.pp.46-52.

King, C.R., Kraus, M.H. & Aaronson, S.A. (1985) Amplification of a novel v-erbB-related gene in a human mammary carcinoma. *Science*, 229 (4717), p.pp.974-6.

Kornberg, R.D. (2005) Mediator and the mechanism of transcriptional activation. *Trends in Biochemical Sciences*, 30 (5), p.pp.235-9.

Kourtidis, A., Jain, R., Carkner, R.D., Eifert, C., Brosnan, M.J. & Conklin, D.S. (2010) An RNA interference screen identifies metabolic regulators NR1D1 and PBP as novel survival factors for breast cancer cells with the ERBB2 signature. *Cancer Research*, 70 (5), p.pp.1783-92.

Kourtidis, A., Srinivasaiah, R., Carkner, R.D., Brosnan, M.J. & Conklin, D.S. (2009) Peroxisome proliferator-activated receptor-gamma protects ERBB2-positive breast cancer cells from palmitate toxicity. *Breast Cancer Research*, 11 (2), p.p.R16.

Kraus, M.H., Issing, W., Miki, T., Popescu, N.C. & Aaronson, S.A. (1989) Isolation and characterization of ERBB3, a third member of the ERBB/epidermal growth factor receptor family: evidence for overexpression in a subset of human mammary tumors. *Proceedings of the National Academy of Sciences of the United States of America*, 86 (23), p.pp.9193-7.

Krey, G., Braissant, O., L'Horset, F., Kalkhoven, E., Perroud, M., Parker, M.G. & Wahli, W. (1997) Fatty acids, eicosanoids, and hypolipidemic agents identified as ligands of peroxisome proliferator-activated receptors by coactivator-dependent receptor ligand assay. *Molecular Endocrinology*, 11 (6), p.pp.779-91.

Lazar, M A, Hodin, R.A., Darling, D.S. & Chin, W.W. (1989) A novel member of the thyroid/steroid hormone receptor family is encoded by the opposite strand of the rat c-erbA alpha transcriptional unit. *Molecular and Cellular Biology*, 9 (3), p.pp.1128-36.

Lenferink, A.E., Pinkas-Kramarski, R., Poll, M.L. van de, Vugt, M.J. van, Klapper, L.N., Tzahar, E., Waterman, H., Sela, M., Zoelen, E.J. van & Yarden, Y. (1998) Differential endocytic routing of homo- and hetero-dimeric ErbB tyrosine kinases confers signaling superiority to receptor heterodimers. *The EMBO Journal*, 17 (12), p.pp.3385-97.

Lertratanangkoon, K., Wu, C.J., Savaraj, N. & Thomas, M.L. (1997) Alterations of DNA methylation by glutathione depletion. *Cancer Letters*, 120 (2), p.pp.149-56.

Liu, E., Thor, A., He, M., Barcos, M., Ljung, B M & Benz, C. (1992) The HER2 (c-erbB-2) oncogene is frequently amplified in in situ carcinomas of the breast. *Oncogene*, 7 (5), p.pp.1027-32.

Liu, Z., Choi, S.-W., Crott, J.W., Smith, D.E. & Mason, J.B. (2008) Multiple B-vitamin inadequacy amplifies alterations induced by folate depletion in p53 expression and its downstream effector MDM2. *International Journal of Cancer.*, 123 (3), p.pp.519-25.

Malik, S. & Roeder, R.G. (2005) Dynamic regulation of pol II transcription by the mammalian Mediator complex. *Trends in Biochemical Sciences*, 30 (5), p.pp.256-63.

Mato, Jose M., Alvarez, L., Ortiz, P. & Pajares, M.A. (1997) S-adenosylmethionine synthesis: molecular mechanisms and clinical implications. *Pharmacology & Therapeutics*, 73 (3), p.pp.265-80.

Mato, José M. & Lu, S.C. (2007) Role of S-adenosyl-L-methionine in liver health and injury. *Hepatology*, 45 (5), p.pp.1306-12.

Matsumoto, K., Huang, J., Viswakarma, N., Bai, L., Jia, Yuzhi, Zhu, Y.T., Yang, G., Borensztajn, J., Rao, M Sambasiva, Zhu, Y.-J. & Reddy, Janardan K (2010) Transcription coactivator PBP/MED1-deficient hepatocytes are not susceptible to diethylnitrosamine-induced hepatocarcinogenesis in the mouse. *Carcinogenesis*, 31 (2), p.pp.318-25.

McCann, A.H., Dervan, P.A., O'Regan, M., Codd, M.B., Gullick, William J, Tobin, B.M. & Carney, D.N. (1991) Prognostic significance of c-erbB-2 and estrogen receptor status in human breast cancer. *Cancer Research*, 51 (12), p.pp.3296-303.

Meyer, D. & Birchmeier, C. (1995) Multiple essential functions of neuregulin in development. *Nature*, 378 (6555), p.pp.386-90.

Mishra, S.K., Mandal, M., Mazumdar, A. & Kumar, R. (2001) Dynamic chromatin remodeling on the HER2 promoter in human breast cancer cells. *FEBS Letters*, 507 (1), p.pp.88-94.

Miyajima, N., Horiuchi, R., Shibuya, Y., Fukushige, S., Matsubara, K., Toyoshima, K. & Yamamoto, T. (1989) Two erbA homologs encoding proteins with different T3 binding capacities are transcribed from opposite DNA strands of the same genetic locus. *Cell*, 57 (1), p.pp.31-9.

Molina, M.A., Sáez, R., Ramsey, E.E., Garcia-Barchino, M.-J., Rojo, F., Evans, A.J., Albanell, J., Keenan, E.J., Lluch, A., García-Conde, J., Baselga, J. & Clinton, G.M. (2002) NH(2)-terminal truncated HER-2 protein but not full-length receptor is associated with nodal metastasis in human breast cancer. *Clinical Cancer Research*, 8 (2), p.pp.347-53.

Mosharov, E., Cranford, M.R. & Banerjee, R. (2000) The quantitatively important relationship between homocysteine metabolism and glutathione synthesis by the transsulfuration pathway and its regulation by redox changes. *Biochemistry*, 39 (42), p.pp.13005-11.

Mukohara, T. (2011) Mechanisms of resistance to anti-human epidermal growth factor receptor 2 agents in breast cancer. *Cancer Science*, 102 (1), p.pp.1-8.

Panda, S., Hogenesch, J.B. & Kay, S.A. (2002) Circadian rhythms from flies to human. *Nature*, 417 (6886), p.pp.329-35.

Park, K., Han, S., Kim, H.J., Kim, J. & Shin, E. (2006) HER2 status in pure ductal carcinoma in situ and in the intraductal and invasive components of invasive ductal carcinoma determined by fluorescence in situ hybridization and immunohistochemistry. *Histopathology*, 48 (6), p.pp.702-7.

Pascale, R.M., Simile, Maria M., Miglio, M.R. De & Feo, Francesco. (2002) Chemoprevention of hepatocarcinogenesis: S-adenosyl-L-methionine. *Alcohol*, 27 (3), p.pp.193-8.

Pauletti, G., Godolphin, W., Press, M.F. & Slamon, D J (1996) Detection and quantitation of HER-2/neu gene amplification in human breast cancer archival material using fluorescence in situ hybridization. *Oncogene*, 13 (1), p.pp.63-72.

Perou, C M, Sørlie, T., Eisen, M.B., Rijn, M. van de, Jeffrey, S.S., Rees, C.A., Pollack, J.R., Ross, D.T., Johnsen, H., Akslen, L.A., Fluge, O., Pergamenschikov, A., Williams, C., Zhu, S.X., Lønning, P.E., Børresen-Dale, A.L., Brown, P.O. & Botstein, D. (2000) Molecular portraits of human breast tumours. *Nature*, 406 (6797), p.pp.747-52.

Plowman, G.D., Culouscou, J.M., Whitney, G.S., Green, J.M., Carlton, G.W., Foy, L., Neubauer, M.G. & Shoyab, M. (1993) Ligand-specific activation of HER4/p180erbB4, a fourth member of the epidermal growth factor receptor family. *Proceedings of the National Academy of Sciences of the United States of America*, 90 (5), p.pp.1746-50.

Pogribny, I.P., James, S.J., Jernigan, S. & Pogribna, M. (2004) Genomic hypomethylation is specific for preneoplastic liver in folate/methyl deficient rats and does not occur in non-target tissues. *Mutation Research*, 548 (1-2), p.pp.53-9.

Pollack, J.R., Perou, C M, Alizadeh, A.A., Eisen, M.B., Pergamenschikov, A., Williams, C.F., Jeffrey, S.S., Botstein, D. & Brown, P.O. (1999) Genome-wide analysis of DNA copy-number changes using cDNA microarrays. *Nature Genetics*, 23 (1), p.pp.41-46.

Portela, A. & Esteller, M. (2010) Epigenetic modifications and human disease. *Nature Biotechnology*, 28 (10), p.pp.1057-1068.

Quirke, P., Pickles, A., Tuzi, N.L., Mohamdee, O. & Gullick, W J (1989) Pattern of expression of c-erbB-2 oncoprotein in human fetuses. *British Journal of Cancer*, 60 (1), p.pp.64-9.

Raghuram, S., Stayrook, K.R., Huang, P., Rogers, P.M., Nosie, A.K., McClure, D.B., Burris, L.L., Khorasanizadeh, S., Burris, T.P. & Rastinejad, F. (2007) Identification of heme as the ligand for the orphan nuclear receptors REV-ERBalpha and REV-ERBbeta. *Nature Structural & Molecular Biology*, 14 (12), p.pp.1207-13.

Ramaswamy, G., Karim, M.A., Murti, K.G. & Jackowski, S. (2004) PPARalpha controls the intracellular coenzyme A concentration via regulation of PANK1alpha gene expression. *Journal of Lipid Research*, 45 (1), p.pp.17-31.

Ruike, Y., Imanaka, Y., Sato, F., Shimizu, K. & Tsujimoto, G. (2010) Genome-wide analysis of aberrant methylation in human breast cancer cells using methyl-DNA immunoprecipitation combined with high-throughput sequencing. *BMC Genomics*, 11, p.p.137.

Schafer, F.Q. & Buettner, G.R. (2001) Redox environment of the cell as viewed through the redox state of the glutathione disulfide/glutathione couple. *Free Radical Biology & Medicine*, 30 (11), p.pp.1191-212.

Schechter, A.L., Stern, D.F., Vaidyanathan, L., Decker, S.J., Drebin, J.A., Greene, M.I. & Weinberg, R.A. (1984) The neu oncogene: an erb-B-related gene encoding a 185,000-Mr tumour antigen. *Nature*, 312 (5994), p.pp.513-6.

Sharma, S., Kelly, T.K. & Jones, P.A. (2010) Epigenetics in cancer. *Carcinogenesis*, 31 (1), p.pp.27-36.

Shukeir, N., Pakneshan, P., Chen, G., Szyf, M. & Rabbani, S.A. (2006) Alteration of the methylation status of tumor-promoting genes decreases prostate cancer cell invasiveness and tumorigenesis in vitro and in vivo. *Cancer Research*, 66 (18), p.pp.9202-10.

Silva, J.M., Li, M.Z., Chang, K., Ge, W., Golding, M.C., Rickles, R.J., Siolas, D., Hu, G., Paddison, P.J., Schlabach, M.R., Sheth, N., Bradshaw, J., Burchard, J., Kulkarni, A., Cavet, G., Sachidanandam, R., McCombie, W.R., Cleary, M.A., Elledge, S.J. & Hannon, G.J. (2005) Second-generation shRNA libraries covering the mouse and human genomes. *Nature Genetics*, 37 (11), p.pp.1281-8.

Simile, M M, Pascale, R., Miglio, M.R.D., Nufris, A., Daino, L., Seddaiu, M.A., Gaspa, L. & Feo, F (1994) Correlation between S-adenosyl-l-methionine content and production of c-myc, c-Ha-ras, and c-Ki-ras mRNA transcripts in the early stages of rat liver carcinogenesis. *Cancer Letters*, 79 (1), p.pp.9-16.

Slamon, D J, Clark, G.M., Wong, S.G., Levin, W.J., Ullrich, A. & McGuire, W.L. (1987) Human breast cancer: correlation of relapse and survival with amplification of the HER-2/neu oncogene. *Science*, 235 (4785), p.pp.177-82.

Slamon, D J, Godolphin, W., Jones, L.A., Holt, J.A., Wong, S.G., Keith, D.E., Levin, W.J., Stuart, S.G., Udove, J. & Ullrich, A. (1989) Studies of the HER-2/neu proto-oncogene in human breast and ovarian cancer. *Science*, 244 (4905), p.pp.707-12.

Tontonoz, P., Hu, E. & Spiegelman, B.M. (1994) Stimulation of adipogenesis in fibroblasts by PPAR gamma 2, a lipid-activated transcription factor. *Cell*, 79 (7), p.pp.1147-56.

Tzahar, E. & Yarden, Y. (1998) The ErbB-2/HER2 oncogenic receptor of adenocarcinomas: from orphanhood to multiple stromal ligands. *Biochimica et Biophysica Acta*, 1377 (1), p.pp.M25-37.

Vander Heiden, M.G., Cantley, L.C. & Thompson, C.B. (2009) Understanding the Warburg effect: the metabolic requirements of cell proliferation. *Science*, 324 (5930), p.pp.1029-33.

Vazquez-Martin, A, Colomer, R, Brunet, J, Lupu, R. & Menendez, J A (2008) Overexpression of fatty acid synthase gene activates HER1/HER2 tyrosine kinase receptors in human breast epithelial cells. *Cell Proliferation*, 41 (1), p.pp.59-85.

Vazquez-Martin, Alejandro, Colomer, Ramon, Brunet, Joan & Menendez, Javier A (2007) Pharmacological blockade of fatty acid synthase (FASN) reverses acquired autoresistance to trastuzumab (Herceptin by transcriptionally inhibiting "HER2 super-expression" occurring in high-dose trastuzumab-conditioned SKBR3/Tzb100 breast cancer cells. *International Journal of Oncology*, 31 (4), p.pp.769-76.

Venter, D.J., Tuzi, N.L., Kumar, S. & Gullick, W J (1987) Overexpression of the c-erbB-2 oncoprotein in human breast carcinomas: immunohistological assessment correlates with gene amplification. *Lancet*, 2 (8550), p.pp.69-72.

Viswakarma, N., Jia, Yuzhi, Bai, L., Vluggens, A., Borensztajn, J., Xu, Jianming & Reddy, Janardan K. (2010) Coactivators in PPAR-Regulated Gene Expression. *PPAR Research*, 2010, p.pp.1-22.

Vogel, C.L., Cobleigh, M.A., Tripathy, D., Gutheil, J.C., Harris, L.N., Fehrenbacher, L., Slamon, D.J., Murphy, M., Novotny, W.F., Burchmore, M. & others (2002) Efficacy and safety of trastuzumab as a single agent in first-line treatment of HER2-overexpressing metastatic breast cancer. *Journal of Clinical Oncology*, 20 (3), p.p.719.

Wang, J. & Lazar, Mitchell A (2008) Bifunctional role of Rev-erbalpha in adipocyte differentiation. *Molecular and Cellular Biology*, 28 (7), p.pp.2213-20.

Warburg, O. (1956) On respiratory impairment in cancer cells. *Science*, 124 (3215), p.pp.269-70.

Weigelt, B., Hu, Z., He, X., Livasy, C., Carey, L. a, Ewend, M.G., Glas, A.M., Perou, Charles M & Van't Veer, L.J. (2005) Molecular portraits and 70-gene prognosis signature are preserved throughout the metastatic process of breast cancer. *Cancer Research*, 65 (20), p.pp.9155-8.

Weinberg, F. & Chandel, N.S. (2009) Mitochondrial metabolism and cancer. *Annals of the New York Academy of Sciences*, 1177, p.pp.66-73.

Wellen, K.E., Hatzivassiliou, G., Sachdeva, U.M., Bui, T.V., Cross, J.R. & Thompson, C.B. (2009) ATP-citrate lyase links cellular metabolism to histone acetylation. *Science*, 324 (5930), p.pp.1076-80.

Yarden, Y. (2001) Biology of HER2 and its importance in breast cancer. *Oncology*, 61 Suppl 2 (suppl 2), p.pp.1-13.

Yin, L. & Lazar, M. a (2005) The orphan nuclear receptor Rev-erbalpha recruits the N-CoR/histone deacetylase 3 corepressor to regulate the circadian Bmal1 gene. *Molecular Endocrinology*, 19 (6), p.pp.1452-9.

Yin, L., Wu, N., Curtin, J.C., Qatanani, M., Szwergold, N.R., Reid, R.A., Waitt, G.M., Parks, D.J., Pearce, K.H., Wisely, G.B. & Lazar, Mitchell A (2007) Rev-erbalpha, a heme sensor that coordinates metabolic and circadian pathways. *Science,* 318 (5857), p.pp.1786-9.

Zhang, T. & Kraus, W.L. (2010) SIRT1-dependent regulation of chromatin and transcription: Linking NAD(+) metabolism and signaling to the control of cellular functions. *Biochimica et Bophysica Acta,* 1804 (8), p.pp.1666-1675.

Zhang, X., Yang, Z., Khan, S.I., Horton, J.R., Tamaru, H., Selker, E.U. & Cheng, X. (2003) Structural basis for the product specificity of histone lysine methyltransferases. *Molecular Cell,* 12 (1), p.pp.177-85.

Zhu, Y., Qi, C, Jain, S., Rao, M S & Reddy, J K (1997) Isolation and characterization of PBP, a protein that interacts with peroxisome proliferator-activated receptor. *The Journal of Biological Chemistry,* 272 (41), p.pp.25500-6.

Zhu, Y., Qi, C, Jia, Y, Nye, J.S., Rao, M S & Reddy, J K (2000) Deletion of PBP/PPARBP, the gene for nuclear receptor coactivator peroxisome proliferator-activated receptor-binding protein, results in embryonic lethality. *The Journal of Biological Chemistry,* 275 (20), p.pp.14779-82.

4

Antioxidant Enzymes as New Biomarkers for Prediction of Tumor Progression in Breast Cancer

Becuwe Philippe
Henri Poincaré's University-Nancy
France

1. Introduction

Today breast cancer represents the most frequent of all cancer pathologies in the world, with more than one million newly diagnosed cases and about 370000 cancer-related deaths in women each year, even with all the significant progress in its diagnosis and treatment (Ott et al., 2011). The development of breast tumor is a multistep process. It is generally thought that the initiation of breast cancer occurs after accumulation of genetic alterations that result in either activation of oncogenes and/or inactivation of tumor suppressor genes, leading to an abnormal cellular proliferation and promoting the development of tumor in mammary gland. A number of risk factors such as reproductive and hormonal factors, alcohol consumption, cigarette smoking, dietary factors and chronic inflammation have been identified for breast cancer, whose mechanisms by which they increase risk of the disease are not always clear (Mitrunen and Hirvonen, 2003). It has been proposed that the production of reactive oxygen species (ROS) leading to an oxidative stress is the linking factor between these carcinogens. The oxidative stress is defined as an imbalance between production of ROS, and their elimination by antioxidant defense system (redox imbalance). This imbalance leads to damage of important biomolecules and cells, with potential impact on the whole organism. ROS are products of a normal cellular metabolism and play vital roles in the stimulation of signalling pathways in cells in response to changes in intra- and extracellular environmental conditions. During endogenous metabolic reactions, aerobic cells produce ROS such as superoxide anion ($O_2\bullet-$), hydrogen peroxide (H_2O_2), hydroxyl radical ($OH\bullet$), and organic peroxides as normal products of the biological reduction of molecular oxygen. Most ROS are generated in cells by the mitochondrial respiratory chain. Under hypoxic conditions following reoxygenation, the electron transfer at the level of complex III of mitochondrial respiratory chain to molecular oxygen occurs directly, leading to a high level of ROS. Beside oxidative phosphorylation, low levels of ROS are continuously formed by oxidase activities in peroxisomes, and by the cytochrome P450 system in endoplasmic reticulum. ROS as $OH\bullet$ is produced *in vivo* in the presence of reduced transition metals (ions of Fe, Cu) mainly *via* the Fenton reaction in contact with H_2O_2. Under normal metabolic conditions, these ROS are eliminated rapidly in normal cells by the antioxidant defense system. However, ROS may be overproduced when normal cells are exposed to a sustained environmental stress, including ionizing radiation and many xenobiotics (Matés et al., 2008). In addition, during inflammation, neutrophils and macrophages are recruited to the site of damage, which leads to a "respiratory burst" due to an increased uptake of oxygen and, thus, an increased release and accumulation of ROS at the site of damage *via* a plasma membrane bound nicotinamide adenine dinucleotide phosphate, reduced form (NADPH)-oxidase (Reuter et al., 2010). An overproduction of ROS over a long time, associated with an exceeded antioxidant defense system, causes significant oxidative damages by reacting with macromolecules, including proteins, lipids and nucleic acids. These oxidative damages may be deleterious for cell structure and functions, and induce somatic mutations and neoplastic transformation. ROS can generate other reactive species (e.g., reactive aldehydes—malondialdehyde and 4-hydroxynonenal) by inducing excessive lipid peroxidation, which increases the membrane permeability. Oxidation of sensitive amino acids (cysteine, methionine, proline, phenylalanine, tryptophane and tyrosine) or reaction with reactive aldehydes from lipid peroxidation causes denaturation of proteins, leading to disturbance of cell signalling and metabolic pathways (Goetz and Luch, 2008). An excess of ROS causes several types of DNA damage, including depurination and depyrimidination, single and double-stranded DNA breaks, base and sugar modifications and DNA-protein crosslinks (Goetz and Luch, 2008). Permanent modification of genetic material resulting from the oxidative damage is one of the vital steps involved in mutagenesis that leads to carcinogenesis (initiation and progression to the development of cancer). Stimulation of DNA damage can either arrest or induce transcription, signal transduction pathways, replication errors and genomic instability, all of which are associated with carcinogenesis. The most frequent DNA mutations caused during oxidative stress, initiated by ionizing radiation and other environmental carcinogens are 8-dihydro-2 deoxyguanosine or 8-oxoguanosine (8-OHdG). Indeed, this oxidized DNA product is relatively easy to generate during oxidative stress and is mutagenic and carcinogenic. Thus, it is considered as a useful marker of oxidative stress and a potential biomarker of carcinogenesis. In addition to extensive studies devoted to the role of oxidative nuclear DNA damage in neoplasia, there exist several evidence about the involvement of the mitochondrial oxidative DNA damage in the carcinogenesis process. Mutations and altered expression in mitochondrial genes encoding for five complexes involved in the respiratory chain have been identified in various human cancers, including breast cancer (Rohan et al., 2010).

To protect against redox imbalance and to prevent oxidative damages, cells have developed a wide variety of enzymatic and nonenzymatic antioxidant defenses. Primary defense system prevents oxidative damage by scavenging ROS directly and includes superoxide dismutase (SOD), glutathione peroxidase/glutathione reductase (GPX/GR), catalase (CAT) and peroxiredoxins/thioredoxin reductase system (PRX/TRX). SOD destroys the highly reactive superoxide anion by converting into the less reactive hydrogen peroxide, which can be destroyed by CAT, GPX or PRX. The secondary defense system is composed of nonenzymatic and low weight molecules scavenging mainly OH• or chelating reduced metal transition to prevent Fenton reaction (ceruloplasmin for Cu, and transferrin and ferritin for Fe). This antioxidant defense includes tripeptide as glutathione or small proteins as metallothioneins, which are involved in the scavenging of OH•. In the case of glutathione (GSH), the oxidized form is rapidly regenerated by the NADPH-dependent glutathione reductase. The oxidized metallothioneins are rapidly degraded in cell. Dietary vitamins A (β-caroten), C (ascorbic acid) and E (α tocopherol), also have antioxidative properties against

OH•. Beside the antioxidant defense, cells have developed reparative mechanisms comprising enzymes involved in the elimination of oxidative damages. Oxidized proteins are specifically recognized by the 20S proteasome, which degrades them in an ATP and ubiquitin independent manner. Phospholipid hydroperoxides formed during lipid peroxidation are converted into the corresponding alcohol by the Ursini's glutathione peroxidase. Moreover, reactive aldehydes from the lipid peroxidation process may be inactivated in the cell by alpha-, pi-, mu-, and theta-class glutathione transferases (GST), which are able to transfer glutathione to the aldehyde group. Finally, the oxidative DNA damage as 8-OHdG in nuclear DNA is eliminated by a specific DNA repair enzyme as 8-OHdG glycosylase (Matés et al., 2008).

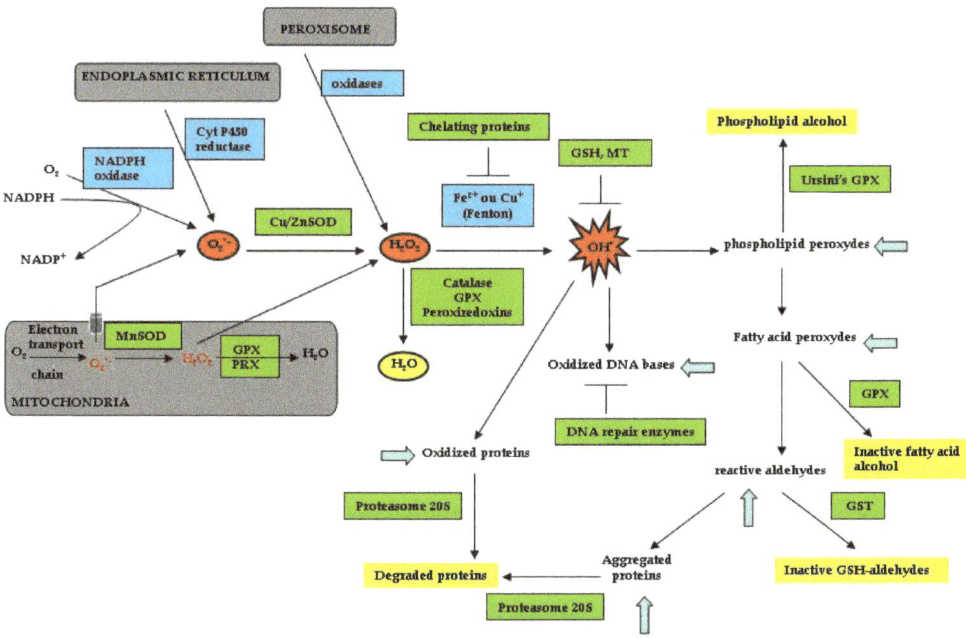

Fig. 1. Intracellular generation of ROS (in red) and main antioxidant defense system (in green). The oxidative damages are indicated by the large blue arrows. Antioxidant defense is constituted of enzymes and nonenzymatic molecules scavenging directly ROS. Antioxidant defense includes repair enzymes involved in the elimination of the oxidative damages (DNA repair enzymes, GPX, GST and proteasome 20S). For more details, see the text above.

During the initiation stage, low and chronic levels of ROS may produce DNA damages by introducing gene mutations and structural alterations into the DNA. In the promotion stage, ROS can contribute to abnormal gene expression, blockage of cell-to-cell communication, and modification of second-messenger systems, thus resulting in an increase in cell proliferation or a decrease in apoptosis of the initiated cell population. Finally, oxidative stress may also participate in the progression stage of the cancer process by adding further

DNA alterations to the initiated cell population. Indeed, carcinoma cells are frequently under persistent oxidative stress, what contribute to render them more aggressive. ROS are constitutively generated in carcinoma cells by altered metabolic pathways, particularly the respiratory chain in mitochondria, by an increase in some enzymatic activity as NADPH oxidase in plasma membrane, as well as by an imbalance in the expression of antioxidant enzymes.

2. Reactive oxygen species (ROS) in breast carcinogenesis and metastatic process

2.1 Breast cancer risk factors generating ROS

Many risk factors of breast cancer are sources of ROS, including caloric intake as fatty acid-enriched diet, cigarette smoking, endogenous and exogenous estrogens, and alcohol. A high caloric intake enriched with fatty acid, is able to modify mitochondrial function. The mitochondria use oxidative phosphorylation to convert dietary calories into usable energy, and they generate ROS as a toxic by-product at the respiratory chain level. These consequences can be exacerbated by polymorphisms in mitochondrial DNA which reduce the efficiency of mitochondrial functioning. Particularly, the A10398G polymorphism, which results in the substitution of threonine for alanine within the NADH dehydrogenase subunit of Complex I in the respiratory chain, has been associated with increased risk of breast cancer (Canter et al., 2005; Setiawan et al., 2008). This polymorphism may lead to impaired respiratory function and so to increased ROS production. The most important carcinogens in tobacco smoke are polycyclic aromatic hydrocarbons and are metabolized by the cytochrome P450 system to generate semiquinone radicals which undergo redox cycling to produce ROS. It is well known that a long-time exposure to estrogens increases the risk for breast cancer. Exposure of breast epithelium to endogenous estrogens is determined by several variables including timing of menarche, age at first full term pregnancy, number of pregnancies, and age at menopause. The serum levels of these endogenous estrogens, such as estrone, estradiol, estriol, have been considered as important risk factors for breast cancer. In addition, exposure of breast epithelium to exogenous estrogens from oral contraception, hormone replacement therapy, or xeno-estrogens (plasticizers, dyes, pollutants, pesticides and food preservatives) represents a potential risks for breast cancer. Indeed, beside their role in the cell proliferation mediated by a nuclear receptor, estrogens have been well described to generate ROS. Estrogen metabolism is mediated by cytochrome P450 reductase, mainly the cytochrome P450 1B1 reductase in human breast tissue, which generates reactive electrophilic estrogen *o*-quinones *via* the formation of hydroxylated estrogens (Mitrunen and Hirvonen, 2003; Gago-Dominguez et al., 2007). These compounds undergo redox cycling with the semiquinone radical, which may react with molecular oxygen to generate $O_2^{\bullet -}$. Women consuming alcohol have been hypothesized to exhibit elevated estrogen levels. Apart from this, alcohol metabolism produces ROS. Alcohol as ethanol is converted to acetate by a simple, two step reaction involving the combined activities of alcohol dehydrogenase, that produces acetaldehyde, and the molybdenum xanthine oxidoreductase and/or aldehyde oxidase, that produce acetate from acetaldehyde. Both xanthine oxidoreductase and aldehyde oxidase can generate ROS from molecular oxygen (Wright et al., 1999; Seitz and Becker, 2007; Kabat et al., 2010).

Chronic inflammation is frequently seen in breast carcinomas and produces notable amounts of ROS, enough to cause additional genetic instability. The sources of inflammation in breast cancer include exposure to allergens, radiation and toxic chemicals, consumption of alcohol or tobacco use. In addition, inflammatory cells also produce soluble mediators, such as metabolites of arachidonic acid, cytokines, and chemokines, which act by further recruiting inflammatory cells to the site of damage and producing more ROS. The main source of ROS, particularly $O_2{\bullet}^-$, is produced by the NADPH oxidase found in the plasma membrane of inflammatory cells. Inflammatory cells may also increase DNA damage by activating procarcinogens to become DNA damaging species; for example, neutrophils can activate aromatic estrogens and polycyclic aromatic hydrocarbons from cigarette smoking by ROS-dependent mechanisms. On the other hand, both neutrophils and macrophages have themselves been shown to release large quantities of $O_2{\bullet}^-$, H_2O_2 and $OH{\bullet}$ after activation of their redox metabolism (Reuter et al., 2010).

2.2 Causes and consequences of persistent oxidative stress in breast carcinoma cells

The oxidative stress exerted by ROS is involved in the breast cancer etiology by the accumulation of oxidative damages resulting to the oxidation of biological molecules, particularly the DNA leading to genomic instability. These events lead to the transformation of normal cells to carcinoma cells. However, the role of ROS may not be limited to early mutagenic events and cell transformation. A number of somatic mutations have been identified in breast cancer (Callahan et al., 1992). These include transversion mutations of p53, the breast cancer susceptibility genes BRCA1 and BRCA2. These key genes have been linked to breast cancer progression and the mutations found in them can be produced by ROS (Elledge et al., 1993; Hussain et al., 1994; Merlo et al., 1994). Although the direct link between ROS modification of DNA and mutation of these genes induced by breast cancer risk factors remains to be established, they should be considered important candidates for the induced carcinogenesis because mutations in these genes could be responsible for tumor initiation as well as tumor progression.

Some altered metabolic pathways have been described in breast carcinoma cells. The majority of the somatic alterations in mitochondrial DNA identified actually may simply represent the consequences of genomic instability and oxidative DNA damage during the multistep carcinogenic process. In humans, several studies have shown a relatively high frequency of mtDNA mutations in breast tumor tissues (range 20%–93%) (Rohan et al., 2010). Among them, we have cited above the A10398G (T114A) polymorphism in the NADH dehydrogenase subunit gene of the mitochondrial genome (Pezzotti et al., 2009). In consequence, a persistent dysfunction of mitochondrial respiratory chain is a source of ROS production in breast carcinoma cells. Actually, no nuclear mutations of mitochondrial proteins, particularly the succinate dehydrogenase proteins, have been associated with breast carcinoma cells, in contrast to some other solid tumors. It has been reported recently that NADPH oxidase contributes to persistent generation of ROS in breast carcinoma cells. This enzyme is overexpressed in breast tumors and carcinoma cell lines when compared to normal breast tissues and cells. Its activity is regulated by binding a partner as the small GTPase Rac1, which is itself downstream of the Ras oncoprotein (Brown and Bicknell, 2001). Carcinoma cell oxidative stress can also be induced by thymidine phosphorylase, an enzyme that is overexpressed in the majority of breast carcinomas. Thymidine phosphorylase catabolizes thymidine to thymine and 2-deoxy-D-ribose-1-phosphate; the latter is a very powerful reducing sugar that rapidly glycates proteins, generating ROS within the carcinoma cell. Thymidine phosphorylase activity has been shown to induce carcinoma cell oxidative stress *in vitro*. The frequent upregulation of thymidine phosphorylase in human

breast tumours suggests that this may be an important cause of oxidative stress in breast cancer (Brown et al., 2000). *In vivo,* an inadequate tumor vascular network can lead to a persistent oxidative stress in breast carcinoma cells. A breast tumor rapidly outgrows its blood supply, leading to glucose deprivation and hypoxia. Glucose deprivation rapidly induces cellular oxidative stress within the breast carcinoma cells because of the depletion of the intracellular antioxidant pyruvate which prevents in part the decomposition of endogenous ROS. Breast carcinomas usually support their growth by stimulating blood vessel development (angiogenesis). Blood flow within these new vessels is often chaotic, causing periods of hypoxia followed by reperfusion. It is well known that the reperfusion of tumor cause the generation of ROS, as observed after myocardial infarction or cerebral ischaemia. This ROS production during reperfusion may therefore be a cause of oxidative stress within breast carcinomas. One additional cause of persistent oxidative stress in carcinoma cells is the fact that breast tumors are frequently infiltrated by large numbers of macrophages (Leek et al., 2002). These may contribute to carcinoma cell oxidative stress, as tumor-associated macrophages have been shown to produce ROS by secreting tumor necrosis factor-alpha. This cytokine is known to induce cellular oxidative stress (Matés et al., 2008). Persistent generation of ROS in breast carcinoma cells is also associated with an alteration in the expression of antioxidant enzymes, those we describe below (see part 3).
Markers of the persistent oxidative stress have been detected in samples from *in vivo* breast carcinomas. For example, 8-OHdG has been reported to be increased 8- to 17-fold in breast primary tumors compared to non-malignant breast tissues (Malins et al. 1996; Matsui et al., 2000b). In addition, lipid peroxidation as evidenced by malondialdehyde (MDA) was enhanced in breast cancer tissues compared to non-malignant Tissues (Tas et al., 2005).
The persistent production of ROS cause additional genomic instability, as well as stimulate the expansion of initiated cell clones through modulating genes and activating signalling pathways (promotion stage of carcinogenesis) related to apoptosis or proliferation. In addition, it creates selection pressure for characteristics such as accelerated growth, invasion and metastasis. ROS are able to play a role as second messengers by activating small G protein, kinases and/or inhibiting phosphatases resulting in stimulation of signalling pathways. Ras oncoprotein can be activated by ROS via oxidative modification of its cysteine 118 residue which leads to the inhibition of GDP-GTP exchange. The effects of ROS occur through targeting a cysteine residues of the active sites of kinases and phosphatases, leading to activation and inactivation, respectively (Klaunig and Kamendulis, 2004). As shown in Figure 2, ROS can stimulate the proliferation of breast tumor cells by activating directly the extracellular signal-regulated kinase in Mitogen-activated protein kinase signalling pathway, as well as c-Src oncoprotein. ROS can stimulate the survival and resistance to apoptosis by activating phosphoinositide 3 kinase/Akt signalling pathway. In addition, these signalling pathways are regulated by the PTEN lipid phosphatase, which is reversely inactivated by ROS (Valko et al., 2006). In addition, ROS are known to induce considerable increase in intracellular calcium, which further may activate proto-oncogenes, such as c-fos, c-jun and c-myc or activate protein kinase C, which enhance tumor cell proliferation (Klaunig and Kamendulis, 2004). Moreover, the oncogenic protein c-Src, which is a nonreceptor tyrosine kinase has been reported to be activated by ROS and is often overexpressed in breast cancers. This oncoprotein binds to cell membranes by myristilation and initiates MAPK and PI3K signalling pathways (Leonard et al., 2004).
ROS are able to modulate the regulation of gene expression, by oxidizing directly a cysteine residues, that this leads to a change in the native conformation promoting an activation of

certain redox sensitive transcription factors. These latter include particularly hypoxia inducible Factor (HIF), Nuclear Factor-kappa B (NF-κB) and Activator protein-1 (AP-1) . ROS generated during hypoxia is responsible for stabilizing HIF. This latter is a heterodimer consisting of a constitutively stable subunit HIF-β and a redox sensitive subunit HIFα, whose the major isoform is HIF-1α. This transcription factor is involved in the tumor growth by activating angiogenesis (Brown and Bicknell, 2001). NF-κB is constitutively activated in many breast tumor cells, because the persistent production of ROS accelerates the degradation of IκB, the cytosolic inhibitory subunit of NF-κB (Nakshatri et al., 1997). This transcription factor is known to regulate target genes involved in proliferation, survival and migration of tumor cells. AP-1 is a heterodimeric transcription factor composed of the c-Jun and c-Fos proteins, which regulates a number of genes involved in the progression of cell cycle, such as cyclins D (Shen and Tergaonkar, 2009).

In addition to regulating tumor growth and survival, ROS also control mechanisms which are associated with the formation of breast tumor metastases. The cellular processes linked to this function are a decrease in the cell adhesion to the basal lamina and an increase in the migratory and invasive potential which favour breast cancer cells to enter the blood vessels. The loss of adhesion of normal cells is always accompanied with a particular type of apoptosis, widely known as anoikis, which is essential for prevention of the dissemination of cells to inappropriate sites. Resistance to anoikis is thus emerging as a hallmark of metastatic cancer cells, mainly because anchorage-independent growth of tumor cells is a classic feature of human malignancies (Storz, 2005).

In this context, increasing blood vessel growth due to hypoxia and reoxygenation increases the risk of blood-borne metastasis. Persistent production of ROS may augment breast tumor invasion and metastasis by increasing the rates of cell migration. As described earlier, the small GTPase Rac1 can activate the NADPH-oxidase in breast tumor cells, causing superoxide production. These ROS have been shown to mediate the role of Rac1 in actin cytoskeleton reorganization which is an important step in the loss of cell-cell adhesion and cell-matrix adhesion to laminin and fibronectin. The resistance to anoikis of cancer cells including breast cancer cells, which is an important step during the metastatic process, has been associated to the oxidation of c-Src by ROS, leading to a sustained activation of pro-survival signals through the ligand-independent phosphorylation of EGFR (Valko et al., 2006). ROS within breast tumors may also facilitate invasion and metastasis by activating MMPs and inhibiting antiproteases, directly or through activation of transcription factors. MMP-2 and -9 are gelatinases, which play a major role in breast cancer invasion and metastasis. High levels of MMP-2 and -9 correlate with poor prognosis in breast cancer patients and active MMP-2 and -9 are detected more frequently in malignant than in benign breast tumors (Jinga et al., 2006). MMP-2 and -9 expressions are regulated by AP-1 and NF-κB, respectively, which can be activated by ROS. In addition, ROS can modulate MMP-2 and -9 activities, by reacting with thiol groups in the protease catalytic domain. Like all MMP, they are secreted in a latent zymogen form in which the cleavage of the pro-domain is ROS dependent (Nelson et al., 2004; Kattan et al., 2008). Due to the expression of cell surface protein ICAM-1 (Intercellular Adhesion protein-1) and CD54 in consequence of the ROS-dependent activation of NF-κB, the trans-endothelial migration of breast tumor cells is favourable for development of metastasis. Protease inhibitors, such as α1-proteinase inhibitor and plasminogen activator inhibitor, may be inactivated by oxidation of methionine residues at their active sites. This facilitates the activity of various proteases, increasing invasion and the likelihood of metastasis. For example, plasminogen activator is believed to play a role in metastasis in breast cancer. The other major regulator of metastasis is the hypoxic microenvironment. The degree of hypoxia correlates positively with metastasis. Hypoxia stimulates the epithelial-mesenchymal transition (EMT), which is characterized by loss of epithelial cell adhesion with repression of E-cadherin, and increased cell mobility. EMT is largely described as a process leading to breast tumor cell dissemination. The ROS-dependent activation of HIF under hypoxia can lead to subsequent activation of the transcription factor Twist, resulting in EMT. In addition, ROS produced during hypoxia can inhibit the activity of glycogen synthase kinase 3β (GSK3β). This results in the up-regulation of the EMT-inducing transcription factor Snail. Together, Twist and Snail are involved in the up-regulation of genes, leading to the breast tumor cell dissemination (Micalizzi et Farabaugh, 2010). From these, it is speculated that ROS are likely to be important regulators of metastasis (Cannito et al., 2010).

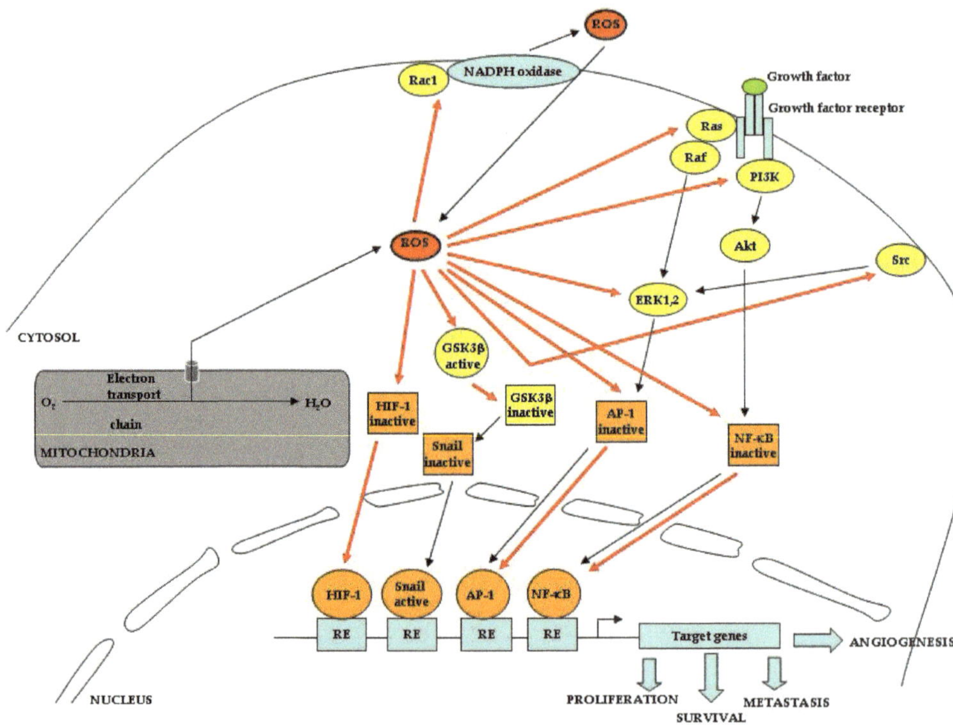

Fig. 2. Interaction between ROS generated from mitochondria and NADPH oxidase activity and signalling pathways leading to proliferation, survival and metastasis of breast tumor cells. Red arrows indicate action of ROS on their targets. RE for response element of transcription factors (in orange) in promoter region of target genes. Small G proteins, kinases and phosphatases in signalling pathways are represented in yellow.

ROS play a role in angiogenesis, which is required for tumor growth as well as metastasis. ROS within the tumor microenvironment may promote metastasis by increasing vascular permeability, either by direct damages to endothelial cells or by the upregulation of inducible nitric oxide synthase (iNOS). By this mechanism, ROS may also increase the blood supply to breast tumor carcinoma by triggering vasodilatation, because the nitric oxide produced would activate cGMP within nearby smooth muscle cells, leading to vasodilatation. In addition, low concentrations of ROS (O_2•− and H_2O_2) produced by breast tumor cells can stimulate endothelial migration and tube formation in an *in vitro* model of angiogenesis, through the activation of the secreted MMP-1, a collagenase that aids vessel growth within the tumor microenvironment. Finally, ROS has been shown to increase production of the angiogenic factor such as vascular endothelial growth factor (VEGF) by tumor cells. As described above, HIF may be increased by ROS, and this transcription factor is known to induce VEGF expression (Ushio-Fukai and Nakamura, 2008).

3. Antioxidant enzymes in breast carcinogenesis and metastatic process

3.1 Relationship between antioxidant enzymes and breast cancer risk factors

As described above, there are three main types of antioxidant defense enzymes: the superoxide dismutases (SOD), including MnSOD and cytosolic CuZnSOD, catalase (CAT), and the peroxidases (GPX1 and GPX4 and peroxiredoxins I to VI). All of them function to protect the cell from damage due to ROS. In addition, several other enzymes are implicated in oxidative damage repair (Figure 3). The reduction of oxidized glutathione (GSSG) produced by action of GPXs is catalyzed by glutathione reductase (GSR). The thioredoxins (TXN and TXN2) and thioredoxin reductases (TXNRD1 and TXNRD2) are also involved in antioxidant defense through the thioredoxin redox cycle which allows the reduction and so the regeneration of peroxiredoxins (Arner and Holmgren, 2006; Matés et al., 2008). Genetic polymorphisms in a number of the genes encoding these enzymes may be important in affecting levels of ROS and oxidative damages when the mammary epithelial cells are exposed to risk factors, and could also have an impact for risk to develop breast cancer.

Common variants in oxidative damage defense and repair genes, including MnSOD, GPX1, catalase, GST and catechol-O-methyl transferase (COMT), may be good candidates for both cancer susceptibility and prognosis. The case of MnSOD will be described in the part 4.

The antioxidant enzyme GPX is involved in the detoxifying hydrogen- and lipid peroxides depending on GSH and GSH redox cycle by GSR. Among GPX, it has been identified a genetic polymorphism in the GPX1 gene at codon 198, resulting in either a proline (Pro) or leucine (Leu) at the corresponding position of the encoded protein, which has drawn increasing attention in the etiology of several cancers, including breast cancer (Hu and Diamond, 2003; Hu et al., 2010). The selenium-dependent activity of GPX198Leu mutant enzyme is lower than for the GPX ^{198}Pro wild-type enzyme, and is associated weakly with higher breast cancer risk, depending on the population (Cox et al., 2004).

Among other primary antioxidant enzymes neutralizing ROS, CAT is the most potent enzyme and inducible by exposure to ROS, particularly hydrogen peroxide (H_2O_2). Located in the peroxisomes of all cells, CAT is a heme enzyme converting H_2O_2 into H_2O and O_2 to directly reduce the production of OH• and lipid hydroperoxides. A C/T substitution at nucleotide position 262 has been identified in the promoter region of the human CAT gene, resulting in reduced enzyme activity. The consequence of the low activity for this polymorphism has been associated with increased breast cancer risk, particularly among low consumers of fruits and vegetables (Ahn et al., 2005).

For other antioxidant enzymes such as GSR, GPX4, Cu/ZnSOD, TXN and TXNRD, no association with a risk of developing of breast cancer was found for any of the polymorphisms reported (Cebrian et al., 2006). In addition, no significant association was observed between common variants in these genes coding for antioxidant defense enzymes (Cu/ZnSOD, MnSOD, CAT, GPX1, GPX4, TXN, TXN2, TXNRD1 and TXNRD2) and susceptibility to breast cancer (Oestergaard et al., 2006).

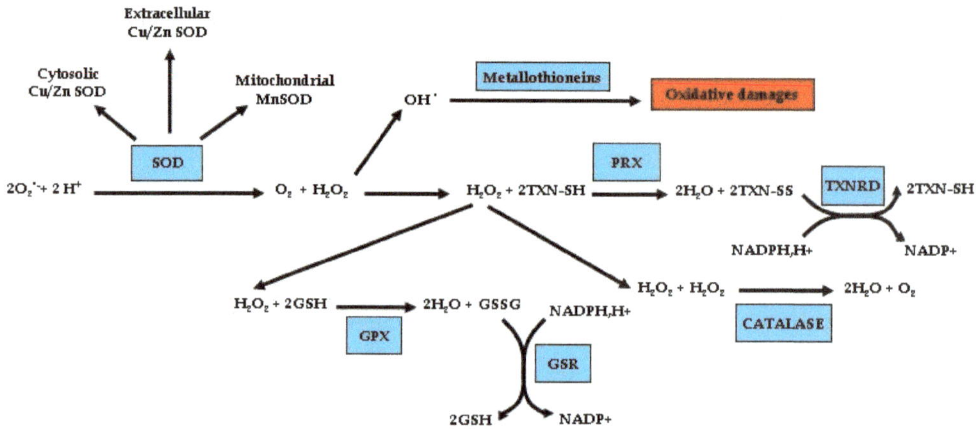

Fig. 3. The main antioxidant enzymes (in blue) involved in the direct elimination of ROS in cells and whose expression is altered in breast cancer cells. The systems involved in the reduction of the cofactor TXN or GSH are indicated with the corresponding enzyme.

Glutathione-associated metabolism is a major mechanism for cellular protection against breast cancer risk factors that generate ROS. GSTs catalyse the conjugation of glutathione to cytotoxic products (aldehydes, lipid hydroperoxides) of lipid peroxidation induced by ROS and thus protect normal mammary epithelial cells (Rundle et al., 2000). These cytosolic and dimeric enzymes are induced under conditions of oxidative stress, and can be differentiated into five classes in mammalian cells termed alpha, mu (M), pi (P), theta (T) and zeta (Di Pietro et al., 2010). Allelic variation has been found in genes encoding for these GST, and the absence of specific isoenzymes affects the tolerance of cells to chemical challenges and may result in increased somatic mutation rate and thereby higher susceptibility to malignancies. In estrogen metabolism, GSTs play a role in the catalysis of glutathione conjugation of catechol estrogen quinones, the reactive intermediates of estrogen metabolism which are able to form DNA adducts. Only GSTM1 and 3 and GSTP1 are expressed in breast tissue and involved in the estrogen metabolism. Several recent studies have examined the GSTM1 and 3 and GSTP1 genotype in relation to individual breast cancer risk. The homozygous deletion (null genotype) of the GSTM1 gene leads to the total absence of the respective enzyme activity. An association has been observed between the GSTM1 null genotype and increased breast cancer risk in some populations, such as postmenopausal Caucasian, French and African-American women, and premenopausal Korean women. It can be noted that the genetic polymorphisms of *GSTM1* have also been found to influence the risk-enhancing effect of alcohol in breast cancer (Zheng et al., 2003). Concerning GSTM3, a variant allele has been reported which differs from the wild-type allele by a three base pair deletion in intron 6. This mutation in the noncoding region of the gene generates a binding site for the YY transcription factor and leading to an expression of the variant allele at different levels with less efficiencies in the metabolism of catechol estrogen quinones. However, only one study has been shown an association between variant allele of GSTM3 and breast cancer risk for women consuming alcohol (Mitrunen et al., 2001). The GSTP1 is the major GST expressed consistently in both normal and breast tumor tissue. Two variant alleles have been detected in addition to the wild-type allele. In both of the variant alleles, a point mutation at position 133 in nucleotide sequence results in a single amino acid change from isoleucine (Ile) to valine (Val) at codon 105. The Ile/Val^{105} polymorphism has been demonstrated lower specific activity. One variant has another point mutation resulting in alanine (Ala) to valine (Val) change at codon 114, which does not modify the enzyme activity. Whereas no significant overall association has been seen between the Ala/Val^{114} polymorphism and breast cancer risk, a significant increase in the risk was observed for former smokers for the homozygous Ile/Val^{105} polymorphism (Millikan et al., 2000).

It is known a genetic polymorphisms in estrogen metabolizing enzymes which can be associated with risk of breast cancer. Estrogens play a crucial role in the development and evolution of human breast cancer, because they are converted by cytochrome P450 1B1 to 4-hydroxyestradiol (4-OHE2), a putative carcinogenic metabolite of estrogen. This catechol estrogen metabolite is oxidized further to produce a reactive quinone *via* semiquinone radical, which can generate ROS by undergoing redox cycling. It exists catechol-O-methyl transferase, a phase II enzyme under soluble or membrane-bound form that inactivates catechol estrogens by transfer of a methyl group. This enzyme is considered as an antioxidant enzyme by preventing the conversion of catechol estrogen metabolite to semiquinones and quinones and, therefore, blocks the generation of ROS. A single G to A base pair change in the COMT-L low activity allele containing genotypes (*HL* or *LL)* results in a valine to methionine amino acid change at codon 108/158 in the cytosolic/membrane-bound form of the protein. This change was associated with a decreased activity of the COMT compared with the wild-type COMT-H allele (Mitrunen and Hirvonen, 2003). It has been observed an increased risk for premenopausal women carrying the *COMT-L* allele-containing genotypes and decreased risk for postmenopausal women with these genotypes. Furthermore, the increase in the risk was confined to never alcohol users and ever smokers (Matsui et al. 2000a).

3.2 Relationship between antioxidant enzymes and persistent oxidative stress in breast carcinoma cells

The persistent oxidative stress in carcinoma cells is often associated with an alteration in the expression of antioxidant defense enzymes (Figure 3). According to the type of antioxidant enzyme has an altered expression, an accumulation of the corresponding ROS ($O_2{\bullet}-$ or H_2O_2) leads to the tumor cell proliferation or migration and invasion.

The case of MnSOD will be described in the part 4. Concerning catalase, it has been observed a relationship between ER status and the enzyme level in breast carcinoma cell lines. It has been reported that catalase expression is higher in ER-positive than in ER-negative breast cancer cells (Kattan et al. 2008). *In vivo,* a decrease in its activity has been found in tumor tissue of breast cancer patients as well as the stage of the tumors (Tas et al., 2005).

In contrast to catalase, an inverse correlation between ER expression and GPX-1 expression has been observed in breast cancer cell lines (Esworthy et al., 1995). However, the GPX level

in breast tumor tissues is relatively low in contrast to the normal counterpart tissue. The GPX-1 being the main mitochondrial and H_2O_2-detoxifying enzyme with peroxiredoxin III, its deficient expression may be associated with the deficient activity of the respiratory chain in aggressive breast cancer cells, explaining in part the high H_2O_2 release from mitochondria, a ROS involved in the metastatic process. In addition, peroxiredoxin III (PRX III) expression may decrease with the aggressiveness of breast cancer cells, which is often associated with a dysfunction in the mitochondrial activity. In addition to PRX III, the other peroxiredoxins, also called thioredoxin peroxidases, are a distinct expression between tumor and normal cells and tissues. These enzymes are characterized by one (PRX VI) or two (PRX I-V) cysteines as their active site and are reduced to the initial state by thioredoxin. In contrast to catalase, PRX are widely distributed subcellularly, with PRX I, II, III, V and VI in cytosol, PRX IV and VI in peroxisomes, endoplasmic reticulum and Golgi apparatus (PRX IV), and mitochondria (PRX III) (Rhee et al., 2005). In response to an increased production of ROS, it has been reported that only PRX III, IV, V and VI is overexpressed in breast cancer cells and tissues in relation to normal cells and tissues. Whereas PRX III, IV and VI overexpression is associated with progesterone and estrogen receptor expression, tumor cell proliferation and with a better prognosis, PRX V was related to the larger tumor size and positive lymph node status and also a shorter survival (Karihtala et al., 2003).
Thioredoxins (TXN), involved in the reduction of PRX, are also overexpressed in breast tumor cells. This overexpression is observed rather in the nuclei of invasive tumor cells or tissues, probably related to the role of these thiol-containing antioxidants in the activation of the transcription factor NF-κB, which is known to play a crucial role in the invasive processes by regulating target genes. In addition, TXN are also a key antioxidant proteins for DNA synthesis by directly serving as an electron donor to ribonucleotide reductase and this redox function is essential for breast cancer cell proliferation (Arner and Holmgren, 2006).
Trx reductase (TRXRD) utilizes NADPH to reduce and activate TRX as well as other proteins. There are three different TRXD proteins in human cells with a distinct localization: TRXD1 are observed in extracellular space, nucleus, cytoplasm and in plasma membrane, while TRXD2 and TRXD3 are present in mitochondria. The TRX and TXRD contribute to maintain a reduced state in cell by maintaining protein thiols in the reduced form, like some active transcription factors which promote breast cancer cell proliferation and invasion (Arner and Holmgren, 2006). Recently, TRX and TXRD have been considered as a tumor growth promoting factors for estrogen-sensitive breast cancer cells (Cadenas et al., 2010). They were identified in a complex associated with the DNA-bound estrogen receptor alpha (ERα) to regulate the expression of estrogen-responsive genes in estrogen-sensitive breast cancer cells (Rao et al., 2009).
Metallothioneins (MTs) are another group of antioxidant proteins which protect cells to the OH• radical production by chelating the transition metal as copper and by scavenging this ROS directly. These MTs are a family of ubiquitous and low molecular weight cysteine-rich proteins encoded by 10 genes which play an important role in tumor cell proliferation (Eckschlager et al., 2009). However, it has been reported in many studies an association between high MT expression, particularly the MT2A isoform, and both poorer prognosis of patients and aggressive histopathological features of tumors (Jin et al., 2004). These observations can be associated with the fact that expression of the MT genes are activated by

hypoxia though the binding of metal response element of their promote region by the metal transcription factor. Thus this molecular mechanism contributes to the survival of hypoxic breast tumor cells which acquire invasive and metastatic abilities.

4. MnSOD in breast carcinogenesis and metastatic process

SODs were the first characterized antioxidant enzymes. Three different types of SOD are expressed in human cells (Figure 3). This part 4 will be focused on MnSOD, which is considered as one of the most important antioxidant enzymes in mammals, for the following reasons. Whereas cytosolic and extracellular Cu/ZnSOD were not essential for survival of mice in knockout studies, mice lacking MnSOD had severe metabolic acidosis, degeneration of neurons and cardiac myocytes and died prenatally of dilated cardiomyopathy (Lebovitz et al., 1996). In addition, the role of MnSOD in cancer has been largely studied even if is still rather ambiguous and is associated with profound alterations in the gene expression of the antioxidant enzyme by different molecular mechanisms (Miao and St Clair, 2009).

4.1 Relationship between MnSOD and breast cancer risk factors

It has been observed a relationship between low MnSOD activity and risk of breast cancer development. The low MnSOD activity depend on a main gene polymorphism identified as a single nucleotide substitution of C to T at the second nucleotide of codon 16 of the MnSOD gene changes which encoded amino acid substitution from alanine (GCT) to valine (GTT) at the position-9 of the mitochondrial targeting sequence of the mature protein. This alteration designated as the MnSOD Ala^{16}Val polymorphism has been found to affect the transport of MnSOD into the mitochondria, thus altering its enzymatic activity. The human MnSOD Ala variant has been found to generate 30-40% more active MnSOD protein compared to the Val variant in mitochondria (Sutton et al., 2003). The MnSOD Val/Val genotype having a low MnSOD activity as consequence could be considered as deleterious for mammary epithelial cells exposed to environmental carcinogens such as alcohol, tobacco smoke or estrogens generating $O_2 \bullet -$ during their metabolism (Bica et al., 2009). However, several epidemiologic studies have looked at the association between a MnSOD gene polymorphism and breast cancer risk. Different studies in diverse populations have resulted in identifying conflicting roles for the Ala/Val^{16} polymorphism and cancer risks. In summary, breast cancer risk is slightly increased in women carrying the MnSOD Ala/Ala genotype compared to those carrying the Val/Val genotype, especially in premenopausal women. This risk is further increased in premenopausal women with low intakes of fruits, vegetables, and various dietary supplements (antioxidant vitamins and selenium). Some other epidemiologic studies reveal a relationship between this Ala/Ala genotype and smoking or alcohol consumption in diverse populations (Wang et al., 2009). Recently, an epidemiological study on a large population of patients has been focused on examining associations between combined gene polymorphisms in antioxidant enzymes and breast cancer risk. An increase in the risk of breast cancer has been observed in patients who carry both the MnSOD Ala/Ala genotype and the GPX-1 Leu/Leu genotype, while neither allele alone show any change in breast cancer risk (Cox et al., 2006).

Another polymorphism in the MnSOD gene has also be identified. MnSOD exists as a homotetramer, and Ile to Thr amino acid change at codon 58 has been shown to result in lower MnSOD activity due to destabilization of the tetrameric structure of the enzyme. However, its frequency seems to be low to have any detectable effect on breast cancer risk (Mitrunen and Hirvonen, 2003).

4.2 Relationship between MnSOD and persistent oxidative stress in breast carcinoma cells

It is known that MnSOD plays a role in breast cancer, depending on its basal expression. *In vitro* studies show that a low MnSOD expression correlates with a high rate of tumor cell growth, whereas high MnSOD content is associated with the invasive and metastatic properties of tumor cells (Nelson et al., 2003). These latter display altered transcription of MnSOD gene, which is also associated with that of H_2O_2-detoxifying enzymes, as compared with the normal counterparts, leading to an imbalance in the redox state by an increase in the level of ROS. Concerning breast cancer cells, the estrogen-sensitive and nonmetastatic tumor MCF-7 cell line exhibits a low basal expression of MnSOD, leading to an accumulation of $O_2{\bullet}^-$, which act as second messenger molecules promoting cell proliferation by activating the Ras-mediated signalling (Li et al., 1995). MnSOD-forced overexpression in these breast cancer cells after transfection of cDNA encoding the antioxidant enzyme reduces cell proliferation and regulates the activation of MMP-2, suggesting a potential modulation of their invasiveness, despite a slower growth rate (Zhang et al., 2002). In contrast, the estrogen-independent and metastatic breast cancer MDA-MB231 and SKBR3 cell lines exhibit a high basal MnSOD expression, which correlates with the invasive and metastatic properties of cells. Up-regulation of MnSOD in estrogen-independent and metastatic cancer cells is associated with an unexplained low expression of catalase, GPX and PRDX3. As a consequence, H_2O_2 from MnSOD activity is overproduced and plays a role in the invasive ability of estrogen-independent and metastatic breast cancer cells, by activating particularly matrix metalloprotease 9 (Kattan et al., 2008). *In vitro* studies are correlated with a clinical investigation which reports that the MnSOD level is positively correlated with the *in vivo* tumor grade in breast carcinomas, and, particularly with the invasive and metastatic phenotypes of advanced breast cancers (Tsanou et al., 2004). Taken together, these observations suggest that an elevated level of MnSOD may reflect tumor progression to a metastatic phenotype in breast cancer cells. The increase of MnSOD expression in breast cancer cells may represent a mechanism by which, by boosting the intracellular concentration of H_2O_2, they reduce their proliferation rate and increase their invasive capacity (Figure 4). In this case, it can be postulated that MnSOD up-regulation would be associated with a poor prognosis in advanced breast cancer. Moreover, the high MnSOD activity may play a role in angiogenesis though the release of H_2O_2, which is able to activate VEGF synthesis (Ushio-Fukai and Nakamura, 2008).

The understanding of the molecular mechanisms involved in the distinct basal expression of MnSOD between nonmetastatic and metastatic breast cancer cells may likely have important clinical implications in predicting tumor progression in breast cancer. Two molecular mechanisms are identified to be involved in the low basal MnSOD expression in nonmetastatic breast cancer cells. Epigenetic processes, such as methylation of CpG islands localized in the proximal gene promoter and a decrease in the histone modifications (methylations and acetylations) are involved in the transcriptional repression of MnSOD gene in some breast cancer cell lines (Hitchler et al., 2006). The other mechanism involves the occupancy of the proximal promoter of MnSOD gene by the both transcription factor Activator protein-2 alpha (AP-2α) and the Damaged DNA binding 2 (DDB2) protein. This latter protein has been described originally for its role in the nucleotide excision repair of DNA lesions (Sugasawa, 2010). It has been described recently that DDB2 regulates negatively the basal MnSOD expression through its binding to a specific and characterized DNA sequence, which is associated with the loss of acetylated histones, and with the recruitment of the AP-2α (Minig et al., 2009). This latter is known to play a role as repressor of MnSOD gene by binding a response element localized in the GC-rich region in the proximal promoter (Zhu et al., 2001).

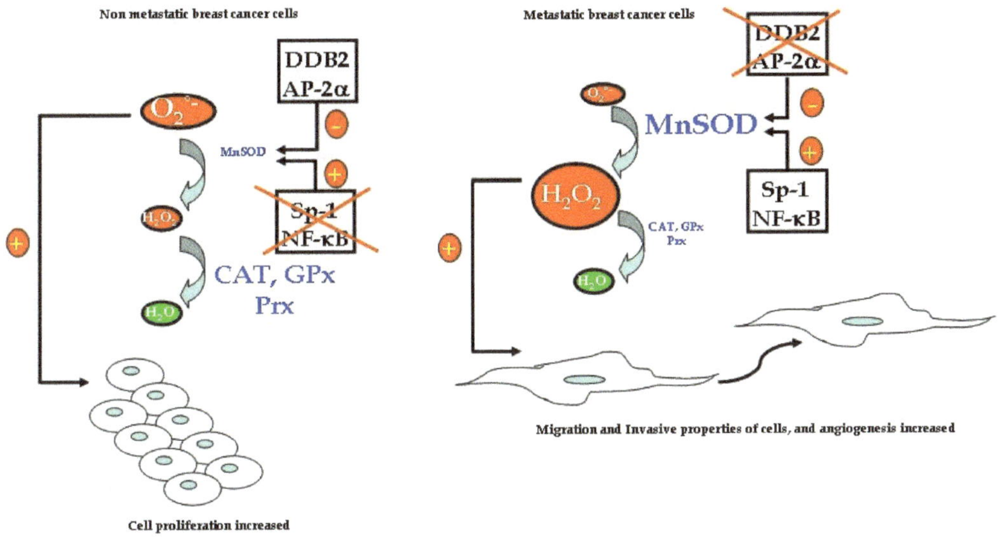

Fig. 4. Role of MnSOD in growth of nonmetastatic and metastatic breast cancer cells. Details are described in the text.

The molecular mechanism, by which the metastatic breast cancer cells exhibit a high basal MnSOD expression, involves essentially the transcription factors Specific-1 (Sp-1) and NF-κB. In absence of DDB2 expression as observed in metastatic breast cancer cells, Sp-1 can bind one of these response elements localized in the GC-rich region in the proximal promoter of MnSOD gene, and cooperates with NF-κB interacting with its binding site localized in intron 2 of the gene and characterized as enhancer element of the transcription (Ennen et al., 2011).

5. Conclusions

In summary, oxidative stress is an important risk factor for cancer development and for disease progression. It seems that polymorphisms in gene encoding the antioxidant enzymes contribute to the accumulation of ROS from the metabolism of risk factors and result in the transformation of normal mammary epithelial cells. Actually, relations between these gene polymorphisms and breast cancer risk are controversial as yet, because of the lack of large case-control studies which need to be drawn, and the difficulties related to the difference between ethnic groups, exposure to environmental factors and the life style. However, reducing ROS by the administration of antioxidants has been considered a good alternative for cancer prevention, since high consumption of fruits and vegetables has been related to the reduction of breast cancer risk. In addition, antioxidant strategy represents the possibility to inhibit in theory some of the stimuli that contribute to cancer transformation and the expression of an aggressive phenotype, minimizing the acquisition of new mutations and the onset of molecular pathways that promote cancer growth, survival and spreading.

The observations showing an alteration in gene expression of antioxidant enzymes in breast carcinoma cells have been pertinent to better understand the role of ROS in the breast tumor progression toward metastatic phenotype. It appears that some antioxidant enzymes represent actually a good potential biomarkers for the breast tumor progression, particularly MnSOD. The overexpression of this latter enzyme, resulting to an altered expression of its gene, seems to be clearly defined and to depend on the malignant phenotype. Finally, it has been already observed that different intracellular antioxidant capacities may determine the ability of metastatic breast carcinoma cells to resist radiotherapy and anticancer drugs whose activity is dependent on the massive ROS production.

6. References

Ahn, J.; Gammon, M.D.; Santella, R.M.; Gaudet, M.M.; Britton, J.A.; Teitelbaum, S.L.; Terry, M.B.; Nowell, S.; Davis, W.; Garza, C.; Neugut, A.I. & Ambrosone, C.B. (2005). Associations between breast cancer risk and the catalase genotype, fruit and vegetable consumption, and supplement use. *American Journal of Epidemiology*, Vol. 162, No. 10, pp. 943-952

Arnér, E.S. & Holmgren, A. (2006). The thioredoxin system in cancer. *Seminars in Cancer Biology*, Vol. 16, No. 6, pp. 420-426

Bica, C.G.; de Moura da Silva, L.L.; Toscani, N.V.; da Cruz, I.B.; Sá, G.; Graudenz, M.S. & Zettler, C.G. (2009). MnSOD gene polymorphism association with steroid-dependent cancer. *Pathology Oncology Research*, Vol. 15, No. 1, pp. 19-24

Brown, N.S.; Jones, A.; Fujiyama, C.; Harris, A.L. & Bicknell, R. (2000). Thymidine phosphorylase induces carcinoma cell oxidative stress and promotes secretion of angiogenic factors. *Cancer Research*, Vol. 60, pp. 6298-6302

Brown, N.S. & Bicknell, R. (2001). Hypoxia and oxidative stress in breast cancer. Oxidative stress: its effects on the growth, metastatic potential and response to therapy of breast cancer. *Breast Cancer Research*, Vol. 3, No. 5, pp. 323-327

Cadenas, C.; Franckenstein, D.; Schmidt, M.; Gehrmann, M.; Hermes, M.; Geppert, B.; Schormann, W.; Maccoux, L.J.; Schug, M.; Schumann, A.; Wilhelm, C.; Freis, E.; Ickstadt, K.; Rahnenführer, J.; Baumbach, J.I.; Sickmann, A. & Hengstler, J.G. (2010). Role of thioredoxin reductase 1 and thioredoxin interacting protein in prognosis of breast cancer. *Breast Cancer Research*, Vol. 12, No. 3, pp. R44

Callahan, R.; Cropp, C.S.; Merlo, G.R.; Liscia, D.S.; Cappa, A.P.M. & Lidereau, R. (1992). Somatic mutations and human breast cancer. *Cancer*, Vol. 69, pp. 1582–1588

Cannito, S.; Novo, E.; di Bonzo, L.V.; Busletta, C.; Colombatto, S. & Parola, M. (2010). Epithelial-mesenchymal transition: from molecular mechanisms, redox regulation to implications in human health and disease. *Antioxidants and Redox Signaling*, Vol. 12, No. 12, pp. 1383-1430

Canter, J.A.; Kallianpur, A.R.; Parl, F.F. & Millikan, R.C. (2005). Mitochondrial DNA G10398A polymorphism and invasive breast cancer in African-American women. *Cancer Research*, Vol. 5, pp. 8028–8033

Cebrian, A.; Pharoah, P.D.; Ahmed, S.; Smith, P.L.; Luccarini, C.; Luben, R.; Redman, K.; Munday, H.; Easton, D.F.; Dunning, A.M. & Ponder, B.A. (2006). Tagging single-nucleotide polymorphisms in antioxidant defense enzymes and susceptibility to breast cancer. *Cancer Research*, Vol. 66, No. 2, pp. 1225-1233

Cox, D.G.; Hankinson, S.E.; Kraft, P. & Hunter, D.J. (2004). No association between GPX1 Pro198Leu and breast cancer risk. *Cancer Epidemiology, Biomarkers & Prevention*, Vol. 13, No. 11 (Pt 1), pp. 1821-1822

Cox, D.G.; Tamimi, R.M. & Hunter, D.J. (2006). Gene x Gene interaction between MnSOD and GPX-1 and breast cancer risk: a nested case-control study. *BMC Cancer*, Vol. 6, pp.217

Di Pietro, G.; Magno, L.A. & Rios-Santos, F. (2010). Glutathione S-transferases: an overview in cancer research. *Expert Opinion on Drug Metabolism and Toxicology*, Vol. 6, No. 2, pp. 153-170

Eckschlager, T. ; Adam, V. ; Hrabeta, J.; Figova, K. & Kizek, R. (2009). Metallothioneins and cancer. Current *Protein Peptide Science*, Vol.10, No. 4, pp. 360-375

Elledge, R.M.; Fuqua, S.A.W.; Clark, G.M.; Pujol, P. & Allred, D. C. (1993). The role and prognostic significance of p53 gene alterations in breast cancer. *Breast Cancer Research and Treatment,* Vol. 27, pp. 95–102

Ennen, M.; Minig, V.; Grandemange, S.; Touche, N.; Merlin, J.L.; Besancenot, V.; Brunner, E.; Domenjoud, L. & Becuwe, P. (2011). Regulation of the high basal expression of the manganese superoxide dismutase gene in aggressive breast cancer cells. *Free Radical Biology & Medicine*, Vol. 50, pp. 1771-1779

Esworthy, R.S.; Baker, M.A. & Chu, F.F. (1995). Expression of selenium-dependent glutathione peroxidase in human breast tumor cell lines. *Cancer Research,* Vol. 55, No. 4, pp. 957-962

Gago-Dominguez, M.; Jiang, X. & Castelao, J.E. (2007). Lipid peroxidation, oxidative stress genes and dietary factors in breast cancer protection: a hypothesis. *Breast Cancer Research*, Vol. 9, No. 1, pp. 201

Goetz, M.E. & Luch, A. (2008). Reactive species: a cell damaging rout assisting to chemical carcinogens. *Cancer Letters*, Vol. 266, No. 1, pp. 73-83

Hitchler, M.J. ; Wikainapakul, K. ; Yu, L. ; Powers, K. ; Attatippaholkun, W. & and Domann, F. E. (2006). Epigenetic regulation of manganese superoxide dismutase expression in breast cancer cells. *Epigenetics,* Vol. 1, pp. 163–171

Hu, Y.J. & Diamond, A.M. (2003). Role of glutathione peroxidase 1 in breast cancer: loss of heterozygosity and allelic differences in the response to selenium. *Cancer Research,* Vol. 63, No. 12, pp. 3347-3351

Hu, J.; Zhou, G.W.; Wang, N. & Wang, Y.J. (2010). GPX1 Pro198Leu polymorphism and breast cancer risk: a meta-analysis. *Breast Cancer Research and Treatment*, Vol. 124, No. 2, pp. 425-431

Hussain, S.P.; Aguilar, F.; Amstad, P. & Cerutti, P. (1994). Oxy-radical induced mutagenesis of hotspot codons 248 and 249 of the human p53 gene. *Oncogene,* Vol. 9, pp. 2277–2281

Jinga, D.C.; Blidaru, A.; Condrea, I.; Ardeleanu, C.; Dragomir, C.; Szegli, G.; Stefanescu, M. & Matache, C. (2006). MMP-9 and MMP-2 gelatinases and TIMP-1 and TIMP-2 inhibitors in breast cancer: correlations with prognostic factors. *Journal of Cellular and Molecular Medicine*, Vol. 10, No. 2, pp. 499-510

Jin, R.; Huang, J.; Tan, P.H. & Bay, B.H. (2004) Clinicopathological significance of metallothioneins in breast cancer. *Pathology Oncology Research*, Vol. 10, No. 2, pp. 74-79

Kabat, G.C.; Kim, M.; Shikany, J.M.; Rodgers, A.K.; Wactawski-Wende, J.; Lane, D.; Powell, L.; Stefanick, M.L.; Freiberg, M.S.; Kazlauskaite, R.; Chlebowski, R.T.; Wassertheil-Smoller, S. & Rohan, T.E. (2010). Alcohol consumption and risk of ductal carcinoma in situ of the breast in a cohort of postmenopausal women. *Cancer Epidemiology, Biomarkers and Prevention*, Vol. 19, No. 8, pp. 2066-2072

Karihtala, P.; Mäntyniemi, A.; Kang, S.W.; Kinnula, V.L. & Soini, Y. (2003). Peroxiredoxins in breast carcinoma. *Clinical Cancer Research*, Vol. 9, No. 9, pp. 3418-3424

Kattan, Z.; Minig, V.; Leroy, P.; Dauça, M. & Becuwe, P. (2008). Role of manganese superoxide dismutase on growth and invasive properties of human estrogen-independent breast cancer cells. *Breast Cancer Research and Treatment*, vol. 108, pp. 203-215

Klaunig, J.E. & Kamendulis, L.M. (2004). The role of oxidative stress in carcinogenesis. *Annual Review of Pharmacology and Toxicology*, Vol. 44, pp. 239-267

Lebovitz, R.M.; Zhang, H.; Vogel, H.; Cartwright, J.Jr.; Dionne, L.; Lu, N.; Huang, S. & Matzuk, M.M. (1996). Neurodegeneration, myocardial injury, and perinatal death in mitochondrial superoxide dismutase- deficient mice. *Proceeding National Academy Sciences USA*, Vol. 93, No. 18, pp. 9782–9787

Leek, R.D.; Talks, K.L.; Pezzella, F.; Turley, H.; Campo, L.; Brown, N.S.; Bicknell, R.; Taylor, M.; Gatter, K.C. & Harris, A.L. (2002). Relation of hypoxia-inducible factor-2 alpha (HIF-2 alpha) expression in tumor-infiltrative macrophages to tumor angiogenesis and the oxidative thymidine phosphorylase pathway in Human breast cancer. Cancer Research, vol. 62, No. 5, pp. 1326-1329

Leonard, S.S.; Harris, G.K. & Shi, X. (2004). Metal-induced oxidative stress and signal transduction. Free Radical Biology and Medicine, Vol. 37, No. 12, pp. 1921-1942

Li, J.J.; Oberley, L.W.; St Clair, D.K.; Ridnour, L.A. & Oberley, T.D. (1995). Phenotypic changes induced in human breast cancer cells by overexpression of manganese-containing superoxide dismutase *Oncogene*, Vol. 10, pp. 1989–2000

Malins, D.C.; Polissar, N.L. & Gunselman, S.J. (1996). Progression of human breast cancers to the metastatic state is linked to hydroxyl radical-induced DNA damage. *Proceeding National Academy Sciences U S A*, Vol. 93, No. 6, pp. 557-563

Matés, J.M.; Segura, J.A.; Alonso, F.J. & Márquez, J. (2008). Intracellular redox status and oxidative stress: implications for cell proliferation, apoptosis, and carcinogenesis. Archives in Toxicology, Vol. 82, No. 5, pp. 273-299

Matsui, A.; Ikeda, T.; Enomoto, K.; Nakashima, H.; Omae, K.; Watanabe, M.; Hibi, T. & Kitajima, M. (2000a). Progression of human breast cancers to the metastatic state is linked to genotypes of catechol-O-methyltransferase. *Cancer Letters*, Vol. 150, No. 1, pp. :23-31

Matsui, A.; Ikeda, T.; Enomoto, K.; Hosoda, K.; Nakashima, H.; Omae, K.; Watanabe, M.; Hibi, T. & Kitajima, M. (2000b). Increased formation of oxidative DNA damage, 8-hydroxy-2'-deoxyguanosine, in human breast cancer tissue and its relationship to GSTP1 and COMT genotypes. *Cancer Letters*, Vol. 151, No. 1, pp. 87-95.

Merlo, G.R.; Venesio, T.; Taverna, D.; Marte, B.M.; Callahan, R. & Hynes, N.E. (1994). Growth suppression of normal mammary epithelial cells by wild-type p53. *Oncogene*, Vol. 9, pp. 443–453

Miao, L. & St Clair, D.K. (2009). Regulation of superoxide dismutase genes: implications in disease. Free Radical Biology and Medicine, Vol. 47, No. 4, pp. 344-356

Micalizzi, D.S.; Farabaugh, S.M. & Ford, H.L. (2010). Epithelial-mesenchymal transition in cancer: parallels between normal development and tumor progression. *Journal of Mammary Gland Biology and Neoplasia*, Vol. 15, No. 2, pp. 117-134

Millikan, R.; Pittman, G.; Tse, C.K.; Savitz, D.A.; Newman, B. & Bell, D. (2000). Glutathione S-transferases M1, T1, and P1 and breast cancer. *Cancer Epidemiology, Biomarkers and Prevention*, Vol. 9, No. 6, pp. 567-573

Minig, V.; Kattan, Z.; van Beeumen, J.; Brunner, E. & Becuwe, P. (2009). Identification of DDB2 protein as a transcriptional regulator of constitutive SOD2 gene expression in human breast cancer cells. *Journal of Biological Chemistry*, Vol. 284, No. 21, pp.14165-14176

Mitrunen, K.; Jourenkova, N.; Kataja, V.; Eskelinen, M.; Kosma, V.M.; Benhamou, S.; Vainio, H.; Uusitupa, M. & Hirvonen, A. (2001). Glutathione S-transferase M1, M3, P1, and T1 genetic polymorphisms and susceptibility to breast cancer. *Cancer Epidemiology, Biomarkers and Prevention*, Vol. 10, No. 3, pp. 229-236

Mitrunen, K. & Hirvonen, A. (2003). Molecular epidemiology of sporadic breast cancer. The role of polymorphic genes involved in oestrogen biosynthesis and metabolism. *Mutation Research*, Vol. 544, No. 1, pp. 9-41.

Nakshatri, H.; Bhat-Nakshatri, P.; Martin, D.A.; Goulet, R.J.Jr.& Sledge, G.W. Jr. (1997). Constitutive activation of NF-kappaB during progression of breast cancer to hormone-independent growth. *Molecular and Cellular Biology*, Vol. 17, No. 7, pp. 3629-3639

Nelson, K.K. ; Ranganathan, A.C.; Mansouri, J.; Rodriguez, A.M.; Providence, K.M.; Rutter, J.L.; Pumiglia, K.; Bennett, J.A. & Melendez, J.A. (2003). Elevated sod2 activity augments matrix metalloproteinase expression: evidence for the involvement of endogenous hydrogen peroxide in regulating metastasis. *Clinical Cancer Research*, Vol. 9, pp. 424–432

Nelson, K.K. & Melendez, J.A. (2004). Mitochondrial redox control of matrix metalloproteinases. *Free Radical Biology Medicine*, Vol. 37, No. 6, pp. 768-784

Oestergaard, M.Z.; Tyrer, J.; Cebrian, A.; Shah, M.; Dunning, A.M.; Ponder, B.A.; Easton, D.F. & Pharoah, P.D. (2006). Interactions between genes involved in the antioxidant defence system and breast cancer risk. *British Journal of Cancer*, vol. 95, No. 4, pp. 525-531

Ott, J.J.; Ullrich, A.; Mascarenhas, M. & Stevens, G.A. (2011). Global cancer incidence and mortality caused by behavior and infection. *Journal of Public Health (Oxford)*, Vol. 33, No. 2, pp. 223-233

Pezzotti, A.; Kraft, P.; Hankinson, S.E.; Hunter, D.J.; Buring, J. & Cox, D.G. (2009). The mitochondrial A10398G polymorphism, interaction with alcohol consumption, and breast cancer risk. *PLoS One*, Vol. 4, No. 4, pp. e5356

Rao, A.K.; Ziegler, Y.S.; McLeod, I.X.; Yates, J.R. & Nardulli, A.M. (2009) Thioredoxin and thioredoxin reductase influence estrogen receptor alpha-mediated gene expression in human breast cancer cells. *Journal of Molecular Endocrinology*, Vol. 43, No. 6, pp. 251-261

Reuter, S.; Gupta, S.C.; Chaturvedi, M.M. & Aggarwal, B.B. (2010). Oxidative stress, inflammation, and cancer: how are they linked? *Free Radical Biology and Medicine*, Vol. 49, No. 11, pp. 1603-1616

Rhee, S.G.; Chae, H.Z. & Kim, K. (2005). Peroxiredoxins: a historical overview and speculative preview of novel mechanisms and emerging concepts in cell signaling. *Free Radical Biology and Medicine*, Vol. 38, No. 12, pp. 1543-1552

Rohan, T.E.; Wong, L.J.; Wang, T.; Haines, J. & Kabat, G.C. (2010). Do alterations in mitochondrial DNA play a role in breast carcinogenesis? Journal of Oncology, Vol. 2010, pp. 604304

Rundle, A.; Tang, D.; Hibshoosh, H.; Estabrook, A. ; Schnabel, F.; Cao, W.; Grumet, S. &, Perera, F.P. (2000). The relationship between genetic damage from polycyclic aromatic hydrocarbons in breast tissue and breast cancer. *Carcinogenesis*, Vol. 21, No. 7, pp. 1281-1289

Seitz HK, Becker P. (2007). Alcohol metabolism and cancer risk. *Alcohol Research in Health*, Vol. 30, No. 1, pp. 38-41

Setiawan, V.W.; Chu, L.H.; John, E.M.; Ding, Y.C.; Ingles, S.A.; Bernstein, L.; Press, M.F.; Ursin, G.; Haiman, C.A. & Neuhausen, S.L. (2008). Mitochondrial DNA G10398A variant is not associated with breast cancer in African-American women. *Cancer Genetics and Cytogenetics*, Vol. 181, No. 1, pp. 16-19

Shen, H.M. & Tergaonkar, V. (2009). NFkappaB signaling in carcinogenesis and as a potential molecular target for cancer therapy. *Apoptosis*. Vol. 14, No. 4, pp. 348-363

Storz, P. (2005). Reactive oxygen species in tumor progression. *Frontiers in Bioscience*, Vol. 10, pp. 1881-1896

Sugasawa, K. (2010). Regulation of damage recognition in mammalian global genomic nucleotide excision repair. Mutation Research, Vol. 685, No. 1-2, pp. 29-37

Sutton, A.; Khoury, H.; Prip-Buus, C.; Cepanec, C.; Pessayre, D. & Degoul, F. (2003). The Ala16Val genetic dimorphism modulates the import of human manganese superoxide dismutase into rat liver mitochondria. *Pharmacogenetics*, Vol. 13, No. 3, pp. 145-157

Tas F, Hansel H, Belce A, Ilvan S, Argon A, Camlica H, Topuz E. (2005). Oxidative stress in breast cancer. Medical Oncology, Vol. 22, No. 1, pp. 11-15.

Tsanou, E.; Ioachim, E.; Briasoulis, E.; Damala, K.; Charchanti, A.; Karavasilis, V.; Pavlidis, N.; Agnantis, N.J. (2004). Immunohistochemical expression of superoxide dismutase (MnSOD) antioxidant enzyme in invasive breast carcinoma. *Histology Histopathology*, Vol. 19, pp. 807–813

Ushio-Fukai, M. & Nakamura, Y. (2008). Reactive oxygen species and angiogenesis: NADPH oxidase as target for cancer therapy. *Cancer Letters*, Vol. 266, No. 1, pp. 37-52

Valko, M.; Rhodes, C.J.; Moncol, J.; Izakovic, M. & Mazur, M. (2006). Free radicals, metals and antioxidants in oxidative stress-induced cancer. *Chemico-Biological Interactions*, Vol. 160, No. 1, pp. 1-40

Wang, S. ; Wang, F.; Shi, X.; Dai, J.; Peng, Y.; Guo, X. ; Wang, X. ; Shen, H. & Hu, Z. (2009). Association between manganese superoxide dismutase (MnSOD) Val-9Ala polymorphism and cancer risk - A meta-analysis. *European Journal of Cancer*, Vol. 45, No. 16, pp. 2874-2881

Wright, R.M.; McManaman, J.L. & Repine, J.E. (1999). Alcohol-induced breast cancer: a proposed mechanism. *Free Radical Biology and Medicine*, Vol. 26, No.3-4, pp. 348-354

Zhang, H.J. ; Zhao, W. ; Venkataraman, S. ; Robbins, M.E. ; Buettner, G.R. ; Kregel, K.C. & Oberley, L.W. (2002). Activation of matrix metalloproteinase-2 by overexpression of manganese superoxide dismutase in human breast cancer MCF-7 cells involves reactive oxygen species. *Journal of Biological Chemistry*, Vol. 277, No. 23, pp. 20919-20926

Zheng, T.; Holford, T.R.; Zahm, S.H.; Owens, P.H.; Boyle, P.; Zhang, Y.; Zhang, B.; Wise, J.P. Sr.; Stephenson, L.P. & Ali-Osman, F. (2003). Glutathione S-transferase M1 and T1 genetic polymorphisms, alcohol consumption and breast cancer risk. *British Journal Cancer*, Vol. 88, pp. 58-62.

Zhu, C.H. ; Huang, Y. ; Oberley, L.W. & Domann, F.E. (2001) A family of AP-2 proteins down-regulate manganese superoxide dismutase expression. *Journal of Biological Chemistry*, Vol. 276, No. 17, pp. 14407-14413

5

Regulation of the Functional Na^+/I^- Symporter (NIS) Expression in Breast Cancer Cells

Uygar Halis Tazebay
Bilkent University Genetics and Biotechnology Research Center (BILGEN) and Department of Molecular Biology and Genetics Faculty of Science, Bilkent University, Ankara Turkey

1. Introduction

Iodide (I^-) is transported from bloodstream to lactating mammary gland tissue and it is secreted to mother's milk (Honour *et al.*, 1952; Grosvenor, 1960; Eskin *et al.*, 1974; Bakheet *et al.*, 1998). I^- in milk is then used by the suckling newborn in thyroid hormone biosynthesis (Brown-Grant, 1957; 1961; Azizi and Smyth, 2009). As the supply of I^- to neonate comes exclusively from milk during first months of its life, I^- uptake by lactocytes and its accumulation in mother's milk is vital for proper development of the nervous system, skeletal muscles, and lungs at those early periods of life (Stanbury, 1992; Delange, 2000; Semba & Delange, 2001).

The activity of the sodium/I^- symporter (Na^+/I^- Symporter, or NIS) expressed in alveolar cells of lactating breast is essential for secretion of I^- to milk (Cho *et al.*, 2000; Tazebay *et al.*, 2000). In fact, by many clinicians and researchers, cellular I^- transport activity was mostly associated with the thyroid gland as the I^- uptake into thyroid follicular cells is the first step in enzymatic synthesis of iodide-containing thyroid hormones triiodothyronine (T_3), and thyroxine (T_4). Molecular investigations following the cloning of NIS gene by Dai *et al.* (1996) have proven that this symporter is not only a key enzyme in I^- uptake in thyroid, but it is also functional in extrathyroidal tissues such as lactating mammary glands, stomach, intestine, salivary glands, kidney, and placenta (Ajjan *et al.*, 1998; Tazebay *et al.*, 2000; Bidart *et al.*, 2000; Mitchell *et al.*, 2001; Spitzweg *et al.*, 2001; Nicola *et al.*, 2009). Therefore, together with its key role in thyrocytes, NIS seems to be the long seeked (Wolff & Maurey, 1961) major I^- transport protein in extrathyroidal tissues as well (De la Vieja *et al.*, 2000). But, as one could expect, the expression and activity of NIS is differentially regulated in thyroid and in above mentioned non-thyroidal tissues (see below).

In human, NIS is encoded by the gene annotated as Solute Carrier 5A5 (SLC5A5) in NCBI databases (www.http://www.ncbi.nlm.nih.gov). Among its other members, SLC5A transporter family includes Na^+/glucose co-transporters 1 and 2, the Na^+/myoinositol transporter, and the Na^+/monocarboxylate transporter (Wright and Turk, 2004). The human NIS gene is located on chromosome 19, mapping to loci 19p13.2-p12 (Smanik *et al.*, 1997). Previous extensive molecular studies carried out by Nancy Carrasco's group at the Albert Einstein College of Medicine have revealed that the transporter is a glycoprotein belonging to the Na^+/solute symporter family, and it is integrated to membrane by 13 hydrophobic trans-membrane domains with N-terminus located extracellularly and C-terminus facing the cytosol (Dai *et al.*, 1996; Levy *et al.*, 1997; 1998). Rat NIS protein is composed of 618 amino acids, while its human homologue contains 643 residues with a relative molecular mass of about 75 kD to 110 kD depending on the glycosylation status of the protein in different tissues (Dai *et al.*, 1996; Smanik *et al.*, 1996; Tazebay *et al.*, 2000).

In order to establish biophysical properties of the transporter, the rat thyroid Na^+/I^- symporter (NIS) was expressed by Eskandari *et al.* (1997) in *Xenopus laevis* oocytes and the symporter was characterized using electrophysiological, tracer uptake, and electron microscopic methods. In this work, I^- transport activity of NIS against its gradient was shown to couple the inward transport of Na^+, occurring in favor of its Na^+/K^+-ATPase-generated electrochemical gradient. Moreover, these authors have clearly shown that the transport activity was electrogenic, and the stoichiometry of cotransport by NIS was 2 Na^+ ions to 1 I^-. Interestingly, this work have also shown that other than I^-, the symporter was capable of transporting a wide variety of anions such as, ClO_3^-, SCN^-, $SeCN^-$, NO_3^-, Br^-, BF_4^-, IO_4^-, BrO_3^- (Eskandari *et al.*, 1997). It also transports radioisotopes such as pertechnetate ($^{99m}TcO_4^-$; Tazebay *et al.* 2000, Van Sande *et al.* 2003), perrhenate ($^{188}ReO_4^-$; Dadachova *et al.* 2002) and astatine ($^{211}At^-$; Lindencrona *et al.* 2001). Binding sites of these substrates on NIS protein, and their molecular interactions during passage through the symporter is not currently known. However, a recent publication on extensive mutational analysis carried out by Antonio De la Vieja and his co-workers indicated that particularly amino acids Thr-351, Ser-353, Thr-354, Ser-356, Thr-357, Asn-360, and Asp-369, all of which either face the same side of the helix in trans-membrane segment IX or close to it at the membrane/cytosol interface (Asp-369) according to their current structural model, are involved in Na^+ binding or translocation activity by NIS (De la Vieja *et al.*, 2007). In fact, T354P mutation in NIS was previously identified as an autosomal recessive mutation resulting in iodide transport defect (ITD), a rare disorder causing congenital hypothyroidism in human (Fujiwara *et al.*, 1998).

In addition to its role in normal breast physiology during lactation, a very significant NIS upregulation as well as increased radioiodide transport activity was reported in large percentage of breast cancers and its metastasis (Tazebay *et al.*, 2000; Wapnir *et al.*, 2003; 2004; Upadhyay *et al.*, 2003; Renier *et al.*, 2009; 2010, and see below). These results indicate that NIS-mediated radionuclide imaging and therapy methods could potentially be used as alternative aproaches, or in combination with existing methodologies, towards a better management of the malignant breast disease, as it is routinely used against thyroid cancer and its metastasis for more than 60 years (Daniel & Haber, 2000; Welcsh & Mankoff, 2000; Spitzweg & Morris, 2002; Boelaert & Franklyn, 2003). Currently, breast cancer management involves adjuvant systemic therapies that are administered before or after mastectomy surgeries with the purpose of ablating micro-metastatic cells and improving disease free overall survival of the patient. In fact, it seems that neo-adjuvant and adjuvant therapies are rather successful, and they reduce recurrences by nearly 50% (Early Breast Cancer Trialist's Collaborative Group, 1998; Citron *et al.*, 2003). The administration of cytotoxic agents used in breast cancer chemotherapy is usually by venal intervention, and it can cause significant side effects, such as loss of healthy blood cells, increased possibilities to get microbial infections, hair loss, tiredness, feeling sick, sore mouth, sore eyes, and diarrhea. Patients and families are looking forward for development of alternative strategies that target breast cancer cells with high specificity, that are less toxic to healthy tissues and with less side-effects. Because of previous, and decades long, clinical work in diagnosing and treating thyroid cancers by radioisotope substrates of NIS ($^{131}I^-$, $^{125}I^-$, $^{123}I^-$, or $^{99m}TcO_4^-$), use of NIS transported radionuclides could offer novel prospective breast cancer treatment modalities with advantages such as, less toxicity to healthy tissues, easier administration procedures, and relatively less side-effects as compared to current chemotherapeutic drugs. However, as discussed in this chapter, a broader knowledge on molecular mechanisms that operate in modulation (upregulation and repression) of functional NIS expression in mammary gland is certainly required in order to achieve a better diagnostic and/or therapeutic effect on breast cancer by using radiolabelled substrates of the symporter.

In this chapter, first, I am going to focus on the biological function of NIS in normal mammary gland epithelia. Then, recent studies on levels of NIS expression in different histopathological types of breast tumours will be analyzed. Subsequently, I will introduce recent findings on regulatory interplays, and small molecular agents that modulate NIS gene expression and activity both in normal mammary gland during gestation and lactation, and in malignant transformation in breast tissue. Recent *in vivo* animal studies, as well as human clinical trials addressing uses of NIS substrate radionuclides for imaging purposes will be introduced in later parts of this review. I will conclude by reviewing current litterature that analyze potential future strategies for the development of NIS radionuclide transport activity based therapeutic and diagnostic methods that could lead to novel clinical approaches in breast cancer management.

2. Regulation of NIS expression during mammary gland development and in lactating breast

I^- accumulation in lactating mammary gland has been recognized for nearly 60 years (Honour *et al.*, 1952; Brown-Grant, 1957; Grosvenor, 1960; Thorpe, 1976; Bakheet *et al.*, 1998). In normal physiology, mammary gland accumulates I^- only at later stages of gestation or pregnancy, and during lactation. An adequate supply of I^- in mother's milk is a must for sufficient thyroid hormone synthesis, which is essential for healthy development of the newborn. With molecular cloning of NIS gene in 1996, and subsequent generation of high affinity antibodies specific for human and rodent NIS proteins, researchers acquired essential tools to investigate whether NIS could have any role in the uptake of I^- in lactating mammary glands. First the group of Spitzweg *et al.* (1998) by relatively simple RT-PCR methods, and later on groups of Cho *et al.* (2000), Tazebay *et al.* (2000), and Perron *et al.* (2001) with more sophisticated immunological and molecular biochemistry techniques have addressed expression of NIS in mammary glands of human or rodent experimental models. From results obtained in above mentioned studies, it is now clear that NIS is not expressed in non-lactating healthy mammary glands, and the expression of symporter rises above detectable limits in the mammary gland tissue only with the onset of gestation. Subsequently, NIS expression is up-regulated at transcription level concomitant to increased proliferation of lactocytes in the gland, and then, after delivery, its expression remain high exclusively in response to hormonal stimuli induced by suckling of nipples by newborn pups.

2.1 Regulation of NIS expression during gestation in mice

In developing mammary glands of healthy CD1(ICR)BR strain pregnant mice, NIS expression starts at mid-gestation, i.e. around days 10 or 11 in a full gestation period of 19 days (Tazebay *et al.*, 2000), and it becomes maximal near the end of gestation (days 18-19) before delivery (Cho *et al.*, 2000; Tazebay *et al.*, 2000). Delivery is not essential for an increased uptake of I- to mammary glands during gestation, and accumulation of radio-labelled substrates of NIS in the gland is observable in pregnant mice (Tazebay *et al.*, 2000). By using immuno-histochemical techniques, NIS protein was detected on the basolateral membranes of alveolar epithelial cells of lactating mammary glands (Cho *et al.*, 2000; Tazebay *et al.*, 2000). These cells take up I- from the bloodstream and secrete it to milk for neonatal nutrition, leading to a concentration of I-up to 15 fold as compared to the plasma I- concentration (Nurnberger & Lippscomb, 1952; Thorpe, 1976). It is also important to note here that, about 20% of transported I- were found to be organified (i.e., inorganic I- conjugated to an organic molecule, or enzyme) by lactoperoxidases in the alveolar cells (Patrick, 2008).

Thyroid gland, mammary glands, salivary glands, and stomach are tissues where most intense NIS expression is observed (Tazebay *et al.*, 2000; Riedel *et al.*, 2001). Even though, these tissues express NIS at relatively high levels, the timing of expression and stimuli for its up or down-regulation are not the same. In thyroid, thyroid stimulating hormone (TSH) that is synthesized and released by thyrotrope cells located in the anterior pituitary gland, is the main regulator of thyroid cell proliferation, differentiation, and endocrine functions, including molecular regulation of NIS expression both at transcriptional and at post-translational levels (Levy *et al.*, 1997; Riedel *et al.*, 2001). The effects of TSH are primarily mediated through the activation of the cAMP cascade via the GTP-binding protein Gs. TSH stimulates iodide accumulation by positively regulating NIS expression at the protein and mRNA level via the cAMP pathway (Levy *et al.*, 1997). Hypophysectomized rats with low circulating levels of TSH have a decreased protein expression of NIS, whereas a single injection of TSH leads to a robust increase in NIS expression. Rats maintained on an iodide-deficient diet or treated with propylthiouracil, an agent blocking iodide organification, have high concentrations of TSH, which correlates with a very significant increase in NIS protein expression (Levy *et al.*, 1997). The reader is advised to refer wonderful reviews by Dohan *et al.* (2003), or by Kogai *et al.* (2006) among many others for detailed information on TSH dependent regulation of thyroid specific genes including NIS. Even though NIS expression is continuous in the thyroid throughout life, in mammary glands it is strictly a gestation/lactation specific event, independent of blood TSH levels (Eskin *et al.*, 1974; Tazebay *et al.*, 2000; Kogai *et al.*, 2006).

In my opinion, a research student who for the first time observes mammary gland development in rodents by animal dissections will certainly be very much surprised in seeing tremendous size differences in mammary glands of virgin and lactating females. In virgin mice/rats, the organ is composed of a thin sheet of tissue close to skin, hard to find and dissect without previous experience. However, in lactating rodents, it is difficult not to notice them, because by size they are comparable to largest internal organs of the animal. This makes mammary glands invaluable experimental models for organ development and morphogenesis. It is branching morphogenesis of mammary gland epithelia that leads to formation of buds and milk ducts, and that characterizes mammary gland growth. In this developmental process, mammary specific molecular networks interpret signals from local cytokines/growth factors in both the epithelial and stromal microenvironments, which is orchestrated by secreted ovarian and pituitary hormones (McNally & Martin, 2011). Because I- transport and functional expression of NIS in the mammary gland is first observed at mid-pregnancy, and during lactation, both us and others have inquired possible roles of ovarian and pituitary lactogenic hormones in regulation of NIS in mammary glands. In two independent studies, steroid hormones estrogen (17-β-estradiol) and progesterone, and two pituitary lactogenic hormones, prolactin and oxytocin were administered to female virgin animals either one by one, or in different combinations, and their effects on NIS upregulation were monitored (Cho *et al.*, 2000; Tazebay *et al.*, 2000). In the study carried out by Tazebay *et al.* (2000), together with normal virgin female mice, the authors have also used ovariectomized females in order to prevent possible interferences between administered and endogenous steroid levels. In these work, it has been demonstrated that estrogen and the two pituitary hormones oxytocin and prolactin have up-regulatory roles in mammary gland NIS expression. Interestingly, estradiol was previously shown to down-regulate NIS expression in FRTL-5 rat thyroid cells under culture conditions (Furlanetto *et al.*, 1999). On the contrary, in mammary gland cell lines in culture, major receptor that interacts with estradiols, estrogen receptor-alpha (ER-α) was shown to be essential for basal expression of NIS in a ligand independent manner, and for its further induction in response to other non-estrogenic extracellular factors (Alotaibi *et al.*, 2006; and see below). Moreover, recently a significant positive correlation was reported between human NIS and ER-α expressions in a cohort of malignant (n=75) or normal breast tissue (n=10) specimens (Ryan *et al.*, 2011).

In fact, the work carried out by Alotaibi *et al.* (2006) could connect these two seemingly conflicting results, and bring possible mechanistic explanations on how estrogens and ER dependent molecular mechanisms (in the presence or absence of their ligands) might have both positive and negative regulatory roles on NIS expression. In this work, first a clear correlation between the transcription factor ER-α and activation of NIS expression was shown in human mammary epithelial cell models. Then, it has been demonstrated that ER-α physically interacts with a novel responsive element (ERE) in NIS gene promoter, occupying this position under conditions where NIS activation is pronounced. It is important to precise here once again that regulation of NIS by ER system has some very uncommon characteristics. Unliganded ER-α (Apo-ER) seems to be functional in basal expression of NIS, and it is shown to be essential to keep the system inducible by other ligands, namely by retinoids (see Part 5 below, for a detailed mechanistic analysis). Another interesting point is that mutations inserted to NIS ERE in a lusiferase reporter gene system have, in fact, increased transcription of the reporter in MCF-7 mammary tumor cells in culture conditions (Hani Alotaibi and U.H.T.; unpublished observations), instead of decreasing the expression of the reporter gene, as one would normally expect in classical ER regulated genes. These results might suggest the presence of a relatively complex and dynamic interplay between ER and other transcription factors (specific or general) operating on NIS gene promoter. Remarkably, the position of this novel functional NIS ERE sequence was precisely conserved in rodent and human genomes, and it was found to be localized only about 9 base pairs far from NIS gene TATA box element (Fig. 1; Alotaibi *et al.*, 2006). The key point in this uncommon regulation of a gene (NIS) by ER may reside at this exceptionally close positioning between NIS ERE and TATA box elements. Speculatively, when concentrations of 17-β-estradiol raises above normal physiological levels (as used in cell culture conditions), over-activated ER-α might create steric effects by continuously disturbing or shielding interaction of general transcription factors with the TATA element of NIS gene, resulting in a negative or down-regulatory effect. According to this hypothesis, among other genetic and epigenetic factors, the amount of ER-α ligands would define the type of interactions (synergistic or antagonistic) and the outcome of interactions (up-regulatory or down-regulatory) between ERE bound ER-α and TATA bound general transcription factors. This might also provide some hints to understand why goiter is more common in females as compared to males, or possible explanations related with molecular mechanisms leading to I^- transport deficiencies (ITD) in females, seen with a higher prevalence during or after pregnancy (Patrick, 2008).

	NIS ERE	TATA Box		
-430	GCGGAGTCGC GGTGACCCGG GAGCCCAATAAATCTGCAAC CCACAATCAC GAGCTGCTCC			
	Transcription start			
-370	CGTAAGCCCC AAGGCGACCT CCAGCTGTCA GCGCTGAGCA CAGCGCCCAG GGAGAGGGAC			

Fig. 1. Functional NIS ERE sequence is located in close proximity of NIS TATA box element in the promoter region. Human NIS gene proximal promoter region sequence is partly shown. Numbers indicate positions of nucleotides relative to NIS start (ATG) codon. The transcription start site is indicated in blue letter (G), TATA box element, and novel ERE sequences are indicated in red, and in writing above these sequences. Two inverted repeats (half sites) of the NIS ERE element located in minus strand are underlined in red.

As mentioned above, NIS expression increases near the end of gestation, and mammary glands start actively transporting I^- before delivery (Tazebay *et al.*, 2000). After delivery, the main physiological regulator of NIS expression is suckling of nipples. In fact, after delivery, in rodent models suckling regulates NIS expression in a reversible way: when pups are separated from the mother for 48 hours, steady-state NIS levels drop below detection levels by Western blots. Subsequently, when pups and mother are reunited for 24 hours, NIS accumulation reaches back to its maximal levels (Cho *et al.*, 2000; Tazebay *et al.*, 2000). Both prolactin and oxytocin, two pituitary hormones that were shown to have up-regulatory effects on NIS expression in breast were released simultaneously in response to suckling (Wakerley *et al.*, 1978). This creates a wonderful regulatory mechanism preventing unnecessary active transport of I^- to mother's milk once grown-up pups stop suckling.

3. NIS expression in human breast cancer

A high prevalence of NIS expression in human breast cancer combined with much lower prevalance in normal extratumoral tissues have been reported in many independent studies, and by using a variety molecular analysis methods. In a pioneering study, Tazebay *et al.* (2000) demonstrated a perchlorate inhibited NIS activity in experimental mammary adenocarcinomas in female transgenic mice carrying Murine Mammary Tumor Virus (MMTV)-promoter driven activated Ras oncogene or over-expressed Neu oncogene. These authors were able to follow in real-time the NIS specific accumulation of radiolabelled I^- isotopes, or another substrate of the symporter, $^{99m}TcO_4^-$, in mammary tumours of animals. These were also the first evidences regarding possible uses of radio-labelled substrates of NIS for imaging of non-thyroid tumours. Importantly, in the same study, also human breast tissue specimens were analyzed by immunobiochemical methods, and it was found that above 80% of invasive and ductal carcinoma *in situ* samples were expressing NIS, whereas only about 20% of non-cancerous samples adjacent to tumours were NIS-positive. Besides, none of the 8 normal specimens obtained by reductive mammoplasties were expressing NIS (Tazebay *et al.*, 2000). In subsequent studies where larger cohorts and variety of molecular techniques were used, results were comparable to initial reports. Wapnir *et al.* (2003) analyzed NIS expression in a total of 202 human breast samples, and they reported a clear

NIS positivity in 76% of invasive breast carcinomas, 88% of ductal carcinomas *in situ*, and 80% of fibroadenoma samples. Only one-out-of eight (13%) normal breast samples analyzed in the same study were weakly expressing NIS. More recently, endogenous NIS expression were analyzed in a subtype of breast carcinomas known as triple-negative breast cancer (Renier *et al.*, 2010). This clinical-pathological subtype with the worst prognosis among breast cancer subtypes is commonly defined by the absence of ER, progesterone receptor (PR), and human epidermal growth factor receptor-2 (HER2) (Sorlie *et al.*, 2003). In this study, Renier *et al.* (2010) demonstrated that 15 specimens out-of 23 were NIS positive (67% positivity), with 11/15 samples being strongly positive (47% of total), suggesting a potential use for NIS-dependent radio-ablative strategies against this aggressive tumour group. Independently, still another research group composed of Beyer and co-workers (2009) has analyzed NIS expression levels in 192 different breast cancer specimens found on tissue microarrays, with a particular focus on sub-cellular localization of NIS protein expressed in those samples. In this study, 72% of samples were found to express -at variable levels- the symporter, and in 28% of tissue samples NIS expression were reported to be null. Beyer *et al.* (2009) argued that according to their visual analysis of stained tissue sections only 27% of NIS-positive tumours the symporter had a cell surface (plasma membrane) localization, and in remaining samples NIS seemed to localize at a cytoplasmic compartment. This is in fact an important observation that could also bring some explanation to the discrepancy between high percentages of NIS positivity (around 80% overall) in breast tumours, whereas relatively low percentage of radionuclide uptake activity in patients (17-25%; see also below). Yet, it is arguable whether immuno-histochemical staining techniques and visual evaluations of stained tissue sections used as main analysis methods in the study of Beyer and co-workers (2009) could be taken as sufficient to comment on sub-cellular localization of a membrane protein. In future, precise cell science techniques with improved microscopy, and quantitative molecular methodologies would be essential in order to better establish quantities of NIS proteins found at variable sub-cellular localizations in breast cancer/normal samples coming from patients.

In a recent and elegantly designed study, both relative levels of NIS expression in breast cancer samples (n=75), in fibroadenomas (n=15), and normal human samples (n=10) coming from premenopausal and postmenopausal patients, as well as correlations between expressions of the symporter gene and that of several proven or putative regulators of NIS [ER-α, retinoic receptors alpha and beta (RAR-α and RAR-β), thyroid hormone receptors alpha and beta (THR-α and THR-β)] were assessed by quantitative molecular techniques by Ryan *et al.* (2011). Furthermore, these authors have tested results of their tissue analysis by treating two distinct mammary cancer cell culture models (ER/PR positive, HER2 negative T47D cells versus ER/PR negative, HER2 positive SK-Br-3 cells) with agonist of those regulators, and thus rigorously validated their findings in tissue analysis. Supporting previous *in vivo* and *in vitro* studies, expression of NIS, RAR-α, RAR-β, and ER-α were found to be higher in breast cancer samples as compared to normal adjacent tissues. Moreover, a significant positive correlation was detected between NIS and these three transcriptional regulators, the highest correlation being between NIS and retinoid inducible factor RAR-β (Ryan *et al.*, 2011). These results were also tested by appropriate ligands used in mammary cell culture experiments, and they were largely validated (see part 5, below). Data obtained by Ryan and co-workers (2011) should certainly be taken into account when deciding on how to better design novel approaches for increasing endogenous mammary cancer NIS expression in different neoplastic growth types by stimulation of appropriate nuclear receptors and other trans-acting regulatory factors.

NIS protein was also demonstrated to be detectable in soft tissue metastasis of breast cancer. Renier and co-workers (2010) have carried-out an immuno-histochemical analysis on 28 archival tumour samples obtained from breast cancer brain metastasis (BCBM). In this analysis, they have studied NIS positivity in BCBM tissues, and correlated it with ER, PR, and HER2/Neu status of specimens. 21/28 cases were reported to be expressing NIS. Among those, 9 were from triple-negative for ER/PR/HER2, and 12 were ER/PR-negative, but HER2 positive. ER/PR-positively stained group of brain metastatic samples did not express NIS protein. Again, these authors argued that only about 24% of NIS positive samples had plasma membrane staining. These studies provided invaluable preliminary results on differences of NIS protein localization in different patient samples, and future scientific studies addressing sub-cellular localization of NIS in BCBM tissues by using appropriate cell biology methods would be essential for a precise characterization of cellular localization of NIS in metastatic tissues. Yet, this study documents about 75% NIS positivity in BCBM, and certainly stands-out with its important implications on possible uses of NIS activity based diagnostic/therapeutic methods in breast cancer soft tissue metastasis cases.

Functional NIS expression was also shown by *in vivo* scintigraphic imaging methods in human breast cancers and its soft tissue metastasis. Recent advances in methodologies and approaches concerning uses of radio-labelled NIS substrates in imaging and diagnosis of malignant tissue are described in the next section below.

4. Human clinical trials on selective targeting of breast cancer by radionuclide substrates of NIS

Specific targeting of tumours with anti-cancer agents is one of the major research areas in cancer biology. Selective targeting of thyroid cancer and its metastasis by radioisotopes of NIS substrates has been successfully developed by nuclear medicine and effectively used as a diagnostic/therapeutic method in fight with malignant thyroid disease. Immediately after the discovery that lactating mammary gland concentrates I^- by the same transport mechanism operating in thyroid, and that the same symporter (NIS) is expressed in more than %80 human of breast cancer cases, there started translational medicine approaches for testing effectiveness of NIS activity based methodologies to diagnose and eradicate malignant breast disease in different groups of patients (Moon *et al.*, 2001; and also see the clinical trial sponsored by Stanford University, entitled: Scintigraphic Assessment of I^- Transport in Metastatic Breast Cancer and Evaluation of Ablative Therapy: Radioiodide Imaging Study; clinicaltrials.gov identifier number NCT00185809, http://www.clinicaltrials.gov). Optimistic results from several studies on uses and effectiveness of radioiodide based therapeutic techniques in non-thyroid cancers that externally received NIS gene by viral delivery methods (Spitzweg *et al.*, 2000; Faivre *et al.*, 2004; Dwyer *et al.*, 2006) gave further hopes to researchers who try to develop NIS based diagnostic/therapeutic tools for breast cancer management.

Several groups have assessed whether NIS substrates were accumulated by breast tumours in human subjects, at high enough concentrations, durations and specificities in order to permit imaging or therapy of malignant tissues by these substances. Moon *et al.* (2001) have investigated the correlation between $^{99m}TcO_4^-$ uptakes and NIS mRNA expressions in breast cancer patients. Among 25 patients studied, $^{99m}TcO_4^-$ scintigraphy revealed positive uptake in 4 patients. There were a positive correlation between $^{99m}TcO_4^-$ uptake and NIS gene mRNA expression levels in tumours, and positive uptake tumours expressed higher levels of NIS as compared to negative uptake breast tumours (Moon *et al.*, 2001). This was an important result indicating that a substrate of NIS, $^{99m}TcO_4^-$, could actually be used in imaging of breast tumours. However, even though in all previous tissue analysis studies NIS positivity in breast cancer samples were reported to be around 80%, in the study carried by Moon et al. (2001) only in 17% of breast cancer patients tumours were visible by $^{99m}TcO_4^-$ imaging. In another study, Upadhyay *et al.* (2003) investigated $^{99m}TcO_4^-$ transport capacities of tumours in a study comprised of 12 female patients (age 33-58 years) with infiltrating ductal carcinomas confirmed by fine needle aspiration cytology (FNAC) and subsequent histopathological analysis. Out of these 12 patients, samples obtained from 5 patients were analyzed by molecular techniques investigating NIS expression at transcriptional and translational levels, and scintigraphic imaging were performed in 4 out-of 5 patients prior to mastectomy. These authors reported both high NIS expression levels in all 4 tumours analyzed by scintigraphy, and high ability to concentrate $^{99m}TcO_4^-$ in tumour tissues. Because of the small sample size used in this study, it is very hard to comment on ratios related with NIS positivity versus radionuclide uptake positivity. Nevertheless, the study indicated possibilities of using $^{99m}TcO_4^-$ for imaging purposes in breast cancer.

So far, only the study of Wapnir *et al.* (2004) addressed whether NIS expressing metastatic breast tumours could be detected by using radioiodides ($^{123}I^-$ and $^{131}I^-$) or $^{99m}TcO_4^-$ in scintigraphic analysis. These authors investigated NIS activity in BCBM tissues of 27 women by administering either $^{99m}TcO_4^-$ or $^{123}I^-$ followed by a whole body scintigraphic analysis. I^- uptake was noted only in 25% of NIS expressing BCBM tissues (2 out-of 8). Apparently, nearly 30% of breast cancer related deaths demonstrate central nervous system involvement on autopsy, and the treatment of BCBM is particularly challenging because many anticancer drugs have limited access to the central nervous system (Renier *et al.*, 2010). Therefore, systemic agents capable of crossing the blood-brain barrier, such as I^- or $^{99m}TcO_4^-$, could especially be important if they are effective against NIS positive breast cancer subtypes that metastasize to the brain.

Importantly, in the investigations carried-out by Wapnir *et al.* (2004), these authors also succeded to suppress thyroidal uptake of radiolabelled tracers by administering thyroxine (T_3) and methimazole (an inhibitor of I^- organification in thyroid) to patients under clinical trials. Suppression of thyroidal uptake in this study by a hormone regiment have in fact answered present discussions on whether it would be possible to protect healthy thyrocytes (which take-up and organify I^-) in case radioiodide based therapies are used to treat non-thyroidal tumours. If thyroidal cells were compromised during administration of radio-labelled NIS substrates, then the patients would need to depend on thyroid hormone medications for the rest of their lives. This is of course not preferable, and it was important to find ways of successfully protecting healthy thyroids of patients under clinical investigations. It seems in future clinical trials, integrity of thyroid cells could be protected by inhibiting thyroidal activity of NIS with hormone treatment regiments similar to the ones used in this study, while the non-thyroid origin tumour is targeted by cytotoxic NIS substrates. There is in fact a pilot radioiodide based breast cancer imaging clinical trial currently carried-out under sponsorship of Stanford University at U.S. where a combination of T_3/methimazole regiment would be used for protection of thyrocytes (Pilot Study to Determine Radioiodide Accumulation and Dosimetry in Breast Cancers Using 124I PET/CT; clinicaltrials.gov identifier number: NCT00725946; http://www.clinicaltrials.gov).

5. Modulation of NIS expression in breast cancer cell models and in xenograft tumors in mice

NIS expression is present in about 80% of breast cancers suggesting that breast cancer patients may benefit from NIS-mediated radioiodide imaging and/or therapeutic methods. Nevertheless, only 17-25% of NIS positive breast tumors had detectable radionuclide transport activity as assessed by scintigraphic imaging (Moon *et al.*, 2001; Upadhyay *et al.*, 2003; Wapnir *et al.*, 2004). Currently, there is a clear need to identify possible mechanisms underlying this discrepancy between NIS expression and NIS-mediated radionuclide uptake activity. Previous studies (reviewed above) based on analysis of breast cancer samples suggested that, in addition to NIS mRNA and protein expression, post-translational modification(s) of the symporter and appropriate membrane targeting are likely to be important for the substrate transport activity of NIS. Differential levels of NIS expression may account for variable cell surface NIS levels among breast cancer samples, and particular hormone combinations may be needed to upregulate expression and activity of the symporter at higher levels for successful future theraputic or diagnostic applications involving NIS activity.

Results from different laboratories have revealed that both the expression of mammary gland NIS gene at the transcriptional level, and the post-translational trafficking/localization of NIS to plasma membrane are tightly regulated in a cellular context and an extracellular stimuli dependent way (Tazebay *et al.*, 2000; Riedel *et al.*, 2001; Kogai *et al.*, 2004; 2008; Dentice *et al.*, 2004; Alotaibi *et al.*, 2006; 2010; Willhauck *et al.*, 2011). The list of hormones that were shown to have an upregulatory effect on NIS expression in a variety of model mammary gland cell lines and in animal experiments (xenografted and normal) include lactogenic hormones (prolactin and oxytocin), steroids (estrogens), retinoids, dexamethasone (Dex), and carbamazepine.

In initial animal experiments, lactogenic hormones prolactin and oxytocin were proven to upregulate NIS expression in the mammary tissue (see above, Cho *et al.*, 2000; Tazebay *et al.*, 2000). Both the two hormones were tested for their upregulatory activities by Cho *et al.* (2000) on human breast cancer cultures kept on collagen gels. In this experimental set-up, individual prolactin (500ng/ml) and oxytocin (100 ng/ml) treatments have positively affected NIS gene regulation by inducing it at the transcriptional level, but a combination of the two hormones failed to do so. A significant induction of NIS gene by prolactin was also reported by Arturi *et al.* (2005) in a mammary cancer cell line, MCF-7. This is a cell line derived from mammary adenocarcinoma metastatic to a pleural effusion of lung, and it is one of the most common ER-positive breast cancer cell line models. This cell line, together with MDA-MB-231 cells which are ER-negative cell models, is used in most of the studies addressing upregulatory effects of a variety of substances on NIS gene regulation (for instance see, Alotaibi *et al.*, 2006; Arturi *et al.*, 2005; Kogai *et al.*, 2006). Using MCF-7 cells, both our group and Kogai *et al.* (2005) have tested the effects of 17-β-estradiol (at 10 nM concentration; one of the most potent estrogens) on NIS gene induction, and neither of the two groups have seen a positive regulatory effect of this estrogen on the induction of the gene when introduced to cell lines in culture (Alotaibi *et al.*, 2006). However, independent of the presence of ligand, ER plays a very critical regulatory role on NIS expression in a number of mammary gland cell models (see above, and also Alotaibi *et al.*, 2006). The fact that some ER-negative tumours have upregulated NIS expression (Tazebay *et al.*, 2000; Ryan *et al.*, 2011) indicate that ER is not absolutely essential for inducibility of NIS in breast tumours, and in tumor milieu *in vivo* other ER-independent molecular mechanisms may operate making NIS induction possible. Recently, in response to 17-β-estradiol administration to ER-negative and ER-positive mammary cancer model cell lines, Ryan and co-workers (2011) have observed a 3 to 6-fold increased NIS expression in T47D cells (ER-positive), and about 5-fold increase in Sk-BR-3 cells (ER-negative). Because they observed estradiol inducible NIS expression in Sk-BR-3 mammary cell line which is an ER-negative cell model, they argued that similar to some breast tumours, ER may not be essential for inducibility of NIS in this cell line model as well, and additional mechanisms which bypass ER dependent regulatory components for activation of NIS gene may be operating in those cells.

Retinoids have a robust effect on functional NIS induction in human MCF-7 cells (Kogai *et al.*, 2000; 2004; 2005; 2008). These compounds are active metabolites of vitamin A, and they have been used in animal models and humans as differentiation agents for various types of cancers including breast cancer (Mark *et al.*, 2006). The typical retinoid pathway involves the ligand-activated nuclear receptors belonging to retinoic acid receptor family (RAR) and retinoid-X-receptor family (RXR). RAR and RXR form heterodimers, and bind corresponding RA or RXR response elements (RARs) at *cis*-acting regulatory DNA sites and activate gene transcription (Mark *et al.*, 2006). All-*trans* retinoic acid (tRA; at 1μM) stimulates NIS induction up to 10-fold above the baseline in ER-positive MCF-7 cells, but it can not induce expression of the symporter in ER-negative model, MDA-MB-231 (Kogai *et al.*, 2000; 2004), and this is because ER-positivity is absolutely essential for retinoid responsive upregulation of NIS virtually in all breast cancer cell line models (Alotaibi *et al.*, 2006), except Sk-BR-3 (Ryan *et al.*, 2011). In fact, Kogai *et al.* (2005) analyzed the isoform specificity of retinoid receptors for the upregulation of NIS gene expression by using isoform selective retinoid receptor ligands. They reported that a RAR-β/γ agonist (AGN190168) is a more potent inducer of NIS than a RAR-α agonist (AGN195183) or a RAR-γ agonist (AGN194433), indicating a central role to RAR-β in upregulation of NIS by retinoids. In line with these results, Ryan *et al.* (2011) have reported a robust positive correlation between NIS upregulation and RAR-β gene expression in human breast tissue samples (n=100) that they have analyzed by quantitative real-time PCR methods.

Even though, RAR and RXR were known to upregulate NIS expression since a while, *cis*-acting elements directly interacting with these nuclear receptors were only identified recently (Alotaibi *et al.*, 2010). This delay in identification of RA responsive elements (RARE) that activate NIS transcription could be due to uncommon positioning of those *cis*-acting sites in multiple intronic positions in NIS gene. In our recent work, we have described that a functional RARE is present in the first intron of human NIS gene, and it seems there are at least six others in other introns of this gene (Alotaibi *et al.*, 2010). In fact, initially we found three putative RAREs in the first intron intron. The first was a perfect DR2-type consensus RARE sequence (AGGTCAggAGTTCA), the second was a DR10-type sequence [AGGTGG(n10)AGGTCA], and the third was again a DR2-type sequence identical to the first one (AGGTCAggAGTTCA), and it was overlapping with the second half-site of the previous putative RARE. By using a series of luciferase reporter constructs containing different fragments of this intronic region, as well as *in vitro* mutagenized versions of these putative RARE sequences, we have demonstrated that the third RARE which is located at +1222 relative to the start codon of NIS was a functional RARE. In MCF-7 cells transfected with a luciferase reporter construct containing this element, tRA treatment resulted in an increase of about 4-fold when compared to cells treated with DMSO vector. We also investigated the potential of this intronic RARE to activate transcription through the native NIS minimal promoter. For this purpose, we constructed reporter plasmids containing the minimal NIS promoter (218 bp of NIS upstream region between -260 bp and +42 bp relative to transcription start site, and capable of initiating transcription as assessed by previous functional reporter assays. As anticipated, the intronic element significantly activated NIS promoter in response to tRA when positioned either at the 5′ or at 3′ of the reporter gene, in agreement with the function of an enhancer. Furthermore, by electromobility shift assays and chromatin immunoprecipitation (ChIP) methods, we have shown that both RARs and RXR interacts with this RARE in response to tRA (Alotaibi *et al.*, 2010). Altogether these findings clearly indicated that the DR2-2 element that is present in the first intron of NIS is an important RARE in regulation of human NIS gene. Similar RARE sequences were also present in introns 5, 7, 8, 12, 13 and 14 of human NIS gene (some having identical sequences with RARE found in intron 1). All these sequences interact with RARs and RXR, and eventually with the RNA Polymerase II (PolII) in ChIP assays at different time points in response to tRA administration to cells (Fig. 2). Earlier work by others, and results obtained by Alotaibi *et al.* (2010) clearly indicate that molecular mechanisms governing NIS expression involve a number of classical and intronic elements that regulate temporal and spatial expression, and they are likely to be more complex than previously anticipated. Future experiments will show whether the activities of intronic enhancers lead also to a tissue or cell-type-specific regulation of NIS.

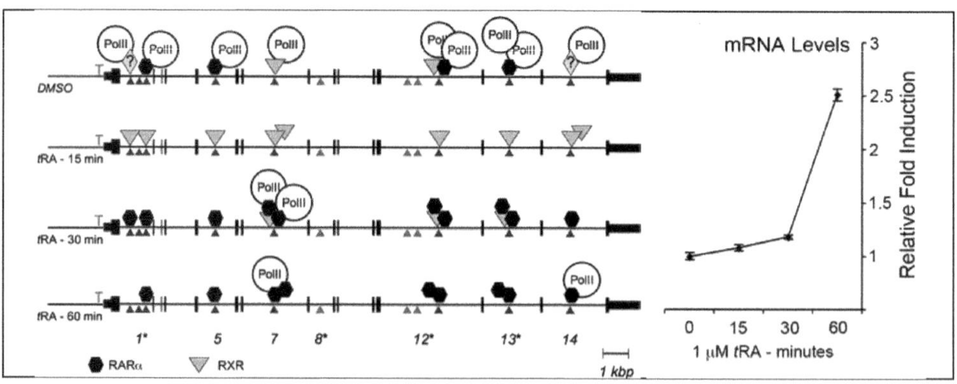

Fig. 2. Nuclear receptors and RNA Pol-II interact with NIS intronic elements in a dynamic manner during the initiation of transcription. MCF-7 cells grown in steroid-free and phenol-red-free DMEM were treated either with DMSO (time 0) or with tRA for 15, 30 and 60 min and used for ChIP analysis using RARa and RXR and RNA Pol-II specific antibodies. mRNA was isolated from a fraction of the cells used for this analysis, NIS expression was normalized to the levels of GAPDH, and presented as relative fold induction compared to DMSO-treated samples. A schematic representation of ChIP data depicting the events of

transcription initiation of NIS in response to tRA stimulation is shown. Numbers indicate introns studied, asterisks above numbers indicate RA responsive elements with identical DNA sequences; AGGTCAnnAGTTCA. Parallelograms with question mark represent unidentified interacting proteins. The figure is reproduced from Alotaibi *et al.*, 2010, Intronic Elements in the NIS Gene Interact with Retinoic Acid Receptors and Mediate Initiation of Transcription. *Nucleic Acids Research*, Vol. 38 (10), pages 3172-3185. Reprinted with permission from The Oxford University Press © 2010.

In vivo studies with MCF-7 xenograft tumours in immunodeficient (CD1 nu/nu) mice have indicated that systemic tRA treatment increases radioiodide ($^{125}I^-$) accumulation capacities of xenografts about 15 fold above background, and this level is sufficient for selective imaging of tumours with $^{125}I^-$. Administration of dexamethasone (Dex), and carbamazepine (CBZ) together with tRA increased both iodide uptake by NIS, and NIS mRNA expression even more. In response to Dex and CBZ administration, tRA induced I^- uptake via NIS have increased about 12 fold in xenograft tumours in experimental animals, clearly indicating that the combination of an RAR isoform selective ligand and Dex and Cbz has a potential to provide a more effective induction of NIS, and it provides an important improvement for the effective use of symporter in theraputic/diagnostic medical approaches (Kogai *et al.*, 2005; Willhauck *et al.*, 2008; 2011).

6. Future strategies for development of NIS activity based diagnostic and therapeutic methods

Detection of radioiodide transport in thyroid cancer tissues at the beginning of 1940's marked the beginning of nuclear medicine as a discipline in medical sciences, by allowing the use of radioiodide and other selective radionuclide substrates of this symporter (for instance, $^{99m}TcO_4^-$) in successful management of thyroid cancers and their metastasis. Similarly, recent detection of functional NIS expression and radioiodide accumulation in breast cancer tissues provide important opportunities for development of novel adjuvant therapies and/or detection methods based on breast cancer specific NIS activity. Routine and successful use of radioiodide in hospitals to evaluate and cure thyroid cancer cases for more than 60 years, make it an even more attractive substance to be worked on for developing future innovative methodologies for implementation to non-thyroidal cancers. Furthermore, as I described in the previous section, a number of substances (especially retinoids and glucocorticoids) modulating NIS expression and enhancing radioiodide transport activities in mammary cancer cell models and xenografted animals were already developed, and these advances in basic research are currently waiting to be brought to "bed side" by translational medicine approaches.

A number of clinical studies have already addressed use of radioiodide in scintigraphic detection of breast tumours, and breast cancer metastasis *in vivo* (see above). Even though data coming from these studies have led to optimistic conclusions on prospective uses of $^{131}I^-$ radioablation techniques on at least some breast cancers and their metastasis, to our knowledge, a clinical trial subjecting breast cancer patients to radioiodide based ablation studies has not yet taken place.

As presented through-out the text above, there are three main problems that have to be solved for effective and routine use of radio-iodide (or other cytotoxic NIS substrates) in management breast cancers: 1) discrepancies in percentages of NIS expressing tumour tissues (around 80%) versus percentages of cancers taking up radio-iodide (17-25%); 2) problems associated with low or insufficient cumulative I^- uptakes in breast cancers (0.00131% ID/ml; Renier *et al.*, 2009), making it difficult to achieve a therapeutic effect; and 3) reported accumulation of radio-iodide in some benign fibroadenoma of breast (Berger *et al.*, 2006), which brings problems of achieving sufficient malignant tissue specificity in diagnosing and targeting breast cancers with NIS substrate radionuclides. A fourth issue may be protection of healthy thyroid from cytotoxicity of agents transported by NIS in imaging or treatment of non-thyroidal tumours, as thyrocytes very robustly and constitutively express functional NIS (for a review see Kogai *et al.*, 2006). In fact, this fourth point was addressed in studies carried out by Wapnir and co-workers (2004), and it has been shown that uptake of solutes to thyroid via NIS could selectively be down regulated by administering a combination of thyroid hormones and I^- organification inhibitor methimazole to imaged patients. Therefore, it seems in future studies this final issue could be at least easily solved with some optimization of hormone/methimazole combinations. However, solutions for the remaining three problems should be rigorously addressed in future clinical, translational, and basic research studies.

Regarding which subtype of breast cancer tissue responds best to, and therefore more suitable for, imaging/treatment with NIS substrate agents, the work of Ryan *et al.* (2011) indicated that cancers expressing RARs and ERs are amenable to radioiodine based imaging techniques. However, it has been shown by their study that the group of tissues that express RARs, ERs, and finally NIS at maximal levels were benign fibroadenoma samples. This suggests that together with radioiodine scintigraphic analysis of the mammary, additional analysis methods would be essential for differentiating radio-iodide transporting benign tissue from the malignant breast cancer. In future prospective approaches, once the possibility of fibroadenoma of the breast is eliminated, radio-iodide uptake in malignant cancerous tissue of the breast could be upregulated by hormone combinations (retinoids, dex, and cbz) as previously suggested by independent works of Kogai *et al.* (2004), and Willhauck *et al.* (2011). That could perhaps solve the problem of discrepancy between NIS expression and NIS-positive tumour radio-iodide uptake, leading to a robust expression of functional NIS in malignant breast tissue, which could then permit use of $^{131}I^-$ dependent ablation strategies for curing the disease. In the meantime, healthy thyroid of the patients could be protected from ablative effects of radionuclides by administering the hormone regiment containing thyroxine and methimazole, as suggested by Wapnir *et al.* (2004).

The beta-emitter radionuclide Rhenium-188-perrhenate ($^{188}RheO_4^-$), and the alpha emitter Astatine-211 (^{211}As) have shorter half lives (17 hours and 10,5 hours, respectively) as compared 8 days half-life of the beta emitter $^{131}I^-$ (Dadachova and Carrasco, 2004). $^{188}RheO_4^-$ have also previously been shown to be effective on NIS expressing mammary cancers of transgenic mice bearing polyoma-middle-T oncoprotein, as this radiosope have significantly inhibited growth of these experimental tumours (Dadachova *et al.*, 2005). Therefore, in future studies, a variety of radionuclides that are transported by NIS could be selected to be used in these possible novel applications targeting malignant breast cancer cells with least possible side-effects, while having high specificity, improved efficiency, and remarkable safety.

7. Conclusion

Breast cancer management involves chemotherapeutic procedures before or subsequent to surgery with the aim of ablating micro-metastatic cells and improving disease free overall

survival of the patient. The administration of cytotoxic agents used in breast cancer chemotherapy is usually by venal intervention, and it can cause significant pain and side effects. Therefore, development and introduction of alternative strategies that target breast cancer cells with high specificity, less toxicity to healthy tissues, and with less overall side-effects is important. Because of previous, and decades long, clinical work in diagnosing and treating thyroid cancers by radioisotope substrates of NIS, use of NIS transported radionuclides could offer novel prospective breast cancer treatment modalities with advantages such as easier administration procedures, and relatively less side-effects as compared to current chemotherapeutic drugs.
Recent scientific studies on molecular biology and regulation of NIS expression in breast cancer models have very clearly shown the important potential of NIS activity based novel radiotherapy techniques in management of malignant breast disease. A number of lactogenic hormones, estradiol, retinoids, and glucocorticoids were shown to enhance radioiodide transport in breast cancer cells, as well as in *in vivo* models. Increased understanding of molecular mechanisms that upregulate NIS expression in response to these hormones and ligands, and enhance the activity of the symporter in breast tissue as well as in breast cancer metastasis will be essential for the development and improvement of methods that will involve use of NIS activity and cytotoxic substrates for imaging and therapeutic purposes in breast cancer clinics.

8. Acknowledgments

I would like to thank Dr. Claudio Scazzocchio, a marvellous scientist, mentor and teacher, who gave me an invaluable opportunity to work in his laboratory during my Ph.D. studies and to focus on regulation of symporters. I thank Dr. Georges Diallinas, a great teacher and close friend who introduced me to the world of transporters. I acknowledge the contribution of Dr. Nancy Carrasco to my career by giving the chance to study the molecular biology of iodide transport in mammary gland cells in the early years of the field. I am indebted to all past and present members of my laboratory at Bilkent who contributed to studies on NIS regulation in the mammary gland, but particularly to Dr. Hani Alotaibi, first a talented research student, and later, a valuable collaborator. My research have been generously supported by the Turkish Scientific and Technological Research Council (TÜBİTAK) grants TBAG-104-T-231, KAMAG-106-G-089, TBAG-109-T-049, TBAG-109-T-925, by Turkish Academy of Sciences-Young Scientist Award (TÜBA-GEBIP/2001-2-18), by Feyzi Akkaya Research Fund for Scientific Activities (FABED), and by Bilkent University research funds.

9. References

Ajjan R.A., Kamaruddin N.A., Crisp M., Watson P.F., Ludgate M., & Weetman A.P. (1998). Regulation and tissue distribution of the human sodium iodide symporter gene. Clin Endocrinol (Oxf), Vol. 49, pp. 517-523.

Alotaibi, H., Yaman, E.C., Demirpençe, E. & Tazebay, U.H. (2006). Unliganded estrogen receptor-alpha activates transcription of the mammary gland Na+/I- symporter gene. *Biochem Biophys Res Commun*, Vol. 345, pp. 1487-1496.

Alotaibi, H., Yaman, E., Salvatore, D., Di Dato, V., Telkoparan, P., Di Lauro, R., & Tazebay, U.H. (2010). Intronic elements in the Na/I Symporter gene (NIS) interact with retinoic acid receptors and mediate initiation of transcription. *Nucl Acids Res*, Vol. 38, pp. 3172-3185.

Arturi F., Ferretti E., Presta I., Mattei T., Scipioni A., Scarpelli D., Bruno R., Lacroix L., Tosi E., Gulino A., Russo D., & Filetti S. (2005). Regulation of iodide uptake and sodium/iodide symporter expression in the mcf-7 human breast cancer cell line. *J Clin Endocrinol Metab*, Vol. 90, pp. 2321-2326.

Azizi, F. & Symth, P. (2009). Breastfeeding and maternal and infant iodine nutrition. *Clin Endocrinol*, Vol. 70, pp. 803-809.

Bakheet S.M., Powe J. & Hammami M.M. (1998). Unilateral radioiodine breast uptake. *Clin Nucl Med*, Vol. 23, pp. 170-171.

Beyer, S.J., Jimenez R.E., Shapiro, C.L., Cho, J.Y., & Jhiang S.M. (2009). Do cell surface trafficking impairments account for variable cell surface sodium iodide symporter levels in breast cancer? *Breast Cancer Res Treat*, Vol. 115, pp. 205-212.

Berger F., Unterholzner S., Diebold J., Knesewitsch P., Hahn K., & Spitzweg C. (2006). Mammary radioiodine accumulation due to functional sodium iodide symporter expression in a benign fibroadenoma. *Biochem Biophys Res Commun*, Vol. 349, pp. 1258-1263.

Bidart J.M., Lacroix L., Evain-Brion D., Caillou B., Lazar V., Frydman R., Bellet D., Filetti S. & Schlumberger M. (2000). Expression of Na+/I- symporter and Pendred syndrome genes in trophoblast cells. *J Clin Endocrinol Metab*, Vol. 85, pp. 4367-4372.

Boelaert K. & Franklyn J.A. (2003). Sodium iodide symporter: a novel strategy to target breast, prostate, and other cancers? *Lancet*, Vol. 361, pp. 796-797.

Brown-Grant, K. (1957) The iodide concentrating mechanism of the mammary gland. *J Physiol*, 135, 644-654.

Bruno R., Giannasio P., Ronga G., Baudin E., Travagli J.P., Russo D., Filetti S., & Schlumberger M. (2004). Sodium iodide symporter expression and radioiodine distribution in extrathyroidal tissues. *J Endocrinol Invest*, Vol. 27, pp. 1010-1014.

Cho J.Y., Léveillé R., Kao R., Rousset B., Parlow A.F., Burak W.E., Mazzaferri E.L., & Jhiang S.M. (2000). Hormonal regulation of radioiodide uptake activity and Na+/I- symporter expression in mammary glands. *J Clin Endocrinol Metab*, Vol. 85, pp. 2936-2943.

Citron M.L., Berry D.A., Cirrincione C., Hudis C., Winer E.P., Gradishar W.J., Davidson N.E., Martino S., Livingston R., Ingle J.N., Perez E.A., Carpenter J., Hurd D., Holland J.F., Smith B.L., Sartor C.I., Leung E.H., Abrams J., Schilsky R.L., Muss H.B., & Norton L. (2003). Randomized trial of dose-dense versus conventionally scheduled and sequential versus concurrent combination chemotherapy as postoperative adjuvant treatment of node-positive primary breast cancer: first report of Intergroup Trial C9741/Cancer and Leukemia Group B Trial 9741. *J Clin Oncol*, Vol. 21, pp. 1431-1439.

Dadachova E., Bouzahzah B., Zuckier L.S. & Pestell R.G. (2002). Rhenium-188 as an alternative to Iodine-131 for treatment of breast tumors expressing the sodium/iodide symporter (NIS). *Nucl Med Biol*, Vol. 29, pp. 13-18.

Dadachova E. & Carrasco N. (2004). The Na/I symporter (NIS): imaging and therapeutic applications. *Semin Nucl Med*, Vol. 34, pp. 23-31.

Dai G., Levy O. & Carrasco N. (1996). Cloning and characterization of the thyroid iodide transporter. *Nature*, Vol. 379, pp. 458-460.

Daniels, G.H. & Haber D.A. (2000). Will radioiodine be useful in treatment of breast cancer. *Nature Med,* Vol. 6, pp. 859-60.

De La Vieja A., Dohan O., Levy O. & Carrasco N. (2000). Molecular analysis of the sodium/iodide symporter: impact on thyroid and extrathyroid pathophysiology. *Physiol Rev,* Vol. 80, pp. 1083-1105.

De la Vieja A., Reed M.D., Ginter C.S. & Carrasco N. (2007). Amino acid residues in transmembrane segment IX of the Na+/I- symporter play a role in its Na+ dependence and are critical for transport activity. *J Biol Chem,* Vol. 282, 2pp. 5290-25298.

Delange, F. (2000). The role of iodine in brain development. *Proc Nutr Soc,* Vol. 59, pp 75-79.

Dentice M., Luongo C., Elefante A., Romino R., Ambrosio R., Vitale M., Rossi G., Fenzi G. & Salvatore D. (2004). Transcription factor Nkx-2.5 induces sodium/iodide symporter gene expression and participates in retinoic acid- and lactation-induced transcription in mammary cells. *Mol Cell Biol,* Vol. 24, pp. 7863-7877.

Dingli D., Russell S.J. & Morris J.C. (2003). In vivo imaging and tumor therapy with the sodium iodide symporter. *J Cell Biochem,* Vol. 90, pp. 1079-1086.

Dohan O., De la Vieja A., Paroder V., Riedel C., Artani M., Reed M., Ginter C.S. & Carrasco N. (2003). The sodium/iodide Symporter (NIS): characterization, regulation, and medical significance. *Endocr Rev,* Vol. 24, pp. 48-77.

Dwyer R.M., Bergert E.R., O'Connor M.K., Gendler S.J. & Morris J.C. (2006). Adenovirus-mediated and targeted expression of the sodium-iodide symporter permits in vivo radioiodide imaging and therapy of pancreatic tumors. *Hum Gene Ther,* Vol. 17, pp. 661-668.

Early Breast Cancer Trialists' Collaborative Group. (1998). Polychemotherapy for early breast cancer: an overview of the randomised trials. *Lancet,* Vol. 352, pp. 930-942.

Elisei R., Vivaldi A. & Pacini F. (2003). Biology and clinical application of the NIS gene. *Tumori,* Vol. 89, 523-528.

Eskandari S., Loo D.D., Dai G., Levy O., Wright E.M. & Carrasco N. (1997). Thyroid Na+/I- symporter. Mechanism, stoichiometry, and specificity. *J Biol Chem,* Vol. 272, pp. 27230-27238.

Eskin B.A., Parker J.A., Bassett J.G. & George D.L. (1974). Human breast uptake of radioactive iodine. *Obstet Gynecol,* Vol. 44, pp. 398-402.

Faivre J., Clerc J., Gérolami R., Hervé J., Longuet M., Liu B., Roux J., Moal F., Perricaudet M. & Bréchot C. (2004). Long-term radioiodine retention and regression of liver cancer after sodium iodide symporter gene transfer in wistar rats. *Cancer Res,* Vol. 64, pp. 8045-8051.

Fujiwara H., Tatsumi K., Miki K., Harada T., Okada S., Nose O., Kodama S. & Amino N. (1998). Recurrent T354P mutation of the Na+/I- symporter in patients with iodide transport defect. *J Clin Endocrinol Metab,* Vol. 83, pp. 2940-2943.

Furlanetto T.W., Nguyen L.Q. & Jameson J.L. (1999). Estradiol increases proliferation and down-regulates the sodium/iodide symporter gene in FRTL-5 cells. *Endocrinology,* Vol. 140, pp. 5705-5711.

Grosvenor C.E. (1960). Secretion of I131 into milk by lactating rat mammary glands. *Am J Physiol,* Vol. 199, pp. 419-422.

Honour A.J., Myant N.B. & Rowlands E.N. (1952). Secretion of radioiodine in digestive juices and milk in man. *Clin Sci,* Vol. 11, pp. 449-462.

Kogai T., Schultz J.J., Johnson L.S., Huang M. & Brent G.A. (2000). Retinoic acid induces sodium/iodide symporter gene expression and radioiodide uptake in the MCF-7 breast cancer cell line. *Proc Natl Acad Sci U.S.A.*, Vol. 97, pp. 8519-8524.

Kogai, T., Kanamoto, Y., Che, L.H., Taki, K., Moatamed, F., Schultz, J.J. & Brent, G.A. (2004) Systemic retinoic acid treatment induces sodium/iodide symporter expression and radioiodide uptake in mouse breast cancer models. *Cancer Res,* 64, 415-422.

Kogai, T., Kanamoto, Y., Li, A.I., Che, L.H., Ohashi, E., Taki, K., Chandraratna, R.A., Saito, T. & Brent, G.A. (2005) Differential regulation of sodium/iodide symporter gene expression by nuclear receptor ligands in MCF-7 breast cancer cells. *Endocrinology,* 146, 3059-3069.

Kogai T., Taki K., Brent G.A. & 2006. Enhancement of sodium/iodide symporter expression in thyroid and breast cancer. *Endocr Relat Cancer,* Vol. 13, pp. 797-826.

Kogai, T., Ohashi, E., Jacobs, M.S., Sajid-Crockett, S., Fisher, M.L., Kanamoto, Y. & Brent, G.A. (2008) Retinoic acid stimulation of the sodium/iodide symporter in MCF-7 breast cancer cells is mediated by the insulin growth factor-I/phosphatidylinositol 3-kinase and p38 mitogen-activated protein kinase signaling pathways. *J Clin Endocrinol Metab,* 93, 1884-1892.

Levy O., Dai G., Riedel C., Ginter C.S., Paul E.M., Lebowitz A.N. & Carrasco N. (1997). Characterization of the thyroid Na+/I- symporter with an anti-COOH terminus antibody. *Proc Natl Acad Sci U.S.A.*, Vol. 94, pp. 5568-5573.

Levy O., De la Vieja A., Ginter C.S., Riedel C., Dai G. & Carrasco N. (1998). N-linked glycosylation of the thyroid Na+/I- symporter (NIS). Implications for its secondary structure model. *J Biol Chem,* Vol. 273, pp. 22657-22663.

Lindencrona U., Nilsson M. & Forssell-Aronsson E. (2001). Similarities and differences between free 211At and 125I- transport in porcine thyroid epithelial cells cultured in bicameral chambers. *Nucl Med Biol,* Vol. 28, pp 41-50.

Mark M., Ghyselinck N.B. & Chambon P. (2006). Function of retinoid nuclear receptors: lessons from genetic and pharmacological dissections of the retinoic acid signaling pathway during mouse embryogenesis. *Annu Rev Pharmacol Toxicol,* Vol. 46, pp. 451-480.

McNally S. & Martin F. (2011). Molecular regulators of pubertal mammary gland development. *Ann Med,* Vol. 43, pp. 214-234.

Mitchell A.M., Manley S.W., Morris J.C., Powell K.A., Bergert E.R. & Mortimer R.H. (2001). Sodium/iodide (NIS) gene expression in human placenta. *Placenta,* Vol. 22, pp. 256-258.

Moon D.H., Lee S.J., Park K.Y., Park K.K., Ahn S.H., Pai M.S., Chang H., Lee H.K. & Ahn I.M. (2001). Correlation between 99mTc-pertechnetate uptakes and expressions of human sodium iodide symporter gene in breast tumor tissues. *Nucl Med Biol,* Vol. 28, pp. 829-834.

Nicola J.P., Basquin C., Portulano C., Reyna-Neyra A., Paroder M. & Carrasco N. (2009). The Na+/I- symporter mediates active iodide uptake in the intestine. *Am J Physiol Cell Physiol,* Vol. 296, pp. C654-C662.

Nurnberger C.E. & Lipscomb A. (1952). Transmission of radioiodine (I131) to infants through human maternal milk. *J Am Med Assoc,* Vol. 150, pp. 1398-1400.

Patrick L. (2008). Iodine: deficiency and therapeutic considerations. *Altern Med Rev*, Vol. 13, pp. 116-127.

Perron B., Rodriguez A.M., Leblanc G. & Pourcher T. (2001). Cloning of the mouse sodium iodide symporter and its expression in the mammary gland and other tissues. *J Endocrinol*, Vol. 170, pp. 185-196.

Renier C., Yao C., Goris M., Ghosh M., Katznelson L., Nowles K., Gambhir S.S. & Wapnir I. (2009). Endogenous NIS expression in triple-negative breast cancers. *Ann Surg Oncol*, Vol. 16, pp. 962-968.

Renier, C., Vogel, H., Offor, O., Yao, C., & Wapnir, I. (2010). Breast cancer brain metastases express the sodium iodide symporter. *J Neurooncol*, Vol. 96, pp. 331-336.

Riedel C., Levy O. & Carrasco N. (2001). Post-transcriptional regulation of the sodium/iodide symporter by thyrotropin. *J Biol Chem*, Vol. 276, pp. 21458-21463.

Riedel C., Dohán O., De la Vieja A., Ginter C.S. & Carrasco N. (2001). Journey of the iodide transporter NIS: from its molecular identification to its clinical role in cancer. *Trends Biochem Sci*, Vol. 26, pp. 490-496.

Ryan J., Curran C.E., Hennessy E., Newell J., Morris J.C., Kerin M.J. & Dwyer R.M. (2011). The sodium iodide symporter (NIS) and potential regulators in normal, benign and malignant human breast tissue. *PLoS ONE*, Vol. 6, e16023.

Semba R.D. & Delange F. (2001). Iodine in human milk: perspectives for infant health. *Nutr Rev*, Vol. 59, pp. 269-278.

Smanik P.A., Liu Q., Furminger T.L., Ryu K., Xing S., Mazzaferri E.L. & Jhiang S.M. (1996). Cloning of the human sodium lodide symporter. *Biochem Biophys Res Commun*, Vol. 226, pp. 339-345.

Sorlie T., Tibshirani R., Parker J., Hastie T., Marron J.S., Nobel A., Deng S., Johnsen H., Pesich R., Geisler S., Demeter J., Perou C.M., Lønning P.E., Brown P.O., Børresen-Dale A.L. & Botstein D. (2003). Repeated observation of breast tumor subtypes in independent gene expression data sets. *Proc Natl Acad Sci U.S.A.*, Vol. 100, pp. 8418-8423.

Spitzweg C., Joba W., Eisenmenger W. & Heufelder A.E. (1998). Analysis of human sodium iodide symporter gene expression in extrathyroidal tissues and cloning of its complementary deoxyribonucleic acids from salivary gland, mammary gland, and gastric mucosa. *J Clin Endocrinol Metab*, Vol. 83, pp. 1746-1751.

Spitzweg C., O'Connor M.K., Bergert E.R., Tindall D.J., Young C.Y. & Morris J.C. (2000). Treatment of prostate cancer by radioiodine therapy after tissue-specific expression of the sodium iodide symporter. *Cancer Res*, Vol. 60, pp. 6526-6530.

Spitzweg C., Dutton C.M., Castro M.R., Bergert E.R., Goellner J.R., Heufelder A.E. & Morris J.C. (2001). Expression of the sodium iodide symporter in human kidney. *Kidney Int*, Vol. 59, pp. 1013-1023.

Spitzweg C. & Morris J.C. (2002). The sodium iodide symporter: its pathophysiological and therapeutic implications. *Clin Endocrinol (Oxf)*, Vol. 57, pp. 559-574.

Stanbury J.B. (1992). Iodine and human development. *Med Anthropol*, Vol. 13, pp. 413-423.

Tazebay U.H., Wapnir I.L., Levy O., Dohan O., Zuckier L.S., Zhao Q.H., Deng H.F., Amenta P.S., Fineberg S., Pestell R.G. & Carrasco N. (2000). The mammary gland iodide transporter is expressed during lactation and in breast cancer. *Nature Med*, Vol. 6, pp. 871-878.

Thorpe S.M. (1976). Increased uptake of iodide by hormone-responsive compared to hormone-independent mammary tumors in GR mice. *Int J Cancer,* Vol. 18, pp. 345-350.

Upadhyay G., Singh R., Agarwal G., Mishra S.K., Pal L., Pradhan P.K., Das B.K. & Godbole M.M. (2003). Functional expression of sodium iodide symporter (NIS) in human breast cancer tissue. *Breast Cancer Res Treat,* Vol. 77, pp. 157-165.

Van Sande J., Massart C., Beauwens R., Schoutens A., Costagliola S., Dumont J.E. & Wolff J. (2003). Anion selectivity by the sodium iodide symporter. *Endocrinology,* Vol. 144, pp. 247-252.

Wakerley J.B., O'Neill D.S. & ter Haar M.B. (1978). Relationship between the suckling-induced release of oxytocin and prolactin in the urethane-anaesthetized lactating rat. *J Endocrinol,* Vol. 76, pp. 493-500.

Wapnir, I.L., van de Rijn, M., Nowels, K., Amenta, P.S., Walton, K., Montgomery, K., Greco, R.S., Dohan, O. & Carrasco, N. (2003). Immunohistochemical profile of the sodium/iodide symporter in thyroid, breast, and other carcinomas using high density tissue microarrays and conventional sections. *J Clin Endocrinol Metab,* Vol. 88, pp. 1880-1888.

Wapnir, I.L., Goris, M., Yudd, A., Dohan, O., Adelman, D., Nowels, K. & Carrasco, N. (2004) The Na+/I- symporter mediates iodide uptake in breast cancer metastases and can be selectively down-regulated in the thyroid. *Clin Cancer Res,* Vol. 10, pp. 4294-4302.

Welcsh, P. L. & Mankoff, D.A. (2000). Taking-up iodide in breast tissue. *Nature,* Vol. 406, pp. 688-689.

Willhauck, M. J., Sharif-Samani, B., Senekowitsch-Schmidtke, R., Wunderlich, N., Göke B., Morris J. C., & Spitzweg C. (2008). Functional sodium iodide symporter expression in brest cancer xenografts in vivo after systematic treatment with retinoic acid and dexamethasone. *Breast Cancer Res Treat,* Vol. 109, pp. 263-272.

Willhauck M.J., O Kane D.J., Wunderlich N., Göke B. & Spitzweg C. (2011). Stimulation of retinoic acid-induced functional sodium iodide symporter (NIS) expression and cytotoxicity of ^{131}I by carbamazepine in breast cancer cells. *Breast Cancer Res Treat,* Vol. 125, pp. 377-386.

Wolff J. & Maurey J.R. (1961). Thyroidal iodide transport. II. Comparison with non-thyroid iodide-concentrating tissues. *Biochim Biophys Acta,* Vol. 47, pp. 467-474.

Wright E.M. & Turk E. (2004). The sodium/glucose cotransport family SLC5. *Pflugers Arch,* Vol. 447, pp. 510-518.

6

Adipokines – Toward the Molecular Dissection of Interactions Between Stromal Adipocytes and Breast Cancer Cells

Pengcheng Fan and Yu Wang*
Department of Pharmacology and Pharmacy,
The University of Hong Kong
Hong Kong SAR,
China

1. Introduction

After more than a half century of efforts, cancer remains the leading cause of death globally, second only to cardiovascular diseases. The World Health Organization estimates that 84 million people will die from cancer in the next ten years if no action is taken (http://www.who.int/cancer). Obesity appears to play important roles not only in cardiovascular and metabolic diseases, but also in cancer etiology (Bray 2004). For example, overweight and obesity account for 25% of the patients with breast cancer, the most frequent cancer and the second leading cause of cancer death among women (Calle et al. 2003; McTiernan 2003). Excess adiposity over the pre- and post-menopausal years is an independent risk factor for breast cancer and its relapse (Alokail et al. 2009; Katoh et al. 1994; McTiernan 2005; Saxe et al. 1999), and is associated with late-stage disease and poor prognosis (Lorincz and Sukumar 2006). On the other hand, information is limited on why excess body fat increases cancer risks and how obesity affects the prognosis and therapy of cancer.

Dysfunctional adipose tissue, characterized by aberrant production of adipokines, is believed to be a key player in obesity-related mammary carcinogenesis. Adipokines are a family of molecules selectively secreted by fat tissue (Deng and Scherer 2010). In obese subjects, the production of adipokines is dysregulated, which in turn contributes to medical conditions associated with obesity (Galic et al. 2010). Evidence from clinical, epidemiological and experimental studies suggest that adipokines are key pathological mediators in obesity-related cancer diseases, although the underlying mechanisms remain to be uncovered and may vary from site to site (Prieto-Hontoria et al. 2010; van Kruijsdijk et al. 2009). The present review is to provide a systemic update on how adipokines affect breast cancer cell function and mammary tumor initiation and development. Specifically, the detailed roles of three adipokines [adiponectin, lipocalin-2 and leptin] in mammary carcinogenesis will be discussed by integrating the information derived from cellular, animal and clinical studies.

* Corresponding Author: yuwanghk@hku.hk

The mechanistic links for each adipokine will be assembled to model the process of breast cancer development under obesity conditions.

2. Stromal adipocytes in obesity-associated mammary carcinogenesis

Mammary gland comprises of epithelial and stromal cells. Stromal tissue regulates the development and differentiation of breast epithelial cells (Creydt et al. 2010; Polyak and Kalluri 2010). Adipocyte is one of the predominant stromal cell types in the microenvironment of mammary tissue. Proper function of adipose tissue plays an important role in mammary gland development and lactation process (Couldrey et al. 2002; Wiseman and Werb 2002). The differentiation/redifferentiation of fat cells apparently regulates epithelial cell cycles and contributes to the maintenance of the mammary epithelial "niche" (Arendt et al. 2010; Hovey and Aimo 2010). The close relationship between adipose tissue and mammary tumor growth has been demonstrated by many *in vitro* and *in vivo* experimental studies (Elliott et al. 1992; Miller et al. 1981; Sheffield and Welsch 1988). Mature adipocytes can promote the growth of breast carcinoma cells in a collagen gel matrix culture (Manabe et al. 2003). Co-transplantation of tumor cells with adipocytes into mice results in increased tumor growth and metastasis (Iyengar et al. 2005). On the other hand, factors derived from mammary tumor cells stimulate the reversion of mammary adipose phenotype and promote the differentiation of adipose stem cells into carcinoma-associated fibroblast (Guerrero et al. 2010; Jotzu et al. 2010). Conditioned media from breast cancer cells facilitates the accumulation of pre-adipocyte cells in the cancer tissue (Meng et al. 2001).

Multiple mechanisms are implicated in linking abnormal adipose tissue with breast cancer development (Figure 1). First, adipocyte is the predominant stromal cell type in mammary tissue responsible for local estrogen production, thus contributing to the development of estrogen-dependent breast cancer in postmenopausal women (Sinicrope and Dannenberg 2011). Obese women are at increased risk of developing estrogen receptor (ER)-positive breast cancer (Cleary and Grossmann 2009). Under obese condition, adipose tissue becomes "inflamed" to produce inflammatory mediators, such as tumor necrosis factor alpha (TNFα) and interleukin (IL)-1β, which promote the expression of cytochrome P450 aromatase, an enzyme responsible for the synthesis of estrogen from androgen, in adipocytes (Subbaramaiah et al. 2011). Second, increased fat mass in obese condition is associated with altered energy metabolism (McTiernan 2005). The concept of a relationship between dysregulated metabolism and carcinogenesis was first enunciated by Otto Warburg more than 80 years ago (Davison and Schafer 2010). There is now a large body of evidence supporting a link between obesity, metabolic syndrome, insulin resistance with increased risk of cancers (Vona-Davis et al. 2007; Wysocki and Wierusz-Wysocka 2010). Type 2 diabetes and high level of circulating blood glucose have been shown to be positively correlated with increased breast cancer mortality (Bjorge et al. 2010; Wolf et al. 2005). Recent studies show that the use of metformin, an oral antidiabetic drug that has been used for many years, is associated with decreased cancer risk (Dowling et al. 2011). Additionally, the increased fat mass is associated with aberrant insulin signaling (insulin resistance) and increased insulin levels, which directly stimulate mammary carcinogenesis (Vona-Davis et al. 2007). During breast cancer progression, the composition of the extracellular matrix is dynamically altered and adipose tissue is critically participated in this process (Erler et al. 2006; Fata et al. 2004). Adipocyte-derived collagen VI could activate the pro-survival and proliferation pathways to promote tumor growth and development (Iyengar et al. 2003). More recently, fat tissue has been recognized as an important secretory organ that can produce various hormones, cytokines and growth factors, collectively called adipokines (Galic et al. 2010). Dys-regulated expression and function of these adipokines play significant roles in the pathogenesis of obesity-related breast cancer diseases (Deng and Scherer 2010; Paz-Filho et al. 2011; Schaffler et al. 2007) (Figure 2). A number of them, including leptin and lipocalin-2, promote breast cancer cell survival, proliferation and tumor development, whereas adiponectin, the anti-inflammatory adipokine, has opposite effects (Jarde et al. 2011; Leng et al. 2011; Wang et al. 2007b; Yang and Moses 2009). Obese women with reduced serum adiponectin levels and low serum adiponectin levels are associated with an increased risk for breast cancer development and mortality (Duggan et al. 2011; Mantzoros et al. 2004). Women with higher adiponectin levels have a reduced risk of breast cancer (Korner et al. 2007; Miyoshi et al. 2003). Moreover, tumors in women with low serum adiponectin levels are more likely to show a biologically aggressive phenotype with poor prognosis (Miyoshi et al. 2003). The level of leptin increases in serum with increasing adiposity. In women diagnosed with breast cancer, the balance of adiponectin and leptin has been indicated to correlate with the disease development (Grossmann et al. 2008b). Serum leptin to adiponectin ratio is increased significantly in breast cancer patients and positively correlated with tumor size (Chen et al. 2006). Adiponectin levels are negatively correlated with leptin, and patients with higher levels of leptin are at increased risk for late stage tumors (Cust et al. 2009). The reduced levels of adiponectin and elevated leptin are associated with lymph node metastasis (Hou et al. 2007). Another adipokine, lipocalin-2, is found to be associated with aggressive types of breast cancers and poor prognosis (Leng et al. 2011).

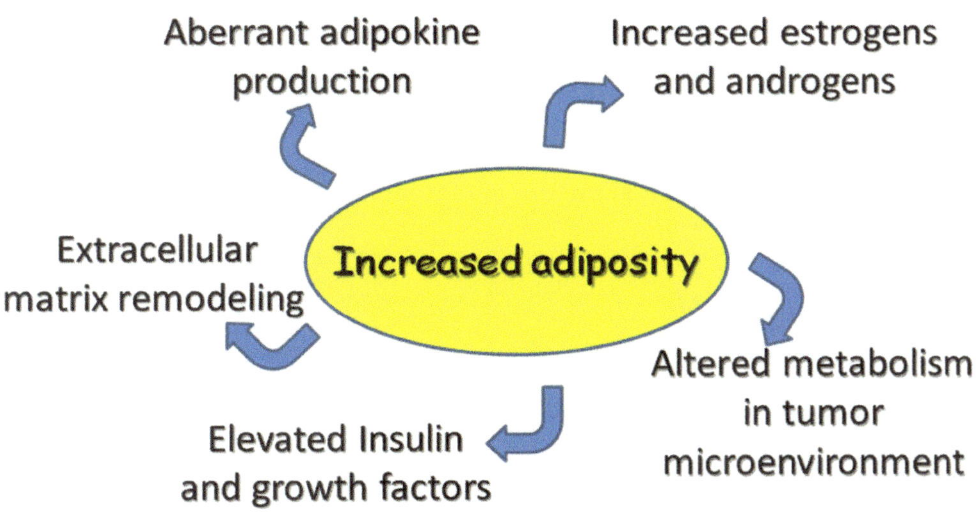

Fig. 1. Multiple mechanisms are implicated in linking increased adiposity with breast cancer development.

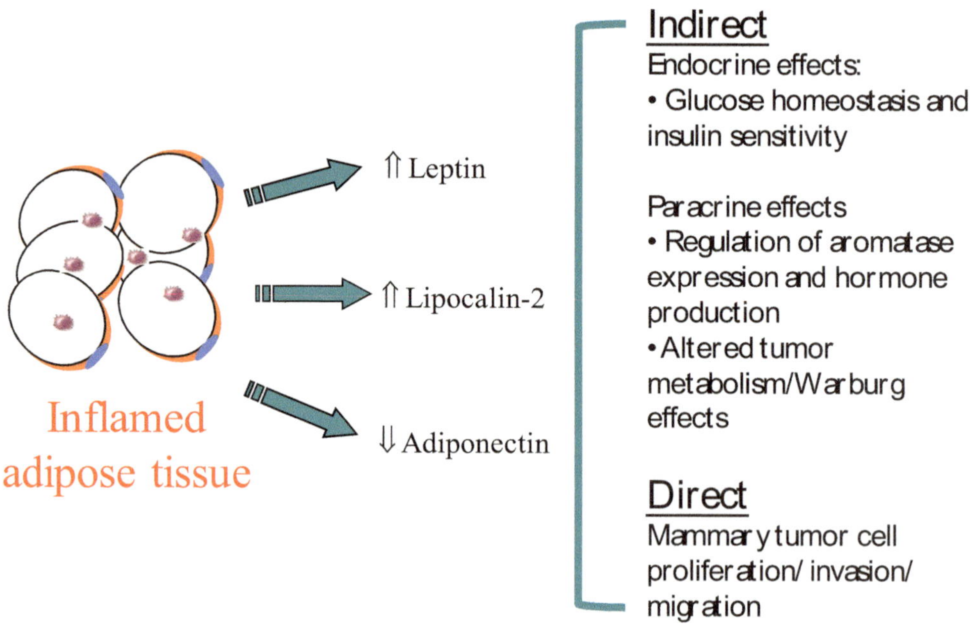

Fig. 2. Dysregulated production of adipokines, such as leptin, lipocalin-2 and adiponectin, from inflamed adipose tissue, contributes to mammary tumor development through both indirect and direct mechanisms.

Taken together, the above experimental and epidemiological evidences suggest that adipose tissue play an important role in breast cancer development and adipokines are key mediators linking obesity with breast cancer disease. The following sections of this chapter will elucidate the detailed role of adipokines, with special focus on the three adipokines, adiponectin, leptin and lipocalin-2, in mediating the stromal-epithelial interactions, in turn influencing the growth and proliferation of breast cancer cells.

3. Adipokines as key stromal factors in regulating mammary carcinogenesis

3.1 Adiponectin

Adiponectin is a 30-kDa glycoprotein exclusively secreted from adipocytes (Scherer et al. 1995). Human adiponectin gene is located on chromosome 3q27 and encodes a 244 amino acids polypeptide (Wang et al. 2008). Circulating concentrations of adiponectin range from 3-30 µg/mL, accounting for ~0.05 % of total human blood proteins (Ryan et al. 2003). Unlike many other adipokines that are up-regulated in obesity, circulating levels of adiponectin are inversely associated with obesity-related disorders (Cnop et al. 2003; Pajvani and Scherer 2003; Wang et al. 2009).

Endogenous adiponectin is predominantly present as several characteristic oligomeric complexes (Wang et al. 2008). The basic building block of the adiponectin complex is a trimer or low molecular weight (LMW) oligomer, which is formed via hydrophobic interactions within its globular domain. Two trimers self-associate to form a disulfide-linked hexamer or middle molecular weight (MMW) oligomer, which further assembles into a bouquet-like high molecular weight (HMW) multimeric complex that consists of 12-18 monomers (Radjainia et al. 2008). Post-translational modifications, including disulfide bond formation at a conserved cysteine residue and glycosylations occurred on several hydroxylated lysine residues within the collagenous domain, are involved in the assembly and stabilization of the oligomeric structures (Wang et al. 2006b; Wang et al. 2005a; Wang et al. 2002). Different oligomeric complexes of adiponectin activate distinct signalling pathways and possess different biological functions.

Two putative adiponectin receptors, termed AdipoR1 and AdipoR2, have been identified. Both receptors are integral membrane proteins containing seven transmembrane spanning domains (Yamauchi et al. 2003). They show unique distributions in various tissues and different affinities for the distinctive forms of circulating adiponectin. T-cadherin, which is highly expressed in endothelium and smooth muscle, has been identified as an adiponectin co-receptor with preference for hexameric and HMW adiponectin multimers (Hug et al. 2004).

Unlike most of the adipokines that are causally linked to obesity-related diseases, adiponectin has potent insulin-sensitizing, anti-inflammatory, anti-atherogenic and anti-tumorigenic activities (Kadowaki et al. 2006; Wang et al. 2007b; Wang et al. 2008; Wang et al. 2009). Notably, adiponectin potently inhibits the proliferation of various types of cells, including aortic smooth muscle cells, myelomonocytic cells, hepatic stellate cells and several types of cancer cells (Arita et al. 2002; Ding et al. 2005; Wang et al. 2005b; Yokota et al. 2000). It selectively binds to various carcinogenic growth factor and prevent the interactions of these growth factors to their respective receptors (Wang et al. 2005a). In addition, adiponectin inhibits the growth and migration of vascular endothelial cells, prevents new blood vessel formation, and attenuates the growth of transplanted fibrosarcoma cell tumors in mice (Brakenhielm et al. 2004).

The stomal effects of adiponectin have been nicely presented in mouse models with spontaneous mammary tumor development. Study by Lam et al demonstrates that insufficient production of adiponectin in adipocyte *per se* promotes tumor onset and development in MMTV-polyomavirus middle T antigen (MMTV-PyVT) transgenic mice (Lam et al. 2009; Landskroner-Eiger et al. 2009). A distinctive basal-like subtype of tumors, characterized by high proliferative activity and unfavorable prognosis, is derived from adiponectin haplodeficient MMTV-PyVT mice (Lam et al. 2009). Histological analysis demonstrated typical morphologic features including markedly elevated geographic tumor necrosis, ribbon-like architecture associated with central necrosis, pushing margin of invasion, and stromal lymphocytic response in tumors (Livasy et al. 2007). In contrast, the original MMTV-PyVT mice showed a well-structured and organized morphology. In more advanced malignant stages, mice lacking adiponectin give rise to a larger tumor burden, an increase in the mobilization of circulating endothelial progenitor cells, and a gene expression fingerprint indicative of more aggressive tumor cells. The potent angio-mimetic properties of adiponectin modulate tumor vascularization and deficiency of this hormone creates a chronically hypoxic microenvironment (Landskroner-Eiger et al. 2009). Breast cancer consists of a heterogeneous group of tumors classified into five types, in which the HER2/neu positive and the basal type (most are ER and HER2 negative) have the worst clinical prognosis. Tumors derived from adiponectin haplodeficient MMTV-PyVT mice show a triple-negative genotype (Lam et al. 2009), which may be aroused from a different origin or subgroups of stem cells that develop tumor more aggressively. The origin of this subtype tumor is unclear, but suggested to be the basal/myoepithelial cells, derived from epithelial-to-mesenchymal transition as a result of dedifferentiation, or from stem cells (Livasy et al. 2007).

In human mammary tumor tissue, adiponectin mRNA expression was observed only in the adipose tissues. On the other hand, AdipoR1 and AdipoR2 mRNA expression was observed in breast cancer cells, adipose tissues and normal breast epithelial cells (Takahata et al. 2007). In breast cancer specimen, a strong positive correlation between insulin as well as IGF1 receptor and AdipoR1 expression, but not AdipoR2 expression, could be observed. AdipoR1 is significantly higher in invasive breast cancer compared to preinvasive DCIS and inversely correlated with tumor size (Pfeiler et al. 2011). AdipoR2 expression is significantly correlated with vascular and lymphovascular invasion of breast cancer (Pfeiler et al. 2009). These results suggest a possibility that adiponectin might modulate the growth of normal breast epithelial cells and breast cancer cells directly through AdipoR1 and AdipoR2 receptors, and that the association of low serum adiponectin levels with a high breast cancer risk might be explained, at least in part, by the direct effect of adiponectin on the breast epithelial cells. The altered expression of AdipoR1 in invasive breast cancer also suggests that adiponectin might exert inhibitory effects on the transformation of preinvasive to invasive breast cancer. Further studies are warranted to investigate the prospective association between the mammary adiponectin levels and the risk of obesity-related breast cancers in humans.

3.2 Leptin

Leptin is a 16-kDa protein hormone abundantly expressed in white adipose tissue (Jarde et al. 2011). The circulating level of leptin is in the range of 5-50 ng/ml (Garofalo and Surmacz 2006). Obese individuals show a much higher plasma level (over 100 ng/ml) (Oksanen et al. 1997). Leptin was originally discovered by positional cloning of the obese (*ob*) gene, which is mutated in the massively obese ob/ob mice (Zhang et al. 1994). Leptin acts in the brain to regulate food intake and energy expenditure (Kelesidis et al. 2011). Treatment with leptin significantly reduces the body weight and food intake of the ob/ob mice. The leptin receptor mutant db/db mice, which are phenotypically similar to ob/ob mice, do not respond to leptin treatment (Campfield et al. 1995). The biological activity of leptin is mediated through the transmembrane leptin receptor ObR, which is expressed as at least six different subtypes in numerous tissues and cell types. Primarily the long isoform (ObRb) is responsible for activating leptin signaling pathways (Ahima and Osei 2004).

In general, higher body weight and/or obesity has been associated with shortened mammary tumor latency and increased incidence for development of spontaneous and carcinogen-induced tumors in animals (Dogan et al. 2007). In two sequential studies, MMTV-transforming growth factor (TGF)-α mice were crossed to genetically obese *ob/ob* and *db/db* mice. Surprisingly, neither type of these mice developed mammary tumors, suggesting that an intact leptin axis is essential for mammary tumorigenesis (Cleary et al. 2004). On the other hand, obesity induced by high fat diet significantly increases the number of tumors and reduces the tumor latency in MMTV-TGF-α mice (Cleary et al. 2010). The involvement of leptin signaling in mammary tumorigenesis was further confirmed by a study using obese Zucker rats, a rat model of genetic leptin receptor deficiency. Administration of chemical carcinogen methylnitrosourea could only induce a smaller number of Zucker rats to develop mammary tumor compared to lean controls (Lee et al.

2001). These findings demonstrate that leptin is a growth factor to support breast cancer development.

Both normal and malignant mammary tissues have been shown to produce leptin and express leptin receptors (Sheffield 2008). Leptin and its receptor are overexpressed in human breast tumor tissues (Garofalo et al. 2006). Expression of ErbB2 promotes high level expression of long-form leptin receptor and response to leptin. In general, the leptin/ObR correlates with higher tumor grade and worse prognosis (Surmacz 2007). Ishikawa et al observed that overexpression of both leptin and leptin receptors in breast cancer tissue are associated with distant metastasis (Ishikawa et al. 2004). The expression of leptin receptor showed a significant positive correlation with the level of leptin expression, suggesting an autocrine regulation of leptin expression in mammary tumor cells (Fiorio et al. 2008; Ishikawa et al. 2004; Revillion et al. 2006). The mRNA levels of leptin and leptin receptor are correlated positively with estrogen (ER) and progesterone receptors (PR), suggesting a possible interaction between leptin and oestrogen systems to promote breast carcinogenesis (Jarde et al. 2008b; Revillion et al. 2006). Analysis of human breast tumor tissues has also suggested an inverse relationship between leptin and adiponectin in breast cancer development (Jarde et al. 2008b). While leptin was expressed in a similar manner in invasive ductal carcinoma and *in situ* lesions, no tissue from *in situ* ductal carcinoma exhibited adiponectin expression. Moreover, myoepithelial cells of normal tissue adjacent to breast cancer exhibited 65% positivity for adiponectin while no cells in this group were positive for leptin expression, suggesting a possible leptin–adiponectin interaction on myoepithelial cells (Jarde et al. 2008b).

3.3 Lipocalin-2

Lipocalin-2, a 25-kDa secretory glycoprotein originally purified from human neutrophils, is constitutively expressed in adipose tissue (Esteve et al. 2009; Law et al. 2010). This protein structurally belongs to the lipocalin superfamily that shares the highly conserved structure of an 8-stranded antiparallel beta-barrel (Goetz et al. 2002). Circulating level of lipocalin-2 is elevated in obese animals and humans (Auguet et al. 2011; Hoo et al. 2008; Wang et al. 2007a; Yan et al. 2007; Zhang et al. 2008). Clinical, animal and cellular studies demonstrate the causal involvement of lipocalin-2 in obesity-associated medical complications (Auguet et al. 2011; Catalan et al. 2009; Esteve et al. 2009; Jin et al. 2010; Kanaka-Gantenbein et al. 2008; Law et al. 2010; Moreno-Navarrete et al. 2010; Sommer et al. 2009; van Dam and Hu 2007; Yan et al. 2007; Zhang et al. 2008). In humans, the serum concentration of lipocalin-2 is associated closely with obesity-related anthropometric and biochemical variables, and represents an independent risk factor for metabolic and cardiovascular disorders (Catalan et al. 2009; Choi et al. 2008; Ding et al. 2010; Esteve et al. 2009; Hemdahl et al. 2006; Lee et al. 2010; Wang et al. 2007a; Yndestad et al. 2009). Role of lipocalin-2 in regulation of cell proliferation, differentiation and apoptosis has been demonstrated (Devireddy et al. 2001). Lipocalin-2 may sequester the intracellular iron causing cell death.

Lipocalins function to transport and present ligands to cell surface receptors and to form macromolecular complexes (Flower 1995). The first identified ligand of lipocalin-2 was bacterial catecholate-type ferric siderophores, such as enterobactin (Goetz et al. 2002). Thus this protein was originally considered as a potent bacteriostatic agent (Berger et al. 2006). A number of studies have reported that lipocalin-2 weakly binds to the tripeptide N-formyl-

Met-Leu-Phe (fMLF), a potent neutrophil chemoattractant, and possibly other lipophilic mediators of inflammation, including platelet activating factor and leukotriene B4 (Strong et al. 1998). Recently, chemical screens combined with crystallography and fluorescence detection reveal a complex of lipocalin-2 that binds iron together with a small metabolic product called catechol (Bao et al. 2010). The formation of the complex blocks the reactivity of iron, permits its transport in the circulation and facilitates recycling in endosomes. The lipocalin-2-catechol-Fe(III) complex represents an unforeseen endogenous siderophore for iron traffic in aseptic tissues. This mammalian siderophore plays a critical role in both cytoplasmic and mitochondrial iron homeostasis. Lacking this siderophore results in the accumulation of abnormally high amounts of cytoplasmic iron and elevated levels of reactive oxygen species (Devireddy et al. 2010).

The promoting effects of lipocalin-2 on mammary tumor development have been signified by two independent studies using MMTV-ErbB2 (V664E) and MMTV-PyVT mouse models (Berger et al. 2010; Leng et al. 2009). Leng et al found that the initiation time of the mammary tumor in MMTV-ErbB2 (V664E) mice complete lacking lipocalin-2 expression was dramatically delayed by ~100 days compared to the mice with two copies of lipocalin-2 alleles (Leng et al. 2009). Furthermore, the tumor burden, the number of tumors per mouse as well as the lung metastasis were dramatically reduced. Another study also showed reduced tumor weight and number of tumors per mouse in MMTV-PyVT mice lacking lipocalin-2 expression (Berger et al. 2010). However, there was no difference observed during early mammary tumorigenesis between the wild type and lipocalin-2 knockout group. Based on this, they concluded that lipocalin-2 played a more important role in the later stage of tumor development in MMTV-PyVT model, which shows a more aggressive phenotype with much shorter tumor latency (Berger et al. 2010).

Positive correlations between the circulating level of lipocalin-2 and the invasive and metastatic status of breast cancer have been reported (Yang and Moses 2009). The expression patterns of lipocalin-2 in mammary tumor samples have been analyzed by a number of studies (Bauer et al. 2008; Stoesz et al. 1998; Yang et al. 2009). Lipocalin-2 positive cells can be identified in the infiltrating carcinomas but not in normal mammary tissues (Bauer et al. 2008). High expression of lipocalin-2 correlates with low ER and PR expression, high-histologic grade, lymph nodes metastasis, high-proliferation index and poor disease-free survival (Leng et al. 2011). The induced expression of lipocalin-2 staining in either the tumor or the stroma area is correlated with the advanced stages and the metastatic status. Orthotopic studies demonstrated that lipocalin-2-expressing breast tumors displayed a poorly differentiated phenotype and showed increased local tumor invasion and lymph node metastasis (Yang et al. 2009).

In summary, animal models have provided unique tools to dissect the roles of individual adipokine in mammary tumor development and to elucidate the multiple pathways responsible for the dialogue between adipocytes and breast cancer cells. The information obtained from the mammary tumor models with deficient adipokine expressions demonstrate that in general, adipokines elicit their activities on tumor progression through regulating a) cancer cell transformation, proliferation and migration; b) local and systemic inflammation; and c) pathological angiogenesis. In addition, the role of adipokines to regulate systematic energy metabolism also impacts the behaviors of breast cancer cells and tumor development.

4. Signaling mechanisms responsible for the regulation of breast cancer cell function by adiponectin, leptin and lipocalin-2

Although adipokines are the key players in obesity-related mammary carcinogenesis, the underlying mechanisms remain largely uncharacterized. Individual adipokines affect mammary tumor development in different manners through distinctive signalling pathways, with concomitant influences on proliferative, inflammatory, and metastatic properties of the tumor cells (Schaffler et al. 2007; Vona-Davis and Rose 2007). Moreover, the mechanistic networks of adipokines in mammary tumor development are usually intertwined with their role in regulating inflammation and angiogenesis (Lorincz and Sukumar 2006; Wang et al. 2007b). Here, the specific signaling mechanisms that are directly involved in regulating the breast cancer cell functions will be discussed and linked with animal and clinical presentations.

4.1 Diversified signaling mechanisms of adiponectin: cross-talking with Wnt/β-catenin pathway

Adiponectin acts as an inhibitory factor for the proliferation of human breast carcinoma cells and mammary tumor development (Arditi et al. 2007; Dieudonne et al. 2006; Grossmann et al. 2008a; Hebbard et al. 2008; Jarde et al. 2008a; Kang et al. 2005; Nakayama et al. 2008; Pfeiler et al. 2008; Wang et al. 2006a). *In vitro* treatment with adiponectin at physiological concentrations attenuates the growth of an ER-negative human breast carcinoma MDA-MB-231 cells by inhibiting cell proliferation and inducing apoptosis (Kang et al. 2005; Wang et al. 2006a). It also inhibits insulin- and growth factors-stimulated proliferation in ER-positive human breast cancer cells (Li et al. 2011; Wang et al. 2006a). These *in vitro* data are supported by animal study demonstrating that adiponectin supplement therapy suppresses the MDA-MB-231 breast tumor development in nude mice (Wang et al. 2006a).

Cell-type dependent signalling mechanisms have been suggested to mediate the growth inhibitory effects of adiponectin (Grossmann et al. 2008a) (Figure 3). In MCF-7 cells, adiponectin induces AMP-activated protein kinase (AMPK) phosphorylation and inactivates p42/p44 MAPkinase (ERK1/2) (Dieudonne et al. 2006). By contrast, the inhibitory effects of adiponectin on T47D cell growth are associated with inactivation of ERK1/2 but not AMPK or p38 MAPK (Korner et al. 2007; Wang et al. 2006a). In MDA-MB-231 cells with ectopic ER over-expression, globular adiponectin inhibits cell proliferation by blocking JNK2 signaling (Grossmann et al. 2008a). A cross-talk between adiponectin and ER signaling exists in breast cancer cells and that adiponectin effects on the growth and apoptosis of breast cancer cells in vitro are partly dependent on the presence of 17-beta estradiol (Pfeiler et al. 2008). In ER-negative MDA-MB-231 cells, adiponectin could modulate the glycogen synthase kinase-3beta (GSK3β)/β-catenin signaling pathway (Wang et al. 2006a). Prolonged treatment with adiponectin markedly reduces serum-induced phosphorylation of Akt and GSK3β, decreases intracellular accumulation and nuclear translocation of β-catenin, and suppresses cyclin D1 expression (Wang et al. 2006a). An increase of protein phosphatase 2A activity has been implicated in the dephosphorylation of Akt by adiponectin treatment in MDA-MB-231 cells (Kim et al. 2009). Although the effects of adiponectin on tumor metastasis are not conclusive, it is suggested that LKB1 is required for adiponectin-mediated inhibition of adhesion, migration and invasion of breast cancer cells (Taliaferro-Smith et al. 2009).

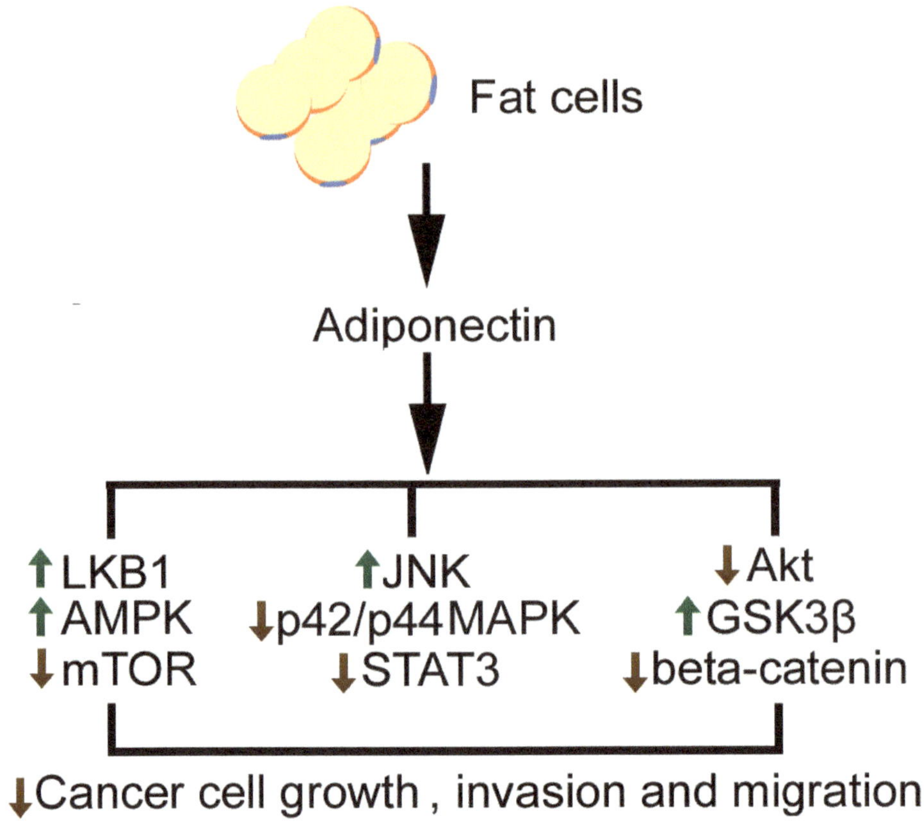

Fig. 3. Signaling pathways that mediate the anti-tumor activities of adiponectin.

Hyperactivation of the canonical Wnt/β-catenin pathway is one of the most frequent signal abnormalities in many types of cancers (Brown 2001; Howe and Brown 2004; Prosperi and Goss 2010). The central event in this pathway is the stabilization and nuclear translocation of β-catenin, where it binds to the transcription factor TCF/LEF and consequently activates a cluster of genes that ultimately establish the oncogenic phenotype (Jin et al. 2008). Stabilization of β-catenin protein and over-expression of cyclin D1 have been observed in over 50% of human breast tumors and increased β-catenin activity was found to be significantly correlated with the poor prognosis of breast cancer patients (Brown 2001). Given the close proximity between mammary gland cells and adipocytes, decreased adiponectin production might be causally linked to increased β-catenin accumulation and cyclin D1 overexpression observed in breast cancer patients. This possibility is supported by animal studies. The isolated mammary tumor cells from adiponectin haplodeficient MMTV-PyVT mice are presented with hyperactivated phosphatidylinositol-3-kinase (PI3K)/Akt/β-catenin signaling, which at least partly attributes to the decreased phosphatase and tensin homolog (PTEN) activities (Lam et al. 2009). PTEN is one of the most frequently mutated tumor suppressors that can prevent the activation of the cell survival PI3K/Akt signaling pathway (Carnero et al. 2008). In MMTV-PyVT animals with reduced production of adiponectin, PTEN is inactivated by a redox-regulated mechanism involving thioredoxin and thioredoxin reductase. Specificity protein 1, a redox-regulated transcription factor, is involved in mediating the effects of adiponectin to stimulate the expression of Wnt inhibitory factor-1, a Wnt antagonist frequently silenced in human breast tumors (Liu et al. 2008). In summary, these findings have not only suggested a cross-talk between adiponectin and Wnt signaling pathway, but also provided a novel mechanistic insight to explain how metabolic alterations in adiponectin haplodeficient tumor may gain a survival advantage.

4.2 Leptin-mediated signaling in breast cancer cells: in relation to other mitogenic receptors

Leptin acts as a mitogen and survival factor for human breast cancer cells (Markowska et al. 2004). Leptin receptors are expressed in various human breast cancer cell lines and in human primary breast carcinoma (Frankenberry et al. 2006; Garofalo et al. 2006; Hu et al. 2002; Laud et al. 2002; Sheffield 2008). Leptin acts through multifaceted signaling pathways, including Jak2/STAT3 (Janus kinase 2/signal transducer and activator of transcription 3), PI3K/Akt, ERK1/2 and SOCS3 (Fusco et al. 2010; Palianopoulou et al. 2011; Saxena et al. 2007; Yin et al. 2004). Different sensitivities to recombinant leptin treatment have been found in distinctive breast carcinoma cell lines. For example, in MCF 7 cells, leptin induces a strong phosphorylation of STAT3 and ERK1/2, leading to an increased cell viability and proliferation (Fusco et al. 2010). This response is not present in MDA-MB 231 cells, in which leptin potentiates the anti-proliferative action of cAMP elevating agents by concurring to cell cycle arrest at G1 phase and inducing apoptosis (Naviglio et al. 2009).
Leptin induces the expression of vascular endothelial growth factor (VEGF) in both human and mouse mammary tumor cells, and promotes angiogenesis, which is related to the worse prognosis of breast cancer (Zhou et al. 2011). HIF-1alpha and NFkappaB are implicated in leptin-regulated VEGF expression through both canonic (MAPK, PI-3K) and non-canonic (PKC, JNK and p38 MAP) signalling pathways (Gonzalez-Perez et al. 2010). Leptin contributes to the elevated circulating estrogen levels in obese women. It stimulates aromatase activity in adipose stromal cells at high concentrations (Magoffin et al. 1999). The action of leptin to enhance the promoter activity of aromatase is mediated by AP-1 in MCF-7 cells (Catalano et al. 2003). These evidence suggest that elevated leptin concentrations may cause locally augmented VEGF and estrogen in the breast and thereby promote tumor formation.
Leptin exerts its activity not only through its own receptors, but also through crosstalks with other signaling systems implicated in tumorigenesis (Ozbay and Nahta 2008). Co-treatment of leptin and insulin-like growth factor (IGF)-I significantly increases proliferation as well as invasion and migration of breast cancer cells (Saxena et al. 2008). A bidirectional crosstalk between leptin and IGF-I signaling exists to synergistically activate the downstream effectors, Akt and ERK1/2. Moreover, leptin and IGF-I treatment transactivates epidermal growth factor receptor (EGFR) to induce invasion and migration of breast cancer cells. In breast cancer cell lines, HER2 and ObR are coexpressed and physically interacted (Fiorio et al. 2008; Ray et al. 2007). Leptin treatment increases HER2 phosphorylation on Tyr 1248 (Fiorio et al. 2008). Coexpression of HER2 and the leptin/ObR system might contribute to enhanced HER2 activity and reduced sensitivity to anti-HER2 treatments. These data suggest indicate the possibility of using EGFR inhibitors to counter the pro-cancerous effects of leptin and IGF-I in breast cancers. Exogenous leptin induces tyrosine phosphorylation of HER2 in SKBR3 cells, which showed marked overexpression of HER2. Leptin-induced HER2 phosphorylation was partially reduced by an EGFR inhibitor, AG1478, or a Jak

inhibitor, AG490. Moreover, leptin-induced phosphorylation of ERK1/2 could be abrogated by a HER2 tyrosine kinase inhibitor, AG825 (Soma et al. 2008). In fact, the influence of leptin on breast cancer development not only relates to the presence or absence of HER2 but also depends on ER status (Ray et al. 2007). Knocking down of ERalpha attenuates leptin-induced activation of STAT3, whereas the enhancement of leptin-mediated STAT3 activity is independent of ERalpha ligands. ERalpha binding to STAT3 and Jak2 might lead to an increased ERalpha-dependent cell viability(Binai et al. 2010). Leptin plays important role in enhancing in situ estradiol production and promoting estrogen-dependent breast cancer progression. The ability of leptin to transactivate ERalpha and mimic the classic features of ERalpha signaling has been observed in MCF-7 breast cancer cell line. MAPK pathway is found to be involved in this process. Moreover, estradiol-induced activation of ERalpha can be potentiated by leptin exposure (Catalano et al. 2004).
Taken together, these findings suggest that the leptin system plays an important role in breast cancer pathogenesis and progression, and that it represents a novel target for therapeutic intervention in breast cancer disease (Cirillo et al. 2008).

4.3 Lipocalin-2: Controversies and role in epithelial to mesenchymal transition

Lipocalin-2 is a putative *in vivo* estrogen target gene and paracrine factor that mediates the growth regulatory effects of estrogen in normal breast epithelium (Seth et al. 2002). It contains an ER response element in its promoter. On the other hand, in T47D breast cancer cells, hormone treatment decreases the mRNA expression of lipocalin-2 (Mrusek et al. 2005), suggesting that normal and cancerous estrogen receptor-positive cells are distinct at the molecular level. Elevated lipocalin-2 may influence the steroid status of the mammary epithelial cells. When ectopically introducing lipocalin-2 into MCF-7 cells, their ER-dependent tumor growth in the xenografted mice is lost and the tumor cells become ER-negative (Yang et al. 2009). These data imply that modulation of lipocalin-2 expression may enable the breast cancer cells to become sensitive to ER therapy, a result that might be translated into clinical usage for ER-targeted therapy.
Both human and mouse mammary tumor cell lines have been used to examine the importance of lipocalin-2 in mammary tumor formation. Overexpression of lipocalin-2 in mouse 4T1 and human MDA-MB-468 cells greatly promoted their ability in cell migration and invasion (Leng et al. 2009; Shi et al. 2008). Moreover, implantation of 4T1 or MDA-MB-468 cells ectopically expressing lipocalin-2 generated a significant more number of lung metastatic nodules compared to those implanted with the unmodified cells. The lung metastasis could be blocked by injection of a polyclonal antibody against lipocalin-2 (Leng et al. 2009). In HER2-positive human breast cancer cell line SKBR3, knocking down lipocalin-2 expression reduced the migration and in and ER-positive MCF-7 cells, These findings are consistent with the study by Fougere et al suggesting that the anti-migration activity of NFAT3 is through inhibition of lipocalin-2 gene expression (Fougere et al. 2010). In human tissue and urine samples, lipocalin-2 levels are consistently associated with invasive breast cancer (Yang et al. 2009).
Lipocalin-2 has been shown to induce the epithelial to mesenchymal transition (EMT) in breast cancer cells (Leng et al. 2011). Cells undergone EMT show increased motility and invasiveness as well as elevated lipocalin-2 expression. When ectopically expressed in MCF-7 cells, lipocalin-2 induces a typical EMT change of the cell morphology, accompanied by a loss of epithelial marker (E-cadherin) and an increased expression of the mesenchymal markers (vimentin and fibronectin) (Yang et al. 2009). Lipocalin-2 silencing in aggressive

breast cancer cells inhibits cell migration and the mesenchymal phenotype. Increased secretion of lipocalin-2 from the tumor cells might directly affect MMP-9 activity to promote cell motility or the transition to a more mesenchymal/aggressive phenotype (Leng et al. 2011). Much higher blood gelatinase activities are found in the tumor-bearing MMTV-ErbB mice with normal lipocalin-2 expression than those deficient of lipocalin-2 expression (Leng et al. 2009). ERalpha is also suggested to participate in lipocalin-2-induced EMT. By contrast, in 4T1 cells lipocalin-2 appears to reverse the EMT process induced by Ras expression (Hanai et al. 2005). Different phases or sites of lipocalin-2 treatment have been suggested for these controversial findings. During EMT, the initial increased lipocalin-2 stimulates epithelial migration and the elevated exogenous lipocalin-2 may facilitate the recovery (Mori et al. 2005; Yang et al. 2002).
In summary, although lipocalin-2 regulates EMT, one of the key processes involved in tumor progression and metastasis, the underlying mechanisms remain to be further elucidated.

5. Concluding remarks

The prevalence of obesity and its associated diseases has posed a huge healthcare impact on our society. During the past two decades, a panel of adipokines critically involved in pathological processes of obesity-associated breast cancer diseases has been discovered. Their contributions to the development of breast cancer and the underlying mechanisms are divergent. For example, adiponectin deficiency is associated with an accelerated mammary tumor development and altered Wnt/β-catenin signaling. On the other hand, the tumors of mice without lipocalin-2 are less metastatic and show slower rate of growth. Clearly, individual adipokines are able to modulate specific oncogenic and metabolic pathways, which synergistically promote or antagonize the development of breast cancer disease under obese conditions. The three adipokines discussed in this chapter not only represent potential therapeutic targets for breast cancer, but can also serve as biomarkers for early diagnosis and disease prevention. Compounds related to leptin that may have therapeutic use are currently being investigated in pre-clinical studies (Gonzalez et al. 2006; Ray and Cleary 2010; Rene Gonzalez et al. 2009; Surmacz 2007). Continued research will undoubtedly provide more insights into the relationship between adipose tissue-derived factors and breast cancer development, as well as the ways to intervene these interactions.

6. Acknowledgement

This work was supported by the grants from Seeding Funds for Basic Research of the HKU and the Area of Excellent Scheme (AoE/P-10-01) established under University Grants Committee, HKSAR.

7. References

Ahima RS, Osei SY (2004) Leptin signaling. Physiol Behav 81:223-41
Alokail MS, Al-Daghri NM, Al-Attas OS, Hussain T (2009) Combined effects of obesity and type 2 diabetes contribute to increased breast cancer risk in premenopausal women. Cardiovasc Diabetol 8:33

Arditi JD, Venihaki M, Karalis KP, Chrousos GP (2007) Antiproliferative effect of adiponectin on MCF7 breast cancer cells: a potential hormonal link between obesity and cancer. Horm Metab Res 39:9-13

Arendt LM, Rudnick JA, Keller PJ, Kuperwasser C (2010) Stroma in breast development and disease. Semin Cell Dev Biol 21:11-8

Arita Y, Kihara S, Ouchi N, Maeda K, Kuriyama H, Okamoto Y, Kumada M, Hotta K, Nishida M, Takahashi M, Nakamura T, Shimomura I, Muraguchi M, Ohmoto Y, Funahashi T, Matsuzawa Y (2002) Adipocyte-derived plasma protein adiponectin acts as a platelet-derived growth factor-BB-binding protein and regulates growth factor-induced common postreceptor signal in vascular smooth muscle cell. Circulation 105:2893-8

Auguet T, Quintero Y, Terra X, Martinez S, Lucas A, Pellitero S, Aguilar C, Hernandez M, Del Castillo D, Richart C (2011) Upregulation of lipocalin 2 in adipose tissues of severely obese women: positive relationship with proinflammatory cytokines. Obesity (Silver Spring)

Bao G, Clifton M, Hoette TM, Mori K, Deng SX, Qiu A, Viltard M, Williams D, Paragas N, Leete T, Kulkarni R, Li X, Lee B, Kalandadze A, Ratner AJ, Pizarro JC, Schmidt-Ott KM, Landry DW, Raymond KN, Strong RK, Barasch J (2010) Iron traffics in circulation bound to a siderocalin (Ngal)-catechol complex. Nat Chem Biol 6:602-9

Bauer M, Eickhoff JC, Gould MN, Mundhenke C, Maass N, Friedl A (2008) Neutrophil gelatinase-associated lipocalin (NGAL) is a predictor of poor prognosis in human primary breast cancer. Breast Cancer Res Treat 108:389-97

Berger T, Cheung CC, Elia AJ, Mak TW (2010) Disruption of the Lcn2 gene in mice suppresses primary mammary tumor formation but does not decrease lung metastasis. Proc Natl Acad Sci U S A 107:2995-3000

Berger T, Togawa A, Duncan GS, Elia AJ, You-Ten A, Wakeham A, Fong HE, Cheung CC, Mak TW (2006) Lipocalin 2-deficient mice exhibit increased sensitivity to Escherichia coli infection but not to ischemia-reperfusion injury. Proc Natl Acad Sci U S A 103:1834-9

Binai NA, Damert A, Carra G, Steckelbroeck S, Lower J, Lower R, Wessler S (2010) Expression of estrogen receptor alpha increases leptin-induced STAT3 activity in breast cancer cells. Int J Cancer 127:55-66

Bjorge T, Lukanova A, Jonsson H, Tretli S, Ulmer H, Manjer J, Stocks T, Selmer R, Nagel G, Almquist M, Concin H, Hallmans G, Haggstrom C, Stattin P, Engeland A (2010) Metabolic syndrome and breast cancer in the me-can (metabolic syndrome and cancer) project. Cancer Epidemiol Biomarkers Prev 19:1737-45

Brakenhielm E, Veitonmaki N, Cao R, Kihara S, Matsuzawa Y, Zhivotovsky B, Funahashi T, Cao Y (2004) Adiponectin-induced antiangiogenesis and antitumor activity involve caspase-mediated endothelial cell apoptosis. Proc Natl Acad Sci U S A 101:2476-81

Bray GA (2004) Medical consequences of obesity. J Clin Endocrinol Metab 89:2583-9

Brown AM (2001) Wnt signaling in breast cancer: have we come full circle? Breast Cancer Res 3:351-5

Calle EE, Rodriguez C, Walker-Thurmond K, Thun MJ (2003) Overweight, obesity, and mortality from cancer in a prospectively studied cohort of U.S. adults. N Engl J Med 348:1625-38

Campfield LA, Smith FJ, Guisez Y, Devos R, Burn P (1995) Recombinant mouse OB protein: evidence for a peripheral signal linking adiposity and central neural networks. Science 269:546-9

Carnero A, Blanco-Aparicio C, Renner O, Link W, Leal JF (2008) The PTEN/PI3K/AKT signalling pathway in cancer, therapeutic implications. Curr Cancer Drug Targets 8:187-98

Catalan V, Gomez-Ambrosi J, Rodriguez A, Ramirez B, Silva C, Rotellar F, Gil MJ, Cienfuegos JA, Salvador J, Fruhbeck G (2009) Increased adipose tissue expression of lipocalin-2 in obesity is related to inflammation and matrix metalloproteinase-2 and metalloproteinase-9 activities in humans. J Mol Med 87:803-13

Catalano S, Marsico S, Giordano C, Mauro L, Rizza P, Panno ML, Ando S (2003) Leptin enhances, via AP-1, expression of aromatase in the MCF-7 cell line. J Biol Chem 278:28668-76

Catalano S, Mauro L, Marsico S, Giordano C, Rizza P, Rago V, Montanaro D, Maggiolini M, Panno ML, Ando S (2004) Leptin induces, via ERK1/ERK2 signal, functional activation of estrogen receptor alpha in MCF-7 cells. J Biol Chem 279:19908-15

Chen DC, Chung YF, Yeh YT, Chaung HC, Kuo FC, Fu OY, Chen HY, Hou MF, Yuan SS (2006) Serum adiponectin and leptin levels in Taiwanese breast cancer patients. Cancer Lett 237:109-14

Choi KM, Lee JS, Kim EJ, Baik SH, Seo HS, Choi DS, Oh DJ, Park CG (2008) Implication of lipocalin-2 and visfatin levels in patients with coronary heart disease. Eur J Endocrinol 158:203-7

Cirillo D, Rachiglio AM, la Montagna R, Giordano A, Normanno N (2008) Leptin signaling in breast cancer: an overview. J Cell Biochem 105:956-64

Cleary MP, Grossmann ME (2009) Minireview: Obesity and breast cancer: the estrogen connection. Endocrinology 150:2537-42

Cleary MP, Grossmann ME, Ray A (2010) Effect of obesity on breast cancer development. Veterinary pathology 47:202-13

Cleary MP, Juneja SC, Phillips FC, Hu X, Grande JP, Maihle NJ (2004) Leptin receptor-deficient MMTV-TGF-alpha/Lepr(db)Lepr(db) female mice do not develop oncogene-induced mammary tumors. Exp Biol Med (Maywood) 229:182-93

Cnop M, Havel PJ, Utzschneider KM, Carr DB, Sinha MK, Boyko EJ, Retzlaff BM, Knopp RH, Brunzell JD, Kahn SE (2003) Relationship of adiponectin to body fat distribution, insulin sensitivity and plasma lipoproteins: evidence for independent roles of age and sex. Diabetologia 46:459-69

Couldrey C, Moitra J, Vinson C, Anver M, Nagashima K, Green J (2002) Adipose tissue: a vital in vivo role in mammary gland development but not differentiation. Dev Dyn 223:459-68

Creydt VP, Sacca PA, Tesone AJ, Vidal L, Calvo JC (2010) Adipocyte differentiation influences the proliferation and migration of normal and tumoral breast epithelial cells. Mol Med Report 3:433-9

Cust AE, Stocks T, Lukanova A, Lundin E, Hallmans G, Kaaks R, Jonsson H, Stattin P (2009) The influence of overweight and insulin resistance on breast cancer risk and tumour stage at diagnosis: a prospective study. Breast Cancer Res Treat 113:567-76

Davison CA, Schafer ZT (2010) Keeping a breast of recent developments in cancer metabolism. Curr Drug Targets 11:1112-20

Deng Y, Scherer PE (2010) Adipokines as novel biomarkers and regulators of the metabolic syndrome. Annals of the New York Academy of Sciences 1212:E1-E19

Devireddy LR, Hart DO, Goetz DH, Green MR (2010) A mammalian siderophore synthesized by an enzyme with a bacterial homolog involved in enterobactin production. Cell 141:1006-17

Devireddy LR, Teodoro JG, Richard FA, Green MR (2001) Induction of apoptosis by a secreted lipocalin that is transcriptionally regulated by IL-3 deprivation. Science 293:829-34

Dieudonne MN, Bussiere M, Dos Santos E, Leneveu MC, Giudicelli Y, Pecquery R (2006) Adiponectin mediates antiproliferative and apoptotic responses in human MCF7 breast cancer cells. Biochem Biophys Res Commun 345:271-9

Ding L, Hanawa H, Ota Y, Hasegawa G, Hao K, Asami F, Watanabe R, Yoshida T, Toba K, Yoshida K, Ogura M, Kodama M, Aizawa Y (2010) Lipocalin-2/neutrophil gelatinase-B associated lipocalin is strongly induced in hearts of rats with autoimmune myocarditis and in human myocarditis. Circ J 74:523-30

Ding X, Saxena NK, Lin S, Xu A, Srinivasan S, Anania FA (2005) The roles of leptin and adiponectin: a novel paradigm in adipocytokine regulation of liver fibrosis and stellate cell biology. Am J Pathol 166:1655-69

Dogan S, Hu X, Zhang Y, Maihle NJ, Grande JP, Cleary MP (2007) Effects of high-fat diet and/or body weight on mammary tumor leptin and apoptosis signaling pathways in MMTV-TGF-alpha mice. Breast cancer research : BCR 9:R91

Dowling RJ, Goodwin PJ, Stambolic V (2011) Understanding the benefit of metformin use in cancer treatment. BMC medicine 9:33

Duggan C, Irwin ML, Xiao L, Henderson KD, Smith AW, Baumgartner RN, Baumgartner KB, Bernstein L, Ballard-Barbash R, McTiernan A (2011) Associations of insulin resistance and adiponectin with mortality in women with breast cancer. J Clin Oncol 29:32-9

Elliott BE, Tam SP, Dexter D, Chen ZQ (1992) Capacity of adipose tissue to promote growth and metastasis of a murine mammary carcinoma: effect of estrogen and progesterone. Int J Cancer 51:416-24

Erler JT, Bennewith KL, Nicolau M, Dornhofer N, Kong C, Le QT, Chi JT, Jeffrey SS, Giaccia AJ (2006) Lysyl oxidase is essential for hypoxia-induced metastasis. Nature 440:1222-6

Esteve E, Ricart W, Fernandez-Real JM (2009) Adipocytokines and insulin resistance: the possible role of lipocalin-2, retinol binding protein-4, and adiponectin. Diabetes Care 32 Suppl 2:S362-7

Fata JE, Werb Z, Bissell MJ (2004) Regulation of mammary gland branching morphogenesis by the extracellular matrix and its remodeling enzymes. Breast Cancer Res 6:1-11

Fiorio E, Mercanti A, Terrasi M, Micciolo R, Remo A, Auriemma A, Molino A, Parolin V, Di Stefano B, Bonetti F, Giordano A, Cetto GL, Surmacz E (2008) Leptin/HER2 crosstalk in breast cancer: in vitro study and preliminary in vivo analysis. BMC Cancer 8:305

Flower DR (1995) Multiple molecular recognition properties of the lipocalin protein family. J Mol Recognit 8:185-95

Fougere M, Gaudineau B, Barbier J, Guaddachi F, Feugeas JP, Auboeuf D, Jauliac S (2010) NFAT3 transcription factor inhibits breast cancer cell motility by targeting the Lipocalin 2 gene. Oncogene 29:2292-301

Frankenberry KA, Skinner H, Somasundar P, McFadden DW, Vona-Davis LC (2006) Leptin receptor expression and cell signaling in breast cancer. Int J Oncol 28:985-93

Fusco R, Galgani M, Procaccini C, Franco R, Pirozzi G, Fucci L, Laccetti P, Matarese G (2010) Cellular and molecular crosstalk between leptin receptor and estrogen receptor-{alpha} in breast cancer: molecular basis for a novel therapeutic setting. Endocr Relat Cancer 17:373-82

Galic S, Oakhill JS, Steinberg GR (2010) Adipose tissue as an endocrine organ. Mol Cell Endocrinol 316:129-39

Garofalo C, Koda M, Cascio S, Sulkowska M, Kanczuga-Koda L, Golaszewska J, Russo A, Sulkowski S, Surmacz E (2006) Increased expression of leptin and the leptin receptor as a marker of breast cancer progression: possible role of obesity-related stimuli. Clin Cancer Res 12:1447-53

Garofalo C, Surmacz E (2006) Leptin and cancer. J Cell Physiol 207:12-22

Goetz DH, Holmes MA, Borregaard N, Bluhm ME, Raymond KN, Strong RK (2002) The neutrophil lipocalin NGAL is a bacteriostatic agent that interferes with siderophore-mediated iron acquisition. Mol Cell 10:1033-43

Gonzalez-Perez RR, Xu Y, Guo S, Watters A, Zhou W, Leibovich SJ (2010) Leptin upregulates VEGF in breast cancer via canonic and non-canonical signalling pathways and NFkappaB/HIF-1alpha activation. Cell Signal 22:1350-62

Gonzalez RR, Cherfils S, Escobar M, Yoo JH, Carino C, Styer AK, Sullivan BT, Sakamoto H, Olawaiye A, Serikawa T, Lynch MP, Rueda BR (2006) Leptin signaling promotes the growth of mammary tumors and increases the expression of vascular endothelial growth factor (VEGF) and its receptor type two (VEGF-R2). J Biol Chem 281:26320-8

Grossmann ME, Nkhata KJ, Mizuno NK, Ray A, Cleary MP (2008a) Effects of adiponectin on breast cancer cell growth and signaling. Br J Cancer 98:370-9

Grossmann ME, Ray A, Dogan S, Mizuno NK, Cleary MP (2008b) Balance of adiponectin and leptin modulates breast cancer cell growth. Cell Res 18:1154-6

Guerrero J, Tobar N, Caceres M, Espinoza L, Escobar P, Dotor J, Smith PC, Martinez J (2010) Soluble factors derived from tumor mammary cell lines induce a stromal mammary adipose reversion in human and mice adipose cells. Possible role of TGF-beta1 and TNF-alpha. Breast Cancer Res Treat 119:497-508

Hanai J, Mammoto T, Seth P, Mori K, Karumanchi SA, Barasch J, Sukhatme VP (2005) Lipocalin 2 diminishes invasiveness and metastasis of Ras-transformed cells. J Biol Chem 280:13641-7

Hebbard LW, Garlatti M, Young LJ, Cardiff RD, Oshima RG, Ranscht B (2008) T-cadherin supports angiogenesis and adiponectin association with the vasculature in a mouse mammary tumor model. Cancer Res 68:1407-16

Hemdahl AL, Gabrielsen A, Zhu C, Eriksson P, Hedin U, Kastrup J, Thoren P, Hansson GK (2006) Expression of neutrophil gelatinase-associated lipocalin in atherosclerosis and myocardial infarction. Arterioscler Thromb Vasc Biol 26:136-42

Hoo RC, Yeung CY, Lam KS, Xu A (2008) Inflammatory biomarkers associated with obesity and insulin resistance: a focus on lipocalin-2 and adipocyte fatty acid-binding protein. . Expert Rev. Endocrinol. Metab. 3:29-41

Hou WK, Xu YX, Yu T, Zhang L, Zhang WW, Fu CL, Sun Y, Wu Q, Chen L (2007) Adipocytokines and breast cancer risk. Chin Med J (Engl) 120:1592-6

Hovey RC, Aimo L (2010) Diverse and active roles for adipocytes during mammary gland growth and function. J Mammary Gland Biol Neoplasia 15:279-90

Howe LR, Brown AM (2004) Wnt signaling and breast cancer. Cancer Biol Ther 3:36-41

Hu X, Juneja SC, Maihle NJ, Cleary MP (2002) Leptin--a growth factor in normal and malignant breast cells and for normal mammary gland development. J Natl Cancer Inst 94:1704-11

Hug C, Wang J, Ahmad NS, Bogan JS, Tsao TS, Lodish HF (2004) T-cadherin is a receptor for hexameric and high-molecular-weight forms of Acrp30/adiponectin. Proc Natl Acad Sci U S A 101:10308-13

Ishikawa M, Kitayama J, Nagawa H (2004) Enhanced expression of leptin and leptin receptor (OB-R) in human breast cancer. Clin Cancer Res 10:4325-31

Iyengar P, Combs TP, Shah SJ, Gouon-Evans V, Pollard JW, Albanese C, Flanagan L, Tenniswood MP, Guha C, Lisanti MP, Pestell RG, Scherer PE (2003) Adipocyte-secreted factors synergistically promote mammary tumorigenesis through induction of anti-apoptotic transcriptional programs and proto-oncogene stabilization. Oncogene 22:6408-23

Iyengar P, Espina V, Williams TW, Lin Y, Berry D, Jelicks LA, Lee H, Temple K, Graves R, Pollard J, Chopra N, Russell RG, Sasisekharan R, Trock BJ, Lippman M, Calvert VS, Petricoin EF, 3rd, Liotta L, Dadachova E, Pestell RG, Lisanti MP, Bonaldo P, Scherer PE (2005) Adipocyte-derived collagen VI affects early mammary tumor progression in vivo, demonstrating a critical interaction in the tumor/stroma microenvironment. The Journal of clinical investigation 115:1163-76

Jarde T, Caldefie-Chezet F, Damez M, Mishellany F, Buechler C, Bernard-Gallon D, Penault-Llorca F, Guillot J, Vasson MP (2008a) Antagonistic proliferative activities of adiponectin and leptin in breast cancer: study on MCF7 cells. Proc Nutr Soc 67:E184

Jarde T, Caldefie-Chezet F, Damez M, Mishellany F, Penault-Llorca F, Guillot J, Vasson MP (2008b) Leptin and leptin receptor involvement in cancer development: a study on human primary breast carcinoma. Oncol Rep 19:905-11

Jarde T, Perrier S, Vasson MP, Caldefie-Chezet F (2011) Molecular mechanisms of leptin and adiponectin in breast cancer. Eur J Cancer 47:33-43

Jin D, Guo H, Bu SY, Zhang Y, Hannaford J, Mashek DG, Chen X (2010) Lipocalin 2 is a selective modulator of peroxisome proliferator-activated receptor-gamma activation and function in lipid homeostasis and energy expenditure. FASEB J 25:754-64

Jin T, George Fantus I, Sun J (2008) Wnt and beyond Wnt: multiple mechanisms control the transcriptional property of beta-catenin. Cell Signal 20:1697-704

Jotzu C, Alt E, Welte G, Li J, Hennessy BT, Devarajan E, Krishnappa S, Pinilla S, Droll L, Song YH (2010) Adipose tissue-derived stem cells differentiate into carcinoma-associated fibroblast-like cells under the influence of tumor-derived factors. Anal Cell Pathol (Amst) 33:61-79

Kadowaki T, Yamauchi T, Kubota N, Hara K, Ueki K, Tobe K (2006) Adiponectin and adiponectin receptors in insulin resistance, diabetes, and the metabolic syndrome. The Journal of clinical investigation 116:1784-92

Kanaka-Gantenbein C, Margeli A, Pervanidou P, Sakka S, Mastorakos G, Chrousos GP, Papassotiriou I (2008) Retinol-binding protein 4 and lipocalin-2 in childhood and adolescent obesity: when children are not just "small adults". Clin Chem 54:1176-82

Kang JH, Lee YY, Yu BY, Yang BS, Cho KH, Yoon do K, Roh YK (2005) Adiponectin induces growth arrest and apoptosis of MDA-MB-231 breast cancer cell. Arch Pharm Res 28:1263-9

Katoh A, Watzlaf VJ, D'Amico F (1994) An examination of obesity and breast cancer survival in post-menopausal women. Br J Cancer 70:928-33

Kelesidis T, Kelesidis I, Chou S, Mantzoros CS (2011) Narrative review: the role of leptin in human physiology: emerging clinical applications. Ann Intern Med 152:93-100

Kim KY, Baek A, Hwang JE, Choi YA, Jeong J, Lee MS, Cho DH, Lim JS, Kim KI, Yang Y (2009) Adiponectin-activated AMPK stimulates dephosphorylation of AKT through protein phosphatase 2A activation. Cancer Res 69:4018-26

Korner A, Pazaitou-Panayiotou K, Kelesidis T, Kelesidis I, Williams CJ, Kaprara A, Bullen J, Neuwirth A, Tseleni S, Mitsiades N, Kiess W, Mantzoros CS (2007) Total and high-molecular-weight adiponectin in breast cancer: in vitro and in vivo studies. J Clin Endocrinol Metab 92:1041-8

Lam JB, Chow KH, Xu A, Lam KS, Liu J, Wong NS, Moon RT, Shepherd PR, Cooper GJ, Wang Y (2009) Adiponectin haploinsufficiency promotes mammary tumor development in MMTV-PyVT mice by modulation of phosphatase and tensin homolog activities. PLoS One 4:e4968

Landskroner-Eiger S, Qian B, Muise ES, Nawrocki AR, Berger JP, Fine EJ, Koba W, Deng Y, Pollard JW, Scherer PE (2009) Proangiogenic contribution of adiponectin toward mammary tumor growth in vivo. Clin Cancer Res 15:3265-76

Laud K, Gourdou I, Pessemesse L, Peyrat JP, Djiane J (2002) Identification of leptin receptors in human breast cancer: functional activity in the T47-D breast cancer cell line. Mol Cell Endocrinol 188:219-26

Law IK, Xu A, Lam KS, Berger T, Mak TW, Vanhoutte PM, Liu JT, Sweeney G, Zhou M, Yang B, Wang Y (2010) Lipocalin-2 deficiency attenuates insulin resistance associated with aging and obesity. Diabetes 59:872-82

Lee WM, Lu S, Medline A, Archer MC (2001) Susceptibility of lean and obese Zucker rats to tumorigenesis induced by N-methyl-N-nitrosourea. Cancer Lett 162:155-60

Lee YH, Lee SH, Jung ES, Kim JS, Shim CY, Ko YG, Choi D, Jang Y, Chung N, Ha JW (2010) Visceral adiposity and the severity of coronary artery disease in middle-aged subjects with normal waist circumference and its relation with lipocalin-2 and MCP-1. Atherosclerosis 213:592-7

Leng X, Ding T, Lin H, Wang Y, Hu L, Hu J, Feig B, Zhang W, Pusztai L, Symmans WF, Wu Y, Arlinghaus RB (2009) Inhibition of lipocalin 2 impairs breast tumorigenesis and metastasis. Cancer research 69:8579-84

Leng X, Wu Y, Arlinghaus RB (2011) Relationships of lipocalin 2 with breast tumorigenesis and metastasis. J Cell Physiol 226:309-14

Li G, Cong L, Gasser J, Zhao J, Chen K, Li F (2011) Mechanisms underlying the anti-proliferative actions of adiponectin in human breast cancer cells, MCF7-dependency on the cAMP/protein kinase-A pathway. Nutr Cancer 63:80-8

Liu J, Lam JB, Chow KH, Xu A, Lam KS, Moon RT, Wang Y (2008) Adiponectin stimulates Wnt inhibitory factor-1 expression through epigenetic regulations involving the transcription factor specificity protein 1. Carcinogenesis

Livasy CA, Perou CM, Karaca G, Cowan DW, Maia D, Jackson S, Tse CK, Nyante S, Millikan RC (2007) Identification of a basal-like subtype of breast ductal carcinoma in situ. Hum Pathol 38:197-204

Lorincz AM, Sukumar S (2006) Molecular links between obesity and breast cancer. Endocr Relat Cancer 13:279-92

Magoffin DA, Weitsman SR, Aagarwal SK, Jakimiuk AJ (1999) Leptin regulation of aromatase activity in adipose stromal cells from regularly cycling women. Ginekol Pol 70:1-7

Manabe Y, Toda S, Miyazaki K, Sugihara H (2003) Mature adipocytes, but not preadipocytes, promote the growth of breast carcinoma cells in collagen gel matrix culture through cancer-stromal cell interactions. J Pathol 201:221-8

Mantzoros C, Petridou E, Dessypris N, Chavelas C, Dalamaga M, Alexe DM, Papadiamantis Y, Markopoulos C, Spanos E, Chrousos G, Trichopoulos D (2004) Adiponectin and breast cancer risk. J Clin Endocrinol Metab 89:1102-7

Markowska A, Malendowicz K, Drews K (2004) The role of leptin in breast cancer. Eur J Gynaecol Oncol 25:192-4

McTiernan A (2003) Behavioral risk factors in breast cancer: can risk be modified? Oncologist 8:326-34

McTiernan A (2005) Obesity and cancer: the risks, science, and potential management strategies. Oncology (Williston Park) 19:871-81; discussion 881-2, 885-6

Meng L, Zhou J, Sasano H, Suzuki T, Zeitoun KM, Bulun SE (2001) Tumor necrosis factor alpha and interleukin 11 secreted by malignant breast epithelial cells inhibit adipocyte differentiation by selectively down-regulating CCAAT/enhancer binding protein alpha and peroxisome proliferator-activated receptor gamma: mechanism of desmoplastic reaction. Cancer research 61:2250-5

Miller FR, Medina D, Heppner GH (1981) Preferential growth of mammary tumors in intact mammary fatpads. Cancer Res 41:3863-7

Miyoshi Y, Funahashi T, Kihara S, Taguchi T, Tamaki Y, Matsuzawa Y, Noguchi S (2003) Association of serum adiponectin levels with breast cancer risk. Clin Cancer Res 9:5699-704

Moreno-Navarrete JM, Manco M, Ibanez J, Garcia-Fuentes E, Ortega F, Gorostiaga E, Vendrell J, Izquierdo M, Martinez C, Nolfe G, Ricart W, Mingrone G, Tinahones F, Fernandez-Real JM (2010) Metabolic endotoxemia and saturated fat contribute to circulating NGAL concentrations in subjects with insulin resistance. Int J Obes (Lond) 34:240-9

Mori K, Lee HT, Rapoport D, Drexler IR, Foster K, Yang J, Schmidt-Ott KM, Chen X, Li JY, Weiss S, Mishra J, Cheema FH, Markowitz G, Suganami T, Sawai K, Mukoyama M, Kunis C, D'Agati V, Devarajan P, Barasch J (2005) Endocytic delivery of lipocalin-siderophore-iron complex rescues the kidney from ischemia-reperfusion injury. J Clin Invest 115:610-21

Mrusek S, Classen-Linke I, Vloet A, Beier HM, Krusche CA (2005) Estradiol and medroxyprogesterone acetate regulated genes in T47D breast cancer cells. Mol Cell Endocrinol 235:39-50

Nakayama S, Miyoshi Y, Ishihara H, Noguchi S (2008) Growth-inhibitory effect of adiponectin via adiponectin receptor 1 on human breast cancer cells through inhibition of S-phase entry without inducing apoptosis. Breast Cancer Res Treat 112:405-10

Naviglio S, Di Gesto D, Romano M, Sorrentino A, Illiano F, Sorvillo L, Abbruzzese A, Marra M, Caraglia M, Chiosi E, Spina A, Illiano G (2009) Leptin enhances growth inhibition by cAMP elevating agents through apoptosis of MDA-MB-231 breast cancer cells. Cancer Biol Ther 8:1183-90

Oksanen L, Ohman M, Heiman M, Kainulainen K, Kaprio J, Mustajoki P, Koivisto V, Koskenvuo M, Janne OA, Peltonen L, Kontula K (1997) Markers for the gene ob and serum leptin levels in human morbid obesity. Hum Genet 99:559-64

Ozbay T, Nahta R (2008) A novel unidirectional cross-talk from the insulin-like growth factor-I receptor to leptin receptor in human breast cancer cells. Mol Cancer Res 6:1052-8

Pajvani UB, Scherer PE (2003) Adiponectin: systemic contributor to insulin sensitivity. Curr Diab Rep 3:207-13

Palianopoulou M, Papanikolaou V, Stefanou N, Tsezou A (2011) The activation of leptin-mediated survivin is limited by the inducible suppressor SOCS-3 in MCF-7 cells. Exp Biol Med (Maywood) 236:70-6

Paz-Filho G, Lim EL, Wong ML, Licinio J (2011) Associations between adipokines and obesity-related cancer. Front Biosci 16:1634-50

Pfeiler G, Hudelist G, Wulfing P, Mattsson B, Konigsberg R, Kubista E, Singer CF (2011) Impact of AdipoR1 expression on breast cancer development. Gynecol Oncol 117:134-8

Pfeiler G, Treeck O, Wenzel G, Goerse R, Hartmann A, Schmitz G, Ortmann O (2009) Influence of insulin resistance on adiponectin receptor expression in breast cancer. Maturitas 63:253-6

Pfeiler GH, Buechler C, Neumeier M, Schaffler A, Schmitz G, Ortmann O, Treeck O (2008) Adiponectin effects on human breast cancer cells are dependent on 17-beta estradiol. Oncol Rep 19:787-93

Polyak K, Kalluri R (2010) The role of the microenvironment in mammary gland development and cancer. Cold Spring Harb Perspect Biol 2:a003244

Prieto-Hontoria PL, Perez-Matute P, Fernandez-Galilea M, Bustos M, Martinez JA, Moreno-Aliaga MJ (2010) Role of obesity-associated dysfunctional adipose tissue in cancer: A molecular nutrition approach. Biochim Biophys Acta

Prosperi JR, Goss KH (2010) A Wnt-ow of opportunity: targeting the Wnt/beta-catenin pathway in breast cancer. Curr Drug Targets 11:1074-88

Radjainia M, Wang Y, Mitra AK (2008) Structural polymorphism of oligomeric adiponectin visualized by electron microscopy. J Mol Biol 381:419-30

Ray A, Cleary MP (2010) Leptin as a potential therapeutic target for breast cancer prevention and treatment. Expert Opin Ther Targets 14:443-51

Ray A, Nkhata KJ, Cleary MP (2007) Effects of leptin on human breast cancer cell lines in relationship to estrogen receptor and HER2 status. Int J Oncol 30:1499-509

Rene Gonzalez R, Watters A, Xu Y, Singh UP, Mann DR, Rueda BR, Penichet ML (2009) Leptin-signaling inhibition results in efficient anti-tumor activity in estrogen receptor positive or negative breast cancer. Breast Cancer Res 11:R36

Revillion F, Charlier M, Lhotellier V, Hornez L, Giard S, Baranzelli MC, Djiane J, Peyrat JP (2006) Messenger RNA expression of leptin and leptin receptors and their prognostic value in 322 human primary breast cancers. Clin Cancer Res 12:2088-94

Ryan AS, Berman DM, Nicklas BJ, Sinha M, Gingerich RL, Meneilly GS, Egan JM, Elahi D (2003) Plasma adiponectin and leptin levels, body composition, and glucose utilization in adult women with wide ranges of age and obesity. Diabetes Care 26:2383-8

Saxe GA, Rock CL, Wicha MS, Schottenfeld D (1999) Diet and risk for breast cancer recurrence and survival. Breast Cancer Res Treat 53:241-53

Saxena NK, Taliaferro-Smith L, Knight BB, Merlin D, Anania FA, O'Regan RM, Sharma D (2008) Bidirectional crosstalk between leptin and insulin-like growth factor-I signaling promotes invasion and migration of breast cancer cells via transactivation of epidermal growth factor receptor. Cancer Res 68:9712-22

Saxena NK, Vertino PM, Anania FA, Sharma D (2007) leptin-induced growth stimulation of breast cancer cells involves recruitment of histone acetyltransferases and mediator complex to CYCLIN D1 promoter via activation of Stat3. J Biol Chem 282:13316-25

Schaffler A, Scholmerich J, Buechler C (2007) Mechanisms of disease: adipokines and breast cancer - endocrine and paracrine mechanisms that connect adiposity and breast cancer. Nature clinical practice. Endocrinology & metabolism 3:345-54

Scherer PE, Williams S, Fogliano M, Baldini G, Lodish HF (1995) A novel serum protein similar to C1q, produced exclusively in adipocytes. J Biol Chem 270:26746-9

Seth P, Porter D, Lahti-Domenici J, Geng Y, Richardson A, Polyak K (2002) Cellular and molecular targets of estrogen in normal human breast tissue. Cancer Res 62:4540-4

Sheffield L (2008) Malignant transformation of mammary epithelial cells increases expression of leptin and leptin receptor. Endocr Res 33:111-8

Sheffield LG, Welsch CW (1988) Transplantation of human breast epithelia to mammary-gland-free fat-pads of athymic nude mice: influence of mammotrophic hormones on growth of breast epithelia. Int J Cancer 41:713-9

Shi H, Gu Y, Yang J, Xu L, Mi W, Yu W (2008) Lipocalin 2 promotes lung metastasis of murine breast cancer cells. J Exp Clin Cancer Res 27:83

Sinicrope FA, Dannenberg AJ (2011) Obesity and breast cancer prognosis: weight of the evidence. J Clin Oncol 29:4-7

Soma D, Kitayama J, Yamashita H, Miyato H, Ishikawa M, Nagawa H (2008) Leptin augments proliferation of breast cancer cells via transactivation of HER2. J Surg Res 149:9-14

Sommer G, Weise S, Kralisch S, Lossner U, Bluher M, Stumvoll M, Fasshauer M (2009) Lipocalin-2 is induced by interleukin-1beta in murine adipocytes in vitro. J Cell Biochem 106:103-8

Stoesz SP, Friedl A, Haag JD, Lindstrom MJ, Clark GM, Gould MN (1998) Heterogeneous expression of the lipocalin NGAL in primary breast cancers. International journal of cancer. Journal international du cancer 79:565-72

Strong RK, Bratt T, Cowland JB, Borregaard N, Wiberg FC, Ewald AJ (1998) Expression, purification, crystallization and crystallographic characterization of dimeric and monomeric human neutrophil gelatinase associated lipocalin (NGAL). Acta Crystallogr D Biol Crystallogr 54:93-5

Subbaramaiah K, Howe LR, Bhardwaj P, Du B, Gravaghi C, Yantiss RK, Zhou XK, Blaho VA, Hla T, Yang P, Kopelovich L, Hudis CA, Dannenberg AJ (2011) Obesity is associated with inflammation and elevated aromatase expression in the mouse mammary gland. Cancer Prev Res (Phila) 4:329-46

Surmacz E (2007) Obesity hormone leptin: a new target in breast cancer? Breast Cancer Res 9:301

Takahata C, Miyoshi Y, Irahara N, Taguchi T, Tamaki Y, Noguchi S (2007) Demonstration of adiponectin receptors 1 and 2 mRNA expression in human breast cancer cells. Cancer Lett 250:229-36

Taliaferro-Smith L, Nagalingam A, Zhong D, Zhou W, Saxena NK, Sharma D (2009) LKB1 is required for adiponectin-mediated modulation of AMPK-S6K axis and inhibition of migration and invasion of breast cancer cells. Oncogene 28:2621-33

van Dam RM, Hu FB (2007) Lipocalins and insulin resistance: etiological role of retinol-binding protein 4 and lipocalin-2? Clin Chem 53:5-7

van Kruijsdijk RC, van der Wall E, Visseren FL (2009) Obesity and cancer: the role of dysfunctional adipose tissue. Cancer Epidemiol Biomarkers Prev 18:2569-78

Vona-Davis L, Howard-McNatt M, Rose DP (2007) Adiposity, type 2 diabetes and the metabolic syndrome in breast cancer. Obes Rev 8:395-408

Vona-Davis L, Rose DP (2007) Adipokines as endocrine, paracrine, and autocrine factors in breast cancer risk and progression. Endocrine-related cancer 14:189-206

Wang Y, Lam JB, Lam KS, Liu J, Lam MC, Hoo RL, Wu D, Cooper GJ, Xu A (2006a) Adiponectin modulates the glycogen synthase kinase-3beta/beta-catenin signaling pathway and attenuates mammary tumorigenesis of MDA-MB-231 cells in nude mice. Cancer Res 66:11462-70

Wang Y, Lam KS, Chan L, Chan KW, Lam JB, Lam MC, Hoo RC, Mak WW, Cooper GJ, Xu A (2006b) Posttranslational modifications on the four conserved lysine residues within the collagenous domain of adiponectin are required for the formation of its high-molecular-weight oligomeric complex. J Biol Chem

Wang Y, Lam KS, Kraegen EW, Sweeney G, Zhang J, Tso AW, Chow WS, Wat NM, Xu JY, Hoo RL, Xu A (2007a) Lipocalin-2 is an inflammatory marker closely associated with obesity, insulin resistance, and hyperglycemia in humans. Clin Chem 53:34-41

Wang Y, Lam KS, Xu A (2007b) Adiponectin as a negative regulator in obesity-related mammary carcinogenesis. Cell Res 17:280-2

Wang Y, Lam KS, Xu JY, Lu G, Xu LY, Cooper GJ, Xu A (2005a) Adiponectin inhibits cell proliferation by interacting with several growth factors in an oligomerization-dependent manner. The Journal of biological chemistry 280:18341-7

Wang Y, Lam KS, Xu JY, Lu G, Xu LY, Cooper GJ, Xu A (2005b) Adiponectin inhibits cell proliferation by interacting with several growth factors in an oligomerization-dependent manner. J Biol Chem 280:18341-7

Wang Y, Lam KS, Yau MH, Xu A (2008) Post-translational modifications of adiponectin: mechanisms and functional implications. Biochem J 409:623-33

Wang Y, Xu A, Knight C, Xu LY, Cooper GJ (2002) Hydroxylation and glycosylation of the four conserved lysine residues in the collagenous domain of adiponectin. Potential role in the modulation of its insulin-sensitizing activity. J Biol Chem 277:19521-9

Wang Y, Zhou M, Lam KS, Xu A (2009) Protective roles of adiponectin in obesity-related fatty liver diseases: mechanisms and therapeutic implications. Arq Bras Endocrinol Metabol 53:201-12

Wiseman BS, Werb Z (2002) Stromal effects on mammary gland development and breast cancer. Science 296:1046-9

Wolf I, Sadetzki S, Catane R, Karasik A, Kaufman B (2005) Diabetes mellitus and breast cancer. Lancet Oncol 6:103-11

Wysocki PJ, Wierusz-Wysocka B (2010) Obesity, hyperinsulinemia and breast cancer: novel targets and a novel role for metformin. Expert Rev Mol Diagn 10:509-19

Yamauchi T, Kamon J, Ito Y, Tsuchida A, Yokomizo T, Kita S, Sugiyama T, Miyagishi M, Hara K, Tsunoda M, Murakami K, Ohteki T, Uchida S, Takekawa S, Waki H, Tsuno NH, Shibata Y, Terauchi Y, Froguel P, Tobe K, Koyasu S, Taira K, Kitamura T, Shimizu T, Nagai R, Kadowaki T (2003) Cloning of adiponectin receptors that mediate antidiabetic metabolic effects. Nature 423:762-9

Yan QW, Yang Q, Mody N, Graham TE, Hsu CH, Xu Z, Houstis NE, Kahn BB, Rosen ED (2007) The adipokine lipocalin 2 is regulated by obesity and promotes insulin resistance. Diabetes 56:2533-40

Yang J, Bielenberg DR, Rodig SJ, Doiron R, Clifton MC, Kung AL, Strong RK, Zurakowski D, Moses MA (2009) Lipocalin 2 promotes breast cancer progression. Proceedings of the National Academy of Sciences of the United States of America 106:3913-8

Yang J, Goetz D, Li JY, Wang W, Mori K, Setlik D, Du T, Erdjument-Bromage H, Tempst P, Strong R, Barasch J (2002) An iron delivery pathway mediated by a lipocalin. Mol Cell 10:1045-56

Yang J, Moses MA (2009) Lipocalin 2: a multifaceted modulator of human cancer. Cell Cycle 8:2347-52

Yin N, Wang D, Zhang H, Yi X, Sun X, Shi B, Wu H, Wu G, Wang X, Shang Y (2004) Molecular mechanisms involved in the growth stimulation of breast cancer cells by leptin. Cancer Res 64:5870-5

Yndestad A, Landro L, Ueland T, Dahl CP, Flo TH, Vinge LE, Espevik T, Froland SS, Husberg C, Christensen G, Dickstein K, Kjekshus J, Oie E, Gullestad L, Aukrust P (2009) Increased systemic and myocardial expression of neutrophil gelatinase-associated lipocalin in clinical and experimental heart failure. Eur Heart J 30:1229-36

Yokota T, Oritani K, Takahashi I, Ishikawa J, Matsuyama A, Ouchi N, Kihara S, Funahashi T, Tenner AJ, Tomiyama Y, Matsuzawa Y (2000) Adiponectin, a new member of the family of soluble defense collagens, negatively regulates the growth of myelomonocytic progenitors and the functions of macrophages. Blood 96:1723-32

Zhang J, Wu Y, Zhang Y, Leroith D, Bernlohr DA, Chen X (2008) The role of lipocalin 2 in the regulation of inflammation in adipocytes and macrophages. Mol Endocrinol 22:1416-26

Zhang Y, Proenca R, Maffei M, Barone M, Leopold L, Friedman JM (1994) Positional cloning of the mouse obese gene and its human homologue. Nature 372:425-32

Zhou W, Guo S, Gonzalez-Perez RR (2011) Leptin pro-angiogenic signature in breast cancer is linked to IL-1 signalling. Br J Cancer 104:128-37

Part 2

Biology – High Throughput Approaches

Comparison of Genome Aberrations Between Early-Onset and Late-Onset Breast Cancer

Ming-Ta Hsu et al.*
Institute of Biochemistry and Molecular Biology, VGH-YM Genome Center, National Yang-Ming University, Taipei, Taiwan

1. Introduction

Breast cancer is the most common cancer and the second leading cause of cancer deaths in women worldwide. Breast cancer statistics in the US shows a bimodal distribution consisting of early-onset and late-onset patients. Although the incidence of early-onset breast cancer in western population is low, the survival rate is significantly poorer before 40 years old (Yankaskas, 2005). Bonnier and his colleagues showed that the breast cancer patients under 35 years old also have poorer prognostic and possess the following characteristics: (1) a higher frequency of undifferentiated tumors, (2) histoprognostic grade-III cancer, (3) microscopic lymph-node involvement and (4) negative hormonal receptor status (Bonnier et al., 1995).

Although incidence rate of breast cancer has been decreasing in the US, this happens only in the late-onset age group (Benz, 2008). Asian women have significant lower incidence rate of breast cancer (about 25/100000 in Eastern Asia) than the western countries (about 90/100000 in Western Europe) but the rate of incidence is increasing steadily with the improvement of economics in the area. In Taiwan, the incidence of breast cancer has dramatically increased from about 13/100000 in 1980 to 49/100000 in 2005 (Chang et al., 2008). The increase in breast cancer in Asia is different from that of western countries in that the incidence of premenopausal breast cancer is proportionally higher in the Asian women. Similar trend of early-onset breast cancer is found in Africa (Kruger et al., 2007).

According to clinical statistics, breast cancer patients in Taiwan are mainly identified 10 years younger than their counterparts in the western countries. Compared with the late-onset group, the early-onset breast cancer (age < or = 40) has a more aggressive clinical behavior, and its five-year survival rate for each stage is much poorer. One unique feature in

*Ching Cheng[1], Chian-Feng, Chen[2],Yiin-Jeng Jong[4], Chien-Yi Tung[3], Yann-Jang Chen[4], Sheng Wang-Wuu[4], Ling-Hui Li[4], Shih-Feng Tsai[4], Mei-Hua Tsou[5], Skye H. Cheng[5], Chii-Ming Chen[5], Andrew T. Huang[5], Chi-Hung Lin[3] and Ming-Ta Hsu[1,2]
[1]*Institute of Biochemistry and Molecular Biology, National Yang-Ming University, Taipei, Taiwan*
[2]*VGH-YM Genome Center, National Yang-Ming University, Taipei, Taiwan*
[3] *Institute of Microbiology and Immunology, National Yang-Ming University, Taipei, Taiwan*
[4]*Institute of Genome Sciences, National Yang-Ming University, Taipei, Taiwan*
[5]*Koo Foundation Sun Yat-Sen Cancer Center, Taipei, Taiwan*

Taiwan is the large proportion of early-onset breast cancer (Cheng et al., 2000). Compared with the late-onset group, the early-onset breast cancer (age < or = 40) has a more aggressive clinical behavior, and its five-year survival rate for each stage is much poorer. The early-onset breast cancer has poorer prognostic features. Standard pathologic factors are not good predictors of their outcome. Several studies have correlated the breast cancer subtypes with early-onset breast cancer recently(Anders et al., 2008; Lin et al., 2009; Sorlie et al., 2003; Sotiriou et al., 2003). The classification of subtypes has been shown to provide prognostic information and etiologic mechanisms of breast cancer. In Taiwan, the young women breast cancer tends to be more luminal A type with higher ER and PR expression and less basal-like subtype than that of the older women (Cheng et al., 2000; Lin et al., 2009), but with higher risk of second primary malignancy and worse prognosis (Lee et al., 2008; Mellemkjaer et al., 2006; Yu et al., 2006). This feature is quite distinct from that of western developed countries with high prevalence of more aggressive basal-like breast cancer in young women. In western populations, younger women are more likely to have biologically aggressive breast cancer as shown by higher proportions of ER-negative and histologic grade III tumors compared with older patients (Anderson et al., 2002; Anderson et al., 2001; Colleoni et al., 2002). Anders and the colleagues also reported that more aggressive subtypes, such as basal-like subtype, would be over-represented among breast cancer arising in early-onset patients, whereas older women would more commonly be diagnosed with luminal tumors in the USA (Anders et al., 2011). The increasing incidence of breast cancer in the young women population is worrisome since they constitute a major labor force and are also potential mothers who need to take care of young children. It is therefore important to understand the epidemiological as well as genetic origin of the rising incidence of early-onset breast cancer with possible implications in prevention as well as diagnostic/prognostic applications.

Etiological factors of breast cancer are complex. Reproductive history, diet, alcohol, and body size among others have been implicated (Jevtic et al., 2010; McTiernan et al., 2010; Phipps et al., 2011). Among these factors reproductive history has been found to be strongly correlated with breast cancer is reproductive history. Since the early observation of high incidence of breast cancer among nuns in eighteenth century nulliparity and older age at first birth have been strongly associated with incidence of breast cancer (Butt et al., 2009; Muti, 2005; Trichopoulos et al., 2008; Wu et al., 2011; Yaghjyan and Colditz, 2011). Both nulliparity and older age pregnancy and child birth are characteristics of developed countries and countries with rapid economic growth as in Taiwan. This may partly explain the rapid rise of this disease here.

The association of reproductive history and breast cancer might be understood from hormone target theory (Adami et al., 1995; Adami et al., 1998; Cerliani et al., 2011; Trepp et al., 2010). Mammary gland formation consists of three stages: *organogenesis,* which grows from terminal end bud (TEB) to non-pregnant primary ductal system with cuboidal epithelial cells and is stimulated by prolactin; mature gland formation, with highly branched ducts and lobular buds; pregnancy gland formation, through the stimulation of several hormones with differentiation of lobular buds into fully differentiated type III lobules with milk secreting columnal cells. These complicated differentiation processes involve temporal controls from hormones, cytokines, specific transcription factors, growth factors as well as contribution from stromal elements including myoepithelial cells, base membrane and a collection of integrins (Ahmad and Kumar, 2011; Chen and Capecchi, 1999; Chodosh et al., 1999; Flucke et al., 2010; Howell and Evans, 2011; Li et al., 2010; Okoh et al.,

2011; Tamimi et al., 2011). As a major organ involved in pregnancy the major player in mammary gland development is hormone. Induction of cell differentiation by hormone during pregnancy provides protection against tumorigenesis because the epithelial cells become fully differentiated and are not susceptible to carcinogens. This explains the role of parity in breast cancer. The better protection for earlier pregnancy can be explained by the smaller hormone targets and the less chance to accumulate deranged cells.

According to the hormone target theory, stimulation of cell growth of undifferentiated epithelial cells in immature mammary gland may provide a mechanism for early-onset breast cancer. The predominance of immature epithelial cells in embryo provides the target for the initiation of tumorigenesis when intrauterine hormone concentration is high. Indeed, animal studies showed that undifferentiated TEB is the most susceptible to carcinogen for the formation of tumor (Bai and Rohrschneider, 2010; Roussos et al., 2010; Russo and Russo, 1994). Recent evidence even points to the immature gland in utero as the target for the initiation of breast cancer (Brisken and O'Malley, 2010; Hardy et al., 2010; Hilakivi-Clarke and Clarke, 1998; Sanderson et al., 1998; Torres-Arzayus et al., 2010).

Although there is intensive study of the genetic pathways involved in breast tumorigenesis, the genetic basis of the breast cancer in young women and the differences between early-onset and late-onset tumors remain largely unknown. The different pathological features of the two types of cancer suggest that they have different genetic origin. In order to explore the genetic basis of early-onset and late-onset breast cancer, we analyzed the candidate genes associated with the chromosomal aberrations in these two types of cancer from data in the public domain as well as from our own array-CGH data from the patients in Taiwan through literature search of involvement of genes in the aberration regions. Furthermore, the differential gene expression of these two types of cancer is analyzed by SAGE technique to deduce the genes that may be specifically related to early-onset cancer.

2. Comparison of genomic aberrations between early- and late-onset breast cancer

Breast cancer frequently contains amplification in several regions of chromosomes. Recent advances in high resolution array-CGH analysis and the availability of human genome sequence enabled finding candidate genes involved in breast cancer from these chromosomal aberration regions. We are interested in studying genes associated with early-onset (age <40) breast cancer which has become a major health concern in Taiwan. Early-onset breast cancer has poor prognosis compared with late-onset (age >70) breast cancer and genomics analysis indicated that they have different chromosomal and genetic aberration profiles, suggesting they have different origins. In this article we summarized the current candidate genes involved in breast cancer from genomic data and presented data on genetic differences between the two types of breast cancer. The possible implication in the genetic differences is discussed.

2.1 Review of chromosome aberrations in early- and late-onset breast cancer and candidate genes associated with tumorigenesis

To explore the genes differentially associated with early-onset and late-onset breast cancers, we first collected the aCGH data in the Progenetix database (www.progenetix.net) (Baudis and Cleary, 2001; Boldt et al., 2010; Fridlyand et al., 2006; Reis-Filho et al., 2005) and reanalyzed the data. All the samples were regrouped based on the age of patients: younger and elder groups were defined as less than 46 and more than 70 years old respectively. Then the frequency of copy number gains or losses (y axis) were plotted with the probes along with the chromosome order (x axis). As the frequency lower than 10% may reflect the randomly change dues to the genomic instability of tumor, we define gain or loss more than 30% as significant aberrations. Early or late onset-specific aberrations were defined as gain or loss more than 30% and higher than the other group at least 15%. When these data are lined up chromosome-by-chromosome (Fig. 1), regions of chromosome aberrations common to both groups as well as specific to each group can be discerned (Table 1). Genes within each regions identified are then examined through literature search to identify candidate genes involved in breast carcinogenesis (Table 2, and 3). Genes that are either down-related or suppress tumorigenesis are in italic.

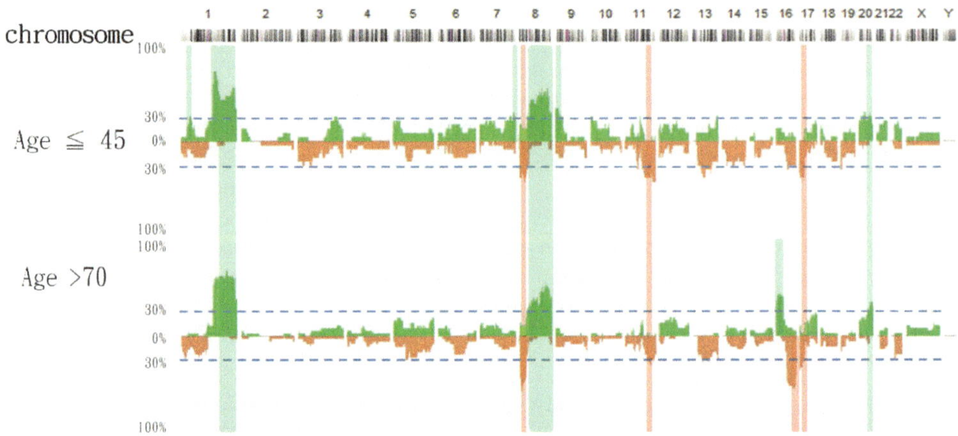

Fig. 1. Chromosome aberrations in early- and late-onset breast cancer.

	Gains		Losses	
Early onset	Ch1	41~42Mb	-	-
	Ch1	148~157Mb	-	-
	Ch3	161~172Mb	-	-
	Ch7	150~151Mb	-	-
	Ch9	0~14Mb	-	-
	Ch13	103~112Mb	-	-
Late onset	Ch16	7~25Mb	Ch16	74~81Mb
Common	Ch1	175~247Mb	Ch8	3~32Mb
	Ch8	48~114Mb	Ch11	108~114Mb
	Ch20	50~51Mb	Ch17	0~9Mb

Table 1. Aberrant chromosomal regions in Breast Cancer Patients.

Early-onset	**GAINS**	Chr1 ***41~42Mb***	MIRN30E
		Chr1 148~157Mb	ECM1, HORMAD1, CTSS, CTSK, ARNT, PRUNE, S100A10, S100A11, FLG, HAX1, PYGO2, CKS1B, ADAM15, MUC1, NES, NTRK1
		Chr3 161~172Mb	PRKCI, SKIL
		Chr7 150~151Mb	ABCF2, RHEB *KCNH2*
		Chr9 0-14Mb	VLDLR
Late-onset	**GAINS**	***Chr16*** *7~25Mb*	CIITA, SOCS1 *MIRN193B, PALB2*
	LOSSES	***Chr16*** *74~81Mb*	CNTNAP4, ADAMTS18, WWOX, HSD17B2

Table 2. Aberrations in early-and late-onset breast cancer.

Totally, there are 6 early-onset specific gains on the chromosomes 1 (41-42Mb; 148-157Mb), 3 (161-172Mb), 7 (150-151), 9 (0-14Mb) and 13 (103-112Mb), one late-onset specific gain on chromosome 16(7-25Mb), three common gains on chromosomes 1 (175-247Mb), 8 (48-114Mb) and 20 (50-51Mb). There is a late-onset specific loss in chromosome 16 (74-81Mb) and common loss on chromosomes 8 (3-32Mb), 11 (108-114Mb) and 17 (0-9Mb). Genes that have been shown to be involved in breast carcinogenesis in these regions through literature search are listed in Table 2 and 3.

Interestingly, the early onset-specific aberrations contain more IGF-1 and ER signaling associated genes than the late onset. Candidate genes present in the IGF-1, ER and TGF-beta pathways in both groups of breast cancer patients are listed in Table 4.

The association of ER genes with early-onset cancer is expected since these patients are premenopausal. Since IGF-1 pathway plays an important role in breast tumorigenesis, the genes specific for the late and early-onset cancer are depicted in Fig. 2 to illustrate their positions in the pathway.

2.2 Clustering of breast cancer related genes in chromosome regions

A striking feature of the analysis of genes associated with gain or loss in breast cancer chromosomes is that the regions often harbor breast cancer related genes in a cluster fashion and demarked by the presence of genes down-regulated or are anti-tumorigenic in breast cancer.

GAINS	***Chr1 175~247Mb***	PTGS2, PLA2G4A, RGS2, KIF14, LAD1, TIMM17A, ELF3, UBE2T, JARID1B, ADIPOR1, ADORA1, PCTK3, IKBKE, MAPKAPK2, CD55, CD46, NEK2, DTL, ATF3, ESRRG, GPATCH2, TGFB2, DUSP10, ENAH, EPHX1, PARP1, WNT9A, WNT3A, ARF1, EXO1, AKT3, SMYD3 *RGSL1, RNASEL, RGS16, BTG2, KISS1, RASSF5, IL10, LAMB3, IRF6, PROX1, PTPN14, TLR5, T53BP2, FH, CHM*
	Chr8 48~144Mb	SNAI2, LYN, SDCBP, ASPH, COPS5, PRDM14, NCOA2, TPD52, FABP5, E2F5, WWP1, CPNE3, MMP16, CCNE2 TSPYL5, MTDH, LAPTM4B, YWHAZ, CTHRC1, ANGPT1, EIF3E, EBAG9, TRPS1, RAD21, TNFRSF11B, HAS2, ATAD2, TRMT12, TATDN1, SQLE, MYC, PVT1, DDEF1, WISP1, PTP4A3 *CEBPD, PRKDC, RB1CC1, SOX17, CRH, VCPIP1, SGK3, SULF1, DECR1, TP53INP1, STK3, UBR5, DPYS, NOV, MTSS1, NDRG1*
LOSSES	***Chr8 3~32Mb***	ANGPT2, CTSB, EGR3, LOXL2, NKX3-1, STC1, CLU, PBK *CSMD1, MCPH1, MSRA, GATA4, DLC1, MTUS1, ASAH1, NAT1, PSD3, LZTS1, PDLIM2, RHOBTB2, BNIP3L, EPHX2, DUSP4, PPP2CB, WRN, NRG1*
	Chr11 108-114Mb	- *PPP2R1B*
	Chr17 0~9Mb	MYBBP1A, PELP1, PLD2, NUP88, *MIRN22, SMYD4, HIC1, MNT, ALOX15, CXCL16, PFN1, XAF1, MIRN195, MIRN497, CLDN7, GPS2, SHBG, ATP1B2, TP53*

Table 3. Aberrations in both early- and late-onset breast cancer.

	IGF-1 Signaling	Estrogen Receptor Signaling	TGF-Beta Signaling
Early onset specific aberrations	IRS2, JAK2, PRKAG2, PRKCI, SHC1	SHC1, HIST2H3C	
Late onset specific aberrations	SOCS1		
Common aberrations	AKT3, NOV, PIK3C2B, PIK3R5, PTK, YWHAE, YWHAZ	H3F3A/H3F3B, HIST3H3, MED30, MED31, NCOA2, PELP1, POLR2A, POLR2K, PRKDC, TAF2, TAF5L	TGFb2

Table 4. The relationship of aberrant genes and IGF-1, ER, and TGF- signal pathways.

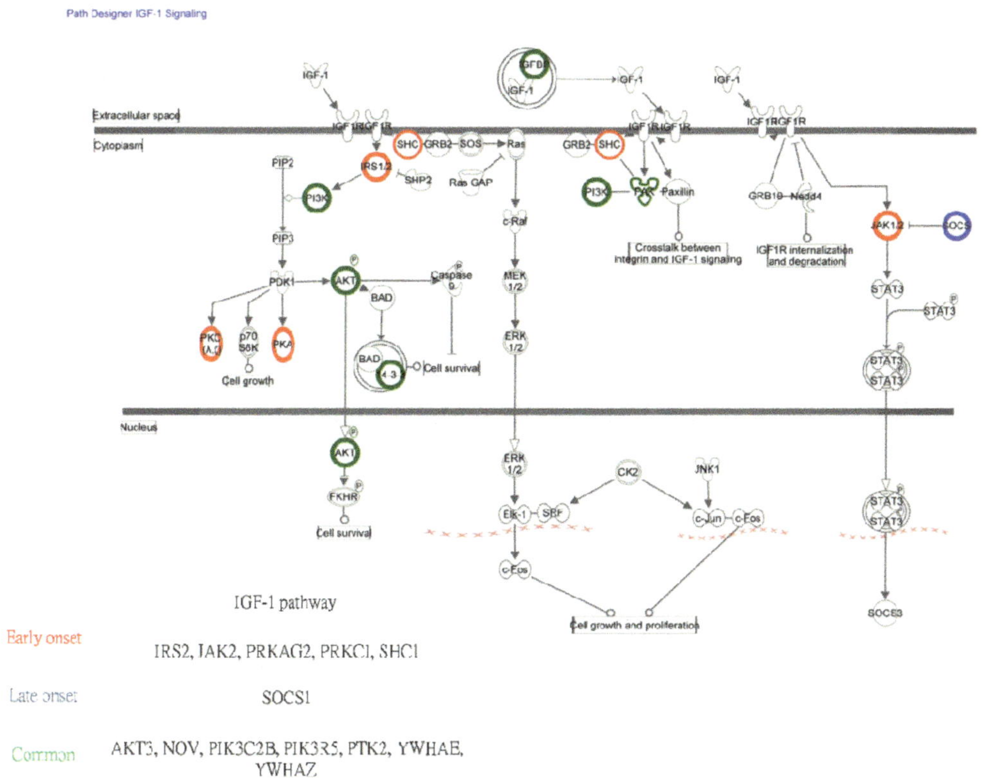

Fig. 2. IGF-1 signal pathway.

For example, 198-201Mb in 1q32.1 contains eight genes related to breast tumorigenesis, KLF14, LAD1, TIMM17A, ELF3, UBE2T, JARID1B, ADIPOR1 and ADORA1 as well as a gene CARP1 that is over-expressed in cancers (Fig. 3 shows the distribution of genes positively correlated with breast cancer as red line and negatively correlated with breast cancer as green). We also observed the clustering of the genes that inhibits breast tumorigenesis or are down-regulated in breast cancer in chr17 0-9Mb region that is often deleted in breast cancer. These are mir-22, SMYD4, HIC1, MNT, ALOX15, CLCX16, PFN1, XAF1, mir-195, mir-497, CLDN7, GPS2, SHBG, ATP1B2, and TP53. The pro- and anti-tumorigenesis genes are often found clustered together in a region of the chromosome.

2.3 Comparison of chromosome aberrations between early-onset and late-onset breast cancers in Taiwan

To investigate the gene aberrations between early-onset and late-onset breast cancer in Taiwan, we have used Vysis GenoSensor ™ Array 300 microarray chip, containing 378 target clone DNA (P1, BAC or PAC clones) representing regions that are important in cytogenetics and oncology, to analyze 15 early-onset and 15 late-onset breast cancer samples. The tissue samples of primary breast cancers were obtained by either biopsies or surgical excision from Koo Foundation Sun Yat- Sen Cancer Center (KF-SYSCC), Taipei, Taiwan. Instead of metaphase chromosome in conventional CGH, BAC or PAC DNAs are used as hybridization template in array- CGH, which can increase resolution up to approximate 100 kb.

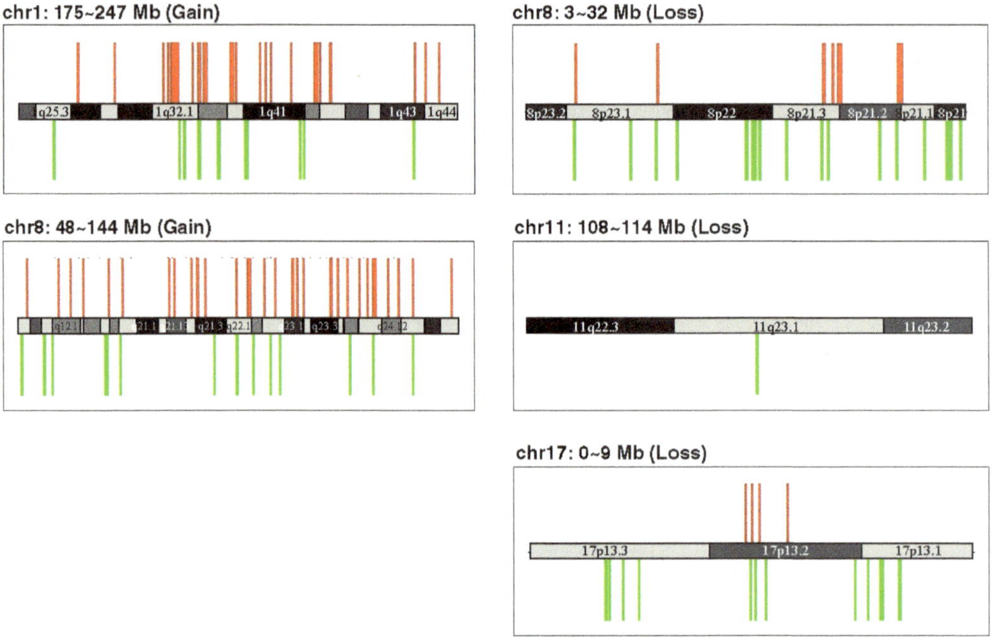

Fig. 3. Common genomic aberration in both early- and late-onset breast cancers. Left panel shows the amplified regions and right panel shows the deleted regions in breast cancers. The red and green lines represent the gene position in the genome. Red lines indicate genes positively correlated with breast cancer and green lines indicate negatively correlated with breast cancer.

The genes present in the most frequent gain or loss regions of early-onset and late-onset breast cancer in Taiwan were analyzed by array-CGH. The genes related to breast cancer in these regions are shown in Table 5. There are two regions differentially gained or loss in late-onset and three regions differentially gained or loss in early-onset. As in the results above, the regions are marked by the presence of both pro- and anti-tumor genes (in *italic*) except 17q23 which is amplified in a subset of early-onset cancer but in none of the late-onset cancer. We analyzed the genes of this region flanking our array-CGH BAC probes. It contains seven genes involved in breast tumorigenesis and represents a region of interest for early diagnosis of breast cancer in young women.

2.4 SAGE analysis of gene expression in early- and late-onset breast cancer in Taiwan

We analyzed 10325 SAGE Taq sequences, and classified SAGE data into two groups (evaluated significance by monte-carol algorthim). There are 460 genes related to the early-onset group, and 214 genes involved in late-onset breast cancer.

SAGE analysis found 12 breast cancer related genes highly prevalent in early-onset than late-onset. Among these genes, cytokeratin 5 and 17 are basal cell markers and are often found in basal-like and triple-negative breast cancer subtypes. Luminal specific cytokeratin KRT8 and KRT19 was also found to be enriched in early-onset cancer. This result suggests that there are two different subtypes, basal-like and luminal groups, of breast cancer in the early-onset samples we analyzed. Both tumor promoting and inhibiting genes are found expressed in the SAGE data. For example, KLK6 inhibits EMT and its expression is negatively correlated with breast cancer metastasis (Pampalakis et al., 2009) and FLNA (filamin A) is known to suppress breast cancer migration and invasion (Xu et al., 2010). The expression of the tumor suppressive CDH1, CDH13, CTNNB1, SFN, NDRG1 and PFN1 in early-onset tumor also suggests the less invasive nature. IGFBP4 is positively correlated with ER and PR but negatively correlated with Her2 and has better disease outcome (Mita et al., 2007). On the other hand, S100P and LCN2 promote breast cancer progression. Whether the expression of tumor suppressive genes reflects the more benign nature of the early-onset breast cancer or due to mutations in these genes remain to be studied. Genes associated with tumor progression, metastasis and poor prognosis such as CXCR4, ERBB2, TOB1, EZH2, HIF1A, S100A7, are found significantly more expressed in the late-onset breast cancer. The overall expression pattern suggests that the late-onset tumors are more advanced in tumorigenesis than that of the early-onset tumors which constitute mostly benign luminal A subtype in Taiwan.

Cyto Location	**Gene related to breast cancer**	**Early-onset (n=15)**	**Late-onset (n=15)**	***P*- value**
Gains				
16p13.3	MSLN, CACNA1H, PDPK1, SRMM2, TRAP1 *STUB1, TSC2, PKD1, ABCA3, DNAJA3*	6.67%	60.00%	0.0026
8q11	PRKDC, SNAI2 *CEBPD, MCM4, ST18, RB1CC1*	6.67%	46.67%	0.0176
16q23.2	-	53.33%	13.33%	0.0251
20q12-q13.1	PLCG1, ADA, WISP2, CD40, NCOA3, SULF2, PREX1 *PTPRT, MYBL2, SDC4, UBE2C*	53.33%	13.33%	0.0251
17q23	RPS6KB1, USP32, PAT1, PPM1D, BCAS3, TBX2, MRC2	26.67%	0.00%	0.0498
Losses				
1p36.22	-	6.67%	53.33%	0.0071
22qtel	*PARVB, PARVG, PRR5, FNLN1, PPARA, GRAMD4*	6.67%	46.67%	0.0176
1p13.1	VANGL1, VTCN1	0.00%	33.33%	0.0211
11q22.3	PDGFD, ALKBH8, RDX *CASP-12, -4, -5, -1, CUL5, ATM*	0.00%	26.67%	0.0498
Xq25	XIAP, SMARCA1, APLN *AIFMI*	0.00%	26.67%	0.0498

Table 5. Significant difference between early- and late-onset breast cancers by array-CGH (aberrant genes correlated with early- or late-onset breast cancers were evaluated by using the Fisher's exact test).

3. Conclusion

In this report we show that early-onset breast cancer has different genetic alterations as compared with that of late-onset cancer, suggesting that different molecular pathways are involved in the generation of these two types of cancer. The genes strongly associated with early-onset breast cancer such as those in 17q23 amplicon may be useful for deducing the molecular mechanism of breast cancer in young women as well as for serving as candidate biomarkers.

Early-onset breast cancer has been a major health concern and had poor prognosis compared with late-onset in Taiwan. We are interested in comparing the genome aberrations between early- and late-onset breast cancers. Although we study the genome aberrations in Taiwan, we also explore the public data which are associated with early-onset and late-onset breast cancers. The findings can help us to address early-onset breast cancer specific gene aberrations and explore the unique tumor biology in Taiwan through this broad view.

4. Acknowledgements

This work is supported by the program for Promoting Academic Excellence of Universities (Phase II, NSC 94-2752-B-010-001-PAE), by a grant from Ministry of Education. Aim for the Top University Plan and by the National Program and a grant from the National Research Program of Genomic Medicine (NSC94-3112-B-010-003 and NSC95-3112-B-010-012) from the National Science Council of Taiwan.

5. References

Adami, H.O., Lipworth, L., Titus-Ernstoff, L., Hsieh, C.C., Hanberg, A., Ahlborg, U., Baron, J., and Trichopoulos, D. (1995). Organochlorine compounds and estrogen-related cancers in women. *Cancer Causes Control* 6: 551-566.

Adami, H.O., Signorello, L.B., and Trichopoulos, D. (1998). Towards an understanding of breast cancer etiology. *Semin Cancer Biol* 8: 255-262.

Ahmad, N., and Kumar, R. (2011). Steroid hormone receptors in cancer development: a target for cancer therapeutics. *Cancer Lett* 300: 1-9.

Anders, C.K., Fan, C., Parker, J.S., Carey, L.A., Blackwell, K.L., Klauber-DeMore, N., and Perou, C.M. (2011). Breast carcinomas arising at a young age: unique biology or a surrogate for aggressive intrinsic subtypes? *J Clin Oncol* 29: e18-20.

Anders, C.K., Hsu, D.S., Broadwater, G., Acharya, C.R., Foekens, J.A., Zhang, Y., Wang, Y., Marcom, P.K., Marks, J.R., Febbo, P.G., *et al.* (2008). Young age at diagnosis correlates with worse prognosis and defines a subset of breast cancers with shared patterns of gene expression. *J Clin Oncol 26*: 3324-3330.

Anderson, W.F., Chatterjee, N., Ershler, W.B., and Brawley, O.W. (2002). Estrogen receptor breast cancer phenotypes in the Surveillance, Epidemiology, and End Results database. *Breast Cancer Res Treat 76*: 27-36.

Anderson, W.F., Chu, K.C., Chatterjee, N., Brawley, O., and Brinton, L.A. (2001). Tumor variants by hormone receptor expression in white patients with node-negative breast cancer from the surveillance, epidemiology, and end results database. J Clin Oncol *19*, 18-27.

Bai, L., and Rohrschneider, L.R. (2010). s-SHIP promoter expression marks activated stem cells in developing mouse mammary tissue. *Genes Dev* 24: 1882-1892.

Baudis, M., and Cleary, M.L. (2001). Progenetix.net: an online repository for molecular cytogenetic aberration data. *Bioinformatics* 17: 1228-1229.

Benz, C.C. (2008). Impact of aging on the biology of breast cancer. *Crit Rev Oncol Hematol* 66: 65-74.

Boldt, V., Stacher, E., Halbwedl, I., Popper, H., Hultschig, C., Moinfar, F., Ullmann, R., and Tavassoli, F.A. (2010). Positioning of necrotic lobular intraepithelial neoplasias (LIN, grade 3) within the sequence of breast carcinoma progression. *Genes Chromosomes Cancer* 49: 463-470.

Bonnier, P., Romain, S., Charpin, C., Lejeune, C., Tubiana, N., Martin, P.M., and Piana, L. (1995). Age as a prognostic factor in breast cancer: relationship to pathologic and biologic features. *Int J Cancer 62*: 138-144.

Brisken, C., and O'Malley, B. (2010). Hormone action in the mammary gland. *Cold Spring Harb Perspect Biol 2*: a003178.

Butt, S., Borgquist, S., Anagnostaki, L., Landberg, G., and Manjer, J. (2009). Parity and age at first childbirth in relation to the risk of different breast cancer subgroups. *Int J Cancer 125*: 1926-1934.

Cerliani, J.P., Guillardoy, T., Giulianelli, S., Vaque, J.P., Gutkind, J.S., Vanzulli, S.I., Martins, R., Zeitlin, E., Lamb, C.A., and Lanari, C. (2011). Interaction between FGFR-2, STAT5 and progesterone receptors in breast cancer. *Cancer Res.*

Chang, K.J., Kuo, W.H., and Wang, M.Y. (2008). The epidemiology of breast cancer in Taiwan. *J. Chinese Oncol. Soc.* 24: 85-93.

Chen, F., and Capecchi, M.R. (1999). Paralogous mouse Hox genes, Hoxa9, Hoxb9, and Hoxd9, function together to control development of the mammary gland in response to pregnancy. *Proc Natl Acad Sci U S A* 96: 541-546.

Cheng, S.H., Tsou, M.H., Liu, M.C., Jian, J.J., Cheng, J.C., Leu, S.Y., Hsieh, C.Y., and Huang, A.T. (2000). Unique features of breast cancer in Taiwan. *Breast Cancer Res Treat* 63: 213-223.

Chodosh, L.A., D'Cruz, C.M., Gardner, H.P., Ha, S.I., Marquis, S.T., Rajan, J.V., Stairs, D.B., Wang, J.Y., and Wang, M. (1999). Mammary gland development, reproductive history, and breast cancer risk. *Cancer Res* 59: 1765-1771s; discussion 1771s-1772s.

Colleoni, M., Rotmensz, N., Robertson, C., Orlando, L., Viale, G., Renne, G., Luini, A., Veronesi, P., Intra, M., Orecchia, R., *et al.* (2002). Very young women (<35 years) with operable breast cancer: features of disease at presentation. *Ann Oncol 13*: 273-279.

Flucke, U., Flucke, M.T., Hoy, L., Breuer, E., Goebbels, R., Rhiem, K., Schmutzler, R., Winzenried, H., Braun, M., Steiner, S., *et al.* (2010). Distinguishing medullary carcinoma of the breast from high-grade hormone receptor-negative invasive ductal carcinoma: an immunohistochemical approach. *Histopathology* 56: 852-859.

Fridlyand, J., Snijders, A.M., Ylstra, B., Li, H., Olshen, A., Segraves, R., Dairkee, S., Tokuyasu, T., Ljung, B.M., Jain, A.N., *et al.* (2006). Breast tumor copy number aberration phenotypes and genomic instability. *BMC Cancer* 6: 96.

Hardy, K.M., Booth, B.W., Hendrix, M.J., Salomon, D.S., and Strizzi, L. (2010). ErbB/EGF signaling and EMT in mammary development and breast cancer. *J Mammary Gland Biol Neoplasia* 15: 191-199.

Hilakivi-Clarke, L., and Clarke, R. (1998). Timing of dietary fat exposure and mammary tumorigenesis: role of estrogen receptor and protein kinase C activity. *Mol Cell Biochem* 188: 5-12.

Howell, A., and Evans, G.D. (2011). Hormone replacement therapy and breast cancer. *Recent Results Cancer Res* 188: 115-124.

Jevtic, M., Velicki, R., Popovic, M., Cemerlic-Adjic, N., Babovic, S.S., and Velicki, L. (2010). Dietary influence on breast cancer. *J BUON 15*: 455-461.

Kruger, W.M., and Apffelstaedt, J.P. (2007) Young breast cancer patients in the developing world: incidence, choice of surgical treatment and genetic factors. *SA Fam. Pract.* 49: 18-24.

Lee, K.D., Chen, S.C., Chan, C.H., Lu, C.H., Chen, C.C., Lin, J.T., Chen, M.F., Huang, S.H., Yeh, C.M., and Chen, M.C. (2008). Increased risk for second primary malignancies in women with breast cancer diagnosed at young age: a population-based study in Taiwan. *Cancer Epidemiol Biomarkers Prev* 17: 2647-2655.

Li, S., Han, B., Liu, G., Ouellet, J., Labrie, F., and Pelletier, G. (2010). Immunocytochemical localization of sex steroid hormone receptors in normal human mammary gland. *J Histochem Cytochem* 58: 509-515.

Lin, C.H., Liau, J.Y., Lu, Y.S., Huang, C.S., Lee, W.C., Kuo, K.T., Shen, Y.C., Kuo, S.H., Lan, C., Liu, J.M., *et al.* (2009). Molecular subtypes of breast cancer emerging in young women in Taiwan: evidence for more than just westernization as a reason for the disease in Asia. *Cancer Epidemiol Biomarkers Prev* 18: 1807-1814.

McTiernan, A., Irwin, M., and Vongruenigen, V. (2010). Weight, physical activity, diet, and prognosis in breast and gynecologic cancers. *J Clin Oncol 28*: 4074-4080.

Mellemkjaer, L., Friis, S., Olsen, J.H., Scelo, G., Hemminki, K., Tracey, E., Andersen, A., Brewster, D.H., Pukkala, E., McBride, M.L., *et al.* (2006). Risk of second cancer among women with breast cancer. *Int J Cancer 118*: 2285-2292.

Mita, K., Zhang, Z., Ando, Y., Toyama, T., Hamaguchi, M., Kobayashi, S., Hayashi, S., Fujii, Y., Iwase, H., and Yamashita, H. (2007). Prognostic significance of insulin-like growth factor binding protein (IGFBP)-4 and IGFBP-5 expression in breast cancer. *Jpn J Clin Oncol* 37: 575-582.

Muti, P. (2005). The role of endogenous hormones in the etiology and prevention of breast cancer: the epidemiological evidence. *Recent Results Cancer Res 166*: 245-256.

Okoh, V., Deoraj, A., and Roy, D. (2011). Estrogen-induced reactive oxygen species-mediated signalings contribute to breast cancer. *Biochim Biophys Acta* 1815: 115-133.

Pampalakis, G., Prosnikli, E., Agalioti, T., Vlahou, A., Zoumpourlis, V., and Sotiropoulou, G. (2009). A tumor-protective role for human kallikrein-related peptidase 6 in breast cancer mediated by inhibition of epithelial-to-mesenchymal transition. *Cancer Res* 69: 3779-3787.

Phipps, A.I., Chlebowski, R.T., Prentice, R., McTiernan, A., Wactawski-Wende, J., Kuller, L.H., Adams-Campbell, L.L., Lane, D., Stefanick, M.L., Vitolins, M., *et al.* (2011). Reproductive history and oral contraceptive use in relation to risk of triple-negative breast cancer. *J Natl Cancer Inst 103*: 470-477.

Reis-Filho, J.S., Simpson, P.T., Jones, C., Steele, D., Mackay, A., Iravani, M., Fenwick, K., Valgeirsson, H., Lambros, M., Ashworth, A., *et al.* (2005). Pleomorphic lobular carcinoma of the breast: role of comprehensive molecular pathology in characterization of an entity. *J Pathol* 207: 1-13.

Roussos, E.T., Wang, Y., Wyckoff, J.B., Sellers, R.S., Wang, W., Li, J., Pollard, J.W., Gertler, F.B., and Condeelis, J.S. (2010). Mena deficiency delays tumor progression and decreases metastasis in polyoma middle-T transgenic mouse mammary tumors. *Breast Cancer Res* 12: R101.

Russo, J., and Russo, I.H. (1994). Toward a physiological approach to breast cancer prevention. *Cancer Epidemiol Biomarkers Prev* 3: 353-364.

Sanderson, M., Williams, M.A., Daling, J.R., Holt, V.L., Malone, K.E., Self, S.G., and Moore, D.E. (1998). Maternal factors and breast cancer risk among young women. *Paediatr Perinat Epidemiol* 12: 397-407.

Sorlie, T., Tibshirani, R., Parker, J., Hastie, T., Marron, J.S., Nobel, A., Deng, S., Johnsen, H., Pesich, R., Geisler, S., *et al.* (2003). Repeated observation of breast tumor subtypes in independent gene expression data sets. *Proc Natl Acad Sci U S A 100*: 8418-8423.

Sotiriou, C., Neo, S.Y., McShane, L.M., Korn, E.L., Long, P.M., Jazaeri, A., Martiat, P., Fox, S.B., Harris, A.L., and Liu, E.T. (2003). Breast cancer classification and prognosis based on gene expression profiles from a population-based study. *Proc Natl Acad Sci U S A 100*: 10393-10398.

Tamimi, R.M., Colditz, G.A., Wang, Y., Collins, L.C., Hu, R., Rosner, B., Irie, H.Y., Connolly, J.L., and Schnitt, S.J. (2011). Expression of IGF1R in normal breast tissue and subsequent risk of breast cancer. *Breast Cancer Res Treat.*

Torres-Arzayus, M.I., Zhao, J., Bronson, R., and Brown, M. (2010). Estrogen-dependent and estrogen-independent mechanisms contribute to AIB1-mediated tumor formation. *Cancer Res* 70: 4102-4111.

Trepp, R., Padberg, B.C., Varga, Z., Cathomas, R., Inauen, R., and Reinhart, W.H. (2010). Extensive extranodal metastases of basal-like breast cancer with predominant myoepithelial spindle cell differentiation. *Pathol Res Pract* 206: 334-337.

Trichopoulos, D., Adami, H.O., Ekbom, A., Hsieh, C.C., and Lagiou, P. (2008). Early life events and conditions and breast cancer risk: from epidemiology to etiology. *Int J Cancer 122*: 481-485.

Wu, A.H., McKean-Cowdin, R., and Tseng, C.C. (2011). Birth weight and other prenatal factors and risk of breast cancer in Asian-Americans. *Breast Cancer Res Treat.*

Xu, Y., Bismar, T.A., Su, J., Xu, B., Kristiansen, G., Varga, Z., Teng, L., Ingber, D.E., Mammoto, A., Kumar, R., *et al.* (2010). Filamin A regulates focal adhesion disassembly and suppresses breast cancer cell migration and invasion. *J Exp Med* 207: 2421-2437.

Yaghjyan, L., and Colditz, G.A. (2011). Estrogens in the breast tissue: a systematic review. *Cancer Causes Control 22*: 529-540.

Yankaskas, B.C. (2005). Epidemiology of breast cancer in young women. *Breast Dis 23*: 3-8.

Yu, G.P., Schantz, S.P., Neugut, A.I., and Zhang, Z.F. (2006). Incidences and trends of second cancers in female breast cancer patients: a fixed inception cohort-based analysis (United States). *Cancer Causes Control 17*: 411-420.

8

Circulating Tumour Cells: Implications and Methods of Detection

Nisha Kanwar and Susan Done
Department of Laboratory Medicine and Pathobiology, University of Toronto
Campbell Family Institute for Breast Cancer Research,
University Health Network, Toronto
Canada

1. Introduction

1.1 Breast cancer and metastasis

Despite progressive advances in the fields of screening, radiation and chemotherapy, metastasis remains the leading cause of more than 90% of breast cancer related deaths. In metastasis, a small, select group of cells develops the capacity to disseminate from the primary tumour, and circulate via the blood or lymphatic system to distant organs, developing tumours at these new sites. Metastasis is a highly inefficient process, where less than 0.01% of tumour cells are able to successfully seed at secondary organs (Chiang & Massagué, 2008). In order to emerge as metastatic, tumour cells must progress through all of the steps of metastasis: invasion of tissues surrounding the primary tumour, intravasation into the circulatory system, survival in the circulation by evasion of the immune system or apoptosis, arrest in a distant capillary, extravasation, and finally proliferation in a distant organ (Fidler, 2003). These cells have often been referred to as decathlon athletes because of their aggressive biology. Once metastasis has occurred, conventional therapies are rendered less effective due to the nature of these cells. They are heterogeneous in their metastatic potentials, growing at different rates, with different invasive abilities and varying responses to drugs and treatment. It is also particularly difficult to detect the early stages of metastasis and assess the presence of minimal residual disease after treatment, owing to the microscopic routes of progression. Current methods used to predict the risk of metastasis and determine suitable treatment regimens are based on evaluation of tumour characteristics such as size, histological grade, lymph node involvement, and expression of treatment response markers like ER, PR and Her2 receptors (Weigelt et al., 2005). These practices however, are invasive and limited in their prognostic value. They are able to identify only 30% of breast cancer patients with a high risk for metastasis (Weigelt et al., 2005). There is a significant need for the development of new early prognostic markers for metastasis. Ultimately, if the spread of cells from the primary tumour could be stopped, then deaths from metastasis could be prevented. Researchers continue to try and shed more light on the molecular alterations in tumour cells which lead to metastasis.

1.2 Circulating tumour cells

The first observation of circulating tumour cells (CTCs) was made in 1867 by an Australian physician, Thomas R. Ashworth. He showed that cells found in the circulation were identical to those found in the original cancer; and that they may be able to explain the origin of multiple metastatic tumours (Ashworth, 1867). Current research has established that primary tumours themselves have a gene expression signature that is predictive of metastasis, and that the shedding of neoplastic cells into the circulation begins early on (van de Vijver et al., 2002). Furthermore, these tumour cells are able to develop the capacity to metastasize independently from the primary tumour, with a unique set of genetic aberrations (Schardt et al., 2005; Schmidt-Kittler et al., 2003). Targeting only the primary and metastatic tumours is insufficient to tackle breast cancer in a systemic manner. It appears that the 'vehicles' that are responsible for cancer spread may provide the supplementary molecular targets urgently needed. Metastasis has been known to develop in patients with small primary tumours, and even in 2-4% of rare cases of undetectable primary tumours (Weigelt et al., 2005; Hüsemann et al., 2008). Early breast cancer mouse models, as well as human samples show evidence of the spread of circulating tumour cells at early stages, completely independent of tumour size (Hüsemann et al., 2008). The number of tumour cells that enter circulation in mouse models is highest immediately after initial transformation, and these cells will accumulate additional mutations over time to eventually be selected for malignant growth in new organs (Hüsemann et al., 2008). However, not all patients with detectable spread of tumour cells will go on to develop metastasis (36-50% of patients show no detectable metastatic disease up to 22 years later) (Graves & Czerniecki, 2011). Many confounding factors in the secondary organ microenvironment will affect the transformation of these cells from dormant to metastatic. None the less, these findings are indicative of metastasis being an early event. Circulating tumour cells (CTCs) might be the earliest detectable cells with metastatic abilities and are emerging as a promising biomarker for breast cancer progression. CTCs may affect cancer prognosis years before the onset of overt metastasis, and therefore improve risk assessment and help identify patients in need of additional treatment. The cells themselves may provide new targets for therapy to prevent their spread to distant sites.

2. Clinical relevance of CTCs

CTCs are found in the peripheral blood and are separate from disseminated tumour cells or DTCs, which are found in the bone marrow. DTCs are an independent prognostic marker for poor prognosis in breast cancer. In a meta-analysis of prospective studies with at least 10 years of follow up data on 4703 metastatic breast cancer patients, 30.6% of patients had DTCs which were associated with tumour stage, lymph node involvement, tumour grade, and hormone receptor negative status (Braun et al., 2005). The acquisition of DTCs from bone marrow, however, is an invasive procedure, requiring a high standard of quality control for repeated draws from the iliac crest of patients (Pantel et al., 2008). Several studies have shown an association between the occurrence of DTCs and CTCs in early and metastatic breast cancer (Graves & Czerniecki, 2011). Therefore, the collection of blood samples from patients for analysis of CTCs without surgical intervention, is a more attractive alternative for clinical purposes.

CTCs have been extensively characterized as epithelial tumour cells, large in size, with a high nuclear to cytoplasmic ratio, irregular nuclear shape, non-proliferative and in some

cases, apoptotic (Pantel et al., 2008; Aktas et al., 2009; Fehm et al., 2010; Ignatiadis et al., 2011; Wikman et al., 2008). These are not exclusive characteristics however, and a great degree of phenotypic heterogeneity exists within this population of cells.
CTCs have been reported in 70-100% of patients with distant metastatic spread and 46-71% of patients with local nodal involvement (Cristofanilli et al., 2004). A multicenter prospective study of 177 patients compared quantities of CTCs in relation to outcome and showed that metastatic breast cancer patients with more than 5 CTCs per 7.5mL of blood had a shorter progression-free and overall survival (2.7 months vs. 7.0 months and 10.1 months vs. >18 months) (Cristofanilli et al., 2005). In a follow up study with the same group of patients, it was reported that the number of CTCs was a better indicator of disease progression than traditional techniques such as imaging with PET, CT or MRI scans (Cristofanilli et al., 2007; Bidard et al., 2008; Nelson, 2010; Liu et al., 2009). Similar associations have been found in patients with colon and prostate cancer. Notably, decreased levels of CTCs are seen in response to chemotherapy suggesting a role for the measurement of CTCs in treatment monitoring. Chemo-resistant CTCs have been shown to be Her2 positive, although they originated from Her2 negative primary tumours (Flores et al., 2010; Fehm et al., 2010). A proportion of these patients had metastatic tumours which were also Her2 positive. Such discrepancies were also found with ER, PR and EGFR status suggesting a critical role for CTCs in stratifying patients for treatment (Fehm et al., 2009). Furthermore, epithelial-mesenchymal transition (EMT) and stem cell characteristics, such as expression of Twist, and ALDH1 are detectable in CTCs of metastatic breast cancer samples (Aktas et al., 2009). Such markers might be associated with a stem-cell like subpopulation persisting after treatment, capable of survival, self-renewal and aggressive propagation of new tumours. Further exemplifying this hypothesis, it has been shown that some CTCs have a multidrug resistance protein (MRP) expression profile which correlates with ALDH1 expression. CTCs from patients who expressed more than 2 MRPs, had shorter progression-free survival, and resistance to chemotherapy (Gradilone et al., 2011). Both DTCs and CTCs were included in tumour marker assessment for breast cancer by the American Society of Clinical Oncology in 2007 (Harris et al., 2007). The report was based on studies rated at Level of evidence I and II (prospective randomized controlled trials, prospective therapeutic trials, or meta-analyses testing the utility of a marker). While acknowledging the immense research interest and publications in the field, the clinical utility of CTCs and DTCs is yet to be established and requires further large scale studies, especially in early breast cancer (Harris et al., 2007). Clinically, the mere presence of CTCs is indicative of a negative prognostic impact and highlights a role for these cells as biomarkers of disease progression and drug response.

3. Methods for enrichment of CTCs from blood

CTCs are a rare cell population (approximately 1 in 100 million nucleated blood cells of breast cancer patients). Metastatic breast cancer patients have been reported to have a range of 0 to a few thousand CTCs per 1-10 mL of blood (Flores et al., 2010; Talasaz et al., 2009) , compared to early stage breast cancers which from the limited publications to date as well as results from our own laboratory, report a range of 0 to less than 10 CTCs per 7-20 mL of blood (Ignatiadis et al., 2011; Lang et al., 2009; Shaw et al., 2011). A major obstacle is obtaining a sufficient number of CTCs, void of contaminating white blood cells, for downstream purposes such as genome, transcriptome or proteome analysis. Enrichment is usually a pre-requisite to any detection or isolation protocol described. After enrichment, detection of cells is improved at least 10,000-fold, depending on the technique. Several methods for enrichment of CTCs have been described - immunomagnetic bead separation; density centrifugation separation, size based exclusion, and flow cytometric separation. Each of these methods allows for either positive selection by targeting CTCs with epithelial markers (cytokeratin, EpCAM), or negative selection by targeting white blood cells with leukocyte markers (CD45). There is however, a common and significant caveat in these procedures; CTCs are enriched from blood using normal epithelial cell markers due to lack of CTC specific malignant cell markers. Also, there is the possibility that in the process of tumourigenic progression, some CTCs may in fact lose their epithelial markers during epithelial-mesenchymal transition, and thus would not be selected for. To address these shortcomings, different methods of enrichment are combined (double selection) in order to compliment each other, and a panel of markers is used to best ascertain the identity of cells being enriched for.

3.1 Immunomagnetic bead enrichment

In February 2008, the FDA approved the CellSearch® System (developed by Veridex, LLC - Johnson & Johnson, NJ) as the first, validated method to accurately detect and enumerate CTCs in order to monitor metastatic disease in cancer patients (Riethdorf et al., 2007). This system incorporates the interaction of target cells with antibodies conjugated to magnetic nanoparticles or 'immunomagnetic beads'. Once cells are bound to the magnetic beads, they are passed through a magnetic core, where they are selectively retained, while unbound cells flow through. They are then fixed and labeled with fluorescent tags for subsequent analysis and enumeration. The advantage of this system is that it allows the use of multiple markers for CTCs as well as non-CTCs to enable more reliable identification. The standard panel includes CTC labeling antibodies such as EpCAM, and cytokeratins, as well as leukocyte labeling antibodies such as CD45. DAPI stains the nuclei to enable characterization of the multi-lobed nuclei, or low nuclear to cytoplasmic ratio seen in white blood cells compared to mostly high nuclear to cytoplasmic ratio seen in CTCs (Figure 1).

Recently, the Her2 antibody was added to the panel of test markers (Ignatiadis et al., 2011). The entire system is automated, including computerized image analysis and acquisition (Figure 2). It appears to be the gold standard of CTC detection to date, with more studies being published, each validating its sensitivity which has been established as a median of 5 CTC per 7.5mL of blood (Kraan et al., 2011; Ignatiadis et al., 2011; Savitri Krishnamurthy et al., 2010; Sandri et al., 2010; Van der Auwera et al., 2010; Bidard et al., 2010).

Recently, a modified version of this system was released, known as the CellSearch® Profile kit. This system incorporates a fewer number of steps, providing only enrichment of cells with the immunomagnetic beads, followed by elution. This allows for isolation and further processing of viable cells for other purposes such as cytometric or molecular analyses such as IHC, TUNEL assays, FISH, RT-PCR or DNA assays (Flores et al., 2010). Fewer processing steps has also resulted in a greater than 20-fold increase in the yield of CTCs with a range of 4 - 2432 CTCs per 7.5mL of blood (Flores et al., 2010). In addition, a group of researchers at Stanford University, CA have developed their own system based on the immunomagnetic principle, called the Magsweeper (Talasaz et al., 2009). This device incorporates magnetic rods with plastic sheets, which undergo repeated capture-wash-release cycles to enhance specific binding of target cells while non-specifically bound cells are gently washed off.

Another innovative device that has branched out from this technology is the CTC-chip, recently developed by a group of researchers at Harvard University, MA(Figure 3). The CTC-chip uses micro-fluidic principles for the capture of viable CTCs from small volumes of blood. Immunomagnetic nanoparticles are replaced by 78,000 microposts over a surface of 970 mm^2, each coated with antibodies for EpCAM (Nagrath et al., 2007). Capture of CTCs from blood by the microposts is dependent on strict laminar flow and volume conditions, with optimal capture occurring at a flow rate of less than 2.5ml per hour (Nagrath et al., 2007). Once bound to the posts, CTCs may be processed in a similar fashion as the CellSearch® system by fixation and fluorescent labeling for analysis. It appears to be an efficient system, enriching CTCs in the range of 5 - 1281 cells per 1mL of blood (Nagrath et al., 2007).

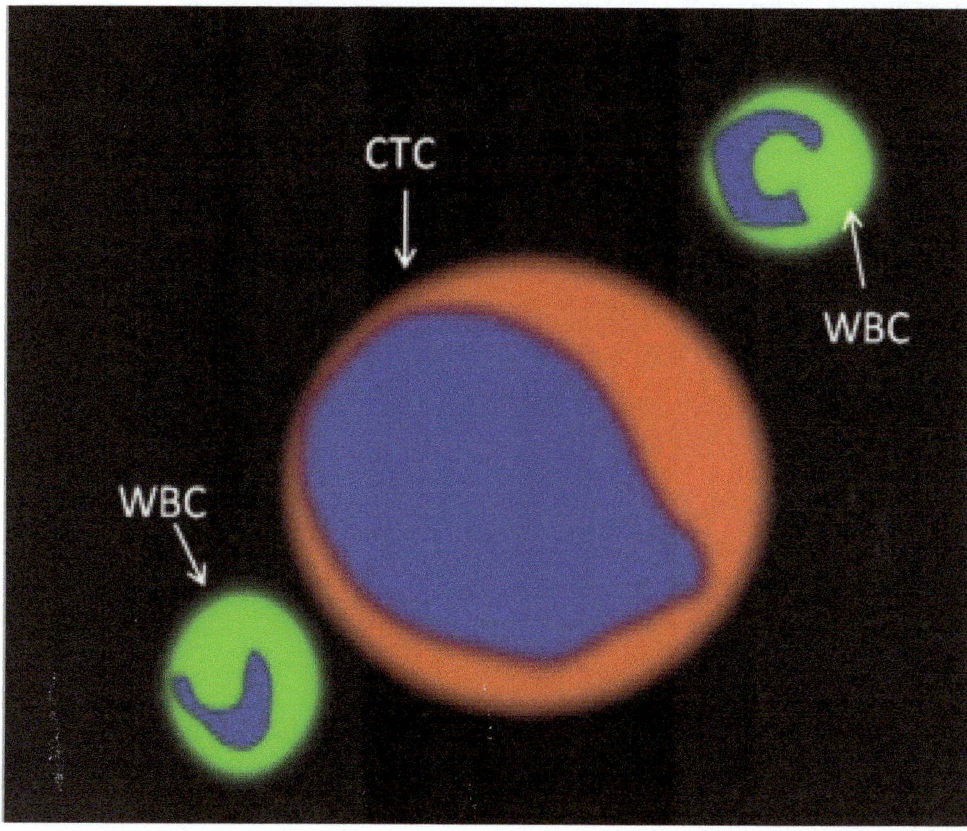

Fig. 1. Schematic of immunofluorescent staining of a CTC (cytokeratin: red, CD45: green, DAPI: blue). Tumour cells (CTC) are identified by high nuclear to cytoplasmic ratio and cytokeratin expression in the cytoplasm. White blood cells (WBC) are identified by smaller cellular size and CD45 expression.

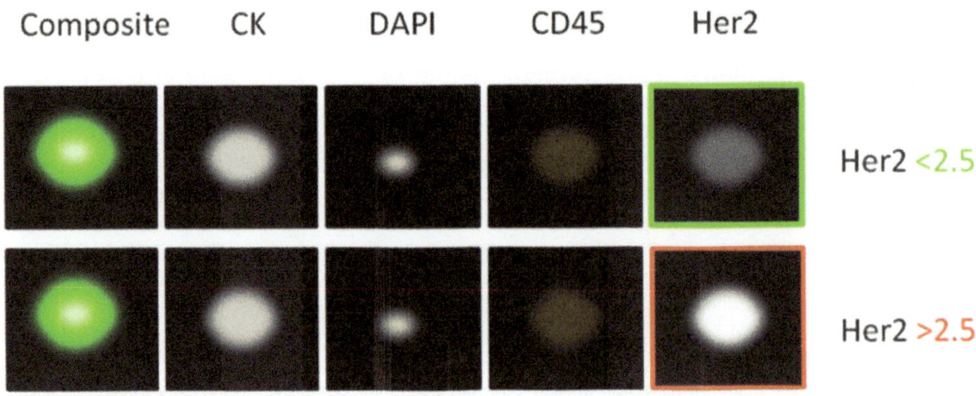

Fig. 2. Schematic of typical results obtained from the CellSearch® analysis of CTCs isolated from metastatic breast cancer patients. Composite analysis of 2 CTCs is displayed; with positive labeling for cytokeratin (CK), DAPI and Her2 (two intensities shown, >2.5 is diagnosed as Her2 positive) and negative labeling for CD45 (leukocyte marker).

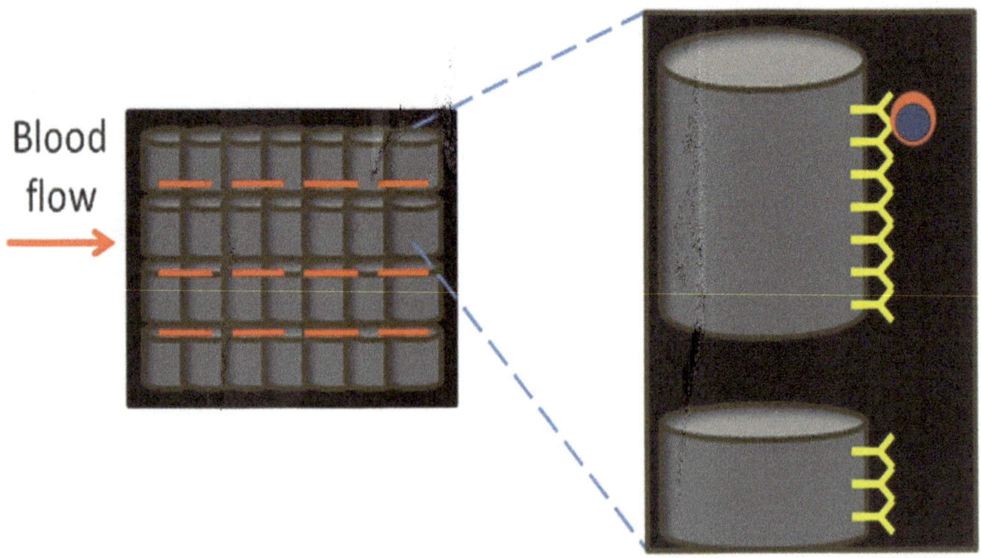

Fig. 3. CTC-chip with microposts; blood flows over and through microposts at designated flow rate and volume for capture of CTCs. Enlarged schematic shows micropost coated with EpCAM antibodies (yellow) interacting with a complementary epitope on the CTC.

The next generation of the CTC-chip is the Herringbone chip, with enhanced capture (26% improvement from the CTC-chip) and higher flow rates (4.8mL of blood per hour) (Figure 4). The improved performance is the result of a platform consisting of angular flow paths or microvortices which allow for passive mixing of blood as it flows through the chip, significantly increasing the number of interactions between CTCs and the antibody coated chip surface (Stott et al., 2010). In addition, the platform of the chip is made up of a transparent material, allowing for improved imaging options, both for transmitted light IHC staining as well as fluorescent staining (Stott et al., 2010).

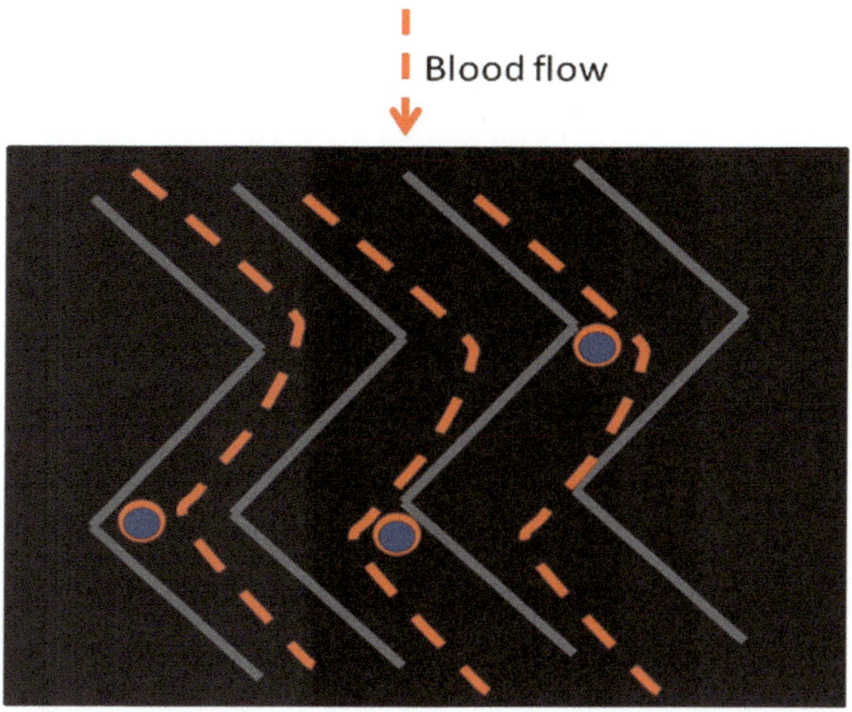

Fig. 4. Magnified representation of the asymmetric, grooved surface of the Herringbone CTC chip. Microvortices allow for enhanced number of interactions between CTCs and the EpCAM antibody coated surface of the chip.

Despite the promise of performance of microfluidic devices, there remain two significant disadvantages to these systems. Firstly, since cells are not fixed, samples must be processed within 2 hours of collection to maintain cell viability and capture by the chip. This complicates multicenter studies or the clinical utility of this system worldwide until this device is made commercially available. Secondly, once captured, CTCs are bound to the chip, and any subsequent analysis must be performed on the chip itself. Although this is beneficial for visualization and enumeration type assays, it is not transferrable to nucleic acid based assays such as RT-PCR or DNA analysis.

3.2 Physical properties based enrichment

CTCs are also enriched based on their physical properties such as density and size. Protocols have been developed for density based separation where tetrameric antibodies aid in the formation of aggregates of white blood cells and red blood cells, called 'immunorosettes' (Gertler et al. 2003). These aggregates are complex structures with a higher density than single CTCs. Centrifugation allows for a fast and convenient pelleting of the blood cells, enriching CTCs in the interphase of blood serum and a separating medium such as Percoll™ or Ficoll™ (Gertler et al., 2003). Size based separation protocols utilize the property of tumour cells being at least twice the size of the majority of leukocytes (>20μm versus 8 - 10μm). Blood is passed through filters which, with the help of a gentle vacuum pressure, exclude CTCs and a small number of larger white blood cells such as macrophages and monocytes (Pinzani et al., 2006).

One obvious advantage of this type of separation is that CTCs are not being selected for by epithelial cell surface markers which might be lost during the aforementioned EMT processes. While both of these methods of separation provide the advantage of enriching for viable CTCs, which may be collected and stained for cytopathological analysis or subjected to RNA or DNA analyses, the technology is quite elementary and imprecise, and fails to give reproducible data. Also, not all CTCs are greater than 8μm, and there will remain a proportion that will be missed by this technique as well.

3.3 Evaluation of two prevalent methods of CTC enrichment

In our laboratory, we have evaluated immunomagnetic and density centrifugation based methods of CTC enrichment using spiking experiments. Quantities of 100, 1000, 10^4 and 10^5 cells from the MCF7 breast cancer cell line were spiked into 10 mL of peripheral blood from healthy volunteers. RossetteSep™ (density centrifugation separation) and EasySep™ (immunomagnetic bead separation) kits from StemCell Technologies Inc. were used for negative selection of spiked MCF7 cells from blood. The RossetteSep™ kit resulted in a purer cell eluate compared with the EasySep™ kit which contained interfering residual magnetic beads, and white blood cell clumps. The disadvantage however, was the lack of sensitivity and automation of both methods. The level for retrieving spiked cells was determined to be less than 60% of 10^4 and 10^5 spiked cells. Cells spiked below this threshold were not retrieved by either method.

We have since validated a method of CTC enrichment from blood using the autoMACS™ cell sorter (Miltenyi Biotec). This machine incorporates negative selection of CTCs and immunomagnetic, automated separation. Immunolabeled cells pass through a magnet containing a column made up of a porous matrix dense enough to allow single cell flow through (Gijs, 2004). Each single cell is analyzed and sorted as labeled (CD45 positive leukocyte) or unlabelled (CD45 negative CTC), and eluted through its respective port. This method parallels the principle of the FDA approved CellSearch® System. Spiking experiments showed a 1000-fold increase in sensitivity of cells recovered compared to previously tested techniques in our laboratory. Sensitivity of the assay was dependent on the volume of blood processed, which corresponded to the number of white blood cells present in the sample. Addition of a red blood cell lysis step served two purposes; (1) to reduce background of interfering red blood cells and enhance immunomagnetic bead-white blood cell interactions; and (2) to pellet the remaining cellular fraction and allow exclusion of non-specific free RNA/DNA. MCF7 breast cancer cells spiked into 3 ml of blood from healthy volunteers showed 70-90% recovery of 10-100 spiked cells, respectively ($R=0.8959$).

4. Genetic profiling of CTCs

Enriched CTCs are subjected to two types of analyses – immunocytometric or RT-PCR based assays. Both methods allow for multiplexing of markers to increase specificity. Markers include cytokeratins, Her2, MET, MUC1, ESR1, TWIST, ALDH1, EGFR, Ki-67 and many more. RT-PCR assays are the most frequently reported method of CTC detection, and have the highest sensitivity (1 CTC in over 1-10 million nucleated blood cells) (Ring et al., 2005; Gerges et al., 2010). RT-PCR assays also have the advantage of high-throughput efficiency and allow for the analysis of larger panels of genes ranging from a few up to 16 genes as was recently published (Sieuwerts et al., 2008). This study showed that the proof of principle experiment was successful for analysis of a panel of 96 genes in one single tumour cell. This result however is affected by a high background of white blood cell RNA in patient samples, and thus was limited to an exploratory set of 16 genes capable of differentiating expression profiles of CTC positive breast cancer patients from CTC negative breast cancer patients (Sieuwerts et al., 2008). Another study aimed to determine the global expression pattern of CTCs, using the Affymetrix GeneChip™ platform, and once again concluded that a different panel of 16 genes was expressed specifically in CTCs from metastatic breast cancer patients (Smirnov et al., 2005). Noticeably, this study also looked at CTCs originating from different cancer tissues, and found that CTCs derived from different cancers had unique expression patterns as well (Smirnov et al., 2005).

The disadvantages of these methods of profiling are false expression signatures created from non-specific primers or staining, lack of expression of the marker of interest on CTCs in the sample, pseudogenes, and low expression of the marker of interest on non-malignant cells. Work done in our own laboratory demonstrated the use of RT-PCR techniques to enumerate CTCs in blood by correcting for a percentage of these types of false signatures (Iakovlev et al., 2007). Blood from healthy human volunteers was spiked with 1-10,000 tumour cells from breast cancer cell lines. Also, free RNA from these same cell lines was spiked separately to determine false positive results from free RNA, and genomic DNA released from dying cells in blood. We were able to show that there is a linear relationship between the number of CTCs in blood, and the amount of CK19 RNA, with a reliable detection limit of 5 cells per mL of blood with Ct values <40 to correct for false positives. We also determined that by including a centrifugation step to pellet CTCs and separate them from other fractions of blood, most of the contaminating free RNA and DNA can be excluded. These techniques may prove useful for high throughput comparative quantification or analyses of CTCs in individual patients during treatment and subsequent follow up for clinical management purposes.

RNA is highly unstable and is readily degraded once it is released from the cell. Comparatively, DNA based assays are much more reliable, robust and less technically demanding. Genomic characterization of CTCs has however been unachievable thus far. Even the most sensitive technique of CTC enrichment from blood does not provide a pure sample void of white blood cell contamination. Furthermore, even if isolation of a pure CTC sample was achieved, genomic analysis would be quite challenging owing to the low numbers of cells in circulation. If the whole genome of CTCs can be profiled, we could identify novel genomic alterations specific to CTCs which may be utilized in the development of specific markers for CTCs in blood. Also, regions of altered DNA in CTCs from early breast cancer patients hold valuable prognostic genetic information for the progression of early breast cancer to metastasis.

4.1 Isolation of single CTCs for DNA extraction

Our laboratory has been involved in the testing and validation of various technologies to address the problem of specificity during isolation of CTCs in order to genomically characterize these cells. We have designed a protocol to isolate single CTCs using immunocytochemical staining and single cell laser capture microdissection (LCM), followed by whole genome amplification (WGA) of DNA for high density copy number analysis (Figure 5).

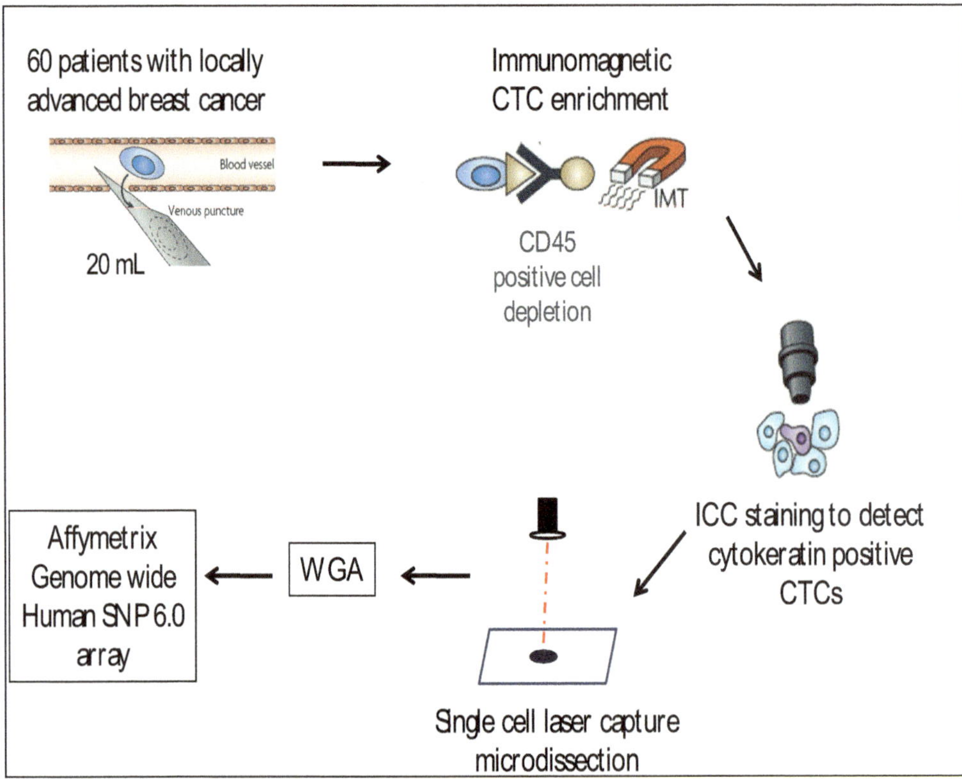

Fig. 5. Flowchart of steps involved in the isolation of single CTCs from the blood of patients with locally advanced breast cancer, for purposes of whole genome amplification (WGA) and high resolution copy number analysis.

We used the autoMACS™ separator for immunomagnetic based enrichment for CTCs from 20mL of blood drawn from patients with locally advanced breast cancer. Each blood sample is processed in 3mL aliquots for optimal enrichment of CTCs from blood, as determined from spiking experiments described earlier. Each aliquot is lysed for red blood cells, pelleted, and then resuspended in separation buffer containing magnetic beads conjugated to CD45 antibodies. The aliquot is then processed, selecting for the CD45 negative fraction which consists of enriched CTCs. The enriched CTC suspension is transferred onto a glass slide using a Cytospin centrifuge. It is then fixed and stained with a pan-cytokeratin AE1/AE3 antibody. This mixture of cytokeratin antibodies recognizes the vast majority of both low and high molecular weight keratins; CK 1-19; except for CK17 and CK18. Once the primary and secondary antibodies are bound, the method of detection that we use is a third antibody conjugated to the enzyme glucose oxidase which is not expressed in mammalian cells (Hard et al., 1989). This property abolishes any non-specific staining that occurs with horseradish peroxidase or alkaline phosphatase methods of detection. These enzymes are expressed endogenously in white blood cells and thus could react with the detection substrate resulting in false positives (Figure 6). Glucose oxidase, however, is absent from white blood cells, and will react with the detection substrate positively staining only those cells that were bound to the primary and secondary antibody. This crucial modification of the staining protocol allows for the certainty of true positives. Positively stained CTCs are then lifted off the slide using single cell laser capture microdissection (Figure 7).

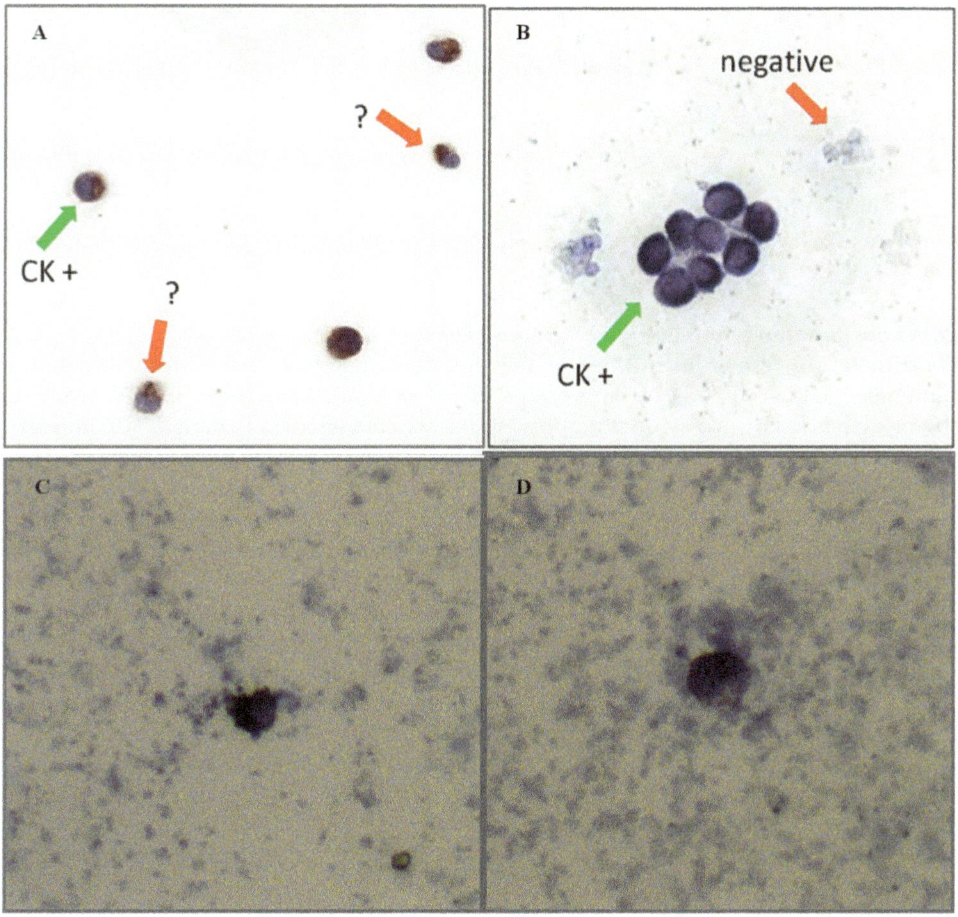

Fig. 6. Enriched cancer cells after spiking of MCF7 cells into blood from healthy human volunteers. (A) Ambiguous staining of CK positive tumour cells and residual white blood cells using horseradish peroxidase detection of antibodies. (B) Specific staining of CK positive tumour cells and negative background of white blood cells using glucose oxidase detection of antibodies. (C) and (D) Enriched single CTCs from locally advanced breast cancer patients using the validated protocol.

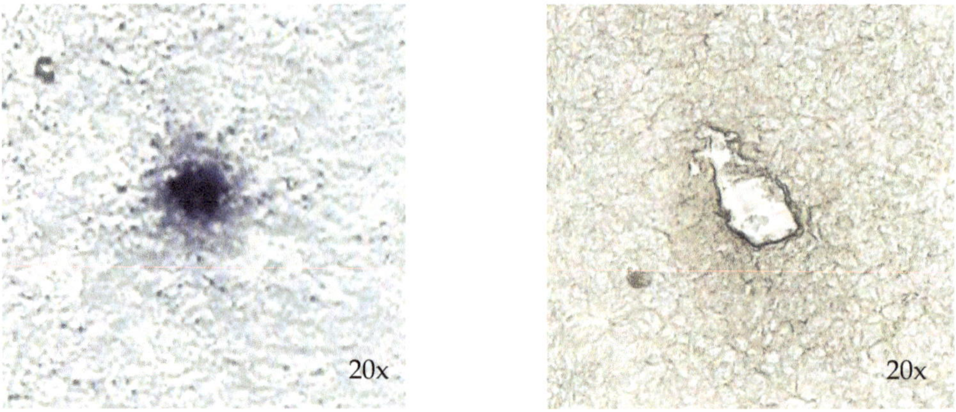

Fig. 7. Cytokeratin positive CTC isolated from the blood of patient with locally advanced breast cancer, before and after lifting off slide using single cell laser capture microdissection.

4.2 Whole genome amplification of single cells

While there are numerous studies in the literature that have successfully isolated and enumerated CTCs; there is no knowledge of the genomic alterations of CTC DNA. Our laboratory has been successful at amplifying the whole genome of single CTCs in order to obtain sufficient amounts of representative DNA for microarray analysis. Most commercial platforms require between 700ng - 1000ng of good quality genomic DNA. We have established a protocol for whole genomic amplification of single cells using a modified protocol of the WGA4 kit (Sigma). We obtained between 1.5 - 3μg of amplified genomic DNA from single cells, which is sufficient for the Affymetrix Genome-Wide Human SNP 6.0 array. This platform currently provides the highest resolution of copy number and loss of heterozygosity data with coverage of greater than 2 million copy number and SNP probes across the entire genome. Our protocol has been validated using MCF7 cell line DNA from as few as 2 single cells. Microarray data was analyzed using Genotyping Console software. Segmented data was analyzed separately for copy number losses and gains (SNP-FASST segmentation algorithm) to identify significant genomic alterations. To begin analysis, we first noted regions of genomic aberrations in the MCF7 cell line that were previously described, and then compared this existing data to regions we obtained with the Affymetrix SNP 6.0 array (Shadeo et al., 2006 & Przybytkowski et al., 2011). Analysis shows expected aberrations in the MCF7 cell line were conserved across samples with amplified single cell starting material when compared to unamplified DNA ($p<0.000001$, 75% concordance). We improved this protocol by introducing a ligation step after genomic amplification. The average size of fragments that probes on the Affymetrix microchip bind to are 700-1000bp long. After WGA however, most DNA fragments are less than 500bp. Ligating these small amplified DNA fragments produces larger fragments of DNA for processing on the microchip, which in turn allows for more SNP and copy number calls to be made. Concordance was improved to greater than 90% after optimization ($p<0.000001$) (Figures 8-10 and Table 1).

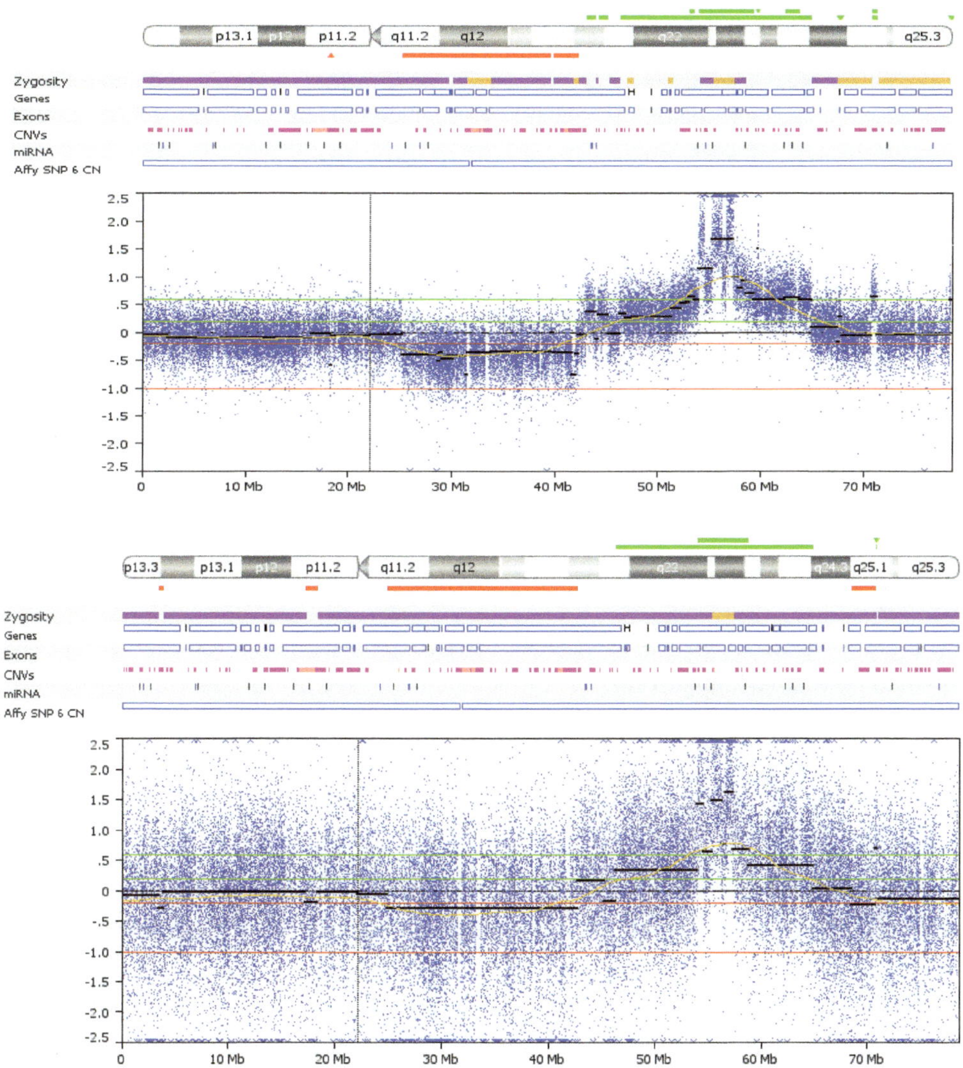

Fig. 8. Comparison of Log2 ratios of copy number between unamplified genomic DNA from MCF7 breast cancer cells (top) and amplified DNA from 2 single MCF7 cells (bottom). Noticeably, although single cells produce more noisy probe calls (blue dots), copy number gains (green) and losses (red), as well as segmentation (black horizontal lines) are significantly conserved across single cell amplification, with 92% concordance. Analysis was performed using Nexus Copy Number software with the following parameters: significance threshold $p<1.0E-6$; maximum contiguous probe spacing = 1Mbp; minimum probes per segment = 10; Log2 ratios: gain >0.2; high gain > 0.6; loss < -0.2; high loss < -1.0.

Unamplified genomic DNA

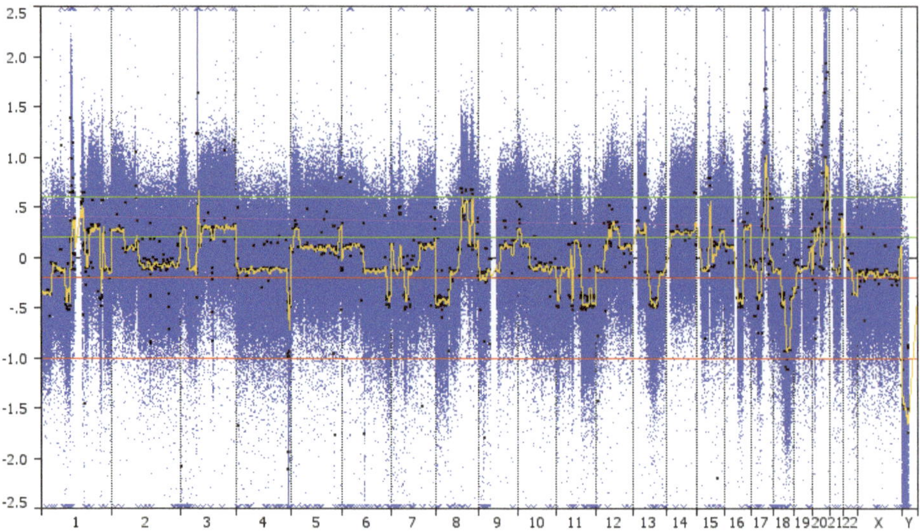

Amplified DNA from 2 single cells

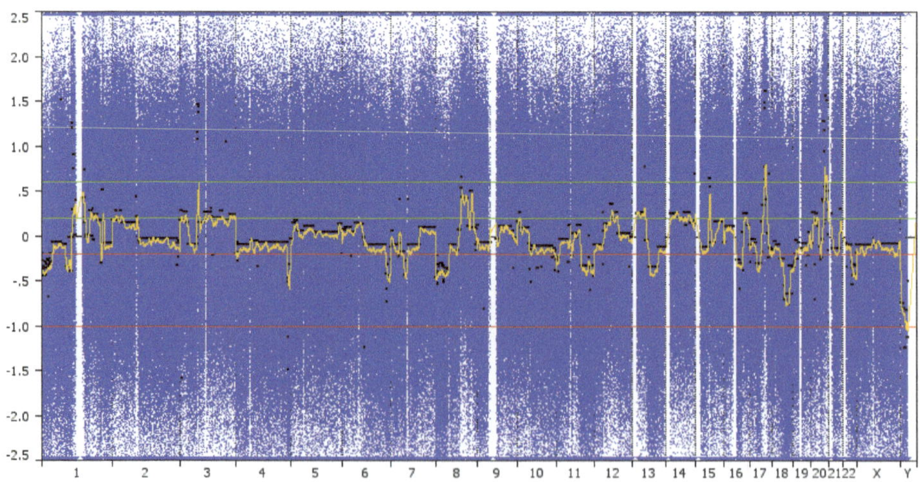

Fig. 9. Moving average of probes (1000 Kb) shows reproducible data between unamplified DNA and amplified single cell DNA from MCF7 breast cancer cells. Analysis was performed using Nexus Copy Number software with the following parameters: significance threshold $p<1.0E-6$; maximum contiguous probe spacing = 1Mbp; minimum probes per segment = 10; Log2 ratios: gain >0.2; high gain > 0.6; loss < -0.2; high loss < -1.0.

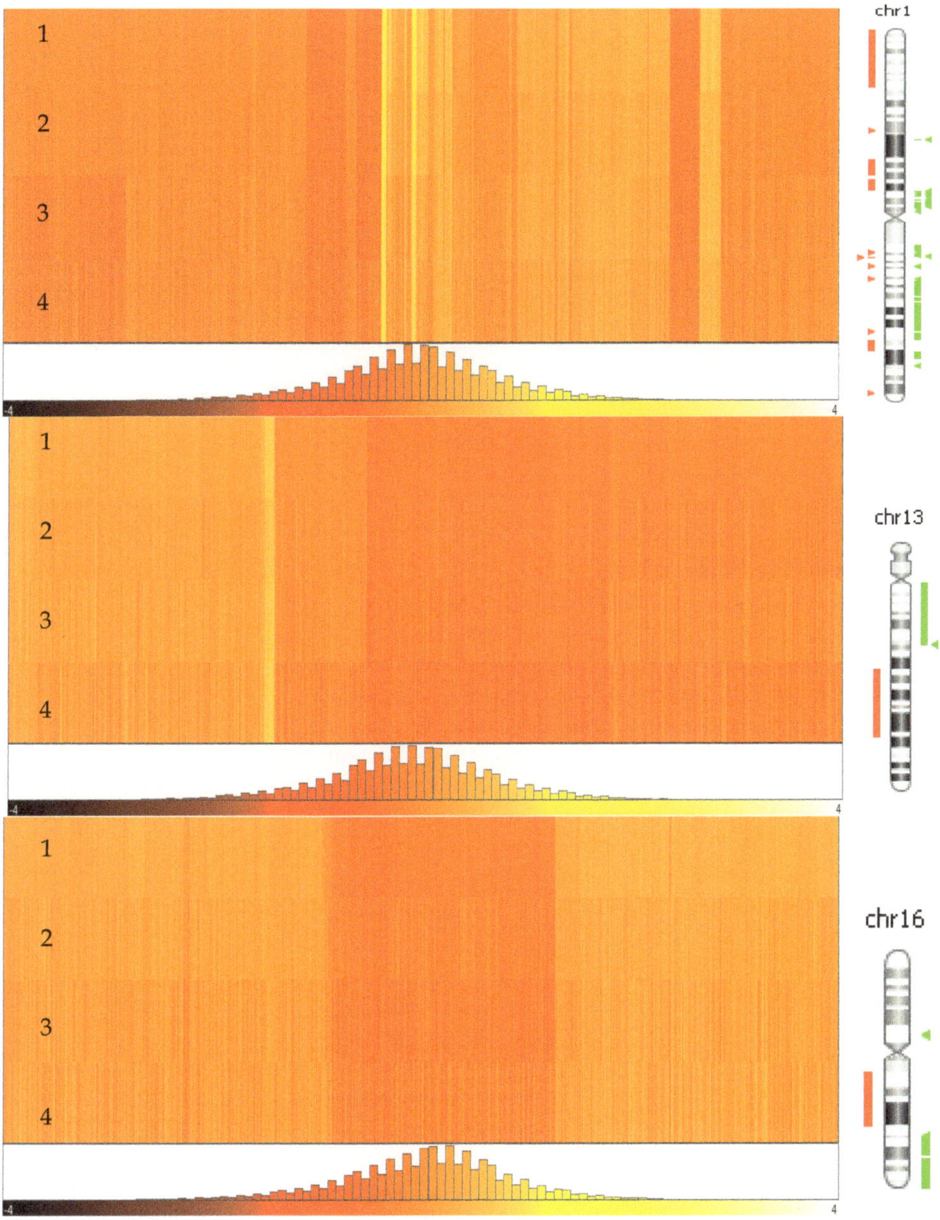

Fig. 10. Copy number heat maps of chromosomes 1, 13 and 16 illustrating genomic gains (yellow) and losses (red) in the MCF7 breast cancer cell line; corresponding chromosomal view showing genomic gains (green) and losses (red), shown to the right. Each row represents one sample (Rows correspond with - 1: unamplified genomic DNA, 2-4: amplified DNA from 2, 3 and 5 single cells, respectively). Analysis was performed with Genotyping Console software.

Subsequently, CTCs isolated from patients with locally advanced breast cancer were processed using this protocol. This is an interesting subgroup of breast cancer patients, as they have locally invasive, larger primary tumours (>5cm) and the cancer has usually metastasized to the lymph nodes but not beyond. Thus they are a subgroup of early metastatic patients, however the cancer is advanced enough for there to be a high likelihood of the presence of detectable numbers of CTCs for genetic analyses. From a total of 31 patients, CTCs were detected in 58% with a range of 1-20 cells per 20 mL of blood. We are currently performing microarray data analyses on these samples, with the goal of addressing some of the research questions discussed below.

Comparison 1	Comparison 2	# SNPs called	# SNPs concordant	SNP concordance (%)
Unamplified genomic	Amplified genomic	733884	700714	96
Amplified genomic	Amplified 2 cells	687896	633305	92
Amplified genomic	Amplified 3 cells	706094	660446	94
Amplified genomic	Amplified 5 cells	663709	567244	86
Amplified 2 cells	Amplified 3 cells	680912	629454	93
Amplified 3 cells	Amplified 5 cells	656417	568087	87
Amplified 2 cells	Amplified 5 cells	644176	558169	87

Table 1. Concordance results of SNP calls made between samples of MCF7 breast cancer cells. SNP call concordance is accurately conserved between the unamplified genomic and amplified genomic samples at 96%. Single cell samples are compared to the amplified genomic sample for concordance so as to control for variability introduced by the WGA protocol. SNP call concordance is accurately conserved in amplified single cell samples (amplified genomic vs 2, 3, and 5 cells). A test for precision and reproducibility of the WGA protocol was also performed by comparing concordance of SNP calls within amplified single cell samples (2vs3, 3vs5, and 2vs5). Analysis performed with Genotyping Console software.

Breast cancer is a heterogeneous disease which can be classified into 5 accepted molecular subtypes. Luminal A tumours tend to be ER+/PR+/Her2-, respond well to hormone therapy and have the most favourable outcome; Luminal B tumours tend to be ER+/PR+/Her+; Her2+ tumours are ER-/PR-; Basal tumours which are ER-/PR-/Her- tend to be the most aggressive, demonstrate the worst prognosis and have limited therapeutic options; and lastly the normal-like tumours are not clearly defined, and display a putative-initiating stem cell phenotype (Perou et al., 1999, 2000; Sørlie et al., 2001, 2006). Using the genomic profiles generated from CTCs, copy number signatures could be configured to determine the predictive power of CTC genomic profiles in the subtyping of breast cancer based on clinical parameters of the primary tumour. Additionally, genomic profiles of matched primary and CTC samples could be analyzed for common and unique regions, to identify alterations involved in disease progression. The utility of CTC genomic profiles could also be extended to the monitoring of patient response to chemotherapy and other treatments. Decrease in CTC numbers is an already established phenomenon in good response and prognosis of patients undergoing treatments. It would be interesting to investigate the idea that CTCs themselves have a genetic signature capable of stratifying patients into responders and non-responders to various treatment regimens. The characterization of genomic signatures of CTCs could pave the way to the development of biomarkers of disease subtype, progression to metastasis and response to treatment. In the future, a simple blood based assay could detect high risk patients, guide treatment options, identify new drug targets, and thus illuminate the process of metastasis.

5. Future directions: Challenges and applications

Although there is substantial evidence showing the prognostic value that CTCs hold in metastatic breast cancer, their clinical significance, especially in early breast cancer remains unclear. There are no reports or studies on the presence of CTCs in ductal carcinoma in situ (DCIS) (Graves & Czerniecki, 2011). Numerous ongoing trials and studies are attempting to shed more light on this field. The Southwest Oncology group aims to determine the clinical value of CTC analyses for monitoring therapies. They are addressing the question of how beneficial serial CTC counts are for non-responding patients to the first-line of chemotherapy to determine if they should be placed on an alternative treatment regimen. If elevated CTCs are indeed informative, then enumeration assays could potentially replace the existing option of waiting for clinically detectable evidence of progressive disease. The DISMAL project hopes to identify new prognostic or therapeutic targets via the molecular characterization of CTCs and primary tumours. They aim to determine if there is a correlation between the profiles of primary tumours and the occurrence of CTCs, and if so are these profiles informative for processes responsible for early tumour cell dissemination? The SUCCESS trial indicates that CTCs do in fact play a prognostic role in early breast cancer, where the presence of just one single CTC has the ability to predict poor disease-free survival, distant disease-free survival, as well as overall survival. Various other ongoing trials are asking questions such as what similarities CTCs have with matched primary cancers, and whether the Her2 status of CTCs can predict a patient's response to trastuzumab, especially in those cases where the primary tumour has been removed and CTCs persist (Pantel et al., 2008)?

The current state of technologies in this field does not allow for the differentiation between CTCs of prognostic value or metastatic potential from those that are merely in circulation for a few hours destined for apoptosis or destruction by the immune system. Less than 0.01% of CTCs in circulation will lead to overt metastasis. CTCs that escape immune surveillance, or adjuvant treatments are believed to be a more aggressive subpopulation of chemoresistant, stem-cell like (CD44+/CD24-) tumour cells. There have been reports on the low concordance between markers such as Her2, ER/PR and EGFR expression in CTCs compared to primary tumours from the same patient. Furthermore, EMT and stem cell characteristics, such as expression of Twist, and ALDH1 are detectable in some CTCs of metastatic breast cancer patients. Expression of EMT markers is what allows cells to evade apoptosis, migrate to distant sites and develop resistance to therapies (Kasimir-Bauer 2009). The property of heterogeneity seen in primary tumours seems to apply to CTCs as well and has very important implications with respect to treatment alterations over the course of the disease. The other side of this argument however is that if breast cancer is heterogeneous, how useful is information derived from a single CTC? Essentially, this question is not too different from one that is asked of small biopsy samples taken from one area of a heterogeneous primary tumour. How representative is a biopsy of the true systemic cancer? Discrepant HER2 amplification found between primary tumours, metastatic tumours, and CTCs raise further questions about the current protocols used in diagnosis and treatment decisions. New technologies like deep sequencing might enable us to delve into the true heterogeneity between single cancer cells. It will also allow us to study cancer cell line models, and determine how similar single cells from cancer cell lines really are, are they different when grown as tumours in vivo and do they produce genetically different tumours? Molecular profiling studies will help researchers to investigate this issue further.

Overall, we are not yet at a point where we can clearly list the biological or molecular characteristics that define a CTC. We first need to standardize methods of analyses of CTCs to advance its utility in the clinic. There is a substantial amount of research interest in this field, and newer, better technologies enter the market steadily. It is entirely possible that different technologies are currently detecting different subsets of the CTC population (Nelson, 2010). What role does time of sampling, amount of sample drawn or individual patient characteristics have on the quality of the assay, are a few of the questions that will need to be tackled. More studies need to be developed around CTCs present in early breast cancer, and their presence and usefulness should be correlated with clinicopathological data, and gene expression data derived from currently recommended breast cancer prognostic markers and tests, for eg: Mammaprint and Oncotype Dx (Krishnamurthy et al., 2010). CTCs have the potential of being established as a reliable prognostic or diagnostic biomarker for early breast cancer, progression to metastasis, response to treatment, and development of anti-metastatic drugs. Given the current interest and impetus in CTC research and technology, this milestone could be reached in the near future.

6. Acknowledgement

We acknowledge the Canadian Breast Cancer Foundation, Ontario Region, for funding the research project grants of SJD and the doctoral fellowship of NK, to work on the characterization of the early molecular events and circulating tumour cells associated with breast cancer metastasis. We would like to thank Dr. Mark Clemons, Dr. Philippe Bedard, Dr. Robert Buckman and Manoj Mathew for their contribution in recruiting and consenting patients to our study. Our deep gratitude goes out to all of the patients at the Princess Margaret Hospital, Toronto, that have, and continue to enthusiastically provide us with blood samples for our study. We would also like to acknowledge all of the members of Susan Done's laboratory for their encouragement and supportive conversations that were essential in the development of our project.

7. References

Aktas, B. et al., 2009. Stem cell and epithelial-mesenchymal transition markers are frequently overexpressed in circulating tumor cells of metastatic breast cancer patients. *Breast Cancer Research: BCR*, 11(4), p.R46.

Ashworth, T.R., 1869. A case of cancer in which cells similar to those in the tumours were seen in the blood after death. *Australian Medical Journal*, 14, pp146-147.

Bidard, F.-C. et al., 2010. Single circulating tumor cell detection and overall survival in nonmetastatic breast cancer. *Annals of Oncology: Official Journal of the European Society for Medical Oncology / ESMO*, 21(4), pp.729-733.

Bidard, F.-C. et al., 2008. Prognosis of women with stage IV breast cancer depends on detection of circulating tumor cells rather than disseminated tumor cells. *Annals of*

Oncology: Official Journal of the European Society for Medical Oncology / ESMO, 19(3), pp.496-500.

Braun, S. et al., 2005. A pooled analysis of bone marrow micrometastasis in breast cancer. *The New England Journal of Medicine*, 353(8), pp.793-802.

Chiang, A.C. & Massagué, J., 2008. Molecular basis of metastasis. *The New England Journal of Medicine*, 359(26), pp.2814-2823.

Cristofanilli, M. et al., 2007. Circulating tumor cells in metastatic breast cancer: biologic staging beyond tumor burden. *Clinical Breast Cancer*, 7(6), pp.471-479.

Cristofanilli, M. et al., 2004. Circulating tumor cells, disease progression, and survival in metastatic breast cancer. *The New England Journal of Medicine*, 351(8), pp.781-791.

Cristofanilli, M. et al., 2005. Circulating tumor cells: a novel prognostic factor for newly diagnosed metastatic breast cancer. *Journal of Clinical Oncology: Official Journal of the American Society of Clinical Oncology*, 23(7), pp.1420-1430.

Fehm, T. et al., 2009. Detection and characterization of circulating tumor cells in blood of primary breast cancer patients by RT-PCR and comparison to status of bone marrow disseminated cells. *Breast Cancer Research: BCR*, 11(4), p.R59.

Fehm, T. et al., 2010. HER2 status of circulating tumor cells in patients with metastatic breast cancer: a prospective, multicenter trial. *Breast Cancer Research and Treatment*, 124(2), pp.403-412.

Fidler, I.J., 2003. The pathogenesis of cancer metastasis: the "seed and soil" hypothesis revisited. *Nature Reviews. Cancer*, 3(6), pp.453-458.

Flores, L.M. et al., 2010. Improving the yield of circulating tumour cells facilitates molecular characterization and recognition of discordant HER2 amplification in breast cancer. *British Journal of Cancer*, 102(10), pp.1495-1502.

Gerges, N., Rak, J. & Jabado, N., 2010. New technologies for the detection of circulating tumour cells. *British Medical Bulletin*, 94, pp.49-64.

Gertler, R. et al., 2003. Detection of circulating tumor cells in blood using an optimized density gradient centrifugation. *Recent Results in Cancer Research. Fortschritte Der Krebsforschung. Progrès Dans Les Recherches Sur Le Cancer*, 162, pp.149-155.

Gijs, A.M., 2004. Magnetic bead handling on-chip: new opportunities for analytical applications. *Microfluid Nanofluid*. 1.pp 22-40.

Gradilone, A. et al., 2011. Circulating tumor cells (CTCs) in metastatic breast cancer (MBC): prognosis, drug resistance and phenotypic characterization. *Annals of Oncology: Official Journal of the European Society for Medical Oncology / ESMO*, 22(1), pp.86-92.

Graves, H. & Czerniecki, B.J., 2011. Circulating tumor cells in breast cancer patients: an evolving role in patient prognosis and disease progression. *Pathology Research International*, 2011, p.621090.

Hard, R.C., Jr, Miller, W.G. & Romagnoli, G., 1989. A background-free assay for cells forming antibody to glucose oxidase coupled with an enzyme-linked immunosorbent assay (ELISA) to quantitate antibody secretion. *The Journal of Histochemistry and Cytochemistry: Official Journal of the Histochemistry Society*, 37(6), pp.909-912.

Harris, L. et al., 2007. American Society of Clinical Oncology 2007 update of recommendations for the use of tumor markers in breast cancer. *Journal of Clinical Oncology: Official Journal of the American Society of Clinical Oncology*, 25(33), pp.5287-5312.

Hüsemann, Y. et al., 2008. Systemic spread is an early step in breast cancer. *Cancer Cell*, 13(1), pp.58-68.

Iakovlev, V.V. et al., 2007. Quantitative detection of circulating epithelial cells by Q-RT-PCR. *Breast Cancer Research and Treatment*, 107(1), pp.145-154.

Ignatiadis, M. et al., 2011. HER2-positive circulating tumor cells in breast cancer. *PloS One*, 6(1), p.e15624.

Kasimir-Bauer, S., 2009. Circulating tumor cells as markers for cancer risk assessment and treatment monitoring. *Molecular Diagnosis & Therapy*, 13(4), pp.209-215.

Kraan, J. et al., 2011. External quality assurance of circulating tumor cell enumeration using the CellSearch(®) system: a feasibility study. *Cytometry. Part B, Clinical Cytometry*, 80(2), pp.112-118.

Krishnamurthy, Savitri et al., 2010. Detection of minimal residual disease in blood and bone marrow in early stage breast cancer. *Cancer*, 116(14), pp.3330-3337.

Liu, M.C. et al., 2009. Circulating tumor cells: a useful predictor of treatment efficacy in metastatic breast cancer. *Journal of Clinical Oncology: Official Journal of the American Society of Clinical Oncology*, 27(31), pp.5153-5159.

Marrinucci, D. et al., 2007. Case study of the morphologic variation of circulating tumor cells☆. *Human Pathology*, 38(3), pp.514-519.

Nagrath, S. et al., 2007. Isolation of rare circulating tumour cells in cancer patients by microchip technology. *Nature*, 450(7173), pp.1235-1239.

Nelson, N.J., 2010. Circulating tumor cells: will they be clinically useful? *Journal of the National Cancer Institute*, 102(3), pp.146-148.

Pantel, K., Brakenhoff, R.H. & Brandt, B., 2008. Detection, clinical relevance and specific biological properties of disseminating tumour cells. *Nature Reviews. Cancer*, 8(5), pp.329-340.

Perou, C.M et al., 1999. Distinctive gene expression patterns in human mammary epithelial cells and breast cancers. *Proceedings of the National Academy of Sciences of the United States of America*, 96(16), pp.9212-9217.

Perou, C.M. et al., 2000. Molecular portraits of human breast tumours. *Nature*, 406(6797), pp.747-752.

Pinzani, P. et al., 2006. Isolation by size of epithelial tumor cells in peripheral blood of patients with breast cancer: correlation with real-time reverse transcriptase–polymerase chain reaction results and feasibility of molecular analysis by laser microdissection. *Human Pathology*, 37(6), pp.711-718.

Przybytkowski, E. et al. 2011. The use of ultra-dense array CGH analysis for the discovery of micro-copy number alterations and gene fusions in the cancer genome. *BMC Medical Genomics*, 4(16).

Riethdorf, S. et al., 2007. Detection of circulating tumor cells in peripheral blood of patients with metastatic breast cancer: a validation study of the CellSearch system. *Clinical*

Cancer Research: An Official Journal of the American Association for Cancer Research, 13(3), pp.920-928.

Ring, A.E. et al., 2005. Detection of circulating epithelial cells in the blood of patients with breast cancer: comparison of three techniques. *British Journal of Cancer*, 92(5), pp.906-912.

Sandri, M.T. et al., 2010. Changes in circulating tumor cell detection in patients with localized breast cancer before and after surgery. *Annals of Surgical Oncology*, 17(6), pp.1539-1545.

Schardt, J.A. et al., 2005. Genomic analysis of single cytokeratin-positive cells from bone marrow reveals early mutational events in breast cancer. *Cancer Cell*, 8(3), pp.227-239.

Schmidt-Kittler, O. et al., 2003. From latent disseminated cells to overt metastasis: genetic analysis of systemic breast cancer progression. *Proceedings of the National Academy of Sciences of the United States of America*, 100(13), pp.7737-7742.

Shadeo, A. et al., 2006. Comprehensive copy number profiles of breast cancer cell model genomes. *Breast Cancer Research*. 8(1),R9.

Sieuwerts, A.M. et al., 2008. Molecular characterization of circulating tumor cells in large quantities of contaminating leukocytes by a multiplex real-time PCR. *Breast Cancer Research and Treatment*, 118(3), pp.455-468.

Smirnov, D.A. et al., 2005. Global gene expression profiling of circulating tumor cells. *Cancer Research*, 65(12), pp.4993-4997.

Sørlie, T. et al., 2001. Gene expression patterns of breast carcinomas distinguish tumor subclasses with clinical implications. *Proceedings of the National Academy of Sciences of the United States of America*, 98(19), pp.10869-10874.

Sørlie, T. et al., 2006. Distinct molecular mechanisms underlying clinically relevant subtypes of breast cancer: gene expression analyses across three different platforms. *BMC Genomics*, 7, p.127.

Stott, S.L. et al., 2010. Isolation of circulating tumor cells using a microvortex-generating herringbone-chip. *Proceedings of the National Academy of Sciences of the United States of America*, 107(43), pp.18392-18397.

Talasaz, A.H. et al., 2009. Isolating highly enriched populations of circulating epithelial cells and other rare cells from blood using a magnetic sweeper device. *Proceedings of the National Academy of Sciences of the United States of America*, 106(10), pp.3970-3975.

Van der Auwera, I. et al., 2010. Circulating tumour cell detection: a direct comparison between the CellSearch System, the AdnaTest and CK-19/mammaglobin RT-PCR in patients with metastatic breast cancer. *British Journal of Cancer*, 102(2), pp.276-284.

van de Vijver, M.J. et al., 2002. A gene-expression signature as a predictor of survival in breast cancer. *The New England Journal of Medicine*, 347(25), pp.1999-2009.

Weigelt, B., Peterse, J.L. & van 't Veer, L.J., 2005. Breast cancer metastasis: markers and models. *Nature Reviews. Cancer*, 5(8), pp.591-602.

Wikman, H., Vessella, R. & Pantel, K., 2008. Cancer micrometastasis and tumour dormancy. *APMIS: Acta Pathologica, Microbiologica, Et Immunologica Scandinavica,* 116(7-8), pp.754-770.

9

Proteomic Analysis of Potential Breast Cancer Biomarkers

Hsiu-Chuan Chou[1] and Hong-Lin Chan[2]
[1]*Department of Applied Science, National Hsinchu University of Education, Hsinchu,*
[2]*Institute of Bioinformatics and Structural Biology and Department of Medical Science, National Tsing Hua University, Hsinchu,*
Taiwan

1. Introduction

1.1 Cell signalling and tumorigenesis

In multi-cellular organisms, cells have to communicate with each other in order to control their proliferation, differentiation, survival and to perform diverse physiological functions. Cells release and receive signals to induce these different states of growth either by direct cell-to-cell interaction or via secreted molecules. This communication is elicited through so-called signaling molecules such as transmembrane receptors that are embedded in cell membrane and can activate intracellular signal transduction cascades which ultimately lead to gene activation or repression and a cellular response. According to the specificity, strength and duration of the signal received, the cell will proliferate, differentiate, change shape, migrate, and enter into growth arrest or undergo apoptosis. These complex signaling networks are highly regulated and alterations of the normal intracellular signals can lead to the development of diseases such as cancer. It is now known that a series of genetic mutations are required for the progressive conversion of normal human cells into cancerous cells. Hanahan and Weinberg have proposed a model of tumorigenesis, whereby several physiological conditions are required before cells become tumorigenic (Hanahan and Weinberg, 2011). These include self-sufficiency in growth signals, insensitivity to growth-inhibitory signals, evasion of programmed cell death, limitless replicative potential, sustained angiogenesis, tissue invasion and metastasis. In proliferative signaling pathways for example, numerous proto-oncogenes or tumor suppressors have been identified, the mutation of which cause amplification of signaling or loss of negative regulation resulting in over-proliferation and eventual tumor formation. Unlike normal cells, which tightly regulate extracellular ligand levels, receptor expression and secondary signaling molecules, cancer cells often lose the ability to regulate these signaling events. For example, overexpression of receptor tyrosine kinases (RTKs) (Libermann et al., 1985), mutation of RAt Sarcoma (Ras) protein (Marshall, 1996) or the overexpression of PI3K (phosphatidylinositol 3-kinase) (Sulis and Parsons, 2003) are thought to lead to cell transformation.

1.2 Correlation between tumor secreted proteins and cancer

During tumor metastasis, cell-cell interactions are decreased leading to cell dissociation and detachment from the primary tumor. On the other hand, cell-extracellular matrix interactions are increased facilitating tumor cell migration and metastasis. Thus, during tumorigenesis and metastasis, the secreted proteins in the extracellular space are majorly responsible for growth control, cell adhesion/migration, matrix-degradation, invasion and angiogenesis (Mbeunkui et al., 2006b). Importantly, these tumor cell secreted proteins majorly enter body fluid system such as blood, urine, lymph fluid and can be measured by non-invasive tests. Thus, analysis the tumor secreted proteins is a promising strategy to discover cancer biomarkers.

1.3 Detection of breast cancer markers with high-throughput technologies

Breast cancer is one of the leading causes of death among women around the world. The 5-year survival rate for breast cancer is near 97% when tumors are confined to breast tissue, but decrease dramatically to 23% when tumors have metastasized to other organs at the time of diagnosis (Kulasingam and Diamandis, 2007b; Jemal et al., 2004). Previous studies indicated that the transformation and metastasis of normal breast cells are correlated to altered expression in both transcription and translation levels (Nuyten and van de Vijver, 2008; Morrow, 2007; Lee et al., 2007; Kulasingam and Diamandis, 2007a; Hondermarck et al., 2002). To better understand the molecular mechanisms associated with tumorigenesis and metastasis, it is necessary to identify gene expression signatures and protein expression markers among non-tumorigenic breast cells, non-invasive breast cancer cells, and invasive breast cancer cells. At the transcription level, microarray strategies have been used to classify breast tumors as highly invasive and non-invasive cancer (Sorlie et al., 2003; Nagaraja et al., 2006). At the translation level, proteomic strategies have been used to discern cancer markers from non-invasive and invasive breast cells (Nagaraja et al., 2006; Pawlik et al., 2006; Pucci-Minafra et al., 2002; Varnum et al., 2003). Nagaraja *et al.* compared the proteomic profiling of cell lines corresponding to healthy breast cells, non-invasive breast cancer cells, and invasive breast cancer cells using two-dimensional gel electrophoresis (2-DE). Pucci-Minafra *et al.* compared a ductal infiltrating carcinoma-derived cell line with a non-tumoral mammary epithelial cell line using 2-DE, silver staining, immunodetection, and N-terminal sequencing and identified 58 differentially expressed proteins. In contrast to these cell line based studies, Pawlik *et al.* and Varnum *et al.* analyzed differentially expressed proteins among nipple aspirate fluid samples from tumor-bearing and disease-free breasts. Although these identified proteins are primarily abundant proteins, few of them have been validated as biomarkers.

During tumorigenesis and metastasis, secreted proteins in the extracellular space are major factors in growth control, cell motility, cell invasion, angiogenesis and matrix-degradation (Mbeunkui et al., 2006a). Consequently, the analysis of tumor secreted proteins is a promising strategy for identifying cancer biomarkers. In the past few years, researchers have used proteomic analysis to identify some secreted biomarker candidates for human cancer using 2-dimensional differential in-gel electrophoresis (2D-DIGE) and liquid chromatography-tandem (LC-tandem) mass spectrometry. These markers have been found in lung cancer, liver cancer, pancreatic cancer and colorectal cancer (Xue et al., 2008b). In breast cancer research, Kulasingam and Diamandis used a liquid chromatography-mass spectrometry/mass (LC-MS/MS) strategy to analyze and compare the expression of extracellular and membrane-bound proteins in conditioned media of three breast cell types corresponding to a normal control and cell lines derived from stage 2 and stage 4 patients. Their studies identified numerous marker proteins from conditioned media (Kulasingam and Diamandis, 2007b).

1.4 Utilization of 2D-DIGE / MALDI-TOF MS-based strategies in the global analysis of breast cancer markers

2-DE is currently a key technique in profiling thousands of proteins within biological samples and plays a role complementary to LC/MS-based proteomic analysis (Timms and Cramer, 2008a). However, reliable quantitative comparisons between gels and gel-to-gel variations remain the primary challenge in 2-DE analysis. A significant improvement in the gel-based analysis of protein quantitation and detection was achieved by the introduction of 2D-DIGE, which can co-detect numerous samples in the same 2-DE. This approach minimizes gel-to-gel variations and compares the relative amount of protein features across different gels using an internal fluorescent standard. Moreover, the 2D-DIGE technique has the advantages of a broader dynamic range, higher sensitivity, and greater reproducibility than traditional 2-DE. This innovative technology relies on the pre-labeling of protein samples with fluorescent dyes (Cy2, Cy3 and Cy5) before electrophoresis. Each dye has a distinct fluorescent wavelength, allowing multiple experimental samples with an internal standard to be simultaneously separated in the same gel. The internal standard, which is a pool of an equal amount of the experimental protein samples, helps provide accurate normalization data and increase statistical confidence in relative quantitation among gels (Timms and Cramer, 2008b; Westermeier and Scheibe, 2008; Marouga et al., 2005; Lai et al., 2010; Chou et al., 2010; Huang et al., 2010; Chan et al., 2005; Chan et al., 2009).

Followed the separation of the proteins from biological samples by 2-DE and proteolysis of interested spots by a specific protease, subsequently mass spectrometry is an accurate and sensitive tool to identify these interesting proteins/peptides. Basically, there are two major types of approach used in the identification of proteins and peptides. The first one is matrix-assisted laser-desorption/ionization mass spectrometry (MALDI-TOF-MS) (Karas and Hillenkamp, 1988) and the other one is electrospray ionization mass spectrometry (ESI-MS) (Fenn et al., 1989; Whitehouse et al., 1985). MALDI-TOF-MS relies on ions generated from a solid phase using laser pulses. The sample is usually applied in a matrix solution [eg. 2,5-dihydroxybenzoic acid (DHB) and alpha-cyano-4-hydroxycinnamic acid (CHCA)] that facilitates the ion formation by absorption of photon energy from a laser source. ESI-MS generates ions from a liquid phase. The sample, in a solvent mixture is directly sprayed into the mass spectrometry where an electrostatic field is formed between the capillary and the walls of the mass spectrometer. As the droplets form and travel, they evaporate and the resulting charged particles enter into the gas phase. Each ion is separated in the mass spectrometry according to its mass-to-charge ratio (m/z ratio). Protein identification by mass spectrometry can be carried out by peptide mass mapping using MALDI-TOF-MS or by further peptide fragmentation to generate sequence data using tandem mass spectrometry (MS/MS) (Henzel et al., 1993; James et al., 1993; Mann et al., 1993; Yates, III et al., 1993).

1.5 Application of luminal epithelial cell models with various invasive stages in the discovery of breast cancer markers

A direct comparison of cancer tissue with normal tissue is the best theoretical method of obtaining protein expression signatures during tumor progression. However, a direct comparison of clinical samples increases the amount of false positives due to the heterogeneity of tumor specimens, which interferes with the identification of tumor-specific markers. For this reason, well-characterized model cell lines established from normal and tumor tissue are recognized as more informative in cancer proteomics research. In the field of breast cancer research, MCF-10A, MCF-7 and MDA-MB-231 are widely used to represent non-tumorigeneic breast luminal epithelial cells, non-invasive breast cancer cells derived from the luminal duct and metastatic breast cancer cells derived from the same tissue, respectively (Singh et al., 2006; Lu et al., 2006). Accordingly, we are introduced a proteomics strategy to discover the putative diagnostic markers and therapeutic targets from this cell model system. To achieve these goals, it is necessary to identify potential biomarkers that reflect the progression of tumorigenesis. Thus, we compared the proteomic profiles of total cellular proteins and secreted proteins of this cell model system using 2D-DIGE to quantitatively identify putative transformation markers in breast cancer.

2. 2D-DIGE and MALDI-TOF MS analysis of secretomes across MCF-10A, MCF-7 and MDA-MB-231 cells

Secreted proteins, plasma membrane bound proteins and extracellular proteins mediate cell attachment, cell motility, cell-cell interactions and cell invasion. These proteins have the highest possibility of being found in the circulation system, including the blood, and thus serve as cancer markers or important markers involved in cancer formation (Xue et al., 2008a). To identify potential proteins that may be involved in tumor formation and metastasis, this study develops a strategy for preparing secreted proteins from normal and cancer cell lines with minimal cytosolic protein contamination. Although these cell lines are generally grown in serum-supplemented media, a serum-free conditioned medium is necessary to prevent serum protein contamination and to allow accurate detection of proteins secreted by cells. A serum-free medium is believed to affect the growth of cells and the production of secreted proteins; however, recent studies indicate that the serum-free condition does not significantly affect the composition of the secreted proteins (Yamaguchi et al., 1990; Inoue et al., 2000). In addition, it is impossible to prevent cell death, and the release of considerable amounts of cytosolic proteins into culture media in either the serum-free condition or the serum-supplemented medium. Accordingly, an intensive wash step was performed prior to incubating these cells in serum-free media to remove both cytosolic proteins and serum proteins. Meanwhile, the incubation time in serum-free media was optimized in advance, minimizing the serum-free induced autolysis of the cells, and enabling the recovery of an adequate amount of secreted proteins for 2D-DIGE analysis. The concentration of secreted proteins in this study was extremely low at approximately 1~2 μg / ml. For this reason, a concentration step was essential to enrich secreted proteins enough for proteomics analysis, and a desalt step was also required for the 2D-DIGE experiment. In this secretomic analysis, MCF-10A, MCF-7 and MDA-MB-231 were grown on cell culture dishes and the confluency of cells was checked prior to incubation in serum-free culture media to ensure that no other exogenous proteins were present. To minimize cell autolysis induced by starvation and to maximize secreted protein concentration in the media, the starvation time of each cell line has to be optimized. Through immunoblotting, the lactate dehydrogenase (LDH) and β-tubulin levels were detected in the 1000-fold concentrated serum-free media starting at 48~60 hrs and at 60~72 hrs, respectively (Figure 1). LDH and β-tubulin are both cytoplasmic proteins and their levels in the media represent the amount of cell death taking place in cell culture. Accordingly, a starvation period of 30 hrs was chosen for further 2D-DIGE based secretomic analysis.

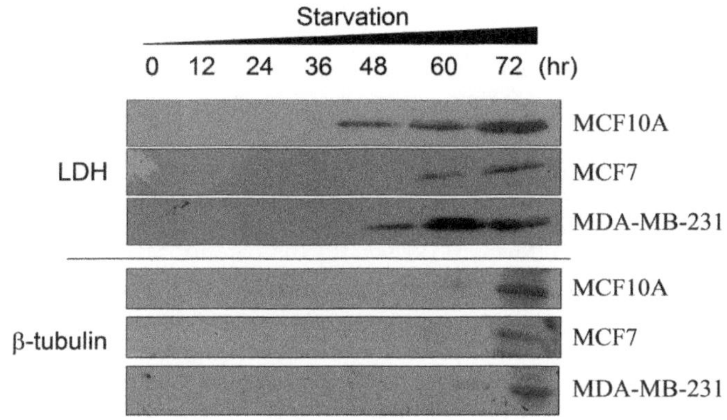

Fig. 1. Optimization of starvation time for secretomic analysis. MCF-10A, MCF-7 and MDA-MB-231 on cell culture dishes were used to check starvation induced cell autolysis by detecting the release of cytoplasmic proteins, LDH and β-tubulin in serum-free media. The serum-free media were harvested and concentrated 1000-fold at indicative starvation periods prior to performing immunoblotting analysis.

Subsequently, proteins secreted from each cell type were enriched from the serum-free medium followed by labeling with CyDyes for 2D-DIGE analysis. The secretomic profiling of MCF-10A, MCF-7 and MDA-MB-231 were visualized using a fluorescence scanner and the images were superimposed using ImageQuant software (Figure. 2). To investigate the potential involvement of secreted proteins in tumorigenesis and metastasis for human breast cancer, biological variation analysis of spots showing greater than 1.5-fold change in expression with a *t*-test score of less than 0.05 were visually checked before confirming the alterations for protein identification. MALDI-TOF MS identification revealed 50 unique differentially expressed proteins across MCF-10A, MCF-7 and MDA-MB-231 (Table 1). Of the proteins identified, 42 were differentially expressed between MCF-7 / MCF-10A, 44 of them were differentially expressed between MDA-MB-231 / MCF-10A, and 37 proteins were differentially expressed between MDA-MB-231 and MCF-7. In the three cell lines investigated, 39% of the total proteins identified were extracellular and plasma membrane-anchored proteins (Figure 3A) indicating that these membrane-associated proteins might be trimmed off the plasma membrane by proteases or might not be completely integrated into the plasma membrane. Most of the identified proteins were involved in signaling transduction, redox-regulation and metabolism (Figure 3B). To our knowledge, 14 out of these identified spots, including tetratricopeptide repeats 3 (IFIT3), have not been reported in any breast cancer related studies. Consequently, these proteins might have the potential to be putative breast cancer markers. As expected, this 2D-DIGE experiment also identified a number of reported breast cancer markers, including Cathepsin D (Zhang et al., 2007) and Insulin-like growth factor-binding protein 4 (IGFBP4) (Mita et al., 2007). These results demonstrate that the proposed approach significantly enriches secreted proteins and membrane proteins in comparison with the previous report that only 2% of the entire mammary epithelial cell proteomes are classified as secreted and membrane proteins (Jacobs et al., 2004). On the other hand, 61% of the total identified proteins in the medium were neither secreted proteins nor membrane-bound proteins. Most of them were sub-located in the cytoplasma, implying that some level of cell necrosis or autolysis was taking place.

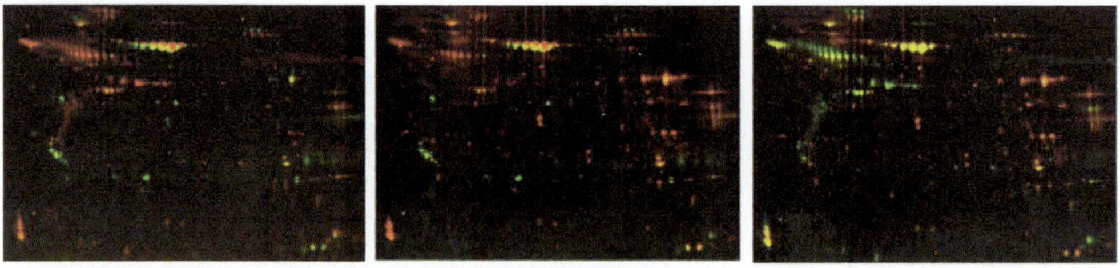

MCF7 (Red) / MCF10A (Green) MDA231 (Red) / MCF10A (Green) MDA231 (Red) / MCF7 (Green)

Fig. 2. **Secretomic comparisons across MCF-10A, MCF-7 and MDA-MB-231 cells using 2D-DIGE.** Protein samples (50μg each) enriched from serum-free media were labeled with CyDyes and separated using 24 cm, pH 3-10 non-linear IPG strips. 2D-DIGE images of MCF-10A, MCF-7, and MDA-MB-231 at appropriate excitation and emission wavelengths were pseudo-colored and overlaid with ImageQuant Tool (GE Healthcare).

Secretomic profiles of MCF7 cells compared to MCF10A cells	
upregulated	*downregulated*
Cell cycle	***Biosynthesis***
E3 ubiquitin-protein ligase CCNB1IP1	Inositol monophosphatase
Cell motility	***Cell motility / protease inhibitor***
Merlin / Neurofibromin-2	Arfaptin-1
Cytoskeleton	Moesin
Actin	***Membrane trafficking***
Alpha-actinin-4	Rab GTPase-binding effector protein 2
Dynein heavy chain 6	***Metabolism***
Electron transport	Alpha-enolase
NADH dehydrogenase iron-sulfur protein 6	Carbonic anhydrase 2
Metabolism	***Protease Inhibitor***
Aldose reductase	SERPIN B1
Cytosolic non-specific dipeptidase / Peptidase	SERPIN B5
Protease inhibitor	SERPIN 1
SERPIN A3	***Redox regulation***
Protein folding	Glutathione S-transferase P
Heat shock protein beta-1	Superoxide dismutase [Mn], mitochondrial
Redox regulation	***Signal transduction***
Glutathione S-transferase Mu 3	14-3-3 protein beta/alpha
Peroxiredoxin-1	14-3-3 protein zeta/delta
Peroxiredoxin-2	IFIT3
Signal transduction	***Transport***
Insulin-like growth factor-binding protein 4	Plasma membrane calcium-transporting ATPase 2
Rab GDP dissociation inhibitor alpha	***Vascular Transport***
TNFAIP3-interacting protein 2	Vacuolar protein sorting-associated protein 54
MAGUK p55 subfamily member 2 / MPP2	
Signal transduction /Ca regulation	
Protein S100-A14	
Transport	
Bestrophin-3	
Unknown	
GRAM domain-containing protein 2	

Secretomic profiles of MDA-MB-231 cells compared to MCF10A cells	
upregulated	*downregulated*
Biosynthesis	***Cell motility /Ca regulation***
3'(2'),5'-bisphosphate nucleotidase 1	Plastin-2 / L-plastin
Inositol monophosphatase	***Immune regulation***
Cell cycle	Complement C3
Cyclin-dependent kinase inhibitor 1B	***Membrane trafficking***
E3 ubiquitin-protein ligase CCNB1IP1	Rab GTPase-binding effector protein 2
Cytoskeleton	***Metabolism***
Dynein heavy chain 6	Carbonic anhydrase 2
Electron transport	***Protease Inhibitor***
NADH dehydrogenase iron-sulfur protein 6	SERPIN B1
Metabolism	SERPIN B5
Aldose reductase	SERPIN 1
Cytosolic non-specific dipeptidase / Peptidase A	***Protein folding***
Phosphoglycerate mutase 1	Heat shock protein beta-1
Purine nucleoside phosphorylase	***Redox regulation***
Signal transduction	Glutathione S-transferase P
Insulin-like growth factor-binding protein 4	***Signal transduction***
Rab GDP dissociation inhibitor alpha	14-3-3 protein beta/alpha
TNFAIP3-interacting protein 2	14-3-3 protein zeta/delta
MAGUK p55 subfamily member 2 / MPP2	IFIT3
Signal transduction /Ca regulation	***Transport***
Annexin A5	Selenium-binding protein 1 / SELENBP1
Transport	Plasma membrane calcium-transporting ATPase 2
Bestrophin-3	***Vascular Transport***
Unknown	Vacuolar protein sorting-associated protein 54
GRAM domain-containing protein 2	

Table 1. Identification of differentially expressed secreted proteins across MCF-10A, MCF-7, and MDA-MB-231 breast cells obtained after 2D-DIGE coupled with MALDI-TOF mass spectrometry analysis. The functional classes of identified proteins were obtained from the Uniprot website (http://www.uniprot.org/). The average ratio (≧2 fold) of differentially expressed proteins across MCF-7 / MCF-10A and MDA-MB-231 / MCF-10A were calculated considering 3 replica gels ($p < 0.05$) and listed in this table.

A

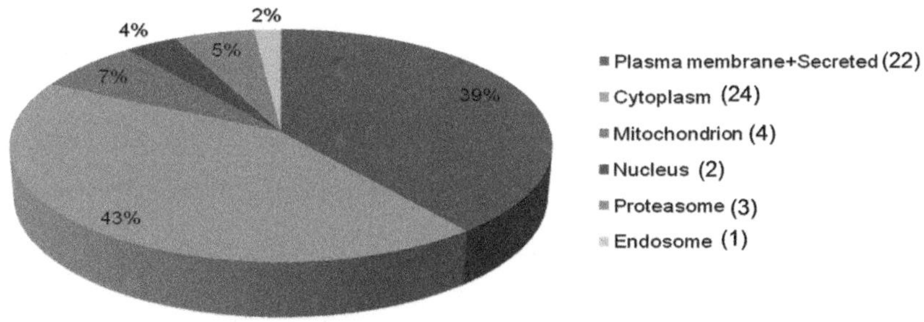

B

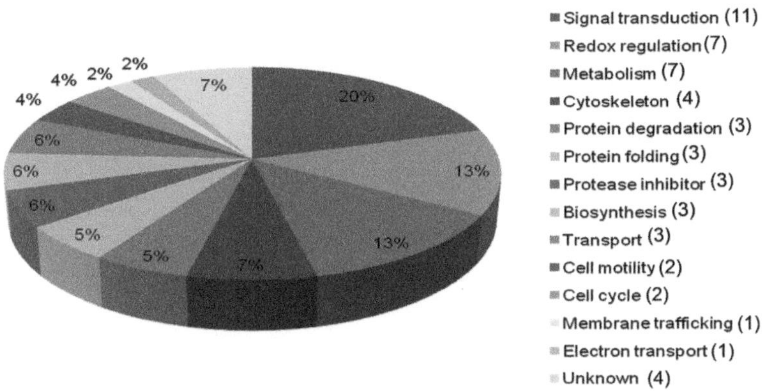

Fig. 3. Percentage of secreted proteins identified from serum-free media by 2D-DIGE / MALDI-TOF MS for MCF-10A, MCF-7 and MDA-MB-231 cells according to their sub-cellular locations (A) and biological functions (B).

3. 2D-DIGE and MALDI-TOF MS analysis of total intracellular proteomes across MCF-10A, MCF-7 and MDA-MB-231 cells

To identify the altered abundances of proteins and relate them to the tumorigenesis of breast cancer, the proteomic profiles of MCF-10A, MCF-7 and MDA-MB-231 were analyzed. Triplicates of the three different cell lysates were compared using 2D-DIGE to obtain an overview of breast cell tumorigenesis. Image analysis using DeCyder v7.0 clearly defined more than 2500 protein spots (Figure 4). To reduce the intrinsic variability derived from protein samples and gel-to-gel variation, only those protein spots that appeared in all of the triplicate gel images were used for statistical analysis. Furthermore, biological variation analysis of spots showing greater than 1.5-fold change in expression with a *t*-test score of less than 0.05 were visually checked before confirming the alterations for protein identification. MALDI-TOF MS identification revealed 133 unique differentially expressed proteins across MCF-10A, MCF-7, and MDA-MB-231 (Table 2). Of the 133 proteins

Proteomic profiles of MCF7 cells compared to MCF10A cells		Proteomic profiles of MDA-MB-231 cells compared to MCF10A cells	
upregulated	*downregulated*	*upregulated*	*downregulated*
Carbohydrate Metabolism	***Carbohydrate Metabolism***	***Cytoskeleton***	***Cell motility***
Fructose-bisphosphate aldolase A	L-lactate dehydrogenase B chain	Vimentin	Rho-associated protein kinase 2
Glucose-6-phosphate 1-dehydrogenase	Pyruvate kinase isozymes M1/M2	***Gene regulation***	F-actin-capping protein subunit beta
Triosephosphate isomerase	***Cytoskeleton***	Achaete-scute homolog 4	Cofilin-1
Cell motility	Glial fibrillary acidic protein	Serine-threonine kinase receptor-associated protein	***Cytoskeleton***
Rho GTPase-activating protein 5	***Metabolism***	***Growth Regulation***	Glial fibrillary acidic protein
Rho-associated protein kinase 2	Leukotriene A-4 hydrolase	Prohibitin	***Gene regulation***
Gene regulation	Phosphoserine aminotransferase	***Metabolism***	Heterogeneous nuclear ribonucleoproteins A2/B1
Zinc finger protein 433	Carbonic anhydrase 2	Lactoylglutathione lyase	Alpha-1-fetoprotein transcription factor
Nuclear receptor subfamily 5 group A member 2	***Protein metabolism***	Aldose reductase	***Growth Regulation***
Growth Regulation	Aminopeptidase B	Alpha-enolase	***Metabolism***
Protein CASC2, isoform 3	***Protein folding***	***Protein metabolism***	Carbonic anhydrase 2
Metabolism	Protein disulfide-isomerase A3	Elongation factor 1-delta	***Protein metabolism***
Lactoylglutathione lyase	cyclophilin A	Elongation factor 1-gamma	Aminopeptidase B
Protein metabolism	***Redox regulation***	***Protein degradation***	***Protein degradation***
Elongation factor 2	Glutathione S-transferase P	***Protein folding***	Cathepsin D
Elongation factor 1-gamma	***Signal transduction***	Endoplasmic reticulum protein ERp29	***Protein folding***
Protein degradation	Inhibitor of apoptosis-like protein 2	Nucleophosmin	cyclophilin A
Cathepsin D	***Signal transduction /Ca regulation***	***Redox regulation***	Heat shock protein beta-1 / HSP 27
Protein folding	Calcium-dependent protease small subunit	Flavin reductase	***Redox regulation***
HSP 27	Annexin A2	Glutathione S-transferase Mu3	Peroxiredoxin-6
Endoplasmic reticulum protein ERp29	Annexin A5	***Signal transduction***	Glutathione S-transferase P
FK506-binding protein 4	***Transport***	Growth factor receptor-bound protein 2 (Grb2)	***Signal transduction***
Heat shock protein 75 kDa	Chloride intracellular channel protein 4	***Transport***	ATP synthase subunit beta
Redox regulation	Voltage-dependent anion-selective channel protein 1	Chloride intracellular channel protein 1	PI3-kinase p110 subunit alpha
Flavin reductase	Voltage-dependent anion-selective channel protein 2		Inhibitor of apoptosis-like protein 2
Glutathione S-transferase Mu3	***Cell-cell interaction***		***Signal transduction /Ca regulation***
Peroxiredoxin-4	Galectin-1		Calcium-dependent protease small subunit
Signal transduction	***Protease inhibitor***		Annexin A2
Rab GDP dissociation inhibitor beta	Serpin B5		Annexin A3
PI3-kinase p110 subunit alpha			Annexin A4
Growth factor receptor-bound protein 2			***TCA cycle***
MAGUK p55 subfamily member 2			Malate dehydrogenase
Prostaglandin E synthase 3			***Transport***
Rho-related BTB domain-containing protein 2			Voltage-dependent anion-selective channel protein 1
Signal transduction /Ca regulation			Voltage-dependent anion-selective channel protein 2
Annexin A3			Chloride intracellular channel protein 4
Annexin A6			Cellular retinoic acid-binding protein 2
Transport			***Cell-cell interaction***
Selenium-binding protein 1			Galectin-1
Cellular retinoic acid-binding protein 2			***Protease inhibitor***
ALG-2-interacting protein 1			Serpin B5

Table 2. Identification of differentially expressed total cellular proteomes across MCF-10A, MCF-7, and MDA-MB-231 breast cells obtained after 2D-DIGE coupled with MALDI-TOF mass spectrometry analysis. The functional classes of identified proteins were obtained from the Uniprot website (http://www.uniprot.org/). The average ratio ($\geqq 2$ fold) of differentially expressed proteins across MCF-7 / MCF-10A and MDA-MB-231 / MCF-10A were calculated considering 3 replica gels ($p < 0.05$) and listed in this table.

identified, 107 of them had differential expressions between MCF-7 / MCF-10A, 63 were differentially expressed between MDA-MB-231 / MCF-10A and 96 had differential expressions between MDA-MB-231 and MCF-7. Almost half of the total proteins identified in this breast cell model were cytosolic proteins (Figure 5A), and most of the identified proteins were involved in signaling transduction, metabolism, protein folding, and cell motility (Figure 5B). To our knowledge, 51 of these identified spots, including calumenin, have not been reported in any breast cancer related studies. As such, these proteins might have the potential to be putative breast cancer markers. As expected, some well-known breast cancer markers, such as 14-3-3 proteins (Danes et al., 2008), annexins (Cao et al., 2008a), calmodulin (Gallo et al., 2008), anterior gradient homolog 2 (AGR-2) (Zweitzig et al., 2007; Fritzsche et al., 2006), Galectin-1 (Jung et al., 2007) and Rho-associated protein kinase-2

(ROCK2) (Fu et al., 2008b), were also identified in this 2D-DIGE experiment, lending credence to the reliability of early phase biomarker detection using this experimental strategy.

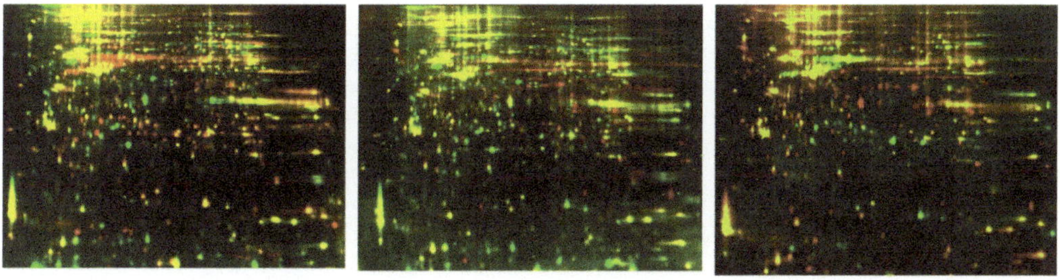

Fig. 4. **Proteomic comparisons across MCF-10A, MCF-7 and MDA-MB-231 cells using 2D-DIGE.** Protein samples (150μg each) purified from total cell lysates were labeled with Cy-dyes and separated using 24 cm, pH 3-10 non-linear IPG strips. 2D-DIGE images of MCF-10A, MCF-7 and MDA-MB-231 at appropriate excitation and emission wavelengths were pseudo-colored and overlaid with ImageQuant Tool (GE Healthcare).

4. Validation of characterized breast cancer markers through immunoblotting and immunofluorescence

The secretomic study indentified some of the well-characterized breast cancer related cytosolic proteins such as Cyclophilin A, 14-3-3delta and peroxiredoxin 2 in culture media (Harding and Handschumacher, 1988; Aitken, 2006; Fujii and Ikeda, 2002). It is essential to validate the levels of these cytosolic proteins in the medium from independent experiments. To this end, the expression level of cyclophilin A, 14-3-3delta and peroxiredoxin 2 from the culture media of MDA-MB-231, MCF-7 and MCF-10A were validated with immunoblotting. The results indicate that both the proteomic and immunoblot analysis showed cyclophilin A and 14-3-3 delta down-regulated in MCF-7 in comparison to the levels in MCF-10A. In contrast, peroxiredoxin 2 showed up-regulation in MCF-7 in comparison to the levels in MCF-10A. Comparing the secreted protein levels between MCF-10A and MDA-MB-231 indicates that the peroxiredoxin 2 and 14-3-3 delta expression levels increased in MDA-MB-231 and MCF-10A, respectively; however, the cyclophilin A level showed no significant change (Figure 6 A~C). This observation confirmed that cyclophilin A, 14-3-3delta and peroxiredoxin 2 were differentially secreted across the breast cells.

Immunoblot and immunofluorescence analysis were carried out to further confirm the differential protein levels observed in total cellular proteins (annexin-2, cathepsin D, profilin, protein disulfide isomerase A1 and Histone deacetylase 1 (HDAC1)) across MDA-MB-231, MCF-7 and MCF-10A (Figure 6 D~H). These proteins have been reported to play important roles in cytoskeleton regulation, proteolysis, calcium regulation, protein disulfide bond rearrangement and chromatin assembly during tumorigenesis (Feldner and Brandt, 2002; Liaudet-Coopman et al., 2006; Sharma and Sharma, 2007; Fu et al., 2008a; Kawai et al., 2003). The results of the immunoblotting indicate that cathepsin D and protein disulfide isomerase (PDI) showed up-regulation in MCF-7 cells but down-regulation in MDA-MB-231 compared to the two protein expressions in MCF-10A. The expression levels of the profilin and annexin 2 proteins showed down-regulation in MCF-7 but no significant changes in MDA-MB-231 compared to the levels in MCF-10A. These immunoblotting results demonstrate a positive correlation with the 2D-DIGE results (Figure 6 D~G). In addition to immunoblotting, validation was also performed with immunofluorescent analysis. Figure 6H shows that most of the HDAC1 signal was distributed within the nucleus, which is consistent with the subcellular location of HDAC1 in cells. As expected, the fluorescent intensity with the same exposure indicates that HDAC1 showed increased expressions in MCF-7 and MDA-MB-231 compared to its expression in MCF-10A. Altogether, the results from immunoblotting and immunofluorescent agreed with the results from 2D-DIGE data.

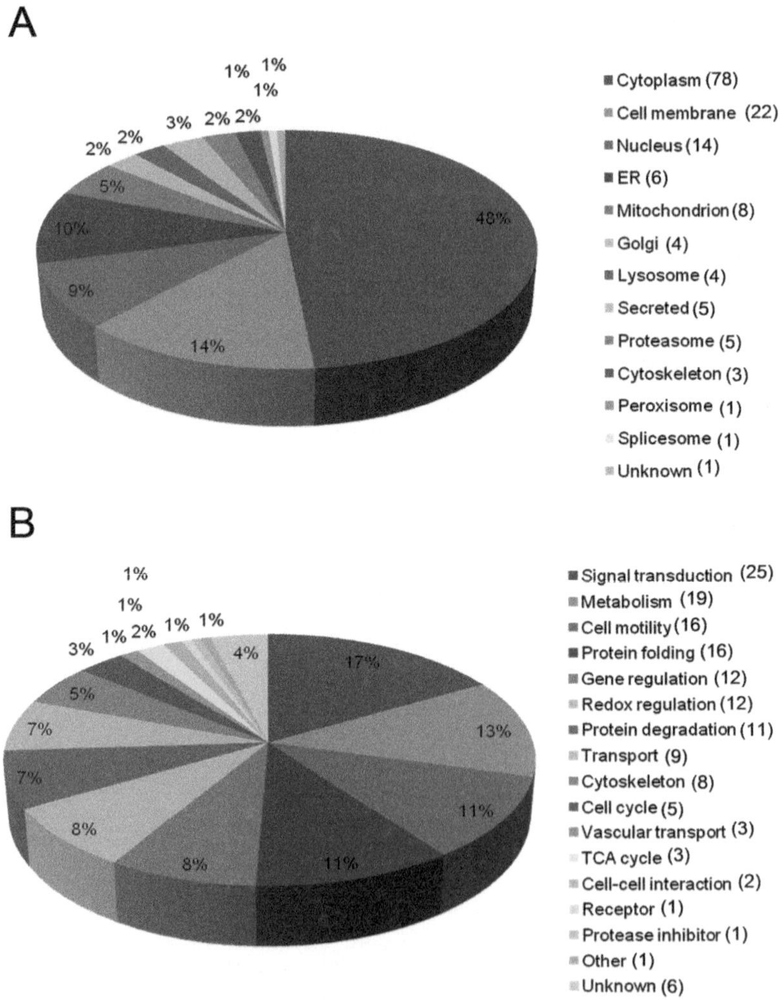

Fig. 5. Percentage of total cellular proteins identified by 2D-DIGE / MALDI-TOF MS for MCF-10A, MCF-7 and MDA-MB-231 cells according to their sub-cellular locations (A) and biological functions (B).

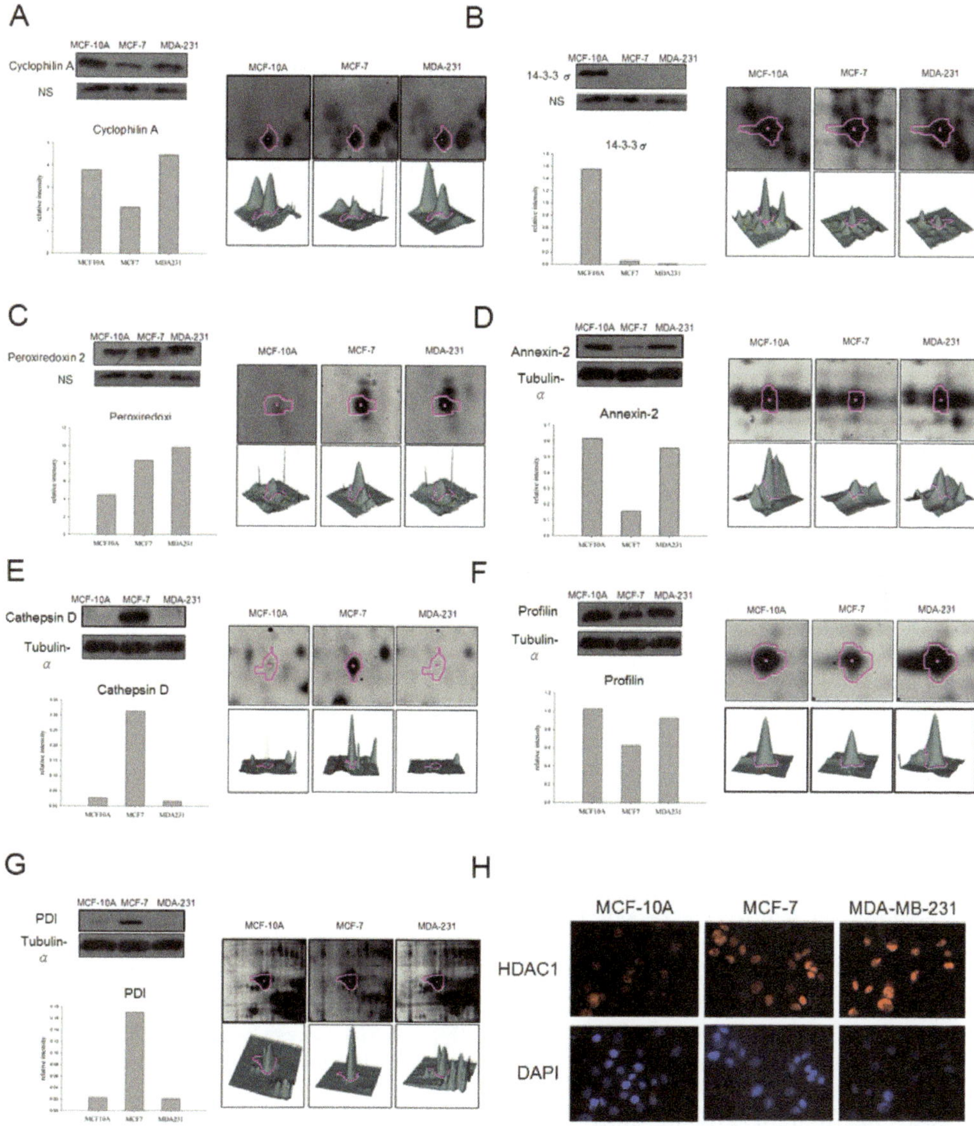

Fig. 6. Representative immunoblotting and immunofluorescent analyses for selected differentially expressed proteins identified by proteomic analysis in MCF-10A, MCF-7 and MDA-MB-231 cells. The levels of identified proteins in serum-free media, (A) Cyclophilin A, (B) 14-3-3 delta and (C) Peroxiredoxin 2 and total cellular proteins, (D) Annexin-2, (E) Cathepsin D, (F) Profilin and (G) Protein disulfide isomerase A1 in MDA-MB-231 and MCF-7 versus MCF-10A confirmed by immunoblot (left top panels), densitometry results with normalized values using nonspecific bands (NS) of secreted proteins and α-tubulin as loading controls (left bottom panels), protein expression map (right top panels) and three-

dimensional spot image (right bottom panels). (H) MCF-10A, MCF-7 and MDA-MB-231 cells were fixed and incubated with anti-HDAC antibody and stained with a Texas Red-conjugated secondary antibody (Red). Nuclei were stained with DAPI (Blue). Each set of three fields was taken using the same exposure, and images are representative of three different fields. Scale bar = 20μm.

5. Validation of unreported identified putative tumorigenic markers through immunoblotting and immunofluorescence

The cellular proteomic and secretomic analyses above reveal that a number of unreported identified proteins may be putative breast cancer markers (Tables 1 and 2). To verify this observation, immunoblotting and immunofluorescence were used to validate these differentially expressed proteins including bestrophin 3, membrane protein, palmitoylated 2 (MPP2), parvalbumin, PDZ and LIM domain protein 1 (PdLIM1), IFIT3 and barrier to autointegration factor 1 (BANF1) as these proteins showed relatively significant changes (> 3 fold) in comparison with most of the unreported identified proteins across MCF-10A, MCF-7 and MDA-MB-231. The immunoblotting analysis of concentrated serum-free media shows that more bestrophin 3 was secreted in the cell lines of MCF-7 and MDA-MB-231 than MCF-10A, while MPP2 was only detected in MDA-MB-231. Notably, the bestrophin 3 blotting result did not completely agree with the 2D-DIGE data, where levels in MCF-7 were higher than MDA-MB-231 (Figure 7A). Using immunofluorescent staining, the robust increase of parvalbumin signal in both the MCF-7 and MDA-MB-231 cells was first confirmed after comparison with the signal in MCF-10A. Parvalbumin was primarily localized in the nucleus, which coincided with the DAPI stained nucleus. Further investigation of parvabumin expression in other breast cancer cell lines indicates that parvabumin was over-expressed in MDA-MB-453, a line of non-invasive breast cancer cells, and slightly up-regulated in MDA-MB-361, an adenocarcinoma with metastatic ability (Figure 7B). These results imply that parvabumin might have the potential to be a breast cancer marker. In contrast, PdLIM1, a cytosolic protein, was down-regulated in all breast cancer lines: MCF-7, MDA-MB-231, MDA-MB-453 and MDA-MB-361 (Figure 7B). In addition, IFIT3, a plasma membrane protein, was down-regulated in transformed cells, especially in MCF-7 and MDA-MB-231, and was consistent with the proteomic data from 2D-DIGE (Figure 7B). Interestingly, BANF1, a major nucleus-located protein, was distributed in the cytoplasma of the MCF-10A cells, but was confined within the nucleus in MCF-7, MDA-MB-231 and MDA-MB-453 cells; in addition, BANF1 was distributed within the cytoplasma and nucleus in MDA-MB-361 (Figure 7B). These results indicate that the BANF1 levels were different between healthy breast cells and breast cancer cells, and that the subcellular locations of the protein may account for tumorigenesis.

Nuclear distribution protein nudE homolog 1 (NDE1), GRAM domain containing 2 (GRAMD2), Parvabumin and bestrophin 3 (Best3), have not been reported in previous breast cancer studies, implying that these proteins need to be further investigated to confirm them as valuable breast cancer markers. In order to examine the expression levels of the newly identified breast cancer markers in clinical specimens, we had used plasma specimens from healthy donors and breast cancer patients to compare the expression levels of the markers including NDE1, GRAMD2, Parvabumin and Best3. The results showed that these identified markers were significantly increased in breast cancer patients rather than in the healthy donors and these increases were observed in both non-metastatic and metastatic breast cancers (Figure 8).

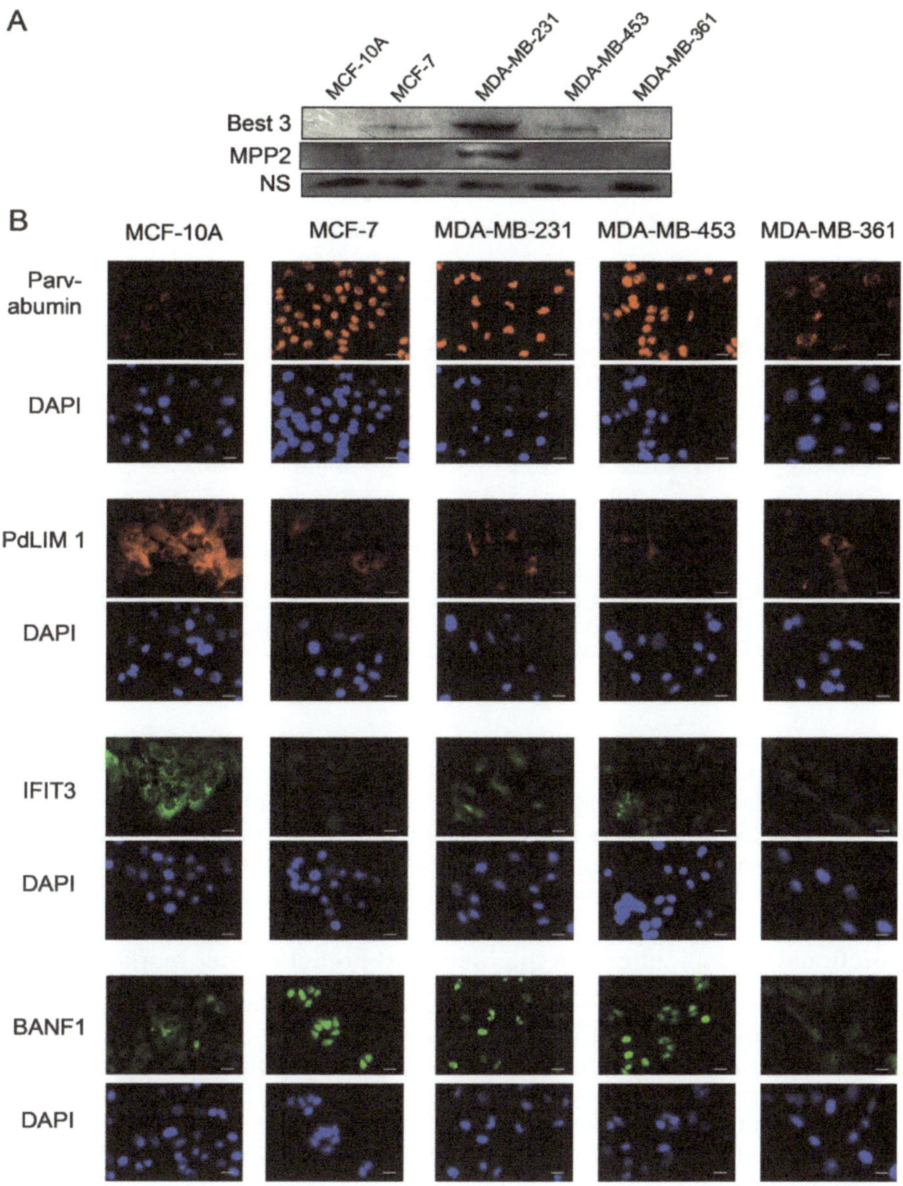

Fig. 7. Immunoblotting and immunofluorescence analyses of the expression and protein localization changes of newly identified putative breast cancer markers across MCF-10A, MCF-7, MDA-MB-231, MDA-MB-453 and MDA-MB-361 cells. (A) The profile of the secreted proteome changes across MCF-10A, MCF-7, MDA-MB-231, MDA-MB-453 and MDA-MB-361 cells. The serum-free media from the cell lines was concentrated and 10μg of the total protein was resolved using SDS-PAGE and immunoblotted for MPP2 and Bestrophin 3. NS represents a nonspecific band used to show equal loading of secreted proteins. (B) 5 x 10^4

MCF-10A, MCF-7, MDA-MB-231, MDA-MB-453 and MDA-MB-361 cells were seeded on cover slips before fixation and staining for Parvabumin, BANF1, PdLIM1 and IFIT3. Each set of three fields was taken using the same exposure, and images are representative of three different fields. Scale bar = 20μm.

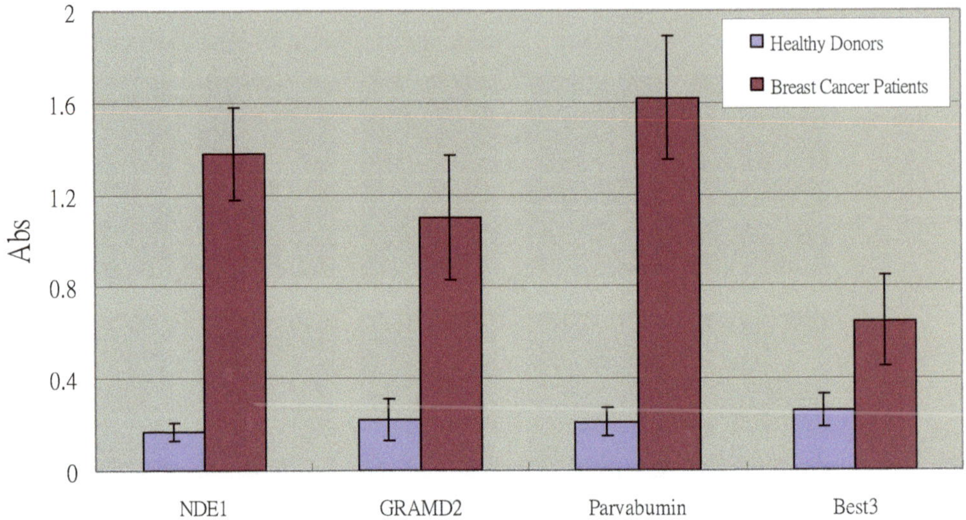

Fig. 8. ELISA analysis of plasma NDE1, GRAMD2, pavabumin and best3 levels in healthy donors, breast cancer patients. Plasma samples were obtained from 30 healthy individuals, 30 breast cancer patients (15 without detectable metastasis and 15 breast cancer patients presenting metastasis) at the time of serum collection. 50 μg of plasma samples were coated onto each well of 96-well plate for ELISA analysis and the absorbance was measured at 450 nm using Stat Fax 2100 microtiterplate reader.

6. Functional classifications of the identified breast cancer markers

With the basis of a Swiss-Prot search and KEGG pathway analysis, numerous potential biological functions of the identified proteins across MCF-10A, MCF-7 and MDA-MB-231 were determined. The information should be useful for studying the mechanisms of breast cancer tumorigenesis and metastasis. Figure 9 compares the expression profiles of the identified differentially expressed proteins in these 3 cell lines. Proteins known to regulate cell cycle are found to be upregulated in both MCF-7 and MDA-MB-231 (Figure 9A), and are associated with the promotion of tumorigenesis (Dictor et al., 1999). In addition, the expression of proteins linked to redox-regulation increased in the MCF-7 cells in comparison to the levels in MCF-10A (Figure 9B). Induced expression of these proteins may be able to account for cancer development and progression. For example, Noh *et al.* showed that peroxiredoxins are greatly over-expressed in most breast cancer tissues (Noh et al., 2001). Proteomic analysis also reveals that proteins involved in carbohydrate metabolism are significantly over-expressed in MCF-7 cells (Figure 9C). This demonstrates that cancer cells rely heavily on glycolysis to obtain ATP for proliferation and tumorigenesis in the presence of adequate oxygen levels (Lopez-Lazaro, 2008); this mechanism has been implicated in numerous cancer therapies (Gatenby and Gillies, 2007; Rivenzon-Segal et al., 2003). Figures 9D~F show the downregulated profiles of proteins in both MCF-7 and MDA-MB-231 cells. These proteins are involved in calcium regulation, vascular transport and protease inhibition. Calcium-binding proteins, such as annexin-1, whose function is modulated by an estrogen receptor, have been reported to show decreased expression in correlation with breast cancer development and progression(Ang et al., 2009; Cao et al., 2008b; Shen et al., 2006; Shen et al., 2005). The S100 protein family is a family of low molecular weight calcium-binding proteins that is responsible for the regulation of protein phosphorylation, intracellular calcium homostasis, the dynamics of cytoskeleton constituents and cell proliferation (Donato, 2003). The S100 family has become a major interest because of its deregulated expression in human diseases, especially in cancer. According to Ji *et al.* (2004), S100 families exhibit significantly reduced expression in esophageal squamous cell carcinoma (Ji et al., 2004) and are hence recognized as a prognostic esophageal cancer marker. In here, S100A14 was identified as downregulated in MCF-7 and MDA-MB-231, suggesting their potential roles in breast cancer. Interestingly, proteins involved in vascular transport, including Rab GTPase-binding effector protein and vacuolar protein sorting-associated protein 54, were decreased in expression in MCF-7 and MDA-MB-231 (Figure 9F). This may be explained by a previous report indicating that the downregulation of Rab5 GDP/GTP exchange factor enhances receptor tyrosine kinase signaling and promotes the growth factor-directed migration of tumor cells (Hu et al., 2008). However, there are few studies on tumorigenesis regarding the roles of the Rab GTPase-binding effector protein and the vacuolar protein sorting-associated protein 54. Serpin is a group of proteins able to inhibit protease and block the growth, invasion, and metastatic properties of breast tumors. Hence, serpin families function as tumor suppressors in cancer research (Sager et al., 1997). The downregulation of serpin is well-correlated with the progression of breast cancer (Webber et al., 2008) and our own observations in MCF-7 and MDA-MB-231 cells (Figure 9F).

Other differentially expressed proteins of interest across MCF-10A, MCF-7 and MDA-MB-231 include cathepsin D, bestrophin-3 and interferon-induced protein with IFIT3. Cathepsin D, a lysosomal aspartic protease, is over-expressed in estrogen receptor positive breast cancer cells (Rochefort, 1999) and is generally of good prognostic value in comparison with estrogen receptor negative breast cancer in clinical studies (Rochefort, 1998). Our study indicates that cathepsin D is highly expressed in MCF-7, both in total cellular proteins or in secreted fraction. In contrast, cathepsin D is significantly down-regulated in MDA-MB-231 cells compared with MCF-7. Thus, our proteomic results display good correlation with these reports. To our knowledge, bestrophin-3, a cGMP-dependent calcium-activated chloride channel, has not been reported to be associated with cancer and shows upregulation in MCF-7 and MDA-MB-231 in this study. Nevertheless, the related study in bestrophin-1 shows the protein improves intracellular Ca^{2+} signaling and increases cell growth rate in colonic carcinoma cells. The proliferation of the cells is significantly suppressed by bestrophin-1 RNA interference treatment (Spitzner et al., 2008). This indicates bestrophin-3 may be a potential target for breast cancer therapy. IFIT3 plays a key role in the antiproliferative activity of the interferon-related signaling pathway through inducing expression of cell cycle inhibitors, p21 and p27 proteins (Xiao et al., 2006). The 2D-DIGE results in this study show that IFIT3 is downregulated in both MCF-7 and MDA-MB-231 cells, implying that breast cancer cells may maintain a high level of proliferative activity by downregulating the expression of IFIT3.

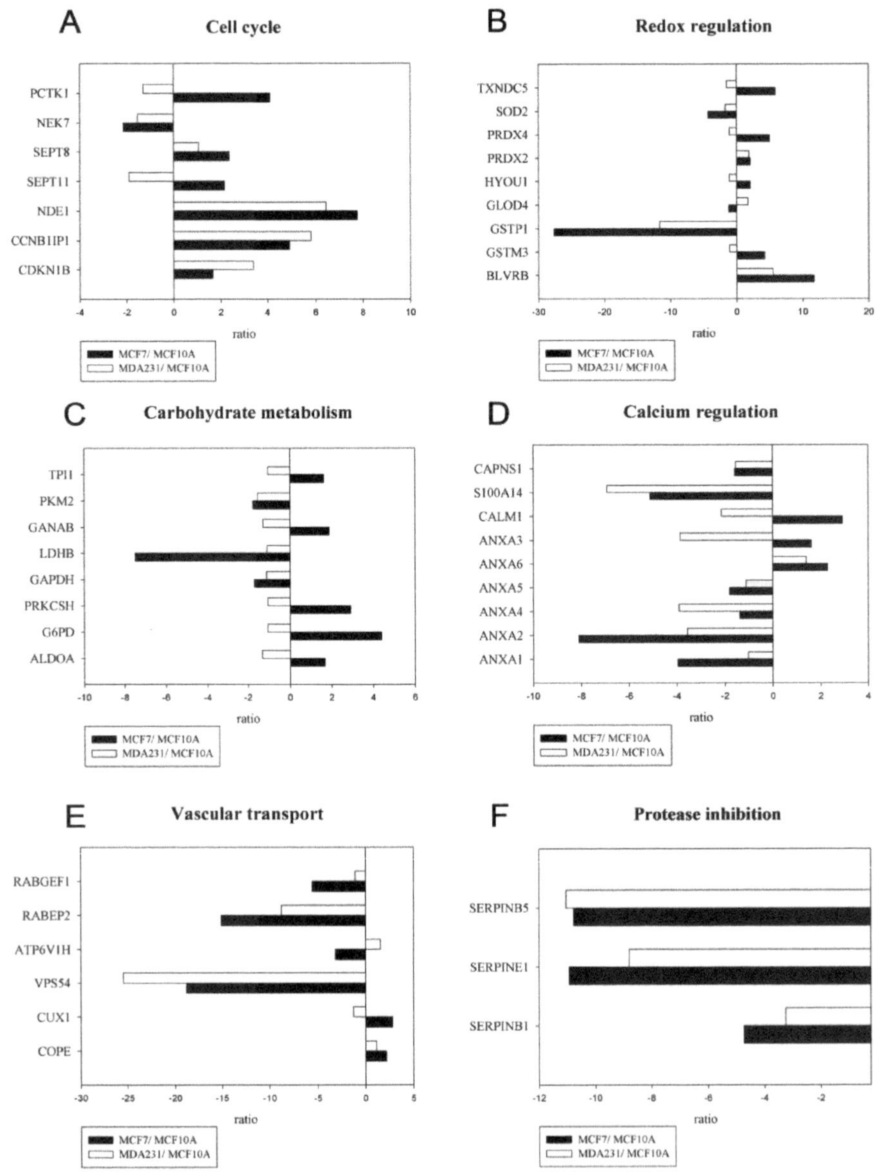

Fig. 9. Expression profiles for proteins potentially contributing to (A) cell cycle (B) redox regulation (C) carbohydrate metabolism (D) calcium regulation (E) vascular transport (F) protease inhibition in comparing MCF-7 and MDA-MB-231 with MCF-10A. White bars represent fold change in protein expression in MDA-MB-231 versus MCF-10A. Black bars represent fold change in protein expression in MCF-7 versus MCF-10A. The vertical axis indicates the identified proteins; the horizontal axis indicates the fold change in protein expression. Additional details for each protein can be found in Table 1 and Table 2.

7. Different proteomic approaches in the study of breast cancer markers

Results of this study include the differentially expressed protein profiles of intracellular proteins and extracellular secreted proteins in non-transformed and transformed breast cell lines. The 2D-DIGE strategy is powerful enough to identify numerous breast cancer signatures and offers a complementary role to LC/MS-based proteomic analysis. Even though the global coverage of protein mixtures identified by LC-MS based analysis is generally higher than that of 2-DE based analysis, 2-DE based analysis offers some distinct advantages, such as direct protein quantification at protein isoform levels instead of peptide levels to reduce analytical variations (Timms and Cramer, 2008a). Using the LC-MS/MS strategy, Kulasingam and Diamandis analyzed and compared the expressions of extracellular and membrane-bound proteins in conditioned media of three breast cells corresponding to the normal control cells and cell lines derived from stage 2 and stage 4 patients, respectively (Kulasingam and Diamandis, 2007b). Their study identified 1062 differentially expressed proteins across these three cell lines. A comparison between Kulasingam's study and our 2D-DIGE secretomic study shows that 25 out of 50 identified differentially expressed secreted proteins coincide with Kulasingam's study, indicating that both LC-MS/MS and 2D-DIGE are potential tools for discovering breast cancer markers with reasonable reproducibility. However, another 25 out of these 50 identified proteins have never been published in Kulasingam's study or any other studies, demonstrating that 2D - DIGE, compared with LC-MS/MS, plays a complementary role in the discovery of biomarkers.

In previous research, Nagaraja *et.al.* used traditional 2-DE with post-stains (silver stain and coomassie blue stain) to reveal 26 differentially expressed proteins among transformed breast cells with different levels of invasiveness and normal cells which were the same cell lines used in the present study (Nagaraja et al., 2006). Their study showed no evidence of visualizing protein spots with sensitive strategies, and protein expression changes were not quantifiable because no broader linear-ranged methods and statistical analysis were employed. Only six out of those 26 proteins coincide with our statistical 2D-DIGE data, which implies that differences might have derived from artificial variations or from results with no statistical analysis.

Mitochondria are key organelles in mammary cells in responsible for several cellular functions including growth, division and energy metabolism. In our recent works, mitochondrial proteins were enriched for proteomics analysis with the state-of-the-art 2D-DIGE and matrix-assistant laser desorption ionization time-of-flight mass spectrometry (MALDI-TOF MS) strategy to compare and identify the mitochondrial protein profiling changes between three breast cell lines with different tumorigenesity and metastatic potential. The mitochondrial proteomics demonstrate more than 1500 protein features from equal amount pooled of mitochondrial proteins of these three breast cancer lines and 125 differentially expressed protein spots were identified by peptide fingerprintings. In which, 33 identified proteins belong to mitochondrial proteins. 18 out of these 33 identified mitochondrial proteins such as short calcium-binding mitochondrial carrier protein-1 (SCaMC-1) have not been reported in breast cancer research in our knowledge. Additionally, mitochondrial protein prohibitin has shown to be differentially distributed in mitochondria and in nucleus for healthy breast cells and breast cancer cell lines, respectively. This approach provides comprehensive studies examining mitochondrial proteins in various stages of breast cancer progression and these identified proteins may be further evaluated as potential breast cancer risk factors for breast cancer initiation and progression.

8. Conclusion

The transformation of a normal cell into a cancer cell has been correlated with alterations in gene regulation and protein expression. To identify altered proteins and link them to the tumorigenesis of breast cancer, non-tumorigenic breast epithelial cells (MCF-10A) were used to distinguish their proteomes from non-invasive breast cancer cells (MCF-7) and invasive breast cancer cells (MDA-MB-231) for the identification of the potential breast cancer markers in transformed breast cells. Using the 2D-DIGE and MALDI-TOF MS techniques, the differentially expressed extracellular secreted proteins and total cellular proteins across MCF-10A, MCF-7 and MDA-MB-231 were quantitatively identified. More than 180 unique differentially expressed secreted and intracellular proteins from these three different cell lines have been identified by proteomic analysis. In which, 14 of the secreted proteins and 51 of the total cellular proteins have not been previously reported in breast cancer research. Some of these unreported proteins have further been verified in other breast cancer cell lines, such as MDA-MB-453 and MDA-MB-361 cells, and clinical specimens. Although breast cell lines have been used widely to study the biological and molecular heterogeneity of breast cancer, it is important to assess their relation to *in vivo* genotypes and phenotypes of breast cancer. According to gene and protein expression profiling, breast cell lines were recently better classified to five major subtypes: luminal-A, luminal-B, ERBB2, basal-like and normal-like, which may not completely correspond to biological reality but have shown a direct correlation with clinical outcomes of this disease (Kao et al., 2009; Charafe-Jauffret et al., 2006; Perou et al., 2000; Chin et al., 2006). It is thus possible to predict the differences in proteins identified among MCF-10A (normal-like), MCF-7 (luminal) and MDAMB-231 (basal-like/post-epithelial mesenchymal transition) are due to the cell lines representing different molecular subtypes of breast cancer in addition to reflect different stages of breast cancer development. Moreover, these three mammary epithelium cells have been commonly selected to compare in many studies as MCF-7 is estrogen receptor positive while MDA-MB-231 is estrogen receptor negative. Therefore, the identified protein signatures in MCF-7 are possible link to estrogen-stimulated progression of non-invasive breast cancer. To sum up, proteomics strategy has offered opportunity to investigate the putative breast cancer markers from various breast cell lines and may aid in developing identified proteins as useful diagnostic and therapeutic candidates in research on cancer and proteomics.

9. Acknowledgments

This work was supported by NSC grant (99-2311-B-007-002 and 100-2311-B-007-005) from National Science Council, Taiwan, NTHU and CGH grant (100N2723E1) from National Tsing Hua University, NTHU Booster grant (99N2908E1) from National Tsing Hua University, Toward Word-Class University project from National Tsing Hua University (100N2051E1) and VGHUST grant (99-P5-22) from Veteran General Hospitals University System of Taiwan. The authors thank Dr. Wun-Shaing Wayne Chang (National Health Research Institute, Taiwan) for providing the MCF-10A cell line.

10. References

Aitken, A. (2006). 14-3-3 proteins: a historic overview. Semin. Cancer Biol. *16*, 162-172.

Ang, E.Z., Nguyen, H.T., Sim, H.L., Putti, T.C., and Lim, L.H. (2009). Annexin-1 regulates growth arrest induced by high levels of estrogen in MCF-7 breast cancer cells. Mol. Cancer Res. *7*, 266-274.

Cao, Y., Li, Y., Edelweiss, M., Arun, B., Rosen, D., Resetkova, E., Wu, Y., Liu, J., Sahin, A., and Albarracin, C.T. (2008b). Loss of annexin A1 expression in breast cancer progression. Appl. Immunohistochem. Mol. Morphol. *16*, 530-534.

Cao, Y., Li, Y., Edelweiss, M., Arun, B., Rosen, D., Resetkova, E., Wu, Y., Liu, J., Sahin, A., and Albarracin, C.T. (2008a). Loss of annexin A1 expression in breast cancer progression. Appl. Immunohistochem. Mol. Morphol. *16*, 530-534.

Chan, H.L., Chou, H.C., Duran, M., Gruenewald, J., Waterfield, M.D., Ridley, A., and Timms, J.F. (2009). Major role of EGFR and SRC kinases in promoting oxidative stress-dependent loss of adhesion and apoptosis in epithelial cells. J. Biol. Chem. *285*, 4307-4318.

Chan, H.L., Gharbi, S., Gaffney, P.R., Cramer, R., Waterfield, M.D., and Timms, J.F. (2005). Proteomic analysis of redox- and ErbB2-dependent changes in mammary luminal epithelial cells using cysteine- and lysine-labelling two-dimensional difference gel electrophoresis. Proteomics. *5*, 2908-2926.

Charafe-Jauffret, E., Ginestier, C., Monville, F., Finetti, P., Adelaide, J., Cervera, N., Fekairi, S., Xerri, L., Jacquemier, J., Birnbaum, D., and Bertucci, F. (2006). Gene expression profiling of breast cell lines identifies potential new basal markers. Oncogene *25*, 2273-2284.

Chin, K., DeVries, S., Fridlyand, J., Spellman, P.T., Roydasgupta, R., Kuo, W.L., Lapuk, A., Neve, R.M., Qian, Z., Ryder, T., Chen, F., Feiler, H., Tokuyasu, T., Kingsley, C., Dairkee, S., Meng, Z., Chew, K., Pinkel, D., Jain, A., Ljung, B.M., Esserman, L., Albertson, D.G., Waldman, F.M., and Gray, J.W. (2006). Genomic and transcriptional aberrations linked to breast cancer pathophysiologies. Cancer Cell *10*, 529-541.

Chou, H.C., Chen, Y.W., Lee, T.R., Wu, F.S., Chan, H.T., Lyu, P.C., Timms, J.F., and Chan, H.L. (2010). Proteomics study of oxidative stress and Src kinase inhibition in H9C2 cardiomyocytes: A cell model of heart ischemia reperfusion injury and treatment. Free Radic. Biol. Med. *49*, 96-108.

Danes, C.G., Wyszomierski, S.L., Lu, J., Neal, C.L., Yang, W., and Yu, D. (2008). 14-3-3 zeta down-regulates p53 in mammary epithelial cells and confers luminal filling. Cancer Res. *68*, 1760-1767.

Dictor, M., Ehinger, M., Mertens, F., Akervall, J., and Wennerberg, J. (1999). Abnormal cell cycle regulation in malignancy. Am. J. Clin. Pathol. *112*, S40-S52.

Donato, R. (2003). Intracellular and extracellular roles of S100 proteins. Microsc. Res. Tech. *60*, 540-551.

Feldner, J.C. and Brandt, B.H. (2002). Cancer cell motility--on the road from c-erbB-2 receptor steered signaling to actin reorganization. Exp. Cell Res. *272*, 93-108.

Fenn, J.B., Mann, M., Meng, C.K., Wong, S.F., and Whitehouse, C.M. (1989). Electrospray ionization for mass spectrometry of large biomolecules. Science *246*, 64-71.

Fritzsche, F.R., Dahl, E., Pahl, S., Burkhardt, M., Luo, J., Mayordomo, E., Gansukh, T., Dankof, A., Knuechel, R., Denkert, C., Winzer, K.J., Dietel, M., and Kristiansen, G.

(2006). Prognostic relevance of AGR2 expression in breast cancer. Clin. Cancer Res. *12*, 1728-1734.

Fu, X., Wang, P., and Zhu, B.T. (2008a). Protein disulfide isomerase is a multifunctional regulator of estrogenic status in target cells. J. Steroid Biochem. Mol. Biol. *112*, 127-137.

Fu, X.D., Giretti, M.S., Baldacci, C., Garibaldi, S., Flamini, M., Sanchez, A.M., Gadducci, A., Genazzani, A.R., and Simoncini, T. (2008b). Extra-nuclear signaling of progesterone receptor to breast cancer cell movement and invasion through the actin cytoskeleton. PLoS. ONE. *3*, e2790.

Fujii, J. and Ikeda, Y. (2002). Advances in our understanding of peroxiredoxin, a multifunctional, mammalian redox protein. Redox. Rep. *7*, 123-130.

Gallo, D., Jacquot, Y., Laurent, G., and Leclercq, G. (2008). Calmodulin, a regulatory partner of the estrogen receptor alpha in breast cancer cells. Mol. Cell Endocrinol. *291*, 20-26.

Gatenby, R.A. and Gillies, R.J. (2007). Glycolysis in cancer: a potential target for therapy. Int. J. Biochem. Cell Biol. *39*, 1358-1366.

Hanahan, D. and Weinberg, R.A. (2011). Hallmarks of cancer: the next generation. Cell *144*, 646-674.

Harding, M.W. and Handschumacher, R.E. (1988). Cyclophilin, a primary molecular target for cyclosporine. Structural and functional implications. Transplantation *46*, 29S-35S.

Henzel, W.J., Billeci, T.M., Stults, J.T., Wong, S.C., Grimley, C., and Watanabe, C. (1993). Identifying proteins from two-dimensional gels by molecular mass searching of peptide fragments in protein sequence databases. Proc. Natl. Acad. Sci. U. S. A *90*, 5011-5015.

Hondermarck, H., Dolle, L., Yazidi-Belkoura, I., Vercoutter-Edouart, A.S., Adriaenssens, E., and Lemoine, J. (2002). Functional proteomics of breast cancer for signal pathway profiling and target discovery. J. Mammary. Gland. Biol. Neoplasia. *7*, 395-405.

Hu, H., Milstein, M., Bliss, J.M., Thai, M., Malhotra, G., Huynh, L.C., and Colicelli, J. (2008). Integration of transforming growth factor beta and RAS signaling silences a RAB5 guanine nucleotide exchange factor and enhances growth factor-directed cell migration. Mol. Cell Biol. *28*, 1573-1583.

Huang, H.L., Hsing, H.W., Lai, T.C., Chen, Y.W., Lee, T.R., Chan, H.T., Lyu, P.C., Wu, C.L., Lu, Y.C., Lin, S.T., Lin, C.W., Lai, C.H., Chang, H.T., Chou, H.C., and Chan, H.L. (2010). Trypsin-induced proteome alteration during cell subculture in mammalian cells. J. Biomed. Sci. *17*, 36.

Inoue, Y., Kawamoto, S., Shoji, M., Hashizume, S., Teruya, K., Katakura, Y., and Shirahata, S. (2000). Properties of ras-amplified recombinant BHK-21 cells in protein-free culture. Cytotechnology *33*, 21-26.

Jacobs, J.M., Mottaz, H.M., Yu, L.R., Anderson, D.J., Moore, R.J., Chen, W.N., Auberry, K.J., Strittmatter, E.F., Monroe, M.E., Thrall, B.D., Camp, D.G., and Smith, R.D. (2004). Multidimensional proteome analysis of human mammary epithelial cells. J. Proteome. Res. *3*, 68-75.

James, P., Quadroni, M., Carafoli, E., and Gonnet, G. (1993). Protein identification by mass profile fingerprinting. Biochem. Biophys. Res. Commun. *195*, 58-64.

Jemal, A., Tiwari, R.C., Murray, T., Ghafoor, A., Samuels, A., Ward, E., Feuer, E.J., and Thun, M.J. (2004). Cancer statistics, 2004. CA Cancer J. Clin. *54,* 8-29.

Ji, J., Zhao, L., Wang, X., Zhou, C., Ding, F., Su, L., Zhang, C., Mao, X., Wu, M., and Liu, Z. (2004). Differential expression of S100 gene family in human esophageal squamous cell carcinoma. J. Cancer Res. Clin. Oncol. *130,* 480-486.

Jung, E.J., Moon, H.G., Cho, B.I., Jeong, C.Y., Joo, Y.T., Lee, Y.J., Hong, S.C., Choi, S.K., Ha, W.S., Kim, J.W., Lee, C.W., Lee, J.S., and Park, S.T. (2007). Galectin-1 expression in cancer-associated stromal cells correlates tumor invasiveness and tumor progression in breast cancer. Int. J. Cancer *120,* 2331-2338.

Kao, J., Salari, K., Bocanegra, M., Choi, Y.L., Girard, L., Gandhi, J., Kwei, K.A., Hernandez-Boussard, T., Wang, P., Gazdar, A.F., Minna, J.D., and Pollack, J.R. (2009). Molecular profiling of breast cancer cell lines defines relevant tumor models and provides a resource for cancer gene discovery. PLoS. One. *4,* e6146.

Karas, M. and Hillenkamp, F. (1988). Laser desorption ionization of proteins with molecular masses exceeding 10, 000 daltons. Anal. Chem. *60,* 2299-2301.

Kawai, H., Li, H., Avraham, S., Jiang, S., and Avraham, H.K. (2003). Overexpression of histone deacetylase HDAC1 modulates breast cancer progression by negative regulation of estrogen receptor alpha. Int. J. Cancer *107,* 353-358.

Kulasingam, V. and Diamandis, E.P. (2007b). Proteomics analysis of conditioned media from three breast cancer cell lines: a mine for biomarkers and therapeutic targets. Mol. Cell Proteomics. *6,* 1997-2011.

Kulasingam, V. and Diamandis, E.P. (2007a). Proteomics analysis of conditioned media from three breast cancer cell lines: a mine for biomarkers and therapeutic targets. Mol. Cell Proteomics. *6,* 1997-2011.

Lai, T.C., Chou, H.C., Chen, Y.W., Lee, T.R., Chan, H.T., Shen, H.H., Lee, W.T., Lin, S.T., Lu, Y.C., Wu, C.L., and Chan, H.L. (2010). Secretomic and Proteomic Analysis of Potential Breast Cancer Markers by Two-Dimensional Differential Gel Electrophoresis. J. Proteome. Res. *9,* 1302-1322.

Lee, W.Y., Huang, S.C., Tzeng, C.C., Chang, T.L., and Hsu, K.F. (2007). Alterations of metastasis-related genes identified using an oligonucleotide microarray of genistein-treated HCC1395 breast cancer cells. Nutr. Cancer *58,* 239-246.

Liaudet-Coopman, E., Beaujouin, M., Derocq, D., Garcia, M., Glondu-Lassis, M., Laurent-Matha, V., Prebois, C., Rochefort, H., and Vignon, F. (2006). Cathepsin D: newly discovered functions of a long-standing aspartic protease in cancer and apoptosis. Cancer Lett. *237,* 167-179.

Lopez-Lazaro, M. (2008). The warburg effect: why and how do cancer cells activate glycolysis in the presence of oxygen? Anticancer Agents Med. Chem. *8,* 305-312.

Lu, T.J., Lai, W.Y., Huang, C.Y., Hsieh, W.J., Yu, J.S., Hsieh, Y.J., Chang, W.T., Leu, T.H., Chang, W.C., Chuang, W.J., Tang, M.J., Chen, T.Y., Lu, T.L., and Lai, M.D. (2006). Inhibition of cell migration by autophosphorylated mammalian sterile 20-like kinase 3 (MST3) involves paxillin and protein-tyrosine phosphatase-PEST. J. Biol. Chem. *281,* 38405-38417.

Mann, M., Hojrup, P., and Roepstorff, P. (1993). Use of mass spectrometric molecular weight information to identify proteins in sequence databases. Biol. Mass Spectrom. *22,* 338-345.

Marouga, R., David, S., and Hawkins, E. (2005). The development of the DIGE system: 2D fluorescence difference gel analysis technology. Anal. Bioanal. Chem. *382*, 669-678.

Mbeunkui, F., Fodstad, O., and Pannell, L.K. (2006a). Secretory protein enrichment and analysis: an optimized approach applied on cancer cell lines using 2D LC-MS/MS. J. Proteome. Res. *5*, 899-906.

Mbeunkui, F., Fodstad, O., and Pannell, L.K. (2006b). Secretory protein enrichment and analysis: an optimized approach applied on cancer cell lines using 2D LC-MS/MS. J. Proteome. Res. *5*, 899-906.

Mita, K., Zhang, Z., Ando, Y., Toyama, T., Hamaguchi, M., Kobayashi, S., Hayashi, S., Fujii, Y., Iwase, H., and Yamashita, H. (2007). Prognostic significance of insulin-like growth factor binding protein (IGFBP)-4 and IGFBP-5 expression in breast cancer. Jpn. J. Clin. Oncol. *37*, 575-582.

Morrow, T. (2007). Gene expression microarray improves prediction of breast cancer outcomes. Manag. Care *16*, 51-52.

Nagaraja, G.M., Othman, M., Fox, B.P., Alsaber, R., Pellegrino, C.M., Zeng, Y., Khanna, R., Tamburini, P., Swaroop, A., and Kandpal, R.P. (2006). Gene expression signatures and biomarkers of noninvasive and invasive breast cancer cells: comprehensive profiles by representational difference analysis, microarrays and proteomics. Oncogene *25*, 2328-2338.

Noh, D.Y., Ahn, S.J., Lee, R.A., Kim, S.W., Park, I.A., and Chae, H.Z. (2001). Overexpression of peroxiredoxin in human breast cancer. Anticancer Res. *21*, 2085-2090.

Nuyten, D.S. and van de Vijver, M.J. (2008). Using microarray analysis as a prognostic and predictive tool in oncology: focus on breast cancer and normal tissue toxicity. Semin. Radiat. Oncol. *18*, 105-114.

Pawlik, T.M., Hawke, D.H., Liu, Y., Krishnamurthy, S., Fritsche, H., Hunt, K.K., and Kuerer, H.M. (2006). Proteomic analysis of nipple aspirate fluid from women with early-stage breast cancer using isotope-coded affinity tags and tandem mass spectrometry reveals differential expression of vitamin D binding protein. BMC. Cancer *6*, 68.

Perou, C.M., Sorlie, T., Eisen, M.B., van de, R.M., Jeffrey, S.S., Rees, C.A., Pollack, J.R., Ross, D.T., Johnsen, H., Akslen, L.A., Fluge, O., Pergamenschikov, A., Williams, C., Zhu, S.X., Lonning, P.E., Borresen-Dale, A.L., Brown, P.O., and Botstein, D. (2000). Molecular portraits of human breast tumours. Nature *406*, 747-752.

Pucci-Minafra, I., Fontana, S., Cancemi, P., Alaimo, G., and Minafra, S. (2002). Proteomic patterns of cultured breast cancer cells and epithelial mammary cells. Ann. N. Y. Acad. Sci. *963*, 122-139.

Rivenzon-Segal, D., Boldin-Adamsky, S., Seger, D., Seger, R., and Degani, H. (2003). Glycolysis and glucose transporter 1 as markers of response to hormonal therapy in breast cancer. Int. J. Cancer *107*, 177-182.

Rochefort, H. (1998). [Estrogens, cathepsin D and metastasis in cancers of the breast and ovary: invasion or proliferation?]. C. R. Seances Soc. Biol. Fil. *192*, 241-251.

Rochefort, H. (1999). [Estrogen-induced genes in breast cancer, and their medical importance]. Bull. Acad. Natl. Med. *183*, 955-968.

Sager, R., Sheng, S., Pemberton, P., and Hendrix, M.J. (1997). Maspin. A tumor suppressing serpin. Adv. Exp. Med. Biol. *425*, 77-88.

Sharma, M.C. and Sharma, M. (2007). The role of annexin II in angiogenesis and tumor progression: a potential therapeutic target. Curr. Pharm. Des *13*, 3568-3575.

Shen, D., Chang, H.R., Chen, Z., He, J., Lonsberry, V., Elshimali, Y., Chia, D., Seligson, D., Goodglick, L., Nelson, S.F., and Gornbein, J.A. (2005). Loss of annexin A1 expression in human breast cancer detected by multiple high-throughput analyses. Biochem. Biophys. Res. Commun. *326*, 218-227.

Shen, D., Nooraie, F., Elshimali, Y., Lonsberry, V., He, J., Bose, S., Chia, D., Seligson, D., Chang, H.R., and Goodglick, L. (2006). Decreased expression of annexin A1 is correlated with breast cancer development and progression as determined by a tissue microarray analysis. Hum. Pathol. *37*, 1583-1591.

Singh, B., Berry, J.A., Vincent, L.E., and Lucci, A. (2006). Involvement of IL-8 in COX-2-mediated bone metastases from breast cancer. J. Surg. Res. *134*, 44-51.

Sorlie, T., Tibshirani, R., Parker, J., Hastie, T., Marron, J.S., Nobel, A., Deng, S., Johnsen, H., Pesich, R., Geisler, S., Demeter, J., Perou, C.M., Lonning, P.E., Brown, P.O., Borresen-Dale, A.L., and Botstein, D. (2003). Repeated observation of breast tumor subtypes in independent gene expression data sets. Proc. Natl. Acad. Sci. U. S. A *100*, 8418-8423.

Spitzner, M., Martins, J.R., Soria, R.B., Ousingsawat, J., Scheidt, K., Schreiber, R., and Kunzelmann, K. (2008). Eag1 and Bestrophin 1 are up-regulated in fast-growing colonic cancer cells. J. Biol. Chem. *283*, 7421-7428.

Timms, J.F. and Cramer, R. (2008a). Difference gel electrophoresis. Proteomics. *8*, 4886-4897.

Timms, J.F. and Cramer, R. (2008b). Difference gel electrophoresis. Proteomics. *8*, 4886-4897.

Varnum, S.M., Covington, C.C., Woodbury, R.L., Petritis, K., Kangas, L.J., Abdullah, M.S., Pounds, J.G., Smith, R.D., and Zangar, R.C. (2003). Proteomic characterization of nipple aspirate fluid: identification of potential biomarkers of breast cancer. Breast Cancer Res. Treat. *80*, 87-97.

Webber, B.A., Lawson, D., and Cohen, C. (2008). Maspin and Mutant p53 expression in malignant melanoma and carcinoma: use of tissue microarray. Appl. Immunohistochem. Mol. Morphol. *16*, 19-23.

Westermeier, R. and Scheibe, B. (2008). Difference gel electrophoresis based on lys/cys tagging. Methods Mol. Biol. *424*, 73-85.

Whitehouse, C.M., Dreyer, R.N., Yamashita, M., and Fenn, J.B. (1985). Electrospray interface for liquid chromatographs and mass spectrometers. Anal. Chem. *57*, 675-679.

Xiao, S., Li, D., Zhu, H.Q., Song, M.G., Pan, X.R., Jia, P.M., Peng, L.L., Dou, A.X., Chen, G.Q., Chen, S.J., Chen, Z., and Tong, J.H. (2006). RIG-G as a key mediator of the antiproliferative activity of interferon-related pathways through enhancing p21 and p27 proteins. Proc. Natl. Acad. Sci. U. S. A *103*, 16448-16453.

Xue, H., Lu, B., and Lai, M. (2008b). The cancer secretome: a reservoir of biomarkers. J. Transl. Med. *6*, 52.

Xue, H., Lu, B., and Lai, M. (2008a). The cancer secretome: a reservoir of biomarkers. J. Transl. Med. *6*, 52.

Yamaguchi, N., Yamamura, Y., Koyama, K., Ohtsuji, E., Imanishi, J., and Ashihara, T. (1990). Characterization of new human pancreatic cancer cell lines which propagate in a protein-free chemically defined medium. Cancer Res. *50*, 7008-7014.

Yates, J.R., III, Speicher, S., Griffin, P.R., and Hunkapiller, T. (1993). Peptide mass maps: a highly informative approach to protein identification. Anal. Biochem. *214*, 397-408.

Zhang, Y.G., DU, J., Tian, X.X., Zhong, Y.F., and Fang, W.G. (2007). Expression of E-cadherin, beta-catenin, cathepsin D, gelatinases and their inhibitors in invasive ductal breast carcinomas. Chin Med. J. (Engl.) *120*, 1597-1605.

Zweitzig, D.R., Smirnov, D.A., Connelly, M.C., Terstappen, L.W., O'Hara, S.M., and Moran, E. (2007). Physiological stress induces the metastasis marker AGR2 in breast cancer cells. Mol. Cell Biochem. *306*, 255-260.

10

Genomic and Proteomic Pathway Mapping Reveals Signatures of Mesenchymal-Epithelial Plasticity in Inflammatory Breast Cancer

Fredika M. Robertson et al.*,
[1]*The Department of Experimental Therapeutics, The University of Texas M.D. Anderson Cancer Center, Houston, TX,*
[2]*The Morgan Welch Inflammatory Breast Cancer Research Program, The University of Texas MD Anderson Cancer Center, Houston, TX,*
[3]*The University of Texas Graduate School of Biomedical Sciences, Houston, TX, USA*

1. Introduction

1.1 Inflammatory breast cancer as a distinct clinicopathologic entity

There are several clinically distinct types of breast cancer, which include early stage breast cancer, locally advanced breast cancer (LABC) and metastatic breast cancer. The most rare but lethal form of LABC is inflammatory breast cancer (IBC) (reviewed in 1). This type of breast cancer accounts for an estimated 2- 5% of all breast cancers in the United States and up to 20% of all breast cancers globally (2-4). Although primary IBC is less commonly diagnosed than other types of breast cancer, IBC is responsible for a disproportionate number of breast cancer-related deaths that occur each year world-wide due to its propensity to rapidly metastasize. (2-4). Women diagnosed with IBC have a significantly shorter median survival time (~ 2.9 years) than women with either LABC (~ 6.4 years) or non-LABC breast cancer (>10 years). The clinical diagnosis of IBC is based on the combination of the physical appearance of the affected breast, a careful medical history, physical examination, and pathological findings from a skin biopsy and/or needle or core

* Chu Khoi[1], Rita Circo[4,5], Julia Wulfkuhle[5], Savitri Krishnamurthy[6], Zaiming Ye[1], Annie Z. Luo[1], Kimberly M. Boley[1], Moishia C. Wright[1], Erik M. Freiter[1], Sanford H. Barsky[7], Massimo Cristofanilli[8] Emanuel F. Petricoin[5] and Lance A. Liotta[5]
[1]*The Department of Experimental Therapeutics, The University of Texas M.D. Anderson Cancer Center, Houston, TX, USA*
[2]*The Morgan Welch Inflammatory Breast Cancer Research Program, The University of Texas MD Anderson Cancer Center, Houston, TX, USA*
[3]*The University of Texas Graduate School of Biomedical Sciences, Houston, TX,USA*
[4]*Istituto Superiore di Sanità, Rome Italy,*
[5]*The Center for Applied Proteomics and Molecular Medicine, George Mason University, Manassas, VA,USA*
[6]*The Department of Pathology, The University of Texas M.D. Anderson Cancer Center, Houston, TX, USA*
[7]*The Department of Pathology, The University of Nevada School of Medicine, Reno NV and The Nevada Cancer Institute, Las Vegas, NV, USA*
[8]*The Department of Medical Oncology, Fox Chase Cancer Center, Philadelphia, PA, USA*

biopsy to confirm the diagnosis of carcinoma. The symptoms of IBC include a rapid onset of changes in the skin overlying the involved breast, including edema, redness and swelling involving over one half to two thirds of the breast, which may include a wrinkled, orange peel appearance in the skin, defined as "peau d'orange" (5,6). IBC is diagnosed in women at a younger age and since it does not present as a lump but rather occurs as sheets or nests of cells defined as tumor emboli, IBC is difficult to detect using mammography and requires more sophisticated imaging modalities such as magnetic resonance imaging (MRI) and positron emission tomography (PET) (1, 7). Since IBC occurs more rarely than other variants of breast cancer, neither the general public nor primary care physicians are aware of the signs and symptoms of IBC. It is commonly misdiagnosed as an infection, such as mastitis, resulting in delays in initiation of appropriate treatment. Disease progression is very rapid in IBC patients, with symptoms appearing often within days or weeks, and IBC patients commonly have lymph node metastasis at the time of first accurate diagnosis (6).

The skin changes observed in the involved breast of IBC patients are the first clinical signs of IBC and are believed to be associated with the presence of tumor cells that tightly aggregate to form multi-cellular nests of cells, defined as tumor emboli, that invade into the dermis. These tumor emboli are one of the classical histopathological findings in IBC (8, 9). Although the presence of dermal tumor emboli is not a requirement for a diagnosis of IBC, approximately 75% of IBC patients have tumor emboli that are observed in skin punch biopsy tissue and they serve as one of most distinctive characteristic signatures of IBC.

1.2 Models of inflammatory breast cancer

Historically, one of the barriers in research into the mechanisms underlying the aggressive metastasis of IBC has been the lack of sufficient numbers of cell lines and pre-clinical animal models derived from IBC patients with diverse breast cancer subtypes. Although there are *in vitro* and *in vivo* models available for a number of IBC cell lines including SUM149 (10-13), SUM190 (10-13), KPL-4 (14) and MDA-IBC-3 (15) with the associated animal xenograft models, the majority of IBC research has primarily used the SUM149 cell system as a model of IBC. Studies described in this chapter use all available IBC cell lines and animal models, including the only animal model of IBC that recapitulates formation of tumor emboli, Mary-X (16, 17).

When Mary-X tumor cells are propagated *in vitro,* they exhibit the unique characteristic of only existing as tightly adhered cell aggregates that we have defined as tumor spheroids (Figure 1 A). As such, Mary-X tumor spheroids provide a convenient *in vitro* surrogate for IBC tumor emboli that form *in vivo*. When Mary-X tumor spheroids are serially transplanted by subcutaneous injection into female immunocompromised mice, primary Mary-X tumors develop (Figure 1 B). In addition, aggregates of cells bud off from the primary tumor and form local metastatic lesions that appear as tumor emboli that invade into the dermal tissue (Figure 1 C). Mary-X also forms distant metastasis at multiple sites, including the lung (Figure 1 D). Triple color immunofluorescence studies demonstrate the highly proliferative characteristic of Mary-X tumor emboli, as defined by Ki-67 staining (Figure 1 E). These tumor emboli invade into and are encircled by lymphatic endothelium within the dermis, defined by their selective expression of podoplanin, a marker specific for lymphatic endothelial cells (Figure 1 E) (16,17). This is visual evidence of the propensity of IBC tumor emboli to exhibit cohesive invasion and to metastasize locally into the dermal lymphatic vessels, which may be one of the mechanisms underlying the common lymph node metastasis that occurs in IBC patients at the time of first diagnosis.

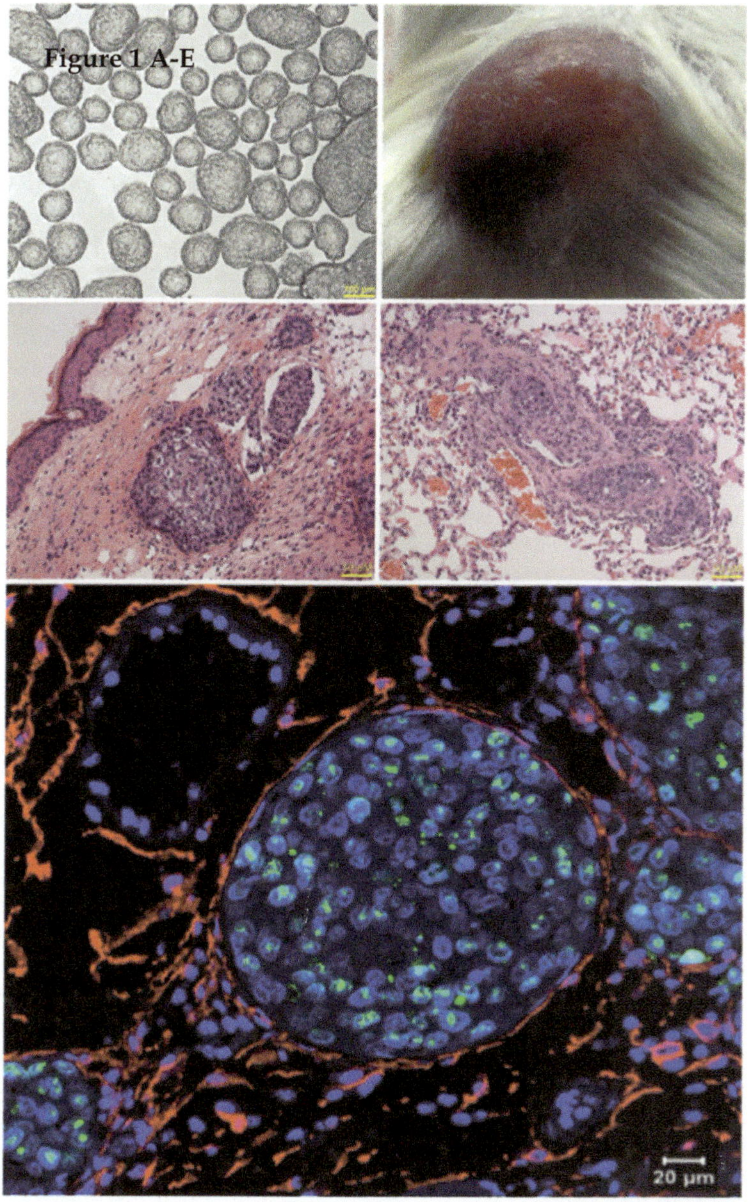

Fig. 1. **A.** Mary-X tumor spheroids can be propagated *in vitro* only as tightly adhered cell aggregates. **B.** Light micrograph image of a primary Mary-X tumor visible as a tumor with redness of the skin following subcutaneous injection of Mary-X spheroids into immunocompromised mice.**C.** Light micrograph of tissue section isolated from a mouse bearing a Mary X primary tumor that has formed local metastases that are visible in dermal tissue as tumor emboli. **D.** Light micrograph of Mary-X tumor emboli that have formed

metastastic lesion in the lung. **E**. Image of Mary-X tumor tissue with highly proliferative Mary-X tumor emboli, as determined by staining with Ki-67 (green fluorescence), that are encircled by lymphovascular endothelium, defined by their selective staining with anti-podoplanin antibodies (red fluorescence), demonstrating their propensity to invade as a cohesive unit of aggregated cells into the dermal lymphatic vessels.

The most recent study that examined the predominant subtypes of inflammatory breast cancers reported that there are approximately equal percentages of basal-like, Her2 amplified and normal like subtypes among IBC patients, with a slightly higher percentage of IBC tumors that are of the luminal B subtype (18). Interestingly, the models of IBC developed thus far are either triple negative basal like, such as the Mary-X and SUM149 IBC cells or are of the luminal B subtypes, such as SUM190 and MDA-IBC-3 cell lines. Based on transcriptional analysis and hierarchical clustering, SUM190, MDA-IBC-3 and KPL-4 cells have characteristics most closely associated with the luminal B subtype and are positive for at least one of the hormone receptors and the Her2 oncogene.
For studies described in this chapter, we examined the SUM149, SUM190, KPL-4, MDA-IBC-3 cell lines and Mary-X tumor spheroids as *in vitro* models of IBC and we also evaluated xenograft tissues generated from animals bearing each of these cell lines/cell systems. This represents the most comprehensive analysis of all available IBC cell lines and animal systems to date.

1.3 E-cadherin as a signature of inflammatory breast cancer

One of the only well characterized histological markers of IBC tumor emboli is their robust expression of the E-cadherin (19-22). In general, the classic cadherins, including E-cadherin, N-cadherin and P-cadherin are transmembrane glycoproteins that are linked to actin cytoskeletal networks and other cytoplasmic and transmembrane proteins by forming complexes with the catenins including α-catenin/vinculin, β-catenin, junction plakoglobin (JUP)/γ–catenin, and p120/δ catenin (23, 24). E-cadherin is considered to be a predominant regulator of what has been defined as "collective cell interactions" (25). Therefore, E-cadherin mediates tight cell:cell homophilic interactions exhibited by epithelial cells (reviewed in 26). Using the Mary-X model of IBC, E-cadherin antibodies were found to induce the loss of integrity of Mary-X spheroids and when injected via the intravenous route into mice bearing Mary-X tumors with known pulmonary metastasis, the metastatic lesions were diminished (16, 17). Additional evidence for the critical role of E-cadherin to survival to tumor emboli came from studies in which Mary-X spheroids containing a dominant-negative E-cadherin mutant (H-2K(d)-E-cad) which lacked the extracellular binding domain but retained the β-catenin binding domain exhibited loss of integrity of the Mary-X tumor spheroids due to inhibition of the tight cell:cell interactions. When injected into mice, these Mary-X tumor spheroids containing dominant-negative mutant constructs were only weakly tumorigenic and inhibited the ability of Mary-X cells to form tumor emboli (16, 17). Using the SUM149 IBC cell line, other studies demonstrated that the presence of dominant negative E-cadherin (H-2kd-E-cad) cDNA blocked SUM149 invasion *in vitro*, which was associated with a decreased expression of the matrix metalloprotease enzymes (27). Recent studies demonstrating that blockade of p120/δ catenin, which anchors E-cadherin within the plasma membrane or inhibition of the translation initiation factor eIF4GI, which regulates translation of specific mRNAs such as p120/δ catenin, resulted in loss of integrity of SUM149 tumor spheroids (28). Taken together, these studies suggest that E-cadherin is critical to the invasive and metastatic phenotype of IBC tumor emboli, and also indicate that E-cadherin and p120/δ catenin may act in concert to maintain the integrity of the tightly aggregated tumor cells that comprise the IBC tumor emboli. These studies suggest that E-cadherin may function not only as part of the signature of IBC but may also serve as a therapeutic target which, when effectively blocked, results in inhibition of the tight cell:cell aggregation of IBC tumor spheroids *in vitro* and abrogates the metastatic potential of IBC tumor emboli *in vivo*.

1.4 Linking E-cadherin as a signature of inflammatory breast cancer and the process of the epithelial mesenchymal transition (EMT) in metastasis

While IBC is a variant of breast cancer that exhibits a program of accelerated metastasis, the robust expression of E-cadherin by aggregates of cells within IBC tumor emboli in patients' tissues and in pre-clinical models of IBC is, at least on first examination, paradoxical to the current hypothesis that the initiation of metastasis occurs through a specific process defined as the epithelial mesenchymal transition (EMT). EMT and the reverse process of mesenchymal epithelial transition (MET) are interlinked programs that are essential to normal embryonic development, as well as to appropriate wound healing and tissue regeneration following injury (29, 30). In these settings, the reversible processes of EMT and MET confer the ability of cells to exhibit plasticity in both their morphology and function (29). In the setting of embryonic development, EMT and MET are highly organized and precisely regulated programs that are critical to appropriate formation of the epithelial, mesoderm and endodermal layers required for organ formation (29). The process of EMT is reactivated as a developmental program in response to injury; as an example, an EMT process is induced in epithelial keratinocytes of surface epithelium at the leading edge of a wound. In this case, the epithelial cells have an intermediate "metastable" phenotype, and acquire an elongated mesenchymal morphology, increase their migratory activity while remaining attached to each other until closure of the wounded area is accomplished (29, 30). In a tumor setting, the process of EMT includes a number of functional changes in tumor cells which include activation of transcription factors including *ZEB1* and *ZEB2, TWIST1, SNAIL, SLUG,* with the associated loss of expression of specific cell-surface proteins that regulate the epithelial phenotype including E-cadherin and zona occludins-1. In addition, there is a concomitant gain of other genes that regulate the mesenchymal phenotype such as N-cadherin, and reorganization and expression of cytoskeletal proteins such as vimentin and alpha smooth muscle actin, production of enzymes that degrade extracellular matrix such as matrix metalloproteinase 2 (MMP-2), also known as gelatinase, and expression or suppression of specific miR families (31). There are several other changes in function of tumor cells undergoing the process of EMT including the acquisition of characteristics that are similar to stem cells including expression of surface markers CD44+/CD24$^{-/low}$ (31, 32).

While IBC is the variant of breast cancer that exhibits the most accelerated metastasis, and has been characterized as being enriched for cells expressing markers of tumor initiating cells/cancer stem cells, including expressing CD44^{+}/CD24$^{-/low}$, aldehyde dehydrogenase 1 (ALDH-1^{+}), and CD133+ (33-35), the robust expression of E-cadherin by IBC tumor emboli is inconsistent with the current hypothesis that initiation of metastatic progression occurs through the process of EMT. This chapter will highlight our studies that have used whole unbiased transcriptional analysis and broad-scale protein pathway activation mapping to define the specific patterns of expression of genes, proteins and miRs, along with functional protein signaling architecture that collectively provide insight into the distinct signature of IBC. It is the changes in the molecular machinery that define the extreme plasticity and collective tumor cell migration patterns exhibited by IBC tumor cells and tumor emboli that are the metastatic lesion of this lethal variant of breast cancer.

2. Defining the signatures of inflammatory breast cancer

2.1 Whole transcriptome analysis and validation of gene signature in IBC cell lines and tumor emboli

Affymetrix microarrays were used to evaluate 56,000+ probe sets expressed by all currently available IBC cell lines and cell systems including SUM149 and Mary-X tumor spheroids which are of the triple negative subtype and the SUM190, MDA-IBC-3, KPL-4, which are of the luminal B molecular subtype. The non-IBC cell lines included in the analysis were MDA-MB-231, SUM159, and MCF-7 human breast cancer cell lines. The MDA-MB-231 and SUM159 cells are both classified as triple negative breast cancer cell lines and MCF-7 cells are of the luminal A molecular subtype.

Whole unbiased transcriptome analysis revealed that, regardless of molecular subtype, the IBC cell lines expressed *CDH1,* which encodes for E-cadherin, compared to non-IBC breast cancer cell lines, with the exception of MCF-7 cells (Figure 2). There was heterogeneity in *CDH1* expression by the different IBC cell lines, with KPL-4 cells having the lowest level of *CDH1* expression. In addition to *CDH1,* IBC cell lines expressed other genes that have previously been shown to be involved with regulating tight cell:cell adhesion of epithelial cells through formation of the adherens junctions including *DSC2,* which encodes for desmocollin 2, and *JUP/*γ catenin and the expression of these two genes by the individual IBC cell lines mirrored that of *CDH1.* Although gene expression of *CTNNA1* and *CTNNB1,* which encode for α catenin and β catenin, respectively, was detectable in IBC cell lines, these genes were not differentially expressed at higher levels by IBC cell lines compared to non-IBC cell lines. One significant difference in the whole transcriptome analysis of IBC cell lines compared to non-IBC cell lines was the striking lack of expression of the zinc finger E-box binding homeobox 1 (*ZEB1*) transcription factor, also previously defined as transcription factor 8 (*TCF8*) and *ZFHX1A* (Figure 2). Analysis of other transcription factors related to the process of EMT revealed that *SNAI2,* which encodes for Slug protein, was expressed by all of the basal like breast cancer cells including SUM149, Mary-X, SUM159 and MDA-MB-231 but was not expressed by SUM190, which are luminal B, suggesting that gene expression of this transcription factor may be subtype dependent. Expression of other transcription factors including *ZEB2* was detectable however the pattern of expression did not appear to be related to molecular subtype or whether cells were IBC or non-IBC.

To validate the results of these transcriptome studies, tissues isolated from mice bearing Mary-X xenografts were assessed for the presence of emboli in tissue sections stained with hematoxylin and eosin (H&E) and the presence of tumor emboli in the dermis was noted (Figure 3 A). Serial sections of this same tissue isolated from Mary-X xenograft were stained with specific antibodies that identified E-cadherin expressed by tumor emboli in the dermis (Figure 3 B). A higher magnification light micrographic image demonstrates the presence of abundant E-cadherin protein on the surface of cells within the Mary-X tumor emboli in the dermis of the skin (Figure 3 C). Figure 3 D shows a micrometastastic lesion of Mary-X within lung tissue stained with E-cadherin antibodies, demonstrating that metastatic lesions of Mary-X have persistant expression of E-cadherin. Triple color immunofluorescence and microscopy defined the specific patterns of co-localization of E-cadherin and JUP/γ catenin (Figure 3 E) in tissue sections of skin isolated from mice bearing Mary-X xenografts containing IBC tumor emboli within the dermis. E-cadherin and JUP/γ catenin both co-localized primarily to the plasma membrane of tumor cells within Mary-X tumor emboli (Figure 3 E). These results are the first to associate the expression of *CDH1,* which encodes for the transmembrane glycoprotein E-cadherin, by Mary-X tumor emboli, with increased expression of other genes, including *JUP/γ* catenin, that collectively regulate tight cell:cell homotypic aggregation by IBC tumor emboli. These results suggest that the upregulation of this specific cassette of genes is part of the distinct signature of IBC tumor emboli that are the local metastatic lesions of IBC.

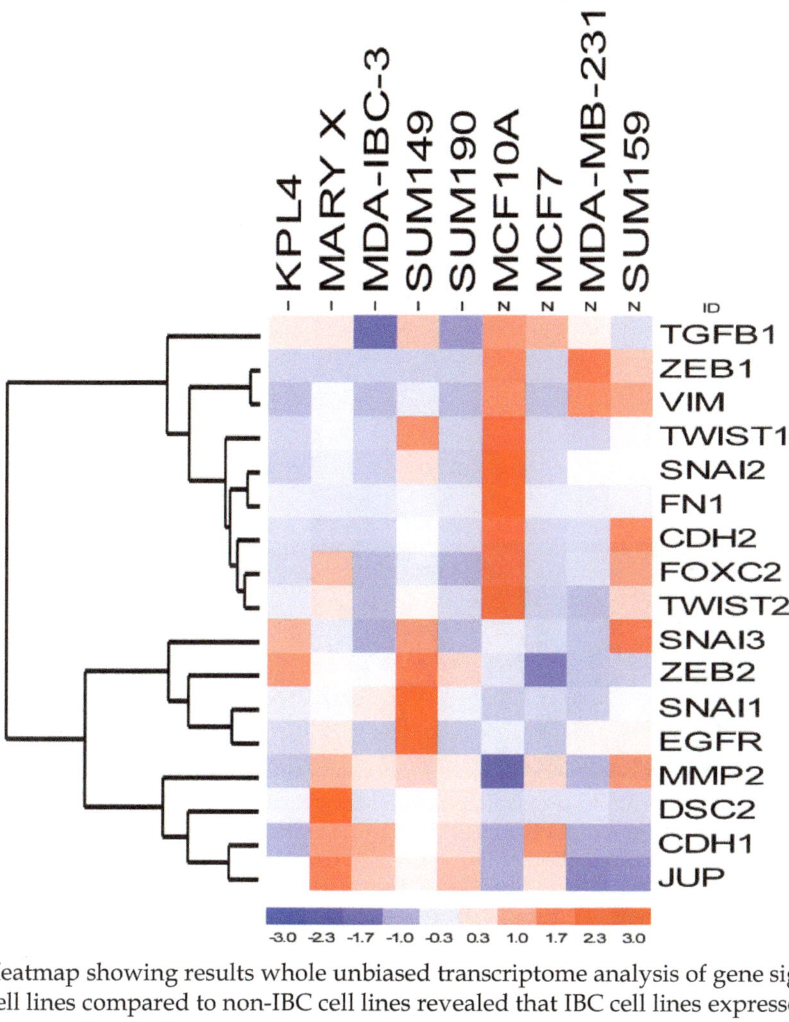

Fig. 2. Heatmap showing results whole unbiased transcriptome analysis of gene signatures of IBC cell lines compared to non-IBC cell lines revealed that IBC cell lines expressed high levels of *CDH1,* JUP/γ, and DCS2, with a lack of expression of *ZEB1* compared to non-IBC breast cancer cell lines.

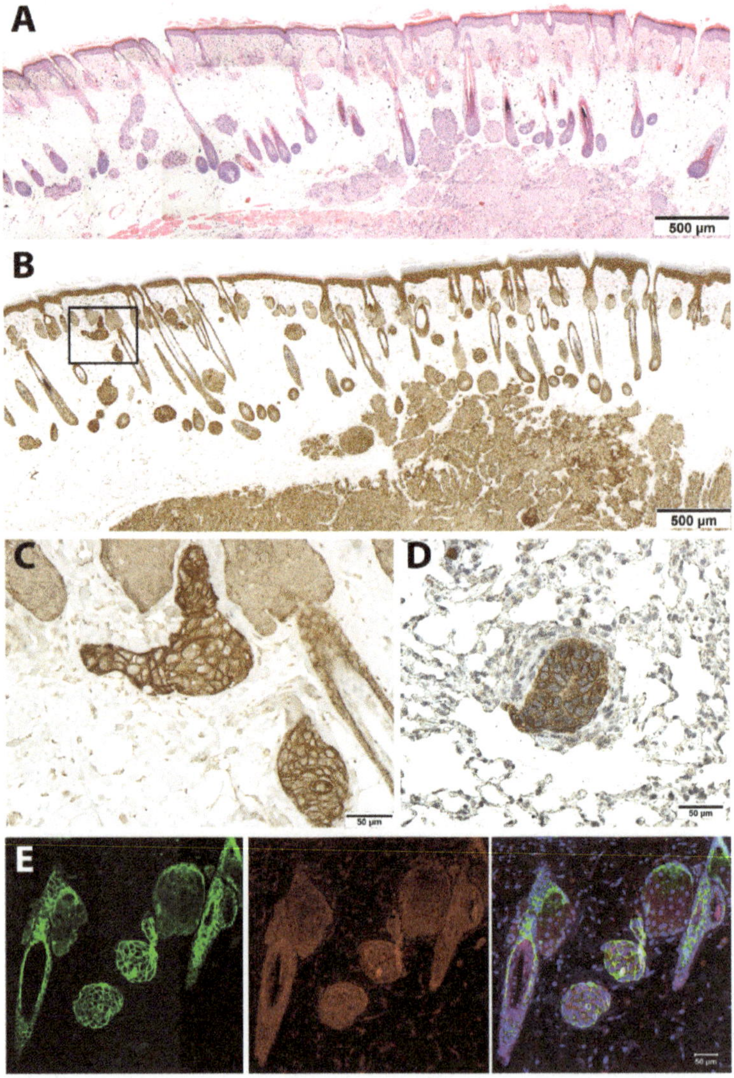

Fig. 3. **A**. H&E stained tissue section isolated from Mary-X xenograft demonstrating the presence of numerous tumor emboli within the dermis of the skin (4x magnification). **B and C.** Light micrographs of a serial section of tissue isolated from Mary-X xenograft as shown in Figure 3 A, stained with E-cadherin antibodies demonstrating that Mary-X primary tumor as well as numerous tumor emboli throughout the dermis express E-cadherin protein (Figure B. 4 x magnification and Figure C. 20X magnification). **D.** Light micrograph of section of lung tissue stained with E-cadherin antibodies demonstrating the presence of E-cadherin in pulmonary micrometastasis lesion (20x magnification). **E.** Triple color immunofluorescence and fluorescence microscopy defined the specific patterns of co-localization of E-cadherin and JUP/γ catenin at the surface of the plasma membrane of Mary-X tumor emboli.

2.2 MicroRNA signatures of inflammatory breast cancer cells

Differential expression of specific microRNAs (miRs) expressed by IBC cell lines compared to non-IBC cell lines was evaluated using a Human Cancer focused PCR array based miRNA analysis (SA Biosciences/Qiagen, Frederick, MD) and were validated by real time PCR. The specific miR identified as being differentially expressed by IBC cell lines was miR200c (Figure 4). The significance of the high expression of miR 200c lies in its reported function as an indirect transcriptional regulator of *CDH1* by *ZEB1/2*. Recent studies report that the reciprocal relationship between *ZEB1/2* and members of the miR 200 family is responsible for the switch between epithelial and mesenchymal states and is driven, in part, by an active autocrine TGF beta signaling network (36). The identification of miR200c as the primary miR expressed by IBC cell lines is consistent with previous studies demonstrating the reciprocal repression of E-cadherin by *ZEB1* through downregulation of miR 200c (37-41). Interestingly, the expression of miR 200c as the primary miRs in IBC cell lines provides independent validation of the observations that IBC cell lines are characterized by a specific gene signature that includes expression of CDH1 and other genes associated with homotypic aggregation and tight cell:cell adhesion, with a lack of expression of *ZEB1* identified using whole transcriptome analysis.

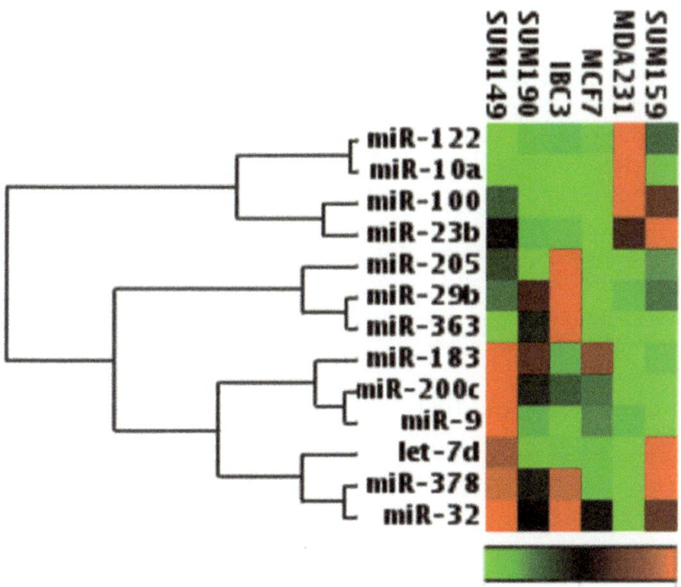

Fig. 4. Heatmap of miRs in SUM149 and SUM190 cells compared to non-IBC cell lines. Analysis of abundantly expressed miRs revealed that IBC cell lines express high levels of miR 200c.

Although the expression of miR 200c in tandem with the robust expression of a cassette of genes associated with homotypic aggregation including *CDH1, DSC2,* and *JUP* appears to be paradoxical to the current understanding of the process of metastatic progression associated with the alternations that occur during EMT, previous studies reported that multi-cellular tumor cell clusters are more efficient at formation of metastasis compared to single cells (42). Moreover, studies that examined primary breast tumors and the corresponding liver, lung and brain metastasis revealed increased E-cadherin expression in the metastatic lesions compared to the primary tumors (43). As an example, the MDA-MB-231 triple negative breast cancer cells have a mesenchymal phenotype and do not express E-cadherin, were demonstrated to re-express E-cadherin protein in spontaneous MDA-MB-231 derived metastatic foci, supporting the hypothesis that the reversion from EMT to exhibit characteristics of the process of MET occurs at sites of metastasis distant from a primary tumor that may exhibit an EMT phenotype (43). Collectively, these studies suggest that IBC, as the most lethal variant of breast cancer, exhibits signatures that point to an ongoing process of MET, which is consistent with the ability of tumor emboli to survive, to undergo what has been defined as "cohesive invasion" and to rapidly colonize organs and tissues distant from the primary tumor (42-44).

2.3 Proteomic pathway mapping of IBC cell lines

Reverse phase microarray (RPMA) technology was developed by our laboratory to address the challenges associated with other types of protein assays, namely the ability to quantitatively measure the levels and activation/phosphorylation state of key signaling proteins in a multiplexed fashion using microscopic quantities of tumor tissue and cells (45-48). We used RPMA in the present studies to identify the specific signal transduction pathways and molecules activated in IBC cell lines compared with non-IBC cell lines. The results of protein pathway mapping identified significant activation of specific pathways in IBC cells including E-cadherin ($p>0.001$) (Figure 5 A) and phospho-focal adhesion kinase (FAK) at Y576/577 ($p>0.015$) (Figure 5 B). Interestingly, recent studies have demonstrated that blocking FAK results in down regulation of the cell:cell adhesion properties of E-cadherin (49). Additionally, histone deacetylase (HDAC) inhibitors have been reported to inhibit FAK protein expression (50). These results provide independent validation of the observations from the whole transcriptome analysis identifying E-cadherin expression as a primary characteristic of IBC and suggests that specific therapeutic molecules, such as HDAC inhibitors that can block the functions of E-cadherin and FAK, may be useful in targeting IBC tumor emboli.

3. Signature based therapeutic targets in inflammatory breast cancer

The whole transcriptome based analysis identified E-cadherin, DSC2, and JUP/γ catenin as gene signatures of the tight cell:cell adhesion exhibited by IBC cells and tumor spheroids. Taken together with the proteomic-based identification of E-cadherin and FAK, these results suggest that these are IBC specific targets appropriate for the activity of HDAC inhibitors. We therefore evaluated the effects of this class of agents on IBC tumor spheroids, which provide an *in vitro* surrogate for IBC tumor emboli. Using fluorescence microscopy, wee demonstrate that the HDAC inhibitor, Suberoylanilide Hydroxamic Acid (SAHA;Vorinostat® Merck, Inc), destroys the integrity of Mary-X tumor spheroids and induce apoptosis as determined by TUNEL staining (Figure 6 A). In addition, SAHA induced the translocation of E-cadherin and JUP/γ catenin from the plasma membrane to the cytoplasm of Mary-X tumor spheroids, resulting in a loss of integrity of the tumor spheroids (Figure 6 B). Using SUM149 IBC tumor spheroids, we previously reported that SAHA induced a loss of integrity and viability of SUM149 tumor spheroids through translocation of E-cadherin protein from the plasma membrane to the cytoplasmic compartment, without altering the amount total E-cadherin protein, suggesting a change in functional activity of E-cadherin (51). We also found that SAHA induced a loss of the tight

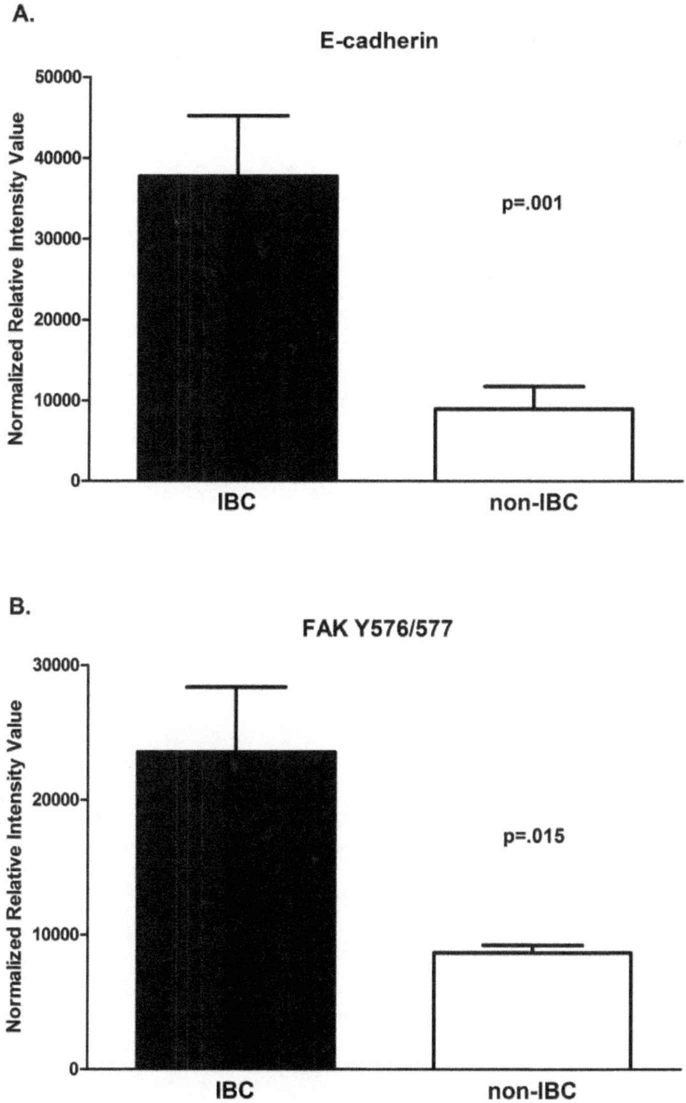

Fig. 5. **A.** RPMA analysis demonstrates significant increase in E-cadherin protein in IBC tumor spheroids including Mary-X, SUM149, SUM190 and MDA-IBC-3 compared to non-IBC cells MDA-MB-231 and SUM159. **B**. RPMA analysis revealed first time evidence for activation of focal adhesion kinase (FAK) protein at Y576/577. Histograms of total E-cadherin and phosphorylated FAK at Y397 and Y576/577 and are shown for both IBC cell lines and non-IBC cell lines (Standard deviations are shown with p values).

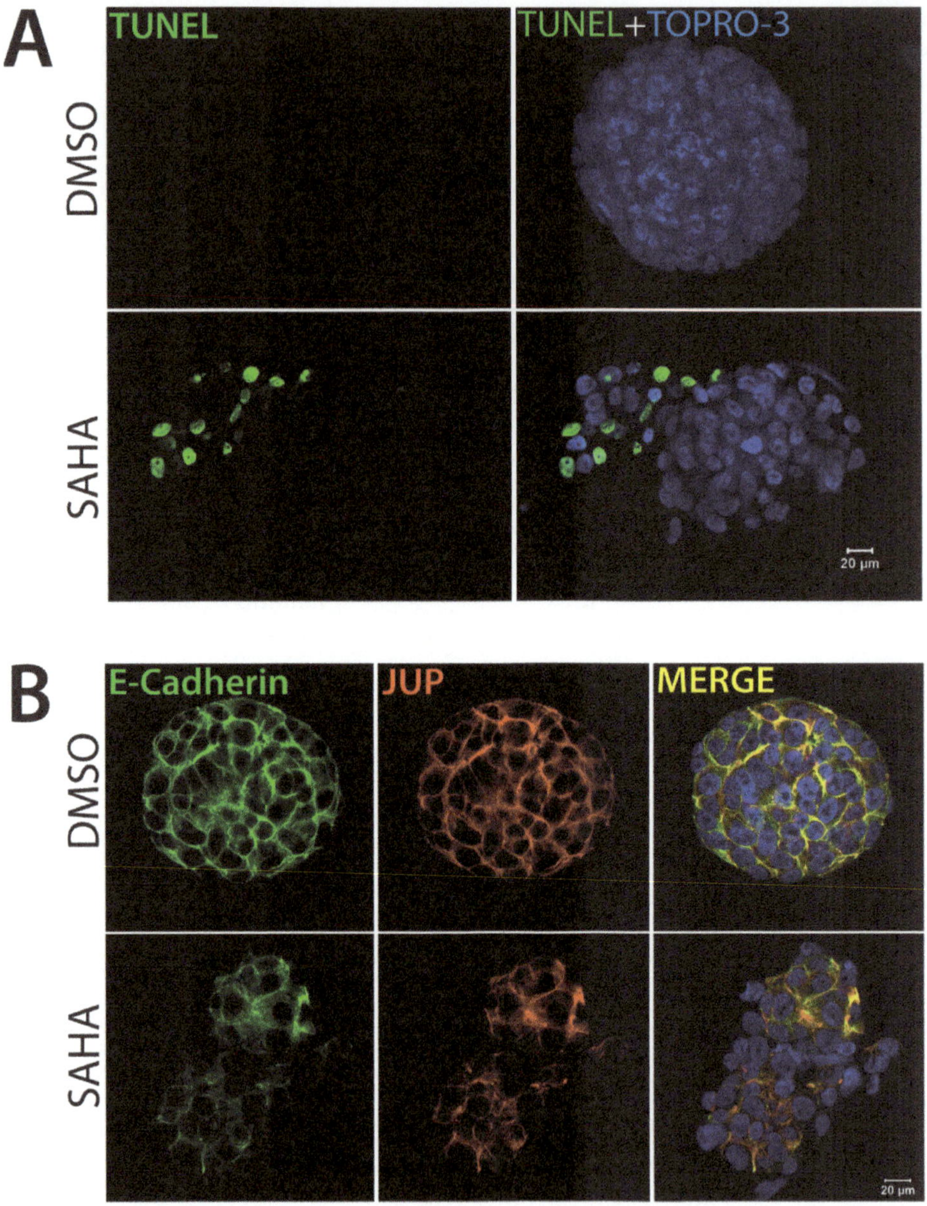

Fig. 6. **A.** Fluorescence microscopy revealed that Suberoylanilide Hydroxamic Acid (SAHA;Vorinostat® Merck, Inc) induced apoptosis in Mary-X tumor spheroids as evaluated by analysis of TUNEL staining. **B.** Flourescence microscopy demonstrated that SAHA induced translocation of E-cadherin (green fluorescence) and JUP/γ catenin (red fluorescence) from the plasma membrane of Mary-X tumor spheroids to reside primarily within the nucleus, resulting in a loss of integrity of the tumor spheroids.

cell: cell aggregation mediated by E-cadherin, resulting in the inhibition of self renewal and clonogenicity of SUM149 tumor spheroids as well as inhibited the tight aggregation of freshly isolated IBC patient tumor cells derived from pleural effusion (51). In non-IBC cell lines, SAHA induces apoptosis and in E-cadherin null cells, SAHA can re-induce E-cadherin, thus reversing EMT. Collectively, these are the first studies to identify the HDAC inhibitors as a class of therapeutic agents that abrogate the functional role of E-cadherin in formation of adherens junctions in IBC tumor spheroids that leads to destruction of these 3 dimensional multi-cellular structures which are surrogates for IBC tumor emboli as the metastatic lesions of this lethal variant of breast cancer. The present results suggest that proteins encoded by the cassette of genes that serve as part of the signature of IBC tumor emboli which specifically regulate the tight cell:cell adhesion of cells within IBC tumor emboli, including E-cadherin, DSC2 and JUP/γ catenin, represent potential therapeutic targets for eliminating IBC tumor emboli. In addition, these studies suggest that HDAC inhibitors are a class of compounds that effectively target the IBC tumor emboli for destruction. Studies are ongoing to determine the potential of HDAC inhibitors for their clinical utility.

4. Summary and conclusions

This chapter provides an overview of newly described IBC-specific molecular alterations expressed in IBC cell lines, tumor spheroids and tumor emboli characterized by a unique plasticity of this distinct variant of breast cancer. The concomitant use of gene and miR expression profiling as well as functional protein pathway activation mapping provides an unprecedented molecular/systems-level view of IBC. While IBC cells, tumor spheroids and tumor emboli express abundant levels of E-cadherin that is expressed in concert with other genes that collectively mediate tight homotypic aggregation of IBC tumor cells, with a loss of *ZEB1*, and express miR 200c, a repressor of *ZEB1*, which is consistent with the process of MET, IBC cells simultaneously express transcription factors that support invasion and metastasis, characteristic of the process of EMT. Proteomic analysis of the signaling architecture of IBC reinforces and expands on the genomic findings of activation of signaling pathways specific to IBC, validating the central role of E-cadherin to IBC tumor emboli. Our observations suggest that, as the most aggressive variant of breast cancer, IBC retains an epithelial phenotype characterized by cell:cell aggregation and cohesive invasion (32), and exhibit a program of accelerated metastasis by IBC tumor emboli distinguished by expression of specific genes, miRs and signaling proteins. The specific function of the genes within this distinct signature of IBC plasticity, which include genes involved in the processes of both MET, such as E-cadherin and FAK activation that may mediate the cohesive invasion of tumor emboli, with lack of *ZEB1*, while simultaneously expressing genes associated with EMT, such as *SNAI1*, *SNAI2* and *TWIST1*, may play important roles in determining the therapeutic agents that will most effectively target IBC tumor emboli for destruction

5. Acknowledgements

Supported by the American Airlines-Komen For the Cure Foundation Promise Grant KGO81287 (FMR, MC) and The State of Texas Fund for Rare and Aggressive Breast Tumors

(FMR). The authors appreciate the generous support of Dr. Vikas Chandhoke and the College of Life Sciences at George Mason University. This work as partially supported by the Italian Istituti Superiore di Sanita within the framework Italy/USA cooperation agreement between the U.S. Department of Health and Human Services, George Mason University and the Italian Ministry of Public Health.

6. References

[1] Robertson FM, Bondy M, Yang W, Yamauchi H, Wiggins S, Kamrudin S, Krishnamurthy S, Le-Petross H, Bidaut L, Player AN, Barsky SH, Woodward WA, Buchholz T, Lucci A, Ueno N, Cristofanilli M. Inflammatory breast cancer: the disease, the biology, the treatment. CA Cancer J Clin. 2010 Nov-Dec;60(6):351-75.

[2] Hance KW, Anderson WF, Devesa SS, Young HA, Levine PH. Trends in inflammatory breast carcinoma incidence and survival: the surveillance, epidemiology, and end results program at the National Cancer Institute. J Natl Cancer Inst. 2005; 97:966-975.

[3] Anderson WF, Schairer C, Chen BE, Hance KW, Levine PH. Epidemiology of inflammatory breast cancer (IBC). Breast Dis. 2005;22:9-23.

[4] Levine PH, Veneroso C. The epidemiology of inflammatory breast cancer. Semin Oncol. 2008;35:11-16.

[5] Cristofanilli M, Valero V, Buzdar AU, Kau SW, Broglio KR, Gonzalez-Angulo AM, Sneige N, Islam R, Ueno NT, Buchholz TA, Singletary SE, Hortobagyi GN. Inflammatory breast cancer (IBC) and patterns of recurrence: understanding the biology of a unique disease. Cancer. 2007 Oct 1;110(7):1436-44.

[6] Singletary SE, Cristofanilli M. Defining the clinical diagnosis of inflammatory breast cancer.Semin Oncol. 2008 Feb;35(1):7-10.

[7] Yang WT. Advances in imaging of inflammatory breast cancer. Cancer. 2010 Jun 1;116(11 Suppl):2755-7.

[8] Vermeulen PB, van Golen KL, Dirix LY. Angiogenesis, lymphangiogenesis, growth pattern, and tumor emboli in inflammatory breast cancer: a review of the current knowledge. Cancer. 2010 Jun 1;116(11 Suppl):2748-54. Review.

[9] Colpaert CG, Vermeulen PB, Benoy I, Soubry A, van Roy F, van Beest P, Goovaerts G, Dirix LY, van Dam P, Fox SB, Harris AL, van Marck EA. Inflammatory breast cancer shows angiogenesis with high endothelial proliferation rate and strong E-cadherin expression. Br J Cancer. 2003 Mar 10;88(5):718-25.

[10] Willmarth NE, Ethier SP. Autocrine and juxtacrine effects of amphiregulin on the proliferative, invasive, and migratory properties of normal and neoplastic human mammary epithelial cells.J Biol Chem. 2006 Dec 8;281(49):37728-37.

[11] Neve, R.M., Chin, K., Fridlyand, J., Yeh, J., Baehner, F., Fevr, T., Clark, L., Bayani, N., Coppe, J.P., Tong, F., Speed, T. Spellman, P.T., DeVries, S., Lapuk, A., Wang, N.J., Kuo, W.-L., Stilwell, J.L., Pinkel, D., Albertson, D.G., Waldman, F.M., McCormick, F., Dickson, R.B., Johnson, M.D., Lippman, M., Ethier, S., Gazdar, A., and Gray, J.W. (2006) A collection of breast cancer cell lines for the study of functionally distinct cancer subtypes. Cancer Cell, 10(6):515-27.

[12] Forozan F, Veldman R, Ammerman CA, Parsa NZ, Kallioniemi A, Kallioniemi OP, Ethier SP: Molecular cytogenetic analysis of 11 new breast cancer cell lines. *Br J Cancer* 1999, 81:1328-1334.

[13] Charafe-Jauffret E, Ginestier C, Monville F, Finetti P, Adélaïde J, Cervera N, Fekairi S, Xerri L, Jacquemier J, Birnbaum D, Bertucci F. Gene expression profiling of breast cell lines identifies potential new basal markers. Oncogene. 2006 Apr 6;25(15):2273-84.

[14] Kurebayashi J, Otsuki T, Tang CK, Kurosumi M, Yamamoto S, Tanaka K, Mochizuki M, Nakamura H, Sonoo H. Isolation and characterization of a new human breast cancer cell line, KPL-4, expressing the Erb B family receptors and interleukin-6. Br J Cancer. 1999 Feb;79(5-6):707-17.

[15] Klopp AH, Lacerda L, Gupta A, Debeb BG, Solley T, Li L, Spaeth E, Xu W, Zhang X, Lewis MT, Reuben JM, Krishnamurthy S, Ferrari M, Gaspar R, Buchholz TA, Cristofanilli M, Marini F, Andreeff M, Woodward WA. Mesenchymal stem cells promote mammosphere formation and decrease E-cadherin in normal and malignant breast cells. PLoS One. 2010 Aug 16;5(8):e12180.

[16] .Alpaugh ML, Tomlinson JS, Shao ZM, Barsky SH. A novel human xenograft model of inflammatory breast cancer. Cancer Res. 1999 Oct 15;59(20):5079-84.

[17] Tomlinson JS, Alpaugh ML, Barsky SH. An intact overexpressed E-cadherin/alpha,beta-catenin axis characterizes the lymphovascular emboli of inflammatory breast carcinoma. Cancer Res. 2001 Jul 1;61(13):5231-41.

[18] Bekhouche I, Finetti P, Adelaïde J, Ferrari A, Tarpin C, Charafe-Jauffret E, Charpin C, Houvenaeghel G, Jacquemier J, Bidaut G, Birnbaum D, Viens P, Chaffanet M, Bertucci F. High-resolution comparative genomic hybridization of inflammatory breast cancer and identification of candidate genes. PLoS One. 2011 Feb 9;6(2):e16950.

[19] Kleer CG, van Golen KL, Braun T, Merajver SD. Persistent E-cadherin expression in inflammatory breast cancer. Mod Pathol. 2001;14:458-464. 561-574.

[20] Van den Eynden GG, Van der Auwera I, Van Laere S, Colpaert CG, van Dam P, Merajver S, Kleer CG, Harris AL, Van Marck EA, Dirix LY, Vermeulen PB.Validation of a tissue microarray to study differential protein expression in inflammatory and non-inflammatory breast cancer. Breast Cancer Res Treat. 2004 May;85(1):13-22.

[21] Colpaert CG, Vermeulen PB, Benoy I, Soubry A, van Roy F, van Beest P, Goovaerts G, Dirix LY, van Dam P, Fox SB, Harris AL, van Marck EA. Inflammatory breast cancer shows angiogenesis with high endothelial proliferation rate and strong E-cadherin expression. Br J Cancer. 2003 Mar 10;88(5):718-25.

[22] Charafe-Jauffret E, Tarpin C, Bardou VJ, Bertucci F, Ginestier C, Braud AC, Puig B, Geneix J, Hassoun J, Birnbaum D, Jacquemier J, Viens P. Immunophenotypic analysis of inflammatory breast cancers: identification of an 'inflammatory signature'. J Pathol. 2004 Mar;202(3):265-73.

[23] Gumbiner BBM. Cell adhesion: the molecular basis of tissue architecture and morphogenesis. Cell 1996;84:345–57.

[24] Kemler R. From cadherins to catenins: cytoplasmic protein interactions and regulation of cell adhesion. Trends Genet 1993;9:317–21.
[25] Friedl P, Gilmour D. Collective cell migration in morphogenesis, regeneration and cancer. Nat Rev Mol Cell Biol. 2009 Jul;10(7):445-57.),
[26] Harris TJ, Tepass U. Adherens junctions: from molecules to morphogenesis. Nat Rev Mol Cell Biol. 2010 Jul;11(7):502-14. Review.
[27] Dong HM, Liu G, Hou YF, Wu J, Lu JS, Luo JM, Shen ZZ, Shao ZM. Dominant-negative E-cadherin inhibits the invasiveness of inflammatory breast cancer cells in vitro. J Cancer Res Clin Oncol. 2007 Feb;133(2):83-92.
[28] Silvera D, Arju R, Darvishian F, Levine PH, Zolfaghari L, Goldberg J, Hochman T, Formenti SC, Schneider RJ. Essential role for eIF4GI overexpression in the pathogenesis of inflammatory breast cancer. Nat Cell Biol. 2009 Jul;11(7):903-8.
[29] Thiery, J.P. 2002. Epithelial-mesenchymal transitions in tumour progression. Nat. Rev. Cancer. 2:442–454.
[30] Thiery JP, Acloque H, Huang RY, Nieto MA. Epithelial-mesenchymal transitions in development and disease. Cell. 2009 Nov 25;139(5):871-90.
[31] Kalluri, R., and Weinberg, R.A. 2009. The basics of epithelial-mesenchymal transition. J. Clin. Invest. 119:1420–1428.
[32] Mani SA, Guo W, Liao MJ, Eaton EN, Ayyanan A, Zhou AY, Brooks M, Reinhard F, Zhang CC, Shipitsin M, Campbell LL, Polyak K, Brisken C, Yang J, Weinberg RA. The epithelial-mesenchymal transition generates cells with properties of stem cells. Cell. 2008 May 16;133(4):704-15.
[33] Charafe-Jauffret E, Ginestier C, Iovino F, Tarpin C, Diebel M, Esterni B, Houvenaeghel G, Extra JM, Bertucci F, Jacquemier J, Xerri L, Dontu G, Stassi G, Xiao Y, Barsky SH, Birnbaum D, Viens P, Wicha MS. Aldehyde dehydrogenase 1-positive cancer stem cells mediate metastasis and poor clinical outcome in inflammatory breast cancer. Clin Cancer Res. 2010 Jan 1;16(1):45-55.
[34] Van Laere S, Limame R, Van Marck EA, Vermeulen PB, Dirix LY. Is there a role for mammary stem cells in inflammatory breast carcinoma?: a review of evidence from cell line, animal model, and human tissue sample experiments. Cancer. 2010 Jun 1;116(11 Suppl):2794-805. Review.
[35] Xiao Y, Ye Y, Yearsley K, Jones S, Barsky SH. The lymphovascular embolus of inflammatory breast cancer expresses a stem cell-like phenotype. Am J Pathol. 2008 Aug;173(2):561-74. Epub 2008 Jul 3.
[36] Gregory PA, Bracken CP, Smith E, Bert AG, Wright JA, Roslan S, Morris M, Wyatt L, Farshid G, Lim YY, Lindeman GJ, Shannon MF, Drew PA, Khew-Goodall Y, Goodall GJ. An autocrine TGF-{beta}/ZEB/miR-200 signaling network regulates establishment and maintenance of epithelial-mesenchymal transition. Mol Biol Cell. 2011 Mar 16. [Epub ahead of print]
[37] Schmalhofer O, Brabletz S, Brabletz T. E-cadherin, beta-catenin, and ZEB1 in malignant progression of cancer. Cancer Metastasis Rev. 2009 Jun;28(1-2):151-66.
[38] Gregory PA, Bracken CP, Bert AG, Goodall GJ. MicroRNAs as regulators of epithelial-mesenchymal transition. Cell Cycle. 2008 Oct;7(20):3112-8.

[39] Hurteau GJ, Carlson JA, Roos E, Brock GJ. Stable expression of miR-200c alone is sufficient to regulate TCF8 (ZEB1) and restore E-cadherin expression. Cell Cycle. 2009 Jul 1;8(13):2064-9.

[40] Park SM, Gaur AB, Lengyel E, Peter ME. The miR-200 family determines the epithelial phenotype of cancer cells by targeting the E-cadherin repressors ZEB1 and ZEB2. Genes Dev. 2008 Apr 1;22(7):894-907.

[41] Korpal M, Lee ES, Hu G, Kang Y. The miR-200 family inhibits epithelial mesenchymal transition and cancer cell migration by direct targeting of E-cadherin transcriptional repressors ZEB1 and ZEB2. J Biol Chem. 2008 May 30;283(22): 14910-4.

[42] Liotta LA, Saidel MG, Kleinerman J. The significance of hematogenous tumor cell clumps in the metastatic process. Cancer Res 1976;36:889–94.

[43] Chao YL, Shepard CR, Wells A. Breast carcinoma cells re-express E-cadherin during mesenchymal to epithelial reverting transition. Mol Cancer. 2010 Jul 7;9:179.

[44] Giampieri S, Manning C, Hooper S, Jones L, Hill CS, Sahai E. Localized and reversible TGFbeta signalling switches breast cancer cells from cohesive to single cell motility. Nat Cell Biol. 2009 Nov;11(11):1287-96.

[45] Speer R, Wulfkuhle J, Espina V, Aurajo R, Edmiston KH, Liotta LA, Petricoin EF 3rd.Molecular network analysis using reverse phase protein microarrays for patient tailored therapy. Adv Exp Med Biol. 2008;610:177-86.

[46] Wulfkuhle JD, Speer R, Pierobon M, Laird J, Espina V, Deng Jm Mammano E, Yang SX, Swain SM, Nitti D, Esserman LJ, Belluco C, Liotta LA and Petricoin EF. Multiplexed Cell Signaling Analysis of Human Breast Cancer: Applications for Personalized Therapy. J of Prot Res. 2008 Apr;7(4):1508-17.

[47] Paweletz, Cloud P; C. P. Paweletz, L. Charboneau, V. E. Bichsel, N. L. Simone, T. Chen, J. W. Gillespie, M.R. Emmert-Buck, M. J. Roth, E. F. Petricoin III, L. A. Liotta (2001). "Reverse phase protein microarrays which capture disease progression show activation of pro-survival pathways at the cancer invasion front". *Oncogene* (Nature publishing group) 20 (16): 1981–1089.

[48] Liotta, LA; L A. Liotta, V. Espina, A I. Mehta, V. Calvert, K. Rosenblatt, D. Geho, P J. Munson, L. Young, J. Wulfkuhle, E F. Petricoin (2003). "Protein microarrays: Meeting analytical challenges for clinical applications". *Cancer Cell* 3 (4): 317–325.

[49] Canel M, Serrels A, Miller D, Timpson P, Serrels B, Frame MC, Brunton VG. Quantitative in vivo imaging of the effects of inhibiting integrin signaling via Src and FAK on cancer cell movement: effects on E-cadherin dynamics. Cancer Res. 2010 Nov 15;70(22):9413-22.

[50] Gould JJ, Kenney PA, Rieger-Christ KM, Silva Neto B, Wszolek MF, LaVoie A, Holway AH, Spurrier B, Austin J, Cammarata BK, Canes D, Libertino JA, Summerhayes IC. Identification of tumor and invasion suppressor gene modulators in bladder cancer by different classes of histone deacetylase inhibitors using reverse phase protein arrays. J Urol. 2010 Jun;183(6):2395-402.

[51] Robertson FM, Woodward WA, Pickei R, Ye Z, Bornmann W, Pal A, Peng Z, Hall CS, Cristofanilli M. Suberoylanilide hydroxamic acid blocks self-renewal and homotypic aggregation of inflammatory breast cancer spheroids. Cancer. 2010 Jun 1;116(11 Suppl):2760-7.

11

Quantitative Organelle Proteomics of Protein Distribution in Breast Cancer MCF-7 Cells

Amal T. Qattan and Jasminka Godovac-Zimmermann
Molecular Cell Dynamics, Division of Medicine, University College London, UK

1. Introduction

In his address on the treatment of breast cancer, delivered in 1894 before the Harveian Society of London, W. Watson Chayne said of breast cancer: the "subject cannot be too often brought before the notice of the medical public. First, because the disease is common, at any rate in certain regions, and seems to be becoming more so"(Cheyne 1894). Although a hundred years of extensive research generated 226 946 scientific publications in the period 1886-2011, breast cancer remains the second leading cause of cancer deaths in women today. Breast cancer is the first human tumor for which targeted therapies have been developed. The most successful therapies include tamoxifen and aromatase inhibitors - both estrogen receptor pathway downregulators - and Herceptin, a HER2 antagonist that prolongs disease remission in selected women, but metastatic breast cancer remains largely an incurable disease (Imyanitov and Hanson 2004).
Breast cancer shares all the hallmarks of cancer postulated by Hanahan and Weinberg (Hanahan and Weinberg 2000) that include sustaining proliferative signaling, evading growth suppressors, resisting cell death, enabling replicative immortality, inducing angiogenesis, and activating invasion and metastasis. In addition, recent progress has added two further hallmarks such as reprogramming of energy metabolism and evading immune destruction (Hanahan and Weinberg 2011). Increasing recognition of the contribution of the tumor microenvironment to tumorigenesis re-affirms the concept of cancer as a systemic disease with very complex, not yet understood biology.
In 2011 more than 7 million humans around the world will die of cancer and 465 000 women will die from breast cancer alone (Mukherjee 2011).
For humanity, cancer is still the "Emperor of all maladies, master of all terrors."(Mukherjee 2011). For scientists it remains a formidable challenge to understanding the complexity of cellular function.

2. Large-scale proteomics analysis of cancer cells

The completion of human genome sequencing and rapid development of DNA-microarray technology led to extensive investigation of gene expression associated with breast cancer. Large-scale screening of mRNA levels showed that multiple and extensive changes in mRNA levels are commonly seen in breast cancer (Ince and Weinberg 2002, Sebastian and Johnson 2006, Sorlie et al. 2001, van de Vijver et al. 2002). However, eukaryotic cell proliferation is known to involve complex molecular choreography of mitogens that stimulate cell growth, membrane receptors, their signaling pathways, and downstream effectors of cell division (Hanahan and Weinberg 2000, Sebastian and Johnson 2006). Such studies clearly indicated an urgent need for complementary, highly parallel studies at the protein level. If genes have "legislative power" much of "executive power" is carried out by proteins. Their spatial and temporal distribution within cells is a very complex, but essential, feature of cellular function. The analysis of such distributions is complicated by the facts that a given protein may have multiple subcellular locations, can exist in multiple transcriptional or post-translational isoforms within the same cell and that the different isoforms may have different spatial and temporal distributions as well as different functional roles (Godovac-Zimmermann et al. 2005, Roberts and Smith 2002). Highly parallel methods such as analysis of mRNA abundance can give information on inputs to cellular protein abundance but the mRNA methods do not always correlate well with direct measurements of protein abundance (Gygi et al. 1999), require additional complexity to measure transcriptional isoforms, do not detect post-translational isoforms, and do not give information on spatial location. Conversely, direct measurements of spatial location by methods such as fluorescence microscopy usually do not distinguish isoforms, are mainly semiquantitative, and are difficult to achieve in highly parallel formats.

2.1 Quantitative proteomics of MCF-7 breast cancer subcellular organelles

In recent years, considerable effort has been devoted to determining the identities of proteins included in different subcellular organelles by proteomics (Au et al. 2007, Rogers and Foster 2007, Simpson and Pepperkok 2006, Xu et al. 2009, Yates et al. 2005). The most common approach has been purification of individual organelles followed by exhaustive determination of the protein content. The main disadvantages of this approach are (a) that the degree of purification/contamination of the organelle is difficult to ascertain conclusively for lower abundance proteins, (b) that the protein content may be altered by the purification process and (c) that the approach is not very suitable for dynamic studies of protein subcellular location. In a few cases, (Dunkley et al. 2004, Foster et al. 2006) an alternative approach of partial purification of organelles in a sucrose gradient has been employed, but the assignment of proteins to individual organelles has been based on matching gradient profiles of proteins to the profiles of presumptive marker proteins. Although this is useful for identifying what might be denominated core proteins of an organelle, it is automatically biased against evaluation of proteins in multiple subcellular locations.

The goal of our work (Qattan et al. 2010) was to establish high throughput proteomics methods that are capable of analyzing dynamically at least some of the complexity involved in subcellular protein distribution. The estrogen-dependent MCF-7 malignant breast epithelial cell line was selected due to the wealth of information available in the literature and its relevance to breast cancer (Lacroix and Leclercq 2004, Soule et al. 1973). Proteomics methods based on mass spectrometry are only suitable for indirect measurements of spatial location and we have therefore concentrated on the distribution of proteins between different subcellular organelles. To avoid the need for multiple purification procedures for many different organelles, partial purification based on sucrose gradient centrifugation was used followed by high throughput proteomics analysis of the protein content of different fractions from the sucrose gradient. Figure 1 illustrates the subcellular proteomics workflow. Following subfractionation of cellular organelles by sucrose gradient centrifugation, the basic functioning of the method was controlled by biochemical assay (Figure 2).

Enzymatic assays and Western blot detection indicated sucrose gradient fractions enriched in cytosol, plasma membrane, endoplasmic reticulum, and mitochondrial proteins, respectively. On the basis of this data obtained, fractions of cytosol, plasma membrane, endoplasmic reticulum and mitochondria from the sucrose gradient fraction were subjected to detailed analysis of protein content by MS methods.

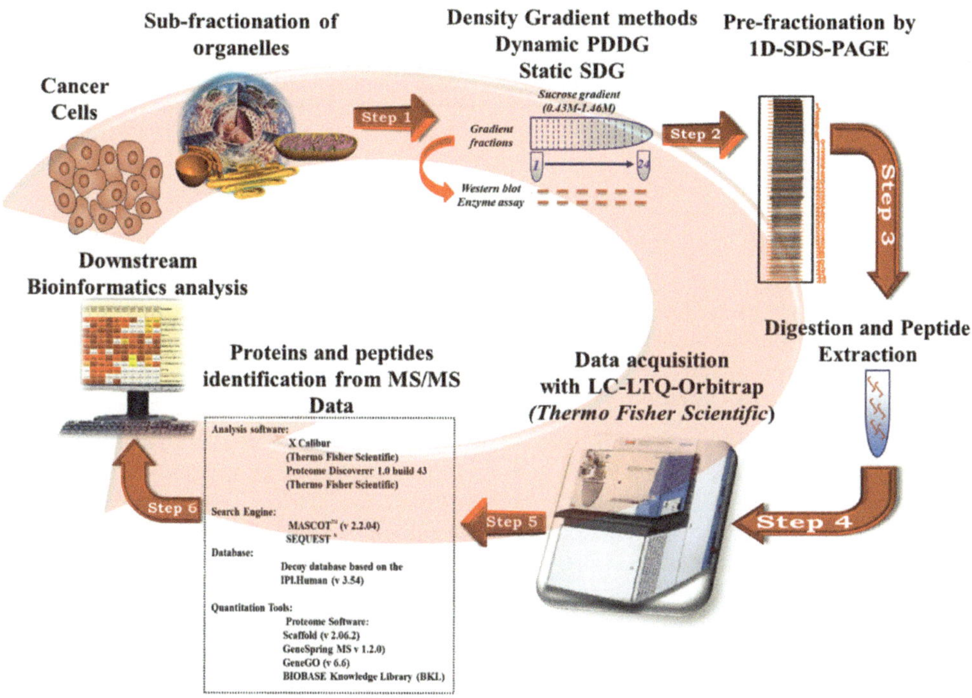

Fig. 1. Subcellular organelle proteomics workflow.

2.1.1 Proteomics data sets show multiple subcellular locations of proteins

Two aspects of the MS analysis are important in the context of the goals of the present work: (1) secure identification of as many proteins as possible in each fraction and (2) accurate measurement of the (relative) amount of any specific protein across the different fractions. We have used direct spectral counts from MS/MS runs for quantitative measurements of the peptides (Usaite et al. 2008). Table 1 shows that that a total of 15 527 different peptides were used to identify 2184 proteins in fractions of cytosol (CT), plasma membrane (PM), endoplasmic reticulum (ER) and mitochondria (MT). The initial set of MS data contained 5514 (protein, fraction, abundance) data points for 2184 proteins: there was an average of 2.5 locations per protein. This *initial data* set contained a substantial number of (protein, fraction, abundance) data points for which in a particular fraction only a single peptide with a small number of spectral counts was observed for some proteins.

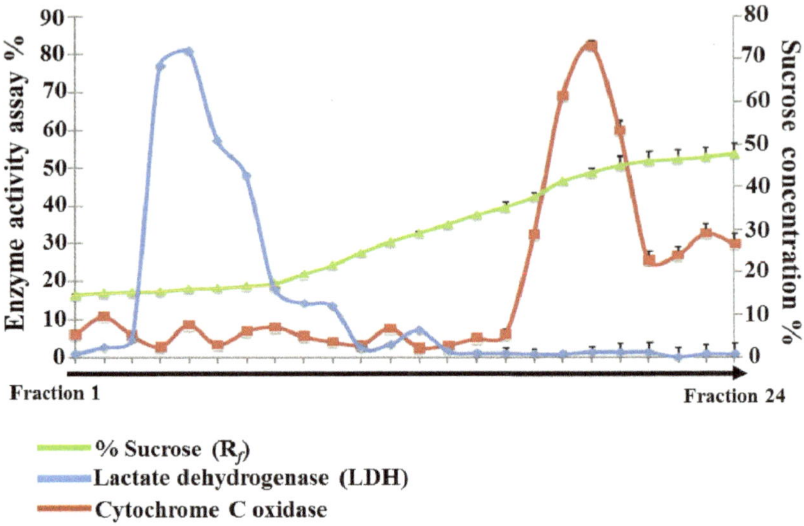

Fig. 2. Subcellular verification of protein markers by enzyme assay and Western blot. A total of 24 fractions was collected from a sucrose-density gradient (0.43-1.46 M) in which fractions 1 and 24 represent the top and the bottom, respectively. Typical density profile of sucrose fractions is calculated by refractive indices. Also shown is the distribution of activity across the gradient for the subcellular enzyme markers LDH and Cytochrome C oxidase.

The assignment of these proteins is less certain for these fractions. Removal of 876 data points for fractions where only a single peptide and 1 or 2 spectral counts were observed gave the *normal data* set in Table 1. 106 (protein, fraction, abundance) data points with only a single peptide in a fraction, but with 3 to 74 spectral counts, were retained to give a total of 4638 data points. The normal data set, which was used for many of the analyses below, corresponds to an average of 2.1 locations per protein. For some of the analyses, we have also removed from the normal data set those (protein, fraction, abundance) data points where less than 4% of the total amount of a given protein was observed in a specific fraction. This *trimmed data* set reduced the number of data points to 4576, that is, an average of 2.1 locations per protein.

In the following we will refer to the three sets of (protein, fraction, abundance) data points used for further analysis as the initial, normal and trimmed data sets (Table 1B), all of which contain a total of 2184 proteins. For individual proteins that were detected in multiple fractions, we will also use the term "primary location" to refer to the (protein, fraction) pair with the highest abundance and the term "secondary location" to refer to other (protein, fraction) pairs with lesser abundances for the same protein.

2.1.2 The observation of the same protein in multiple fractions is not due to "tailing" of the proteins in the sucrose gradient

With the normal data set, many of the proteins were observed in more than one sucrose gradient fraction and hierarchical clustering was used to analyze their distribution over the gradient (Figure 3). This indicated that in many cases the observation of the same protein in multiple fractions was not due to "tailing" of the proteins in the sucrose gradient.

Summary of MS Data				
Distribution Over Sucrose Gradient Fractions				
Fractions				
Total number of	**CT**	**PM**	**ER**	**MT**
Initial Data [a]				
Unique MS Spectra	4393	11435	8628	9654
Unique Peptides	3969	9876	7553	8588
Total Proteins per Fraction	852	1611	1441	1610
Unique Proteins per Fraction [b]	129	116	27	209
Normal Data [c]				
Unique MS Spectra	4233	11233	8341	9427
Unique Peptides	3810	9674	7267	8359
Proteins per Fraction	962	1409	1154	1383
Unique Proteins per Fraction [b]	189	239	69	347
Trimmed Data [d]				
Unique MS Spectra	4092	11223	8320	9375
Unique Peptides	3669	9664	7246	8311
Proteins per Fraction	657	1405	1145	1369
Unique Proteins per Fraction [b]	189	239	69	350

Data Sets		
Data set	**Number of (protein, fraction, abundance) data points**	**Number of proteins**
Initial [a]	5514	2184
Normal [c]	4638	2184
Trimmed [d]	4576	2184

a Includes all (protein, fraction, spectral counts) data points verified by Scaffold.
b Number of proteins found only in one fraction.
c Excludes(protein, fraction, spectral counts) data points where only a single peptide with 1 or 2 spectral counts was observed in a specific fraction.
d After removal from the normal data set of (protein, fraction, abundance) data points for which the proportion of the protein in a specific fraction was less than 4% of the total protein abundance in all four fractions.

Table 1. Summary of MS Data

The data shows numerous examples of bimodal distribution of proteins over two fractions that are not adjacent in the gradient (e.g., cytosol and mitochondria fractions in Figure 3C), as well as examples of proteins with more complicated bimodal distributions over three of the four fractions (Figure 3B) that are highly unlikely to arise from tailing. A Venn diagram (Figure 4) has been used to summarize the observed distribution of the proteins over the four sucrose gradient fractions as determined by the hierarchical clustering. A notable characteristic for the normal data set is that only 844 of the 2184 proteins (38.6%) were uniquely found in a single fraction. A further 296 proteins (13.6%) were found to be ubiquitously distributed over all fractions. The remaining 1044 proteins (47.8%) were consistent with intermediate distribution over multiple, but not all, subcellular locations. Of these 1044 proteins, 248 (11.4% of total proteins) were distributed over two fractions (e.g., cytosol and mitochondria, Figure 3C) or over three fractions (e.g., cytosol, membrane proteins and mitochondria, Figure 3B) in a "bimodal" manner that is inconsistent with inclusion in a single subcellular organelle and "tailing" over the sucrose gradient.

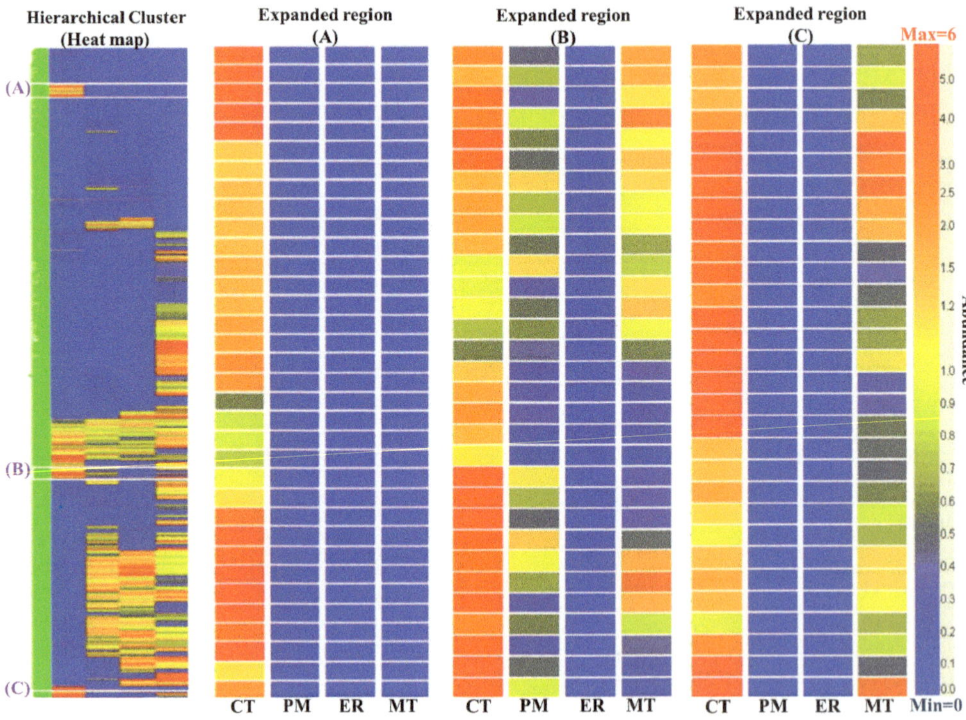

Fig. 3. Hierarchical clustering and heat map across the four fractions. Individual proteins are represented by a single row, each fraction is represented by a single column, and each cell represents the abundance of a single protein in a single fraction. The color scale is for normalized relative abundance from 6.0 (red) to 1.0 (yellow) to 0.0 (blue, not detected). The expansions show typical regions of the heat map corresponding to: (a) proteins observed uniquely in cytosol, (b) "bimodal" proteins (see text) observed in fractions cytosol (CT), plasma membrane (PM), mitochondria (MT), and (c) "bimodal" proteins observed in fractions cytosol and mitochondria.

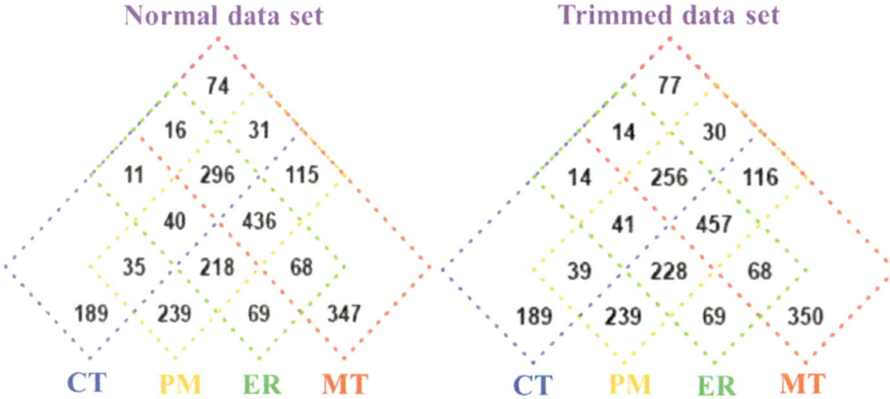

Fig. 4. Four-way Venn diagrams summarizing the distribution of the 2184 proteins over different combinations of the sucrose gradient fractions.

2.1.3 The data represent a good sampling of the distribution over multiple subcellular locations for the observed proteins

Inspection of the distribution of the proteins between primary and secondary locations revealed that they are well dispersed over the regions compatible with a primary location and 1-3 secondary locations (Figure 5). Thus, for example, proteins for which we detected a primary location and a single secondary location must lie on the line from (0.5, 0.5) to (1.0, 0.0) (green plus signs in Figure 5), but are well dispersed along that line. For 2-3 secondary

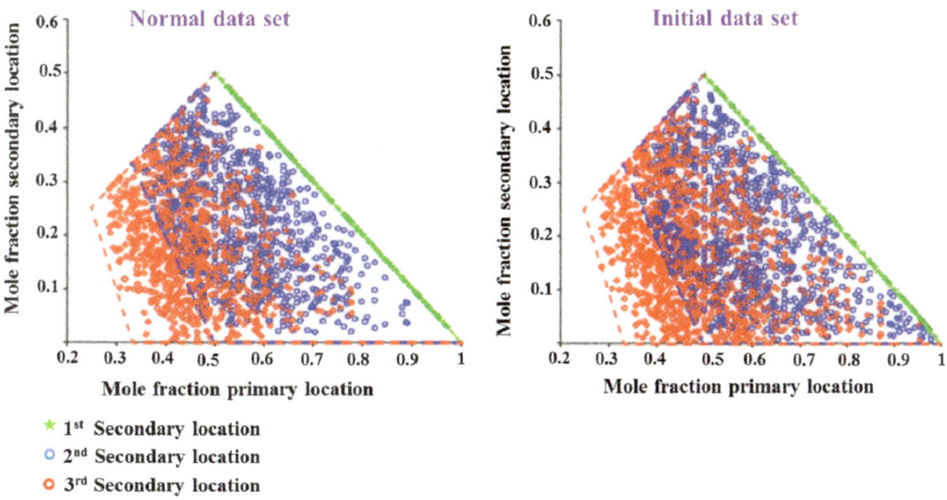

Fig. 5. Distribution of proteins with a primary location and 1 (green), 2 (blue), or 3 (red) secondary locations over compatible areas of a plot of primary mole fractions vs secondary mole fractions. For each protein, the spectral counts observed in a specific gradient fraction were expressed as mole fractions of the total number of spectral counts observed in all four gradient fractions.

locations, the initial data set shows better sampling near the edges of the compatible regions, for example, there are more data points at large values of the primary mole fraction and at very small values of the secondary mole fractions. Many of these data points arise from proteins corresponding to sequencing of only one peptide and only 1-2 spectral counts in a specific fraction. This is a consequence of the sampling properties of spectral counting. The dispersion of the data points in Figure 5 over the compatible areas of the plot is a strong indication that the data represent a good sampling of the distribution over multiple subcellular locations for the observed proteins.

2.1.4 Spurious tailing of proteins in the sucrose gradient does not make any major contributions to the observed multiplicity of locations

A more quantitative evaluation of the possibility of tailing in the gradient was obtained by looking for proteins with high abundance in a given gradient fraction, but with no detectable abundance in the adjacent fractions. For the most abundant proteins, the MS detection method was capable of detecting as little as about 0.2% of the protein in an adjacent fraction. Because the proteins may correspond to different subcellular organelles, tailing between two fractions need not be symmetrical, e.g. tailing from CT to PM may not be the same as tailing from PM to CT. This leads to the six tests for the possibility of tailing shown in Table 2. For all the fractions there are many highly abundant proteins which do not tail into the adjacent fraction (Table 2). The highly abundant proteins also reveal some characteristics which are common in the data set. Some very abundant proteins were found uniquely in a single fraction (e.g., see hepatoma-derived growth factor and Protein S100-A9 in Table 2). Other proteins were detected in only two fractions, but with a bimodal distribution over the fractions (e.g., see sialic acid synthase and pyridoxal kinase in Table 2). Many proteins were distributed over several fractions, with substantial proportions of the protein present in different fractions (e.g., see ATP-citrate synthase in Table 2). Some proteins were primarily present in a single fraction, but small amounts of the protein were found in other fractions (see e.g. Rho GDP-dissociation inhibitor 1 and nucleophosmin in Table 2). We conclude from the data in Table 2 that spurious tailing of proteins in the sucrose gradient does not make any major contributions to the observed multiplicity of locations.

2.1.5 Annotations of subcellular location

We have used previous subcellular location annotations in the UniProtKB database (in the keyword "subcellular location" field and the ontology "subcellular component" field) and in the Locate Subcellular Location database to compare three aspects of the present work with earlier work: (1) the degree to which the individual sucrose gradient fractions are enriched with proteins corresponding to specific subcellular organelles; (2) the extent to which the multiplicity of subcellular locations observed here is reflected in current annotations of subcellular locations; and, (3) the extent to which there are discrepancies between this work and previous annotations of subcellular locations.

In evaluating these comparisons, it is important to keep in mind that there is not an exact mesh between our experimental strategy and the ontological descriptions of subcellular location used in the databases. The top level of our experimental design matches the levels (extracellular region, plasma membrane, cytoplasm, nucleus) in the GO classification scheme, but the experiment excludes the extracellular region and the nucleus. At a lower level we only tried to obtain an approximate resolution of the cytoplasm as (cytosol,

Test for Overlap of Proteins Between Sucrose Gradient Fractions					
	Normalized protein abundance [b]				
Accession number	CT	PM	ER	MT	Proteins name
					Overlap from CT to PM
	Top [c]	*ND* [c]	*all* [c]	*all* [c]	
4758516	15	-	-	-	**Hepatoma-drived growth factor**
157829557	11.92	-	-	0.77	Carbonic anhydrase2
36038	11.76	-	-	0.49	Rho GDP-dissociation inhibitor 1
4502105	10.97	-	-	0.31	Annexin A4
4506387	9.53	-	0.24	1.47	UV excision repair protein RAD23 homologue B
7023053	7.79	-	-	1.95	**Sialic acid synthase**
4505701	7.37	-	-	1.28	**Pyridoxal Kinase**
					Overlap from PM to CT
	ND [c]	*Top* [c]	*all* [c]	*all* [c]	
24307879	-	7.25	1.58	0.42	Cytoplasmic dynein 1 intermediate chain 2
68533125	-	6.55	1.28	0.72	**ATP-citrate synthase**
34366439	-	6.33	1.89	0.11	Cytoplasmic dynein 1 light intermediate chain 1
30749633	-	6	1.78	0.22	Tyrosine-protein phosphatase non receptor type 1
38570062	-	5.81	0.61	0.61	UPF0363 protein C7 or f20
24307879	-	5.35	1.47	0.21	Coatomer subunit beta
	-	7.25	1.58	0.42	UTP-glucose-1-phosphate uridylyltransferase
					Overlap from PM to ER
	all [c]	*Top* [c]	*ND* [c]	*all* [c]	
4506773	-	5.26	-	-	**Protein S100-A9**
18655500	-	4.24	-	-	tr|Q6GMX0|Q6GMX Human Putative uncharacterized protein
12054072	-	3.03	-	-	Ig gamma-1 chain C region
5454024	-	2.99	-	0.37	Ribonuclease P protein subunit p30
4826659	0.36	2.89	-	0.36	F-actin-capping protein subunit beta
22726186	-	2.65	-	0.38	Proteosome assembly chaperone 2
13876386	-	2.51	-	0.73	Epiplakin
					Overlap from ER to PM
	all [c]	*ND* [c]	*Top* [c]	*all* [c]	
4506645	-	-	11.43	-	60S ribosomal protein L38
51036603	-	-	4.17	-	Guanine nucleotide-binding protein G(I)/G(S)/G(O) gamma-12
4506761	-	-	4.12	-	Protein S100-A10
4507129	-	-	4	2	Small nuclear ribonucleoprotein E
5454090	-	-	3.75	2	Translocon- associated protein subunit delta
6005860	-	-	3.2	2	60S ribosomal protein L35
7661728	-	-	3.2	-	Mitogen-activated protein binding protein interacting protein
					Overlap from ER to MT
	all [c]	*all* [c]	*Top* [c]	*ND* [c]	
4506645	-	-	11.43	-	60S ribosomal protein L38
10190712	-	0.96	8.65	-	Protein S100-A14
150010589	-	0.8	7.2	-	Interferon-induced transmembrane protein 1
17933772	-	2	4.8	-	Protein S100-A16
51036603	-	-	4.17	-	Guanine nucleotide-binding protein G(I)/G(S)/G(O) gamma-12
4506761	-	-	4.12	-	Protein S100-A10
3462883	-	1.32	3.51	-	Vesicle transport protein SEC20
					Overlap from MT to ER
	all [c]	*all* [c]	*ND* [c]	*Top* [c]	
1483131	-	0.34	-	12.24	**Nucleophosmin**
8922331	-	-	-	11.49	Protein mago nashi homologue 2
34201	-	-	-	10.91	60S ribosomal protein L35a
399758	-	-	-	9.52	Heterogenous nuclear ribonucleoprotein A3
7706425	-	-	-	9.38	U6 snRNA-associated Sm-like protein LSm8
11037094	-	-	-	8.7	tr|Q9HC85|Q9HC85_Human Metastasis realted protein
1232077	-	1.44	-	8.19	DNA replication licensing factor MCM2

a Proteins where the name is shown in bold correspond to proteins which exemplify general characteristics of the data that are noted in the text.

b Normalized abundances were calculated from the Spectral Abundance Factor using GeneSpring, that is, the abundances have been normalized using a correction for the differing number of amino acids in the proteins. For all proteins, the normalized abundances ranged from 0.018 to 22.25. A dash indicates the protein was not detected.

c Selection criteria. A filter to select non detected proteins was applied to a chosen fraction (ND). In an adjacent fraction in the sucrose gradient, the proteins were sorted according to abundance and the seven most abundant proteins (top) are shown.

Table 2. Test for overlap of proteins between sucrose gradient fractions endoplasmic reticulum, mitochondria), while the databases typically use (cytoplasm/ cytosol, endoplasmic reticulum, mitochondrion, Golgi apparatus). Overall, relative to the UniProtKB subcellular locations, 271 proteins had no annotations, 1388 had annotations at the top level and 525 had annotations at the lower level. For the 481 (22.0%) proteins in the initial data set that were observed in only a single fraction, we compared their locations with previous experimental information about subcellular location in the UniProtKB database. Figure 6 summarizes the proportion of these "unique" proteins which were previously assigned to various subcellular locations. This data provides an overview of the enrichment of the four fractions with cytosolic, plasma membrane, endoplasmic reticulum and mitochondrial proteins respectively. First, all four fractions show a substantial proportion of proteins either for which there is no previous annotation of subcellular location, or for which the previous annotation is only nucleus or extracellular region (from 5 (19%) of proteins in ER to 83 (40%) of proteins in MT). These annotations are compatible with the enrichment of the fractions with their various types of proteins and the present results constitute new annotation information for these proteins. Fraction CT shows three other major slices: (1) proteins which are fully compatible with cytosolic proteins, (2) proteins which have previously been assigned to cytoplasm, but also to other subcellular locations, and (3) proteins which have been previously assigned to other subcellular locations, but not to cytoplasm or cytosol. There is some ambiguity in the second and third groups since cytosol is not distinguished in many experimental strategies and the assigned locations are daughters of cytoplasm (but not of cytosol) in the GO ontology. Overall for the 127 proteins observed only in fraction CT, 119 (93.7%) have annotations that are compatible with enrichment of this fraction with cytosolic proteins. Only 8 proteins (6.3%) appear to be discrepancies that have other, incompatible locations. Of the 119 compatible proteins, 16 proteins have previous annotations that deviate from observation uniquely in fraction CT. For the other sucrose gradient fractions the cytoplasm/cytosol distinction also leads to some ambiguity, but overall the number/proportion of proteins compatible with enrichment of fraction PM (plasma membrane), fraction ER (endoplasmic reticulum) and fraction MT (mitochondrion) with the respective protein types are 94 (78.3%), 18 (67.0%), and 184 (88.9%) respectively. Because there is some inconsistency between the different subcellular location annotation sources , these numbers vary somewhat if the UniProtKB subcellular components or the Subcellular Location database are used, but do not change the overall conclusion. Within the limitations of such comparisons, we conclude that the previous annotations are largely consistent with enrichment of the fractions with the expected protein types. Apparent experimental/ database annotation discrepancies for all 2184 proteins are considered in more detail below. Is the apparent multiplicity of protein subcellular locations observed in our experiments captured in current database annotations? To address this question, we used the set of 163 proteins in the initial data set that showed bimodal, nonadjacent distributions over the sucrose gradient fractions (includes proteins observed only in combinations of non-adjacent fractions CT-ER, CT-MT, PM-MT, CT-PM-MT, and CT-ER-MT, i.e. proteins that clearly have multiple locations) and which also had at least 8 spectral counts. The latter condition ensures that the classification of these proteins as bimodal is not unduly influenced by the dynamic range limitations of MS/MS spectral counting. This set of proteins was compared with (merged) subcellular location annotations from the UniProtKB and LOCATE Subcellular Location databases. Figure 7 shows the distribution over the bimodal combinations of fractions and the annotations of subcellular location for all 163 proteins. As seen above with the proteins identified in only a single fraction, 59 (36.2%) of the bimodal proteins only had annotation at the level (nucleus, extracellular region, no annotation). Furthermore, only 22 (13.5%) of the proteins show multiple locations at the annotation level (cytoplasm/cytosol, plasma membrane, endoplasmic reticulum, Golgi apparatus, mitochondrion). In general these results are consistent with the conclusion that current database annotations of subcellular location are sparse and skewed toward single locations for proteins.

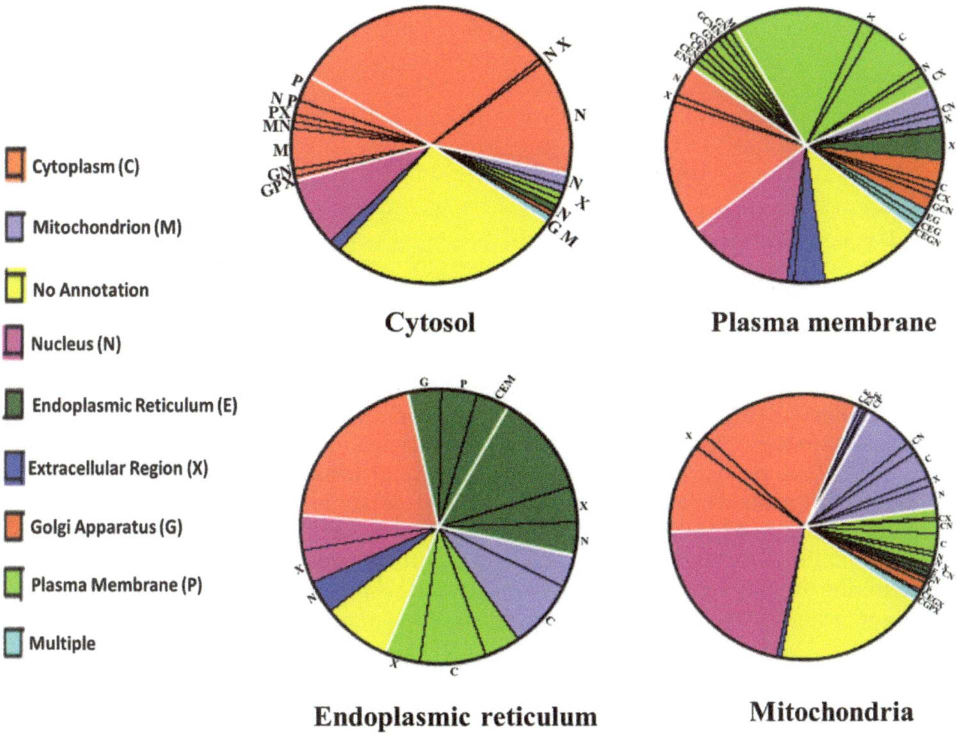

Fig. 6. Distribution of current subcellular location annotations in the UniProtKB database over the proteins observed solely in a single sucrose gradient fraction in the initial data set. The annotations are color coded (legend) according to the GO classification levels compatible with our experimental strategy (upper: extracellular region, plasma membrane, cytoplasm, nucleus; lower: cytosol/cytoplasm, endoplasmic reticulum, Golgi apparatus, mitochondrion). A small number of proteins had multiple lower level annotations and are shown in the region color coded as multiple. Proteins that had multiple annotations that included other locations different from the color code are indicated by the radial letters. The heavy white lines delineate slice regions that have different compatibility with the experimental data.

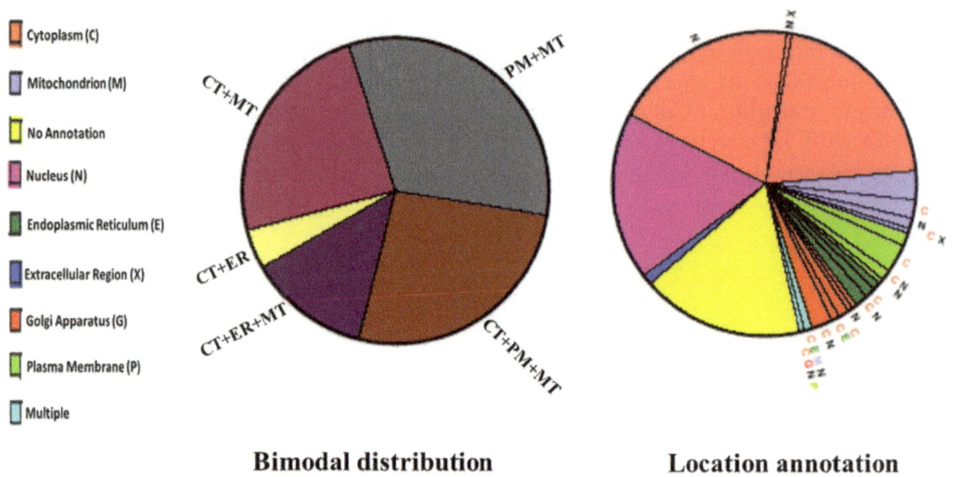

Fig. 7. Comparison of the present data on subcellular location of bimodal proteins with (merged) subcellular location annotations in the UniProtKB subcellular location comments, UniProtKB subcellular component GO terms and LOCATE Subcellular Location database. (left) Distribution of the 299 bimodal proteins in the initial data set over different combinations of sucrose gradient fractions. The indicated combinations of fractions can only arise for proteins with at least two different subcellular locations. (right) Summary of the (merged) subcellular location annotations for all 299 bimodal proteins. The annotations are color coded (legend) according to the GO classification levels compatible with our experimental strategy (upper: extracellular region, plasma membrane, cytoplasm, nucleus; lower: cytosol/cytoplasm, endoplasmic reticulum, Golgi apparatus, mitochondrion). A small number of proteins had multiple lower level annotations and are shown in the region color coded as multiple. Proteins that had multiple annotations that included other locations different from the color code are indicated by the radial letters. Slices that have color coded radial lettering are those corresponding to proteins whose annotations indicate multiple subcellular locations within the GO classification levels of our experimental design.

Over all of the 2184 proteins, the annotations at the subcellular level in the examined databases tend to be to single locations. Given that many previous proteomics studies were biased against detection of proteins in multiple locations (e.g., studies of purified organelles) and that annotations at sub-cytoplasmic levels are clearly still very sparse, we consider that the previously available annotations of experimental data are not inconsistent with the proposal that many, probably a sizable majority, of the proteins have multiple subcellular locations. Using the initial data set of (protein, fraction) pairs, there were a relatively small number of discrepancies between our data and previous annotations of subcellular location in the two databases. Of the 1441 proteins identified in fraction ER, there were a total of 33 proteins previously annotated to endoplasmic reticulum that we did not observe in fraction ER. Similarly for fractions PM (1611 proteins) and MT (1610 proteins), there were a total of 58 and 29 proteins previously annotated to plasma membrane and mitochondrion respectively that we did not observe in the corresponding gradient fraction.

Inconsistencies in the databases might contribute to the apparent discrepancies. For the 2184 proteins identified here, Figure 8 shows the status of annotations of plasma membrane (443 proteins), mitochondrion (168) and endoplasmic reticulum (243) proteins. There is rather little concordance between the annotation sets, which presumably must reflect the inclusion of very different experimental data sets.

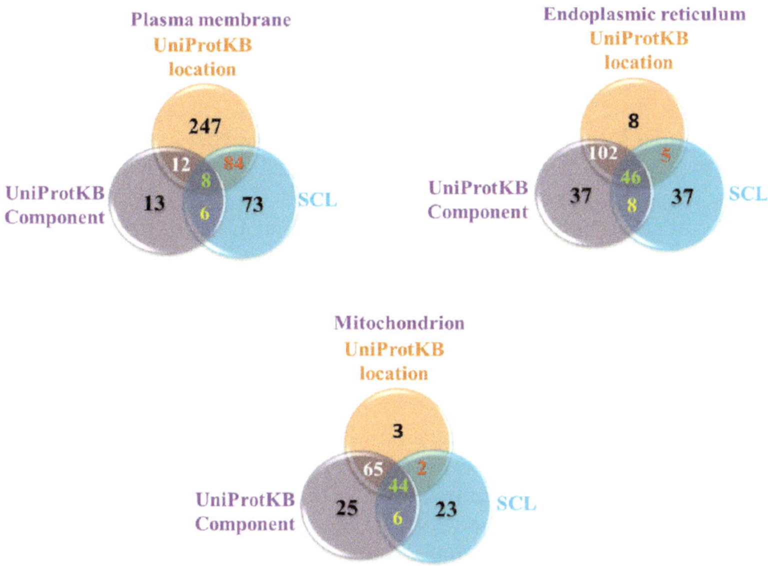

Fig. 8. Venn diagrams comparing the status of annotations of subcellular locations in the UniProtKB subcellular location components, UniProtKB cellular component GO terms and LOCATE Subcellular Location database for proteins observed in this work. 443 proteins annotated as plasma membrane. 168 proteins annotated as mitochondrion. 243 proteins annotated as endoplasmic reticulum.

Only 8 of the 443 proteins with annotations of plasma membrane were so annotated in all three data sets! For the proteins annotated to plasma membrane, endoplasmic reticulum and mitochondrion that we did not observe in the corresponding gradient fractions, our data would suggest different primary locations for these 120 proteins, but does not exclude their presence in the annotated subcellular locations as secondary locations which could not be detected at our sensitivity limits. We believe that some occurrences of apparent discrepancies are almost inevitable for three reasons. First, there is still very little information about whether subcellular distributions of proteins are the same in different cell types or under different cellular conditions. Second, many experiments do not distinguish between different isoforms of the same protein, which may have different subcellular distributions. Indeed, the present data set includes these proteins, which in part show different distributions over subcellular locations for isoforms of the same protein. This data will be analyzed in a separate paper. Third, the databases attempt to aggregate data from experimental strategies with very different sensitivity, selectivity, dynamic range, and coverage of proteins. Targeted searches for individual proteins in purified subcellular fractions with antibody methods probably have the highest sensitivity for detecting trace amounts of proteins in any specified location, even if the trace is a tiny proportion of the total protein abundance. Conversely, some high throughput methods may have limited resolution for some subcellular locations, for example, distinguishing cytosol from cytoplasm, and may have insufficient sensitivity and dynamic range to detect trace amounts of proteins in specific locations. Aggregating subcellular location information from many cell types and conditions obtained with very different experimental strategies, many of which do not distinguish protein isoforms, then becomes a very tricky task which seems likely to produce some discrepancies with any specific experimental method/data set. Although only a few of the fractions from the sucrose density gradient have been analyzed, the normal data set provides clear evidence that a minimum of 543 of the 2184 proteins (24.9%) show multiple locations. The minimum estimate is based on those proteins that are either present in all fractions or show bimodal distributions with abundance peaks in nonadjacent fractions of the sucrose gradient (Figure 3B, C). For the 321 proteins (14.7%) that were found only in adjacent fractions of the gradient (i.e., CT-PM, PM-ER, and ER-MT), the present experiments are insufficient to exclude that this might be due to the presence of a single organelle that occupies an intermediate position between the two fractions. On the other hand, we intentionally spaced the analyzed fractions widely in the sucrose gradient and for the 476 proteins (21.8%) that were found in three adjacent fractions (i.e., CT-PM-ER, or PM-ER-MT), it is improbable that these proteins have single subcellular locations. Especially since other proteins demonstrated lack of overlap (e.g., proteins in fractions CT-ER or PM-MT) and lack of tailing in the sucrose gradient (Table 2). Furthermore, in most cases the relative abundances for the proteins observed in three adjacent fractions were substantial and did not correspond to trace proportions. Thus, the normal data set provides evidence indicating that 38.6% of the proteins may have unique locations, 24.9% certainly have multiple locations, 21.8% most likely have multiple locations and 14.7% may have either unique or multiple locations. We have used the observed set of proteins to examine possible connections between subcellular location and function as related to breast cancer. Many of the proteins observed in our experiments have previously been annotated with functional information.

2.1.6 Breast cancer related proteins

Biological process annotations for 1673 proteins, molecular function annotations for 1980 proteins, Reactome Pathway annotations for 176 proteins and posttranslational modification annotations for 1653 proteins were available in the UniProtKB database. We used the BioBase Biological Databases, BIOBASE Knowledge Library (BKL) and ExPlainTM 2.3 platform to identify 94 proteins in our data set that are known or suspected to be implicated in breast cancer via disease molecular mechanism, diagnostic marker and therapeutic target association. These proteins were examined for common Gene Ontology (http://www.geneontology.org) biological process and molecular function terms and for common Reactome Pathway (http://www.reactome.org) terms, which were then used as lures to obtain the set of proteins identified in this study that share the same terms. A majority of the proteins implicated in breast cancer were related to five high level cellular processes that involved a subset of 519 proteins observed in our experiments: apoptosis (68 proteins), cell growth (127), signaling (131), cell interaction (62), and protein processing (230). 93 proteins were involved in more than one of the five processes. Figure 9 shows how the proteins associated with each cellular process are distributed over the subcellular locations using the initial data set. The striking features are that each process is distributed over all four locations, as might be anticipated for regulated processes, and that for all of the cellular processes there is an appreciable majority of proteins with 3-4 subcellular locations (ranging from 54.8% for cell interaction to 66.5% for protein processing). Furthermore, the latter characteristic was most pronounced for the 93 proteins that were involved in more than one of the high level cellular processes (68.8%)

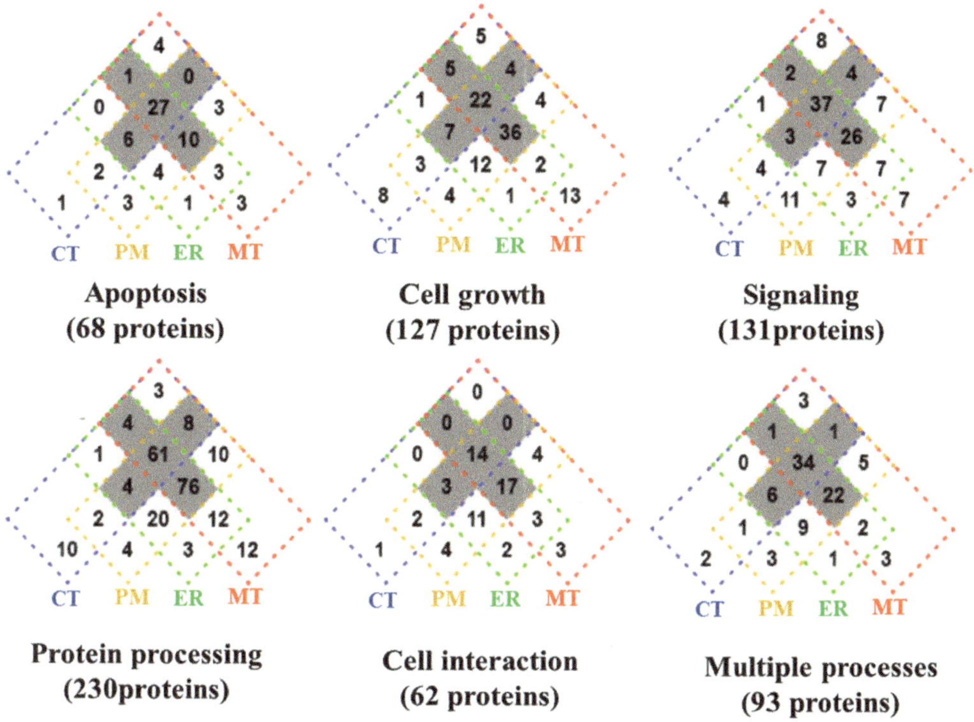

Fig. 9. Four-way Venn diagrams summarizing the distribution of the breast-cancer-related set of 519 proteins over the subcellular locations for the cellular processes: signaling (131 proteins), cell growth (127), protein processing (230), apoptosis (68 proteins), and cell interaction (62), as well as for proteins involved in more than one of these cellular processes (93). The shaded regions of the diagrams correspond to proteins with 3 or 4 locations.

3. Conclusion

Large scale and quantitative proteomics analysis of subcellular organelles revealed 268 nuclear proteins and 22 extracellular region proteins that were found in various sucrose gradient fractions, but which had previously only been annotated experimentally to the nucleus and extracellular region respectively. Another 271 proteins that we detected had no prior annotation at either the upper level (cytoplasm, plasma membrane) or lower level (cytosol, endoplasmic reticulum, mitochondria) of our experimental strategy. The present experiments were not designed to obtain specific annotations at the lower level, e.g. to mitochondrion. Hence, observation of a protein in a Fraction MT that is enriched in mitochondrial proteins should presently only be taken as an indication and not as proof of its presence in mitochondria. Nonetheless, the present experiments gave several hundred new location annotations at the level (plasma membrane, cytoplasm). There are several ways the limits on MS detection sensitivity may influence the number of locations in which the proteins were observed. In particular, for the highest abundance proteins, the sensitivity and dynamic range of the MS spectral counting methods are such that trace amounts as small as about 0.2% of a protein in a secondary location could be detected. As shown above for the normal data set, trace amounts of abundant proteins in secondary locations do not strongly influence estimates of the proportion of proteins with multiple subcellular locations. Conversely, the proportion of a protein which must be present in a secondary location to be detectable increases as the overall abundance of the proteins decreases, for example, for the lowest abundance proteins, only the highest abundance, primary location falls within the detection limits of the MS methods. Furthermore, for lower abundance proteins or for trace proportions of proteins in specific fractions, the sampling constraints on spectral counting that result from MS/MS sequencing of only the more abundant peptides means that only one peptide may be counted in some fractions. For example, there were 847 (38.8%) proteins classified as "unique" (observed in a single fraction) in the normal data set, but only 481 (22.0%) in the initial data set. This difference corresponds to proteins in various gradient fractions that were only counted with a single peptide and 1 or 2 spectral counts. This means that estimations of multiple locations based on the normal data set are very conservative and certainly underestimate, probably strongly, the proportion of proteins with multiple subcellular locations. Given that estimates based on the normal data set provide evidence for multiple locations of at least 46.7% of the observed proteins, we conclude that a substantial majority of the proteins observed have multiple subcellular locations. Given that only 22% of proteins were seen solely in a single fraction in the initial data set, perhaps as much as 75% of the proteins have multiple locations. We noted above that 120 proteins had annotations to subcellular locations that we did not observe in the corresponding sucrose gradient fractions (33 to endoplasmic reticulum, 58 to plasma membrane and 29 to mitochondrion). We suggested that these discrepancies were not inconsistent with our data if the annotations corresponded to secondary locations. On the basis of the observed spectral counts, there are 39 of these proteins for which our data suggest that the previous annotations correspond to proteins with functional significance in a secondary location, but that >80% of the protein is in a different primary location. This kind of analysis can be extended to many other proteins where the functional activity and the measured mole fractions indicate functional roles at secondary locations. Indeed, some of the proteins that we detected at trace amounts (<3%) in secondary locations already have known functions at those locations. The present experiments thus indicate numerous proteins with primary locations which probably differ from current function/location annotations and for which confirmation of the primary location (and potentially of other functional activities) might be profitably sought. The present experiments suggest 1383 (protein, location, function) data points for 519 proteins involved in five major cellular functional processes for which investigation of functional roles might further elucidate mechanisms involved in breast cancer. This is a very promising situation for experiments aimed at investigating dynamic changes in the spatio/temporal location/form of proteins in breast cancer cells, their potential roles in regulation and their potential importance in breast cancer disease. Finally, in summary, we have found evidence that strongly suggests a majority of the detected proteins have multiple subcellular locations in the breast cancer model MCF-7 cells, that even with a fairly simple experiment a wealth of new annotation data can be obtained, that available evidence suggests that for many proteins distribution over multiple subcellular locations can be important to their functional roles, and that large numbers of (protein, location) pairs deserving of further investigation of functional/regulatory roles can be delineated. We are still very far from having good static descriptions of the spatial distributions of cellular proteins, let alone dynamic information on relationships between spatio/temporal distribution and function. However, high-throughput proteomics in combination with other experimental methods seems to offer ways forward.

4. Acknowledgment

We would like to thank Professor Samia M. A. Al-Amoudi (King Abdulaziz University, Jeddah, SA) for generous help and discussions and to the Wellcome Trust, UK, King Faisal Foundation, Riyadh, SA, Sheikh Mohammed Hussien Al-Amoudi Centre Scientific Chair for Breast Cancer Researches, Jeddah, SA, Susan G. Komen for the Cure Breast Cancer Foundation, USA, King Faisal Specialist Hospital and Research Center, Riyadh, SA for their continuous support.

5. References

http://www.ncbi.nlm.nih.gov

Au, C. E., A. W. Bell, A. Gilchrist, J. Hiding, T. Nilsson & J. J. Bergeron (2007) Organellar proteomics to create the cell map. *Curr Opin Cell Biol,* 19, 376-85.

Cheyne, W. W. (1894) An Address on the Treatment of Cancer of the Breast: Delivered before the Harveian Society of London. *Br Med J,* 1, 289-91.

Dunkley, T. P., R. Watson, J. L. Griffin, P. Dupree & K. S. Lilley (2004) Localization of organelle proteins by isotope tagging (LOPIT). *Mol Cell Proteomics,* 3, 1128-34.

Foster, L. J., C. L. de Hoog, Y. Zhang, X. Xie, V. K. Mootha & M. Mann (2006) A mammalian organelle map by protein correlation profiling. *Cell,* 125, 187-99.

Godovac-Zimmermann, J., O. Kleiner, L. R. Brown & A. K. Drukier (2005) Perspectives in spicing up proteomics with splicing. *Proteomics,* 5, 699-709.

Gygi, S. P., Y. Rochon, B. R. Franza & R. Aebersold (1999) Correlation between protein and mRNA abundance in yeast. *Mol Cell Biol,* 19, 1720-30.

Hanahan, D. & R. A. Weinberg (2000) The hallmarks of cancer. *Cell,* 100, 57-70.

Hanahan, D. & R. A. Weinberg (2011) Hallmarks of cancer: the next generation. *Cell,* 144, 646-74.

Imyanitov, E. & K. Hanson (2004) Mechanisms of breast cancer. *Drug Discovery Today: Disease Mechanisms,* 1, 235-245.

Ince, T. A. & R. A. Weinberg (2002) Functional genomics and the breast cancer problem. *Cancer Cell,* 1, 15-7.

Lacroix, M. & G. Leclercq (2004) Relevance of breast cancer cell lines as models for breast tumours: an update. *Breast Cancer Res Treat,* 83, 249-89.

Mukherjee, S. 2011. *The Emperor of All Maladies: A Biography of Cancer.* UK: Fourth Estate Ltd.

Qattan, A. T., C. Mulvey, M. Crawford, D. A. Natale & J. Godovac-Zimmermann (2010) Quantitative organelle proteomics of MCF-7 breast cancer cells reveals multiple subcellular locations for proteins in cellular functional processes. *J Proteome Res,* 9, 495-508.

Roberts, G. C. & C. W. Smith (2002) Alternative splicing: combinatorial output from the genome. *Curr Opin Chem Biol,* 6, 375-83.

Rogers, L. D. & L. J. Foster (2007) The dynamic phagosomal proteome and the contribution of the endoplasmic reticulum. *Proc Natl Acad Sci U S A,* 104, 18520-5.

Sebastian, T. & P. F. Johnson (2006) Stop and go: anti-proliferative and mitogenic functions of the transcription factor C/EBPbeta. *Cell Cycle,* 5, 953-7.

Simpson, J. C. & R. Pepperkok (2006) The subcellular localization of the mammalian proteome comes a fraction closer. *Genome Biol,* 7, 222.

Sorlie, T., C. M. Perou, R. Tibshirani, T. Aas, S. Geisler, H. Johnsen, T. Hastie, M. B. Eisen, M. van de Rijn, S. S. Jeffrey, T. Thorsen, H. Quist, J. C. Matese, P. O. Brown, D. Botstein, P. Eystein Lonning & A. L. Borresen-Dale (2001) Gene expression patterns of breast carcinomas distinguish tumor subclasses with clinical implications. *Proc Natl Acad Sci U S A,* 98, 10869-74.

Soule, H. D., J. Vazguez, A. Long, S. Albert & M. Brennan (1973) A human cell line from a pleural effusion derived from a breast carcinoma. *J Natl Cancer Inst,* 51, 1409-16.

Usaite, R., J. Wohlschlegel, J. D. Venable, S. K. Park, J. Nielsen, L. Olsson & J. R. Yates Iii (2008) Characterization of global yeast quantitative proteome data generated from the wild-type and glucose repression saccharomyces cerevisiae strains: the comparison of two quantitative methods. *J Proteome Res,* 7, 266-75.

van de Vijver, M. J., Y. D. He, L. J. van't Veer, H. Dai, A. A. Hart, D. W. Voskuil, G. J. Schreiber, J. L. Peterse, C. Roberts, M. J. Marton, M. Parrish, D. Atsma, A. Witteveen, A. Glas, L. Delahaye, T. van der Velde, H. Bartelink, S. Rodenhuis, E. T. Rutgers, S. H. Friend & R. Bernards (2002) A gene-expression signature as a predictor of survival in breast cancer. *N Engl J Med,* 347, 1999-2009.

Xu, P., M. Crawford, M. Way, J. Godovac-Zimmermann, A. W. Segal & M. Radulovic (2009) Subproteome analysis of the neutrophil cytoskeleton. *Proteomics,* 9, 2037-49.

Yates, J. R., 3rd, A. Gilchrist, K. E. Howell & J. J. Bergeron (2005) Proteomics of organelles and large cellular structures. *Nat Rev Mol Cell Biol,* 6, 702-14.

Part 3

Diagnosis and Imaging

12

Diagnostic Optical Imaging of Breast Cancer: From Animal Models to First-in-Men Studies

Michel Eisenblätter[1], Thorsten Persigehl[1],
Christoph Bremer[2] and Carsten Höltke[1]
[1]*Dept. of Clinical Radiology, University Hospital Münster*
[2]*Dept. of Radiology, St. Franziskus Hospital Münster*
Germany

1. Introduction

The use of light-driven imaging techniques for the diagnosis of breast cancer dates back to as early as 1929. Transillumination was evaluated for potential differentiation of breast lesions, e.g. to distinguish benign cysts from solid tumours. Cutler summed the technique to be "...a simple procedure and a valuable aid in the interpretation of pathological conditions in the mammary gland. Its use is recommended in the routine examination of the breast..."(Cutler, 1929, 1931).

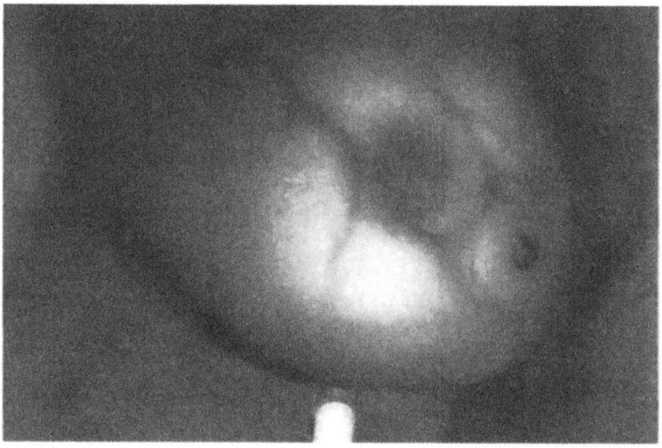

Fig. 1. Opacity on transillumination of a solid tumour in the breast (Cutler, 1931, reproduced with permission from Wolters & Kluwer).

At the same time, x-ray mammography emerged, routinely used for detection and diagnosis of breast cancer from the 1950s (Leborgne, 1951). Only relatively low sensitivity and specificity of mammography findings in combination with significant x-ray exposure though always triggered the parallel search for alternative diagnostic approaches. Over the following years, the use of near infrared (NIR) light was discussed to further facilitate transillumination of breast tissue (Watmough, 1982a; Watmough, 1982b). Its unique characteristics regarding interaction with tissue - low absorption and reduced scattering – enable NIR light to travel through tissue and thus to reach deep tissue sections, therefore defining a valuable tool in diagnostic optical imaging (OI) techniques (Weissleder & Ntziachristos, 2003). Originating from transillumination, diffuse optical tomography (DOT) was initially thought to be capable of identifying tumour formation in anatomical regions accessible to NIR light, as tumour tissue is characterized by distinct optical properties, based on altered tissue architecture, blood flow and oxygen consumption. However, the limitations of this technique, especially the limited spatial resolution, have been illustrated in several publications. Although the advances on the field of instrumentation were significant, first clinical studies in breast cancer patients proved discriminating lesions regarding their malignant potential reflected by their absorption characteristics still to be challenging (Boas, 1997). To further improve the specificity of OI, fluorescence contrast agents, fluorophores operating in the NIR range of the spectrum, have been used. Three different types of optical probes are currently available for clinical or preclinical (basic research) purposes - unspecific, specific and so-called smart probes. The only clinically approved fluorochrome, indocyanine green (ICG) is an unspecific, perfusion-type contrast agent. First promising results of ICG-driven DOT for detection and differentiation of breast lesions have recently been published, confirming sensitivity and specificity (Ntziachristos et al., 2000). So far restricted to preclinical use only, specifically binding optical contrast agents, targeted on key-structures of cancer cells, allow for disease specific imaging and *in vivo* characterization of lesions down to the molecular level. As state of the art anatomical imaging frequently fails in detecting early effects of modern anti-tumour therapy, contrast agents targeted to different tumour cell epitopes have been described and used to sensitively detect the molecular characteristics of malignant lesions and their alteration under therapy (Achilefu, 2004; Achilefu et al., 2000; Becker et al., 2001). So called smart probes even increase sensitivity and specificity of OI. Fluorescence characteristics of these probes change upon interaction with specific target structures, e.g. proteinases, therefore allowing detection of vital, invasive tumour lesions with unrivalled sensitivity (Bremer et al., 2001c; Bremer et al., 2002). This review gives an overview about the approaches, recently made on the field of optical tracer development and evaluation with a focus on targets relevant for breast cancer diagnosis and characterization. Especially the visualization of angiogenesis as a key process in tumour progression is emphasized. Many factors that are involved in angiogenic events have been evaluated over the last decades and are now well understood. Several growth factors, their receptors and diverse pathways triggering their expression, are crucially involved in cancer progression and metastasis. Moreover some proteinases, especially matrix metalloproteinases (MMPs) and cathepsins, proved to contribute to tumour growth by e.g. degradation of extracellular matrix (ECM) components. Clinical translation of the efforts made in the past recent years will be the main challenge for researchers active on the molecular imaging field.

2. Instrumentation

Technically, optical imaging is based on the detection of light and the visualization of photon distribution in tissue. While visible light (380-700 nm) is almost completely absorbed, scattered and reflected in the uppermost sections of tissue already, light of the NIR range of the spectrum can be facilitated for *in vivo* imaging approaches. Light of around

650 - 950 nm is absorbed to a much lesser extent than light of lower wavelengths and can thus be detected in deeper tissue sections (Ntziachristos et al., 2003). Moreover, autofluorescence of tissue is minimal in this so called optical window (Fig. 2), resulting in a higher signal-to-background ratio for near infrared images (Bremer et al., 2001b).

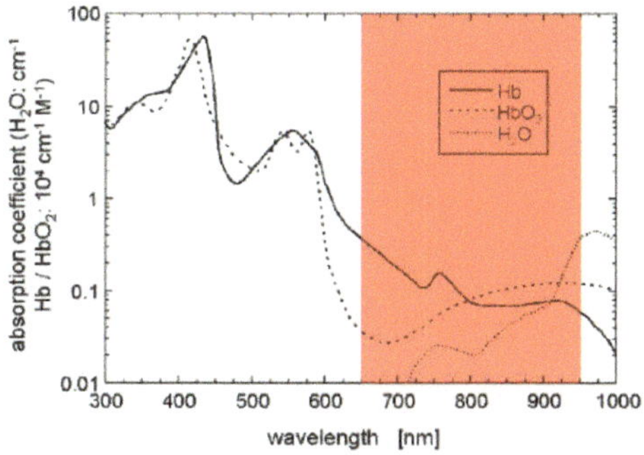

Fig. 2. The optical window between 650 and 950 nm, where absorption by water haemoglobin and deoxyhaemoglobin is minimal.

For non-enhanced optical imaging approaches, simple opposed lightsource detector pairs are used. Light is applied to the scan volume at a distinct place and the detector is used to collect the non-absorbed photons. Highly absorbing lesions (e.g. tumour lesions) are supposed to delineate as negative contrast. Diffuse optical tomography (DOT) is based on the same principle, creating 3D absorption maps from e.g. the female breast (Ntziachristos et al., 2000; O'Leary et al., 1995). Commercially available optical imaging devices use adapted light for dye excitation; in experimental settings ultrasound was alternatively used successfully for the excitation of fluorophores (Razansky et al., 2008; Yuan & Liu, 2010). Fluorescence-producing proteins, encoded by so-called imaging target genes can either be light-excitable or metabolism-dependent, producing fluorescence upon interaction with exogenous substrates (Chudakov et al., 2010; Lukyanov et al., 2010). All dyes regularly used for targeted *in vivo* imaging require excitation with light of distinct wavelength to produce a specific emission. An imaging unit therefore always consists of an excitation light source on the one hand and a signal recording camera on the other (Fig. 3). The animal is placed either between both for optical tomography (Fluorescence Mediated Tomography - FMT) or on the ground of an imaging chamber with light source and camera both on one side (Fluorescence Reflectance Imaging - FRI) (Mahmood et al., 1999; Weissleder et al., 1999). Reflectance imaging approaches in this context basically resemble traditional photography, allowing for acquisition of 2D image data at video rate with highly sensitive CCD cameras. Regularly, cameras are adapted with filter sets for each particular wavelength, virtually blocking diffuse background fluorescence. The image acquisition is preceded by illumination of the whole field of view with either light of distinctive wavelengths - adapted for the applied dye - or unfiltered, multi-wavelength light (Graves et al., 2004). The latter of course results in excitation not only of the applied dye but of virtually all substances capable of producing fluorescence. This circumstance contributes to the background signal and thus requires more sophisticated filter equipment at the signal recording side. Further increase of signal-specificity can be achieved by using excitation light of discrete wavelengths, using e.g. filters or even more precisely laser-light. The main disadvantage of such laser-light equipped units is the reduced flexibility, as upgrading the system for detection of a new spectrum of dyes with different spectral characteristics would always require a new laser-light source, which is usually much more expensive than a new set of filters for multi-wavelength excitation devices. State of the art FRI systems frequently allow for fusion of fluorescence images with white-light and x-ray images.

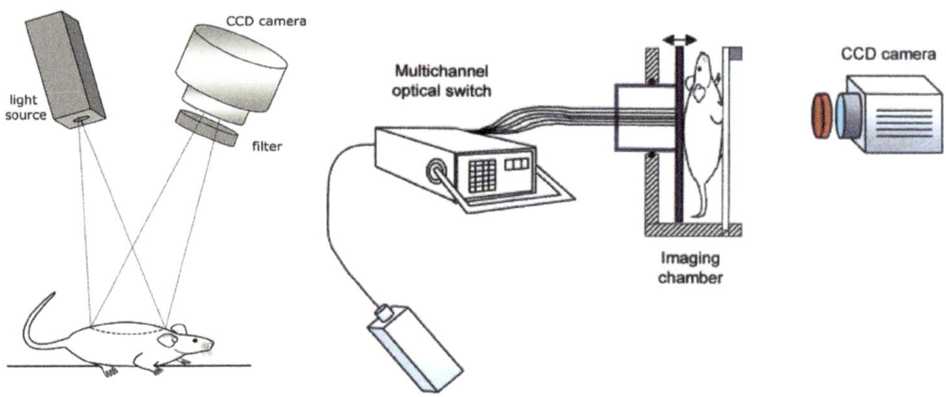

Fig. 3. Left: Typical FRI system for *in vivo* animal investigations. The illumination source and CCD camera are on the same side of the animal. Right: Example of an FMT scanner. The scanner uses multiple light sources and detectors to effectively collect light at multiple projections around the animal's body (from Graves et al., 2004; Ntziachristos et al., 2003; reproduced with permission).

Anatomical correlation of FRI results, though, is limited due to the basic imaging principle. Absorption and scattering of light in tissue hamper detection and correct visualization especially of such signals originating from deeper regions of the scan volume which may thus not be properly reflected by the signals obtained at the scan volume surface (Montet et al., 2005). Multi-angle imaging is frequently regarded as one possible solution for this general FRI limitation. First approaches on this field are promising regarding the propriety of signal-to-source correlation, but are still in a prototype stage. Moreover, multi-angle optical imaging does still not offer anatomical co-information and thus lacks the possibility to correct fluorescence signals for scattering and absorption yet. In first studies, combination of optical tomography and x-ray based computed tomography (CT) is used to overcome this limitation. CT is used to acquire anatomical information and thus to depict optical properties of tissue for more precise prediction of the origin of detected photons (Guo X. et al., 2010b; Nahrendorf et al., 2009). Commercially available FMT systems aim to solve this problem without additional anatomical data acquired by CT or MRI. A 2D scan matrix is excited point by point with dye-adapted laser-light while the resulting fluorescence signals are recorded on the other side of the animal. In a first step, the resulting fluorescence signals are used to calculate a scattering map of the scan volume. In a second step, the specific dye-associated signals are recorded and a 3D dataset is calculated on the basis of the scattering map and presumptions about the optical properties of the examined tissue (Stasic et al., 2003). The mathematical algorithm underlying this reconstruction of a 3D dataset from a matrix of 2D data is based on the Born approximation to solve the wave equation (Vinegoni et al., 2009). The approach has been validated, using surgical implants of known concentrations of fluorescent dyes implanted into animals at defined points (Ntziachristos et al., 2002). The presumptions on optical properties of the heterogeneous tissue on the track of a single photon, though, can only be approximations and may cause inaccurate results in individual cases. Combination with established cross-sectional imaging for the creation of fusion images is on the way and may help to correct for those adverse results. Additionally, anatomical co-information will simplify interpretation of fluorescence signals, especially in complex models of disease.

The more modern translation into patient diagnosis started with the development of the first clinical optical breast imaging systems. Companies and academia put a lot of effort in this task, and in addition to several prototype instruments, three systems are commercially available at the moment. The Computed Tomography Laser Mammography system CTLM®, developed by Imaging Diagnostic Systems Inc., is a fully tomographic system and generates volumetric images of the breast (http://www.imds.com/ctlm/). Poellinger (Poellinger et al., 2008) and Floery (Floery et al., 2005) have used the system for small study groups and concluded that CTLM could be used for the delineation of malignant tissue but should be seen as an adjunct to conventional mammography only. The ComfortScan® system, distributed by Danum International Ltd., is a transillumination system that requires breast compression to generate 2D-images (http://www.danum.com/comfortscan.html). Fournier and colleagues concluded that the system had the potential to distinguish benign from malignant lesions but were not certain about specificity of findings and finally assumed a higher number of false positive results compared to conventional mammography (Fournier et al., 2009). The SoftScan® system by Advanced Research Technologies Inc., is a system that requires slight breast compression but is able to generate tomographic images of the breast (http://www.art.ca/en/clinical/). Using this system, van de Ven performed a phantom study, testing contrast agents of different intensity. It was concluded that the use of such contrast agents, at best in addition to a targeting ligand, would have a great potential in future optical breast cancer diagnosis (van de Ven et al., 2011). Detectors for fluorescence signals can also be minimized and e.g. integrated in endoscopic devices. Jaffer in this context reported the use of intravascular NIRF imaging in murine models of atherosclerosis (Jaffer et al., 2008; Jaffer et al., 2009).

3. Optical imaging of tissue perfusion

Due to the fact that oxy- and deoxyhaemoglobin are mainly responsible for absorption of NIR light in tissue, non-enhanced OI, e.g. transillumination, has been explored for detection of breast cancer, reflected by elevated tissue perfusion (Hawrysz & Sevick-Muraca, 2000). In 1931 already, Cutler described that naive transillumination diaphanography could help to identify breast cancer (Cutler, 1931). Decades later, DOT allowed for 3-D determination of scattering and absorption properties of tissue or turbid material, respectively. Both approaches nevertheless fail to provide sufficient physiological information for safe delineation of malignant lesions. And so, low specificity of imaging findings and reduced sensitivity for lesions in deeper tissue regions always promoted efforts to develop optical contrast agents. Proof-of-concept DOT mammography experiments employing ICG as a contrast-enhancing agent successfully showed that breast lesions could be delineated from healthy tissue, although the poor water-solubility and the resulting rapid liver-uptake hampers the use of ICG in routine breast cancer imaging (Ntziachristos et al., 2000; Riefke et al., 1997). Other carbocyanine-based dyes with a more hydrophilic character were designed and employed in imaging experiments, as well. Especially SIDAG (1,1'-bis-(4-sulfobutyl)indotricarbo-cyanine-5,5'-dicarboxylic acid diglucamide monosodium; Global Drug Discovery, Bayer Schering Pharma AG, Berlin, Germany) shows improved photophysiological and pharmacological characteristics. This dye was developed by Licha and co-workers in the mid-nineties (Licha et al., 1996, 2000; Riefke et al., 1997) and showed good target-to-background contrast in a number of different murine xenograft models (Fig. 4), including breast cancer. A correlation of SIDAG-signal intensity to the vascular volume fraction of the tumour as an MRI-based parameter of angiogenic potential could be shown (Wall et al., 2008).

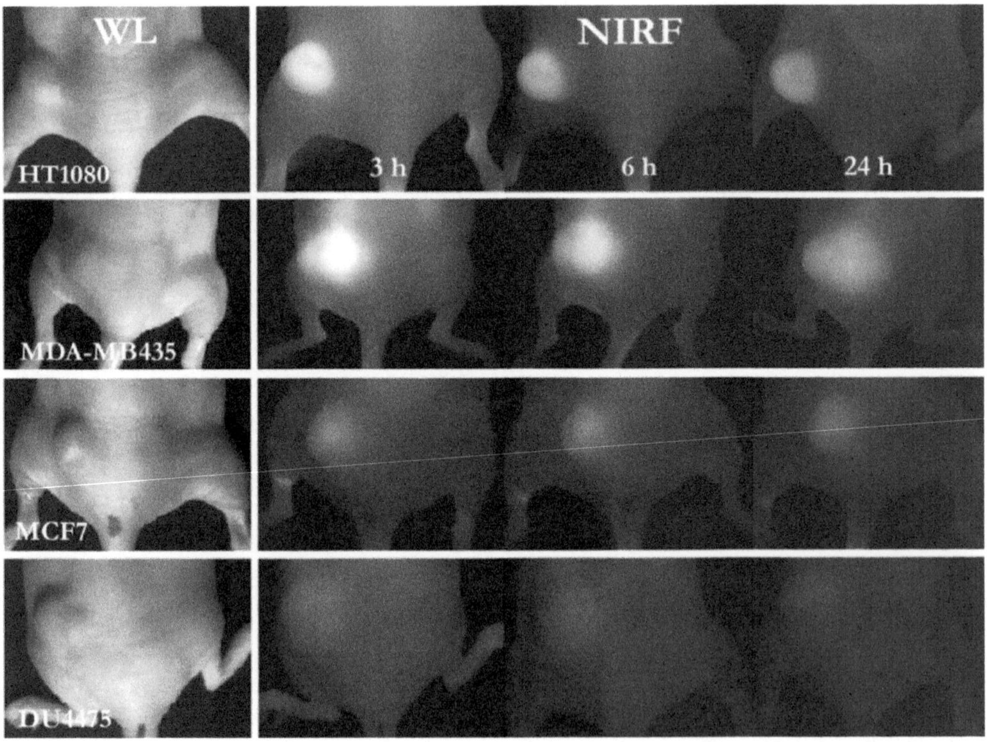

Fig. 4. Comparison of perfusion-type fluorescent dye SIDAG application to differently vascularized tumours. White light images of different tumour xenografts (left row), followed by FRI images taken sequentially after application of 2 μmol/kg body weight SIDAG. There is a strong fluorescence signal in HT-1080 fibrosarcomas and in MDA-MB 435 tumours, whereas MCF-7 and DU-4475 adenocarcinomas exhibit only moderate tumour fluorescence (modified from Wall et al., 2008, courtesy of the author).

Van de Ven et al. evaluated contrast-enhanced DOT, using Omocianine (Bayer Schering Pharma, Berlin, Germany), a novel fluorescent contrast agent, in a first clinical trial of 12 patients suffering from BI-RADS 4–5 breast lesions, using MRI as reference modality and a Philips prototype DOT scanner. They observed dose-dependent enhancement in malignant lesions. The fluorophore allowed for a reliable detection of malignant lesions in the breast (Fig. 5). Limitations of this approach comprised the visualization of lesions close to the chest wall as well as the absence of clear anatomical landmarks for lesion localization (van de Ven et al., 2009, 2010). Just recently, Poellinger et al. in a larger study examined 52 patients with 53 suspicious breast lesions (BI-RADS 4–5) by using the CTLM® system. In this placebo-controlled, dose-escalating trial a detection rate of up to 100% (7 of 7 lesions) after injection of 0.1 mg/kg Omocianine has been reported (Poellinger et al, 2011). Overall, higher detection rates were achieved for larger lesions, at smaller breast sizes, and for cases in which the tumour was located closer to the skin. However, there were also limitations in this study including detection of additional lesions or reconstruction artefacts.

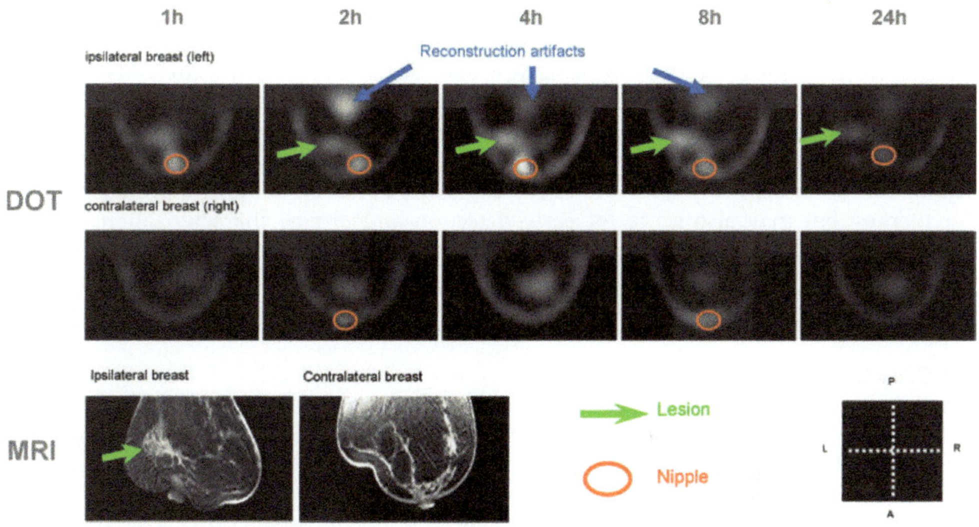

Fig. 5. Contrast-enhanced DOT of the breast: Omocianine-enhanced DOT of a patient with invasive lobular carcinoma in the left breast (first row) with visible contrast agent accumulation in the region of the tumour. The contralateral breast (second row) showed no suspicious contrast enhancement. MRI corroborated the optically detected breast cancer lesions (bottom row) (van de Ven et al., 2010; reproduced with permission from Springer).

In summary, perfusion-type fluorescence contrast agents like ICG, SIDAG or Omocianine (Fig. 6) facilitate a higher target-to-non-target contrast than simple transillumination techniques or non-enhanced DOT. Assuming a linear correlation of signal intensity and local tissue perfusion, contrast enhanced OI could provide quantitative data of tumour vascularization. The future use of these types of contrast agents and imaging procedures in clinical routine, either as an adjunct to or a replacement for x-ray mammography, strongly depends on legal approval and further refinement of this imaging technology.

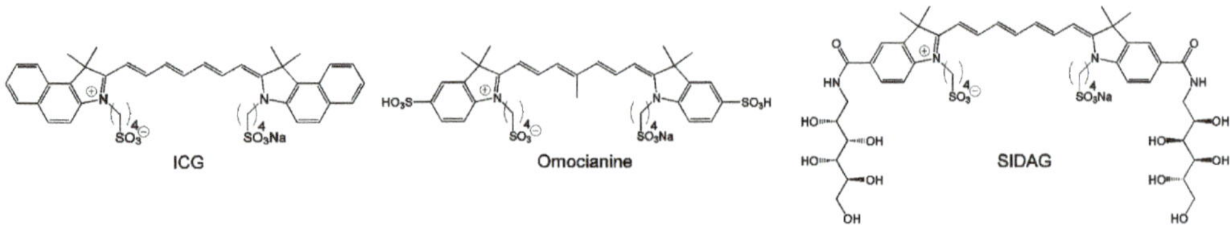

Fig. 6. Molecular structures of ICG, Omocianine and SIDAG.

4. Molecular targets

Breast cancer (BC) is a heterogeneous class of disease, exhibiting a variety of phenotypes and molecular profiles. For selection of the most promising therapy with regard to the molecular profile of a cancer lesion, immunohistochemistry of e.g. biopsies is performed. In this context, identification of e.g. hormone receptor positive (estrogene, ER+, progesterone PR+) or human epidermal growth factor receptor 2 positive (HER-2+) cancers for receptor antagonist driven therapy is frequently possible. Antibody based therapy is routinely combined with classical chemotherapy after surgery for therapy of ER+ and HER-2+ tumours, significantly contributing to therapy success (Alvarez & Price, 2010; Alvarez et al., 2010; Giovannini et al., 2010; Johnson & Brown, 2010; Parker & Sukumar, 2003; Rose & Siegel, 2010). Cancers devoid of the mentioned receptors, so-called triple negative breast cancers (TNBCs), therefore show a relatively poor prognosis due to reduced therapy options (De Laurentiis et al., 2010). Cell surface receptors are, however, not only a promising target for therapy but may also serve for early detection and *in vivo* characterization of breast cancer. Especially growth factors and their receptors, hormone receptors, proteases and integrines have been addressed as targets for diagnostic *in vivo* imaging. This article will give an exemplary overview of successfully performed molecular imaging approaches.

4.1 Growth factors and their receptors

Many cancer cell lines have been shown to produce different types of growth factors, promoting tumour growth and survival. The most prominent of these growth factors is the vascular endothelial growth factor (VEGF). A number of seven different growth factors of this family have been recognized, of which five have been found in human, including placenta growth factor (PlGF), which is responsible for angionenic processes during the menstrual cycle (Fig. 7).

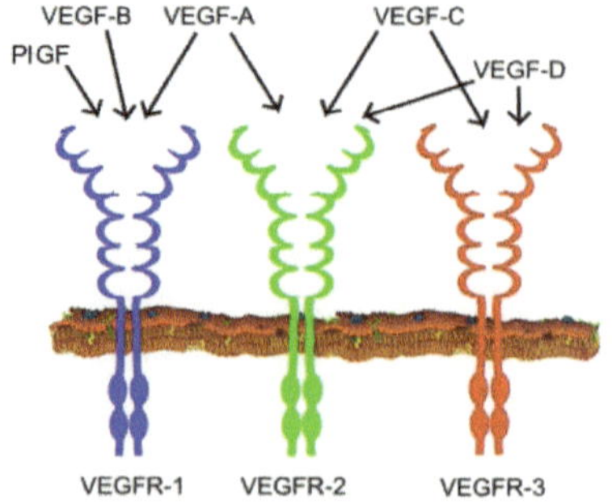

Fig. 7. Human VEGFs and their receptors.

Under physiological conditions, VEGF promotes angiogenesis and vasculogenesis in e.g. wound healing or muscle growth. VEGF expression is to a considerable extent induced by low oxygen supply. Hypoxia inducible factors (HIF-1α and -2α) are the main determinants in this context, inducing VEGF mRNA transcription. Other elements enhancing VEGF expression are intracellular adenosine, interleukin-6 (IL-6) and transforming growth factor β (TGF-β). Signalling of VEGF is mediated by binding of these peptides to three closely related tyrosine kinase (TK) cell surface receptors (VEGFR-1, -2 and -3) which dimerize upon activation and induce endothelial cell (EC) proliferation, vascular remodelling and neovascularization (De Laurentiis et al., 2010; Gasparini, 2000; Giovannini et al., 2010; Guo S. et al., 2010a; Hasan & Jayson, 2001; Hendrix et al., 2000; Hicklin & Ellis, 2005). In patients, elevated expression of VEGF and/or its receptors is often associated with reduced event-free or overall survival. Therefore anti-angiogenic therapy approaches targeting the VEGF system have been developed and tested in first clinical trials. The VEGF system can also be employed for the *in vivo* determination of receptor expression profiles of tumours in preclinical settings. In 2007 Backer et al. facilitated the use of a recombinant single chain protein construct (scVEGF) to image VEGFR expression *in vivo* by OI in combination with single photon emission computed tomography (SPECT) and positron emission tomography (PET). The Cy 5.5 labelled probe (scVEGF/Cy) was used to image human breast cancer cell line MDA-MB 231 and murine mammary tumour cell line 4T1, both transfected for luciferase expression for bioluminescence imaging (BLI), in nude mice. The tracer was shown to bind to tumour vasculature, even in barely palpable lesions, indicating an early influence of the VEGF system in the process of tumour progression. In both tumour models, Cy 5.5 fluorescence could be co-localized with immunofluorescence staining of VEGF receptors and CD31 (Fig. 8) (Backer et al., 2007).

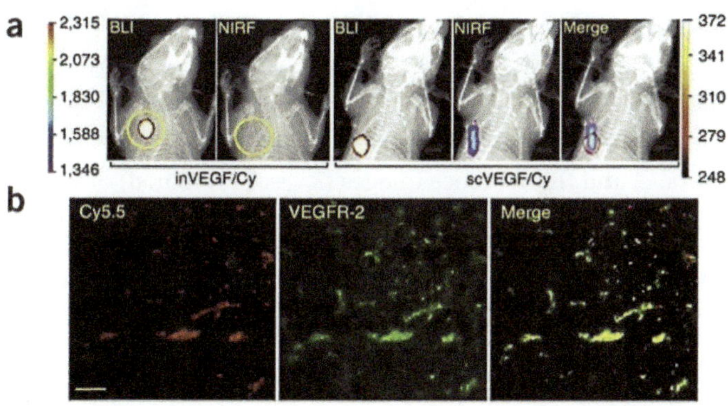

Fig. 8. NIRF imaging with scVEGF/Cy and localization of Cy5.5 on histological sections. (**a**) NIRF imaging and BLI of 4T1luc-tumour-bearing mouse injected intravenously with scVEGF/Cy or inactive control peptide inVEGF/Cy. (**b**) Co-localization of Cy5.5 fluorescence and immunofluorescence staining for VEGFR-2 on 4T1luc tumour cryosections indicates the potency of the CY 5.5 labelled protein conjugate scVEGF/Cy for *in vivo* imaging of VEGF receptors. (Reproduced from Backer et al., 2007 with permission from Nature Publishing Group).

Although the tracer showed a highly heterogeneous accumulation and retention, specific binding and consecutive internalization of the scVEGF-based agent by VEGF receptors in the tumour area was assumed. Generally, it is recognized that the *in vivo* imaging of VEGF receptors will facilitate assessment of angiogenesis-related parameters for personalized treatment in the future. In another approach, the anti-VEGF monoclonal antibody bevacizumab (Avastin®), a therapeutic against diverse metastatic cancers used in the US since 2004, was labelled with a fluorescent dye and explored for the *in vivo* imaging of VEGF. The scintigraphic imaging of VEGF receptors employing ^{111}In- and ^{89}Zr-labelled bevacizumab conjugates is also discussed as a rapid technique to follow therapy response with SPECT and PET (Nagengast et al., 2007).

Epidermal growth factor receptors (EGFRs) are closely related to VEGF-Rs, sharing their tyrosine kinase activity and their frequent presence on the cell surface of tumours, also promoting proliferation and cell-survival. Trastuzumab (Herceptin®) is a monoclonal antibody against human epidermal growth factor receptor 2 (HER-2). In 2004, fluorescently labelled Herceptin® has been used for the stratification of tumour lesions with regard to HER-2-expression. *In vivo* signals after application of the probe reflected the strong or moderate level of HER-2-expression of human breast cancer cell line SK-BR-3 (high HER-2-expression) or human squamous cell carcinoma cell line PE/CA-PJ34 (mild HER-2-expression) (Fig. 9, Hilger et al., 2004).

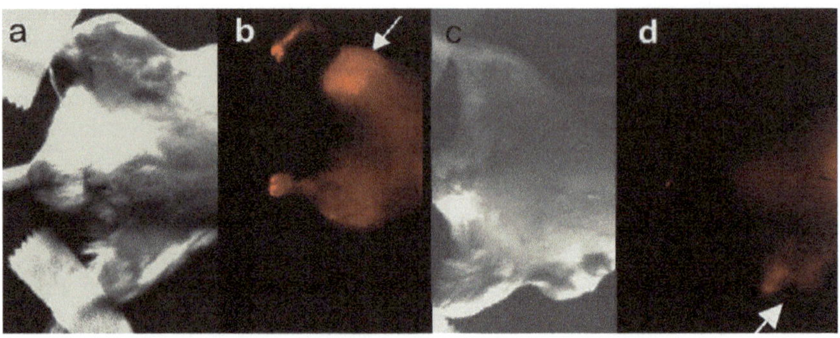

Fig. 9. White light (**a, c**) and fluorescence images (λ_{em}=694 nm, **b, d**) of xenografted mice after application of 100 μg Cy5.5-labelled Herceptin® in an SK-BR-3 tumour (**a, b**) and a PE/CA-PJ34 tumour (**c, d**). The highly expressing SK-BR-3 tumour clearly shows a distinct fluorescence signal compared to the normal expressing PE/CA-PJ34 tumour (arrows, modified from Hilger et al., 2004; reproduced with permission from Springer).

Lee et al. have used engineered affibodies for HER-2 imaging ($Z_{HER2:342}$). Affibodies are highly water-soluble α-helical proteins, which can be produced from bacterial systems and have a high affinity for HER-2 besides a much smaller size compared to antibodies (20x) or antibody fragments (4x). In their study, three different types of HER-2-specific affibody molecules were conjugated with AlexaFluor dyes and compared with AlexaFluor–labelled trastuzumab in terms of affinity and specificity to the HER-2 receptor *in vitro* and *in vivo*. The human breast cancer cell line SK-BR-3 was used as positive control, xenografted in nude mice. Interestingly, in addition to the trastuzumab-AlexaFluor conjugate, only the dimeric form of the affibody coupled to an albumin binding domain (ABD) showed accumulation in the tumour region and could be used for the imaging of HER-2 *in vivo* (Fig. 10). Monomeric or simple dimeric forms of the affibody-AlexaFluor-conjugate showed a rapid renal clearance and therefore failed to accumulate in the tumour (Lee et al., 2008).

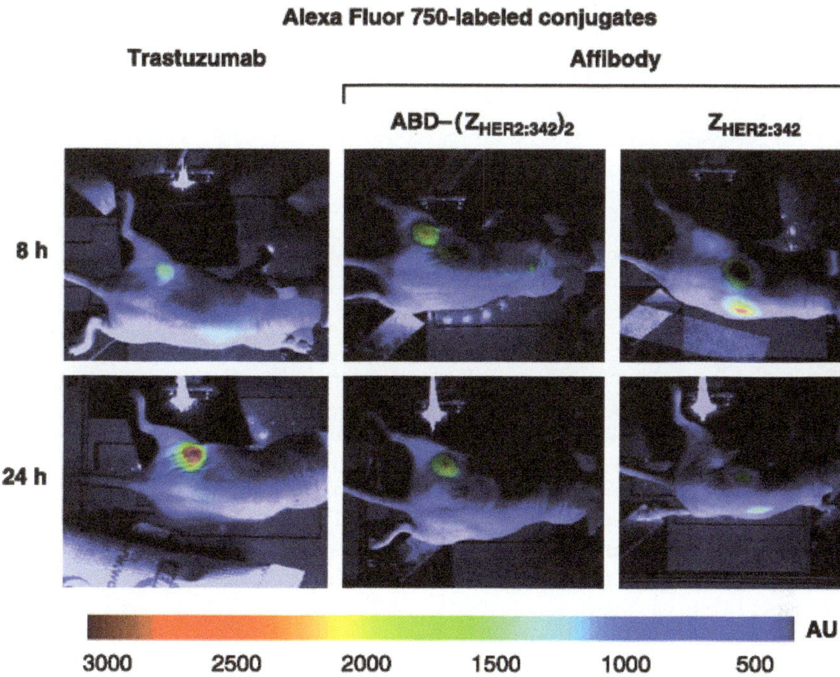

Fig. 10. *In vivo* NIR optical imaging of HER-2-expressing tumour xenografted mice after tail-vein injection of the AlexaFluor 750 labelled conjugates, showing pseudocolor fluorescence images obtained after injecting trastuzumab-AlexaFluor 750, affibodyABD-($Z_{HER2:342}$)$_2$-AlexaFluor 750, or affibody $Z_{HER2:342}$-AlexaFluor 750 conjugates. Images of trastuzumab-Alexa Fluor 750 conjugate were taken 6 hrs after injection instead of 8 hrs (left column)(Modified from Lee et al., 2008; reproduced with permission from AACR).

Human adenocarcinoma cell lines provide a huge variety of cell surface receptors. MDA-MB 468, e.g. is an EGFR-positive cell line, while MDA-MB 435 is EGFR-negative. These two cell lines have been chosen to evaluate the performance of Cy5.5-labelled EGF *in vivo*. Ke et al. used a custom-made imaging device to examine mice bearing xenografts of these tumour types in the chest walls. A fluorescence signal could clearly be visualized in MDA-MB 468 tumours, but not in MDA-MB 435 tumours. Specificity of binding could be confirmed by blocking experiments with anti-EGFR antibody C225 (cetuximab, Erbitux®) (Ke et al., 2003). A similar approach was used by Wang and Chen in 2009 (Wang K. et al., 2009). They labelled the, by now commercially available, antibody to generate Erbitux®-Cy5.5 as an EGFR imaging tracer. The xenograft model they used was also adenocarcinoma-based. MDA-MB 231 and MCF-7 were chosen as strong and moderate EGFR-expressing cell lines, respectively. Murine xenograft models of both tumour entities were imaged and the tracer was shown to specifically accumulate in tumour regions 24 hours after intravenous injection with the EGFR-overexpressing MDA-MB 231 tumour showing an about two-fold higher fluorescence signal than the only moderately EGFR-expressing MCF-7 tumour (Fig. 11). Again, specificity was proven by excess unlabelled antibody treatment (blocking).

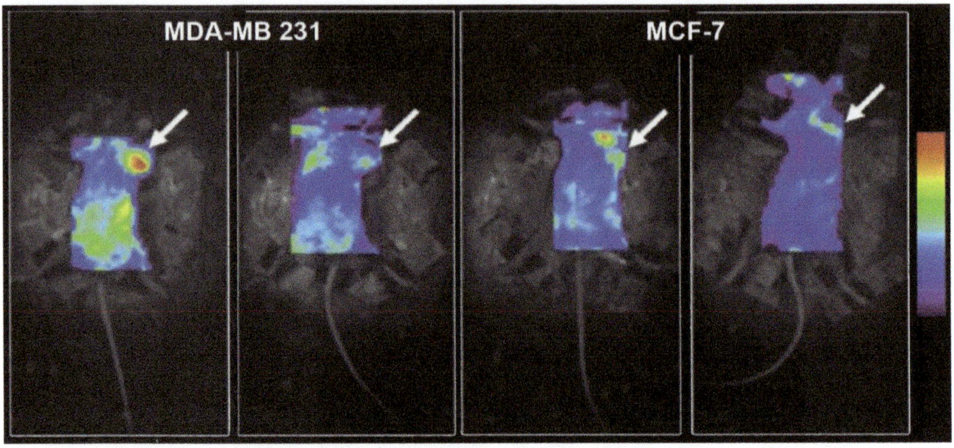

Fig. 11. *In vivo* near-infrared (NIR) images of MDA-MB-231 and MCF-7 xenografted (arrows) nude mice at 24 hours post injection of Erbitux®-Cy5.5. The fluorescence signal is clearly visualized in the left thoracic tumour region of MDA-MB-231 and MCF-7 xenografts. Blocking experiments indicate an apparent decrease of the fluorescent signal by pre-injection of excess Erbitux®, proving specificity (modified from Wang K. et al., 2009; reproduced with permission from InformaHealth).

4.2 Hormone receptors

Estrogen receptors (ERs) are over-expressed in around 70% of breast cancers, which are then referred to as ER-positive or hormone-dependent. Tamoxifen is the most frequently used anti-hormonal drug for treatment of women with hormone-dependent breast cancer. Tamoxifen treatment is very effective in these cases and significantly reduces the mortality of breast cancer patients. Unfortunately, during treatment many tumours develop a resistance to the drug, often accompanied by a reduction or loss of estrogen receptors. Several mechanisms have been discussed to be responsible for this development (Kumar 2007) and a non-invasive imaging technology to detect ER expression *in vivo* could help identifying the underlying process. A recent approach from Jose and co-workers describes the labelling of estradiol with a carbocyanine dye for the evaluation of the hormone receptor status *in vivo* and could therefore help in decreasing the need for unnecessary biopsies. Future research will show the performance of the developed tracer in preclinical models (Jose et al., 2011).

A rather particular system in this context is represented by the endothelin (ET)-axis, which is comprised of the three peptide hormones ET-1, ET-2 and ET-3 and their two associated receptors ET_AR and ET_BR. Endothelin (ET) was first described as a 21-amino acid peptide with vasoactive potency; in fact ET-1 is one of the most vasoconstricting substances currently known (Hickey et al., 1985; Yanagisawa et al., 1988). In addition to its role as a vasoconstrictor, more recently the role of the ET-axis as a progression factor in certain human cancers, including breast and ovarian cancer, has been discussed (Bhalla et al., 2009; Rosano et al., 2010). The influence of the ET-axis is attributed to elevated levels of ET-1 as well as overexpression of ET receptors on tumour cells and tumour associated cells (e.g. fibroblasts, endothelial cells, macrophages). In addition, a close interaction of the ET-axis with EGFR/HER-2 signalling (Fischgräbe et al., 2009) and VEGF-induced angiogenesis (Kandalaft et al., 2010) has been found in breast cancers and consequently ET receptor antagonists as new chemotherapeutic drugs for cancer therapy have been introduced. The evaluation of the ET receptor status *in vivo* would allow for early diagnosis and clarify the impact of e.g. anti-angiogenic therapies. In 2007 our group reported the design of a small-molecular ET_AR antagonist conjugated to a fluorescent dye via a short polyethylene glycol spacer (Fig. 12), capable of imaging tumour-associated ET_AR-expression *in vivo* (Höltke et al., 2007; Höltke et al., 2009).

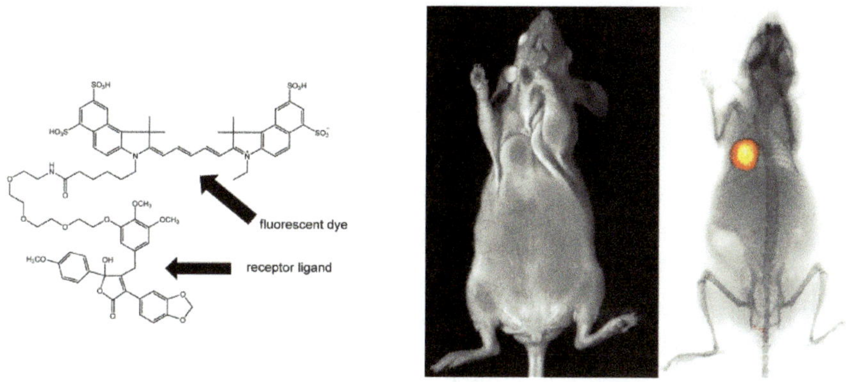

Fig. 12. Molecular structure of the designed fluorescent ET_AR tracer (left). White light (middle) and merged x-ray and fluorescence (FRI) image (right) of tumour-associated ET_AR expression in a murine breast cancer xenograft model 24 hrs after i.v. tracer administration (Höltke, unpublished results).

4.3 Integrins

Integrins are cell-adhesion proteins that mediate cell-cell and cell-extracellular matrix interactions, thereby increasing tumourigenicity and invasiveness of cancer. They are composed of an α and a β subunit. So far 24 α/β combinations (αβI) have been identified, seven of them have been demonstrated to bind the RGD motif, an arginine-glycine-aspartic acid-based peptide sequence (Arnaout, 2002; Arnaout et al., 2002; Hood et al., 2003; Schottelius et al., 2009). Also, the two αβI known to be most active in tumoral neoangiogenesis, the vitronectin receptor αvβ3 and the fibronectin receptor α5β1, bind RGD with high affinity. Integrin αvβ3 is a transmembrane protein, which is specifically expressed on tumour surfaces and on activated and proliferating endothelial cells. In 1998, Gasparini and co-workers introduced vascular αvβ3 as a prognostic factor in breast cancer (Gasparini et al., 1998). Soon after first RGD-based radiotracers for PET or SPECT were developed (Choe & Lee, 2007; Liu, 2006) fluorophore-labelled RGD derivatives were designed for NIR optical imaging approaches (Chen et al., 2004; Cheng et al., 2005; Gurfinkel et al., 2005; Ye et al., 2006). Since linear peptides containing the RGD sequence provide only low integrin subtype selectivity and are furthermore rather unstable under metabolic conditions cyclic RGD peptides were synthesized, which show a higher selectivity for αvβ3 and are characterized by a sufficient metabolic stability (Fig. 13).

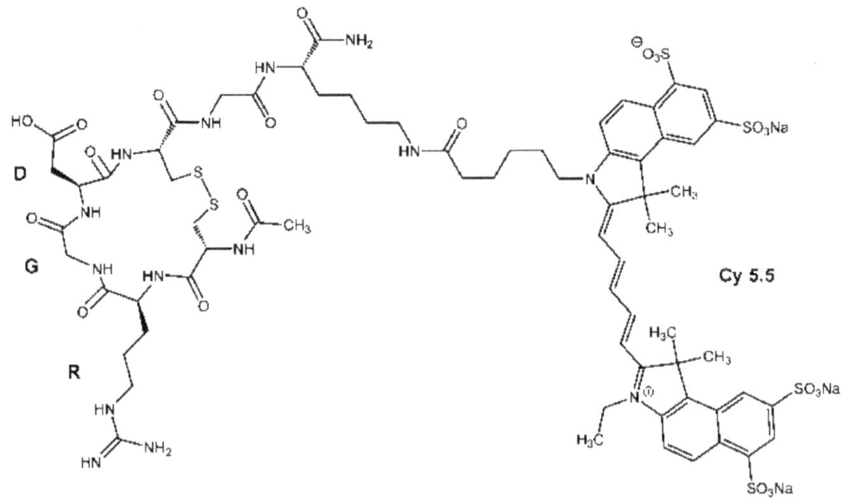

Fig. 13. Molecular structure of a typical cyclic RGD peptide conjugated to a fluorescent dye.

First experiments with Cy 5.5-labelled RGD peptides were published in 2004 (Chen et al., 2004; Wang W. et al., 2004) and aimed at glioblastoma, sarcoma and melanoma tumour entities. Besides the peptidic $\alpha v\beta 3$ ligands derived from RGD, antibodies, nanobodies and small molecular peptidomimetics have been presented (Winter et al., 2003; Winter et al., 2006; Xie et al., 2008). In 2007, von Wallbrunn et al. visualized $\alpha v\beta 3$ activity in three different xenograft models, including breast cancer, using FRI and FMT (von Wallbrunn et al., 2007). Both modalities provided mutually correlating results, confirming histological gold standard measurements (Fig. 14, left). Recently, Mulder et al. presented an RGD-conjugated quantum dot (QD) for visualization of $\alpha v\beta 3$ expression in melanoma-bearing mice (Mulder et al., 2009). The QDs were coated with gadolinium diethylene-triaminepentaacetic acid (Gd-DTPA)-based lipids and therefore serving as bimodal imaging agents for a use in MRI and OI. *In vivo* examinations revealed an attachment of the QDs to tumour vessels after i.v. injection. Interestingly, a labelling of blood vessels as far as 1 cm outside the primary tumour lesion was observed, indicating activation of distant vascular endothelium. Confirming the specificity of binding to tumour vasculature, no significant accumulation of QDs in distant vessels of e.g. muscle was observed. The combination of MRI and fluorescence imaging allowed both exact anatomical localization and evaluation of angiogenic activity. In this study, luciferase-transfected tumour cells were used, providing bioluminescence images of the tumour for additional correlation of the QD-triggered imaging findings (Fig. 14, right).

In summary, a large number of integrin-targeted optical probes have been developed and tested. Most approaches base on RGD-containing small peptides labelled with a fluorophore or conjugated to fluorescent nanoparticles (quantum dots). Many of these show promising results concerning sensitivity and specificity for tumour vasculature, demonstrating the potential of integrin targeting in cancer imaging. A representative review paper on the diverse structures of integrin targeted optical probes has recently been published, also touching the potential of integrin-based therapy (Ye & Chen, 2011).

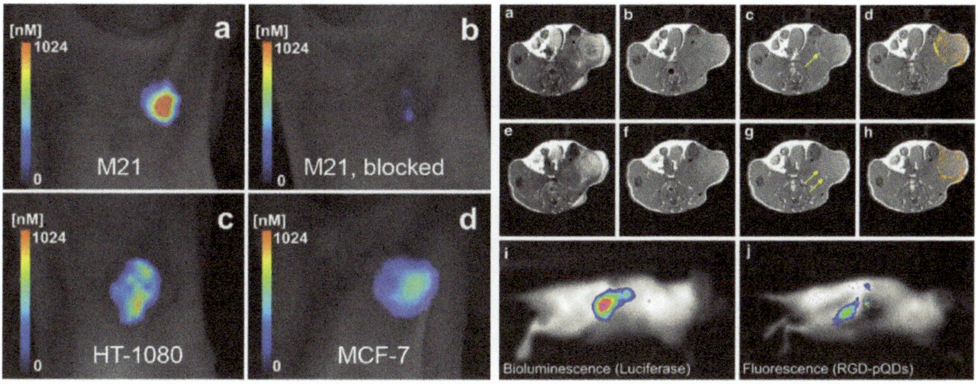

Fig. 14. Two examples of recent integrin imaging approaches. Left: Fluorescence mediated tomography (FMT) images of different tumour entities 60 minutes after injection of a Cy 5.5-labelled cyclic RGD peptide into athymic nude mice (2 nmol/animal), displaying tracer accumulation in the tumour lesion dependent on target structure expression and predosing (modified from von Wallbrunn et al., 2007, courtesy of the author). Right: MRI and OI of tumour-related angiogenesis visualized by αvβ3 integrin-targeted multimodal QDs (pQDs): MRI, bioluminescence and FRI of a C57B16 tumour-bearing mouse before and after injection of RGD-pQDs. T2-weighed MR images (a,e) show the contour of the tumour on the flank. T1-weighted images were measured before (b,f) and 45 min after (c,g) the injection of the RGD-pQDs. The arrows in (c,g) indicate bright (positive contrast) regions in the periphery of the tumour. In d and h strong signal enhancement is colour-coded (red-orange). Correlative FRI (j) shows good co-localization of the signal with bioluminescence (i) of the tumour cells (reproduced from Mulder et al., 2009 with permission from Springer).

4.4 Proteases

Matrix metalloproteinases (MMPs) are closely connected to the pathophysiological properties of integrines, which also makes them relevant factors associated with tumour growth, progression and metastasis (Brooks et al., 1996; Chabottaux & Noel, 2007; Stefanidakis & Koivunen, 2006). Human MMPs are a family of 24 structurally related zinc ion-dependent endopeptidases, able to degrade almost all components of the extracellular matrix (ECM) and the basal membrane. Moreover, they contribute to the morphogenesis of endothelial cells and have been shown to regulate the transcription of growth factors. The large number of MMPs and their diverse routes of involvement in cancer progression have made it difficult to address their activity in therapeutic interventions. First clinical trials with broad-spectrum MMP inhibitors like *Marimastat* or *Batimastat* were discontinued because of poor performance and severe side effects (Dorey, 1999; Renkiewicz et al., 2003). In this respect, especially the gelatinases MMP-2 and MMP-9 were identified as diagnostic factors in breast cancer on both, their local and systemic level, frequently predicting lymph node involvement and metastatic status (Jezierska & Motyl, 2009; Radisky E.S. & Radisky D.C., 2010). The *in vivo* assessment of MMP activity would be highly desirable for diagnosis and the evaluation of therapy. Bremer et al. have developed a fluorescently labelled substrate probe for MMP-2 (Bremer et al., 2001a; Bremer et al., 2001c). A graft copolymer, consisting of a poly-lysine backbone and polyethylene glycol side chains, was equipped with Cy 5.5 labelled specific peptidic substrates cleavable by MMP-2. Due to the close proximity of the dyes their fluorescence is quenched by the transfer of electronic excitation energy between two (or more) molecules (fluorescence resonance energy transfer, FRET) (Kiyokawa et al., 2006). Upon cleavage of the peptidic substrate by MMP-2 the dye molecules are removed from the backbone polymer, their fluorescence is dequenched and a signal can be detected. The resulting signal to background ratio is unrivalled due to virtually absent background fluorescence. (Fig. 15).

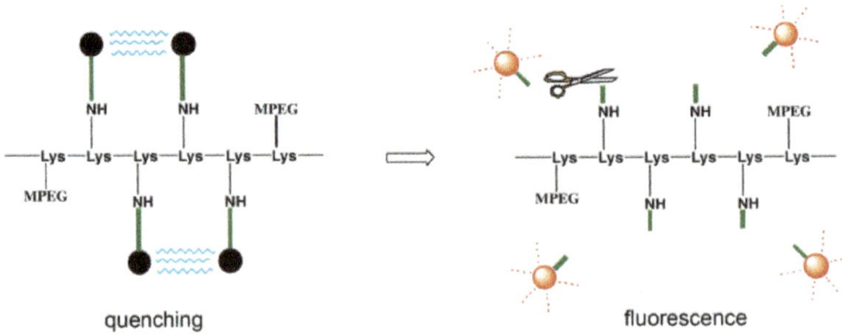

Fig. 15. Principle of the use of FRET for the detection of proteolytic activity. When dye molecules are in close proximity to each other, the fluorescence is quenched by FRET (black circles). After cleavage of the peptide substrate by e.g. MMP-2 (scissors) fluorescence can emerge (red circles). Modified from Bremer et al., 2001a, courtesy of the author.

The probe was applied to xenograft models of human fibrosarcoma HT-1080 and human breast adenocarcinoma BT-20. While HT-1080 cells express a high amount of MMP-2, BT-20 cells show only moderate protease levels. Accordingly, *in vivo* examinations show strong fluorescence signals from HT-1080 tumours, compared to only low signals from BT-20 xenografts (Fig. 16).

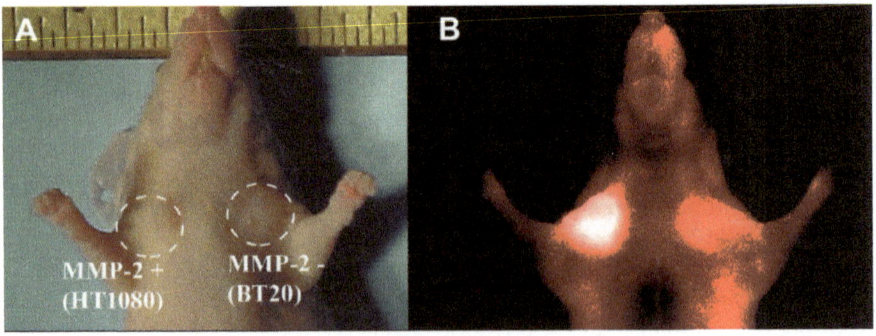

Fig. 16. Demonstration of protease activity by NIRF imaging in murine xenograft models of MMP-2 positive human fibrosarcoma HT-1080 and MMP-2 negative adenocarcinoma BT-20. A: Colour photograph of the implanted nude mouse. Both tumours measured approximately 2 x 3 mm. B: The NIRF image shows that the fibrosarcoma generated strong fluorescent signal intensity 2 hours after i.v. injection of the MMP-2–sensitive probe, but the signal intensity of the BT-20 tumour was only slightly higher than background fluorescence (modified from Bremer et al., 2001a, courtesy of the author).

The method has also been successfully applied for the imaging of cathepsins (Bremer et al., 2002). Cathepsins represent another group of proteases involved in cancer progression and the growth of metastases. Like MMPs, cathepsins comprise a large group of proteins responsible for a variety of processes in the animal/human body. Unlike MMPs, cathepsins do not depend on a Zn-atom at the active site, but are serine, cysteine or aspartate dependent. Most cathepsins are lysosomal proteins, activated by the low pH value inside the organelle. In particular cathepsins B, D, K and L2 have been assigned a role in breast cancer development and metastasis (Duffy, 1996; Nomura & Katunuma, 2005; Radisky E.S., 2010; Rose & Siegel, 2010). In the presented examination, a cathepsin B sensitive probe was designed and used to distinguish a highly invasive (DU-4475) and a well differentiated adenocarcinoma (BT-20). The less invasive tumour showed a significantly lower fluorescence signal (- 35%) than the highly invasive one (Bremer et al., 2002).

5. Conclusion

The successful preclinical application of optical imaging methods for cancer imaging has been extensively demonstrated over the last years. Especially in small animal imaging, techniques for tumour characterization (e.g. surface target expression or vascularization) have been developed and validated. The synthesis of specific tracers for targets arising from the ever-growing pathophysiological understanding of diseases can easily be performed and does not require large-scale laboratory equipment. This enables more and more scientists to accelerate their research on targeted *in vivo* imaging. In addition, OI devices offer quick and convenient image acquisition and reconstruction, especially compared to other small animal imaging technologies. In basic research, OI of breast cancer is a well established part of everyday work. Future use of OI in clinical routine depends on several factors, amongst which probe design and approval and further improvement of the imaging techniques appear the most important. For the elaboration of both factors, industry - either pharmaceutical- or medical technology companies - is required to partner with academic research institutions. On the technical side, spatial resolution and access to deep tissue lesions are the most striking and obvious points, where the refinement of techniques has to focus on. Pioneering work in this area is accomplished by the companies already distributing optical breast scanners. First trials with smaller groups of patients showed promising results, although by today the technique has to be considered an adjunct to conventional x-ray mammography only. On the field of tracer development, simple perfusion tracers, targeted fluorescent ligands, protease-sensitive smart probes and fluorescent nanoparticles or a combination of these still struggle for highest diagnostic accuracy on the one hand versus applicability on the other. It remains to be seen, whether targeted imaging will make the way into clinical routine and which role OI can play in this context. From the vast variety of targets relevant for basic research imaging, the identification of few molecular markers, expressed by a wide range of cancer entities seems to be a promising first step towards targeted molecular imaging, especially with regard to the immense regulatory effort and major investments (toxicology studies, GMP-production facilities etc.), which approval of a contrast agent requires. The existence of ICG on the market, though, substantiates the general possibility and shows that there is a demand for optical imaging contrast agents in the clinics and an increasing interest for further development in this field of alternative imaging technologies.

6. Acknowledgments

Financial support from the German Research Foundation (DFG, SFB 656, subprojects A4 and C8) and the Interdisciplinary Centre for Clinical Research (IZKF, Core-Unit OPTI) of the Medical Faculty at the Westfälische Wilhelms-Universität Münster is gratefully acknowledged.

7. References

Achilefu, S., Dorshow, R.B., Bugaj, J.E., & Rajagopalan, R. (2000). Novel receptor-targeted fluorescent contrast agents for in vivo tumor imaging. *Invest Radiol 35(8)*, 479-485.

Achilefu, S. (2004). Lighting up tumors with receptor-specific optical molecular probes. *Technol Cancer Res Treat 3(4)*, 393-409.

Alvarez, R.H., & Price, J.E. (2010). Biomarkers for breast cancer: the search continues. *Cancer Biol Ther 9(1)*, 31-32.

Alvarez, R.H., Valero, V., & Hortobagyi, G.N. (2010). Emerging targeted therapies for breast cancer. *J Clin Oncol 28(20)*, 3366-3379.

Arnaout, M.A. (2002). Integrin structure: new twists and turns in dynamic cell adhesion. *Immunol Rev 186*, 125-140.

Arnaout, M.A., Goodman, S.L., & Xiong, J.P. (2002). Coming to grips with integrin binding to ligands. *Curr Opin Cell Biol 14(5)*, 641-651.

Backer, M.V., Levashova, Z., Patel, V., Jehning, B.T., Claffey, K., Blankenberg, F.G., & Backer, J.M. (2007). Molecular imaging of VEGF receptors in angiogenic vasculature with single-chain VEGF-based probes. *Nat Med 13(4)*, 504-509.

Becker, A., Hessenius, C., Licha, K., Ebert, B., Sukowski, U., Semmler, W., Wiedenmann, B., & Grötzinger, C. (2001). Receptor-targeted optical imaging of tumors with near-infrared fluorescent ligands. *Nat Biotechnol 19(4)*, 327-331.

Bhalla, A., Haque, S., Taylor, I., Winslet, M., & Loizidou, M. (2009). Endothelin receptor antagonism and cancer. *Eur J Clin Invest 39 Suppl 2*, 74-77.

Boas, D. (1997). A fundamental limitation of linearized algorithms for diffuse optical tomography. *Opt Express 1(13)*, 404-413.

Bremer, C., Bredow, S., Mahmood, U., Weissleder, R., & Tung, C.H. (2001a). Optical imaging of matrix metalloproteinase-2 activity in tumors: feasibility study in a mouse model. *Radiology 221(2)*, 523-529.

Bremer, C., Ntziachristos, V., Mahmood, U., Tung, C.H., & Weissleder, R. (2001b). [Progress in optical imaging]. *Radiologe 41(2)*, 131-137.

Bremer, C., Tung, C.H., & Weissleder, R. (2001c). In vivo molecular target assessment of matrix metalloproteinase inhibition. *Nat Med 7(6)*, 743-748.

Bremer, C., Tung, C.H., Bogdanov, A., Jr., & Weissleder, R. (2002). Imaging of differential protease expression in breast cancers for detection of aggressive tumor phenotypes. *Radiology 222(3)*, 814-818.

Brooks, P.C., Stromblad, S., Sanders, L.C., von Schalscha, T.L., Aimes, R.T., Stetler-Stevenson, W.G., Quigley, J.P., & Cheresh, D.A. (1996). Localization of matrix metalloproteinase MMP-2 to the surface of invasive cells by interaction with integrin alpha v beta 3. *Cell 85(5)*, 683-693.

Chabottaux, V., & Noel, A. (2007). Breast cancer progression: insights into multifaceted matrix metalloproteinases. *Clin Exp Metastasis 24(8)*, 647-656.

Chen, X., Conti, P.S., & Moats, R.A. (2004). In vivo near-infrared fluorescence imaging of integrin alphavbeta3 in brain tumor xenografts. *Cancer Res 64(21)*, 8009-8014.

Cheng, Z., Wu, Y., Xiong, Z., Gambhir, S.S., & Chen, X. (2005). Near-infrared fluorescent RGD peptides for optical imaging of integrin alphavbeta3 expression in living mice. *Bioconjug Chem 16(6)*, 1433-1441.

Choe, Y.S., & Lee, K.H. (2007). Targeted in vivo imaging of angiogenesis: present status and perspectives. *Curr Pharm Des 13(1)*, 17-31.

Chudakov, D.M., Matz, M.V., Lukyanov, S., & Lukyanov, K.A. (2010). Fluorescent proteins and their applications in imaging living cells and tissues. *Physiol Rev 90(3)*, 1103-1163.

Cutler, M. (1929). Transillumination as an aid in the diagnosis of breast lesions. *Surg Gynecol Obstet 48*, 721-730.

Cutler, M. (1931). Transillumination of the Breast. *Ann Surg 93(1)*, 223-234.

De Laurentiis, M., Cianniello, D., Caputo, R., Stanzione, B., Arpino, G., Cinieri, S., Lorusso, V., & De Placido, S. (2010). Treatment of triple negative breast cancer (TNBC): current options and future perspectives. *Cancer Treat Rev 36 Suppl 3*, S80-86.

Dorey, E. (1999). British Biotech settles up. *Nat Biotechnol 17(7)*, 624.

Duffy, M.J. (1996). Proteases as prognostic markers in cancer. *Clin Cancer Res 2(4)*, 613-618.

Fischgräbe, J., Götte, M., Michels, K., Kiesel, L., & Wülfing, P. (2009). Targeting endothelin A receptor enhances anti-proliferative and anti-invasive effects of the HER2 antibody trastuzumab in HER2-overexpressing breast cancer cells. *Int J Cancer 127(3)*, 696-706.

Floery, D., Helbich, T.H., Riedl, C.C., Jaromi, S., Weber, M., Leodolter, S., & Fuchsjaeger, M.H. (2005). Characterization of benign and malignant breast lesions with computed tomography laser mammography (CTLM): initial experience. *Invest Radiol 40(6)*, 328-335.

Fournier, L.S., Vanel, D., Athanasiou, A., Gatzemeier, W., Masuykov, I.V., Padhani, A.R., Dromain, C., Galetti, K., Sigal, R., Costa, A., & Balleyguier, C. (2009). Dynamic optical breast imaging: a novel technique to detect and characterize tumor vessels. *Eur J Radiol 69(1)*, 43-49.

Gasparini, G., Brooks, P.C., Biganzoli, E., Vermeulen, P.B., Bonoldi, E., Dirix, L.Y., Ranieri, G., Miceli, R., & Cheresh, D.A. (1998). Vascular integrin alpha(v)beta3: a new prognostic indicator in breast cancer. *Clin Cancer Res 4(11)*, 2625-2634.

Gasparini, G. (2000). Prognostic value of vascular endothelial growth factor in breast cancer. *Oncologist 5 Suppl 1*, 37-44.

Giovannini, M., Aldrighetti, D., Zucchinelli, P., Belli, C., & Villa, E. (2010). Antiangiogenic strategies in breast cancer management. *Crit Rev Oncol Hematol 76(1)*, 13-35.

Graves, E.E., Weissleder, R., & Ntziachristos, V. (2004). Fluorescence molecular imaging of small animal tumor models. *Curr Mol Med 4(4)*, 419-430.

Guo, S., Colbert, L.S., Fuller, M., Zhang, Y., & Gonzalez-Perez, R.R. (2010a). Vascular endothelial growth factor receptor-2 in breast cancer. *Biochim Biophys Acta 1806(1)*, 108-121.

Guo, X., Liu, X., Wang, X., Tian, F., Liu, F., Zhang, B., Hu, G., & Bai, J. (2010b). A combined fluorescence and microcomputed tomography system for small animal imaging. *IEEE Trans Biomed Eng 57(12)*, 2876-2883.

Gurfinkel, M., Ke, S., Wang, W., Li, C., & Sevick-Muraca, E.M. (2005). Quantifying molecular specificity of alphavbeta3 integrin-targeted optical contrast agents with dynamic optical imaging. *J Biomed Opt 10(3)*, 034019.

Hasan, J., & Jayson, G.C. (2001). VEGF antagonists. *Expert Opin Biol Ther 1(4)*, 703-718.

Hawrysz, D.J., & Sevick-Muraca, E.M. (2000). Developments toward diagnostic breast cancer imaging using near-infrared optical measurements and fluorescent contrast agents. *Neoplasia 2(5)*, 388-417.

Hendrix, M.J., Seftor, E.A., Kirschmann, D.A., & Seftor, R.E. (2000). Molecular biology of breast cancer metastasis. Molecular expression of vascular markers by aggressive breast cancer cells. *Breast Cancer Res 2(6)*, 417-422.

Hickey, K.A., Rubanyi, G., Paul, R.J., & Highsmith, R.F. (1985). Characterization of a coronary vasoconstrictor produced by cultured endothelial cells. *Am J Physiol 248(5 Pt 1)*, C550-556.

Hicklin, D.J., & Ellis, L.M. (2005). Role of the vascular endothelial growth factor pathway in tumor growth and angiogenesis. *J Clin Oncol 23(5)*, 1011-1027.

Hilger, I., Leistner, Y., Berndt, A., Fritsche, C., Haas, K.M., Kosmehl, H., & Kaiser, W.A. (2004). Near-infrared fluorescence imaging of HER-2 protein over-expression in tumour cells. *Eur Radiol 14(6)*, 1124-1129.

Höltke, C., von Wallbrunn, A., Kopka, K., Schober, O., Heindel, W., Schäfers, M., & Bremer, C. (2007). A fluorescent photoprobe for the imaging of endothelin receptors. *Bioconjug Chem 18(3)*, 685-694.

Höltke, C., Waldeck, J., Kopka, K., Heindel, W., Schober, O., Schäfers, M., & Bremer, C. (2009). Biodistribution of a nonpeptidic fluorescent endothelin A receptor imaging probe. *Mol Imaging 8(1)*, 27-34.

Hood, J.D., Frausto, R., Kiosses, W.B., Schwartz, M.A., & Cheresh, D.A. (2003). Differential alphav integrin-mediated Ras-ERK signaling during two pathways of angiogenesis. *J Cell Biol 162(5)*, 933-943.

Jaffer, F.A., Vinegoni, C., John, M.C., Aikawa, E., Gold, H.K., Finn, A.V., Ntziachristos, V., Libby, P., & Weissleder, R. (2008). Real-time catheter molecular sensing of inflammation in proteolytically active atherosclerosis. *Circulation 118(18)*, 1802-1809.

Jaffer, F.A., Libby, P., & Weissleder, R. (2009). Optical and multimodality molecular imaging: insights into atherosclerosis. *Arterioscler Thromb Vasc Biol 29(7)*, 1017-1024.

Jezierska, A., & Motyl, T. (2009). Matrix metalloproteinase-2 involvement in breast cancer progression: a mini-review. *Med Sci Monit 15(2)*, RA32-40.

Johnson, K.A., & Brown, P.H. (2010). Drug development for cancer chemoprevention: focus on molecular targets. *Semin Oncol 37(4)*, 345-358.

Jose, I., Deodhar, K.D., Desai, U.B., & Bhattacharjee, S. (2011). Early Detection of Breast Cancer: Synthesis and Characterization of Novel Target Specific NIR-Fluorescent Estrogen Conjugate for Molecular Optical Imaging. *J Fluoresc.*

Kandalaft, L.E., Motz, G.T., Busch, J., & Coukos, G. (2010). Angiogenesis and the Tumor Vasculature as Antitumor Immune Modulators: The Role of Vascular Endothelial Growth Factor and Endothelin. *Curr Top Microbiol Immunol.*

Ke, S., Wen, X., Gurfinkel, M., Charnsangavej, C., Wallace, S., Sevick-Muraca, E.M., & Li, C. (2003). Near-infrared optical imaging of epidermal growth factor receptor in breast cancer xenografts. *Cancer Res 63(22)*, 7870-7875.

Kiyokawa, E., Hara, S., Nakamura, T., & Matsuda, M. (2006). Fluorescence (Forster) resonance energy transfer imaging of oncogene activity in living cells. *Cancer Sci 97(1)*, 8-15.

Kumar R. (2007). Targeted functional imaging in breast cancer. *Eur J Nucl Med Mol Imaging 34(3)*, 346-353.

Leborgne, R. (1951). Diagnosis of tumors of the breast by simple roentgenography; calcifications in carcinomas. *Am J Roentgenol Radium Ther 65(1)*, 1-11.

Lee, S.B., Hassan, M., Fisher, R., Chertov, O., Chernomordik, V., Kramer-Marek, G., Gandjbakhche, A., & Capala, J. (2008). Affibody molecules for in vivo characterization of HER2-positive tumors by near-infrared imaging. *Clin Cancer Res 14(12)*, 3840-3849.

Licha, K., Riefke, B., & Semmler, W. (1996). Synthesis and characterization of cyanine dyes as contrast agents for near-infrared imaging. *SPIE 927*, 192-198.

Licha, K., Riefke, B., Ntziachristos, V., Becker, A., Chance, B., & Semmler, W. (2000). Hydrophilic cyanine dyes as contrast agents for near-infrared tumor imaging: synthesis, photophysical properties and spectroscopic in vivo characterization. *Photochem Photobiol 72(3)*, 392-398.

Liu, S. (2006). Radiolabeled multimeric cyclic RGD peptides as integrin alphavbeta3 targeted radiotracers for tumor imaging. *Mol Pharm 3(5)*, 472-487.

Lukyanov, K.A., Serebrovskaya, E.O., Lukyanov, S., & Chudakov, D.M. (2010). Fluorescent proteins as light-inducible photochemical partners. *Photochem Photobiol Sci 9(10)*, 1301-1306.

Mahmood, U., Tung, C.H., Bogdanov, A., Jr., & Weissleder, R. (1999). Near-infrared optical imaging of protease activity for tumor detection. *Radiology 213(3)*, 866-870.

Montet, X., Ntziachristos, V., Grimm, J., & Weissleder, R. (2005). Tomographic fluorescence mapping of tumor targets. *Cancer Res 65(14)*, 6330-6336.

Mulder, W.J., Castermans, K., van Beijnum, J.R., Oude Egbrink, M.G., Chin, P.T., Fayad, Z.A., Lowik, C.W., Kaijzel, E.L., Que, I., Storm, G., Strijkers, G.J., Griffioen, A.W., & Nicolay, K. (2009). Molecular imaging of tumor angiogenesis using alphavbeta3-integrin targeted multimodal quantum dots. *Angiogenesis 12(1)*, 17-24.

Nagengast, W.B., de Vries, E.G., Hospers, G.A., Mulder, N.H., de Jong, J.R., Hollema, H., Brouwers, A.H., van Dongen, G.A., Perk, L.R., & Lub-de Hooge, M.N. (2007). In vivo VEGF imaging with radiolabeled bevacizumab in a human ovarian tumor xenograft. *J Nucl Med 48(8)*, 1313-1319.

Nahrendorf, M., Waterman, P., Thurber, G., Groves, K., Rajopadhye, M., Panizzi, P., Marinelli, B., Aikawa, E., Pittet, M.J., Swirski, F.K., & Weissleder, R. (2009). Hybrid in vivo FMT-CT imaging of protease activity in atherosclerosis with customized nanosensors. *Arterioscler Thromb Vasc Biol 29(10)*, 1444-1451.

Nomura, T., & Katunuma, N. (2005). Involvement of cathepsins in the invasion, metastasis and proliferation of cancer cells. *J Med Invest 52(1-2)*, 1-9.

Ntziachristos, V., Yodh, A.G., Schnall, M., & Chance, B. (2000). Concurrent MRI and diffuse optical tomography of breast after indocyanine green enhancement. *Proc Natl Acad Sci U S A 97(6)*, 2767-2772.

Ntziachristos, V., Bremer, C., Graves, E.E., Ripoll, J., & Weissleder, R. (2002). In vivo tomographic imaging of near-infrared fluorescent probes. *Mol Imaging 1(2)*, 82-88.

Ntziachristos, V., Bremer, C., & Weissleder, R. (2003). Fluorescence imaging with near-infrared light: new technological advances that enable in vivo molecular imaging. *Eur Radiol 13(1)*, 195-208.

O'Leary, M.A., Boas, D.A., Chance, B., & Yodh, A.G. (1995). Experimental images of heterogeneous turbid media by frequency-domain diffusing-photon tomography. *Opt Lett 20(5)*, 426-428.

Parker, B., & Sukumar, S. (2003). Distant metastasis in breast cancer: molecular mechanisms and therapeutic targets. *Cancer Biol Ther 2(1)*, 14-21.

Poellinger, A., Martin, J.C., Ponder, S.L., Freund, T., Hamm, B., Bick, U., & Diekmann, F. (2008). Near-infrared laser computed tomography of the breast first clinical experience. *Acad Radiol 15(12)*, 1545-1553.

Poellinger, A., Persigehl, T., Mahler, M., Bahner, M., Ponder, S.L., Diekmann, F., Bremer, C. & Moesta, T., Near-Infrared Imaging of the Breast Using Omocianine as a Fluorescent Dye, Results of a Placebo-Controlled, Clinical, Multicenter Trial. *Invest Radiol* EPub ahead of print.

Radisky, E.S. (2010). Cathepsin D: Regulation in mammary gland remodeling, misregulation in breast cancer. *Cancer Biol Ther 10(5)*, 467-470.

Radisky, E.S., & Radisky, D.C. (2010). Matrix metalloproteinase-induced epithelial-mesenchymal transition in breast cancer. *J Mammary Gland Biol Neoplasia 15(2)*, 201-212.

Razansky, D., Vinegoni, C., & Ntziachristos, V. (2008). Polarization-sensitive optoacoustic tomography of optically diffuse tissues. *Opt Lett 33(20)*, 2308-2310.

Renkiewicz, R., Qiu, L., Lesch, C., Sun, X., Devalaraja, R., Cody, T., Kaldjian, E., Welgus, H., & Baragi, V. (2003). Broad-spectrum matrix metalloproteinase inhibitor marimastat-induced musculoskeletal side effects in rats. *Arthritis Rheum 48(6)*, 1742-1749.

Riefke, B., Licha, K., & Semmler, W. (1997). [Contrast media for optical mammography]. *Radiologe 37(9)*, 749-755.

Rosano, L., Spinella, F., & Bagnato, A. (2010). The importance of endothelin axis in initiation, progression, and therapy of ovarian cancer. *Am J Physiol Regul Integr Comp Physiol 299(2)*, R395-404.

Rose, A.A., & Siegel, P.M. (2010). Emerging therapeutic targets in breast cancer bone metastasis. *Future Oncol 6(1)*, 55-74.

Schottelius, M., Laufer, B., Kessler, H., & Wester, H.J. (2009). Ligands for mapping alphavbeta3-integrin expression in vivo. *Acc Chem Res 42(7)*, 969-980.

Stasic, D., Farrell, T.J., & Patterson, M.S. (2003). The use of spatially resolved fluorescence and reflectance to determine interface depth in layered fluorophore distributions. *Phys Med Biol 48(21)*, 3459-3474.

Stefanidakis, M., & Koivunen, E. (2006). Cell-surface association between matrix metalloproteinases and integrins: role of the complexes in leukocyte migration and cancer progression. *Blood 108(5)*, 1441-1450.

van de Ven, S.M., Elias, S.G., Wiethoff, A.J., van der Voort, M., Nielsen, T., Brendel, B., Bontus, C., Uhlemann, F., Nachabe, R., Harbers, R., van Beek, M., Bakker, L., van der Mark, M.B., Luijten, P., & Mali, W.P. (2009). Diffuse optical tomography of the breast: preliminary findings of a new prototype and comparison with magnetic resonance imaging. *Eur Radiol 19(5)*, 1108-1113.

van de Ven, S., Wiethoff, A., Nielsen, T., Brendel, B., van der Voort, M., Nachabe, R., Van der Mark, M., Van Beek, M., Bakker, L., Fels, L., Elias, S., Luijten, P., & Mali, W. (2010). A Novel Fluorescent Imaging Agent for Diffuse Optical Tomography of the Breast: First Clinical Experience in Patients. *Mol Imaging Biol 12(3)*, 343-348.

van de Ven, S.M., Mincu, N., Brunette, J., Ma, G., Khayat, M., Ikeda, D.M., & Gambhir, S.S. (2011). Molecular Imaging Using Light-Absorbing Imaging Agents and a Clinical Optical Breast Imaging System-a Phantom Study. *Mol Imaging Biol 13(2)*, 232-238.

Vinegoni, C., Razansky, D., Figueiredo, J.L., Fexon, L., Pivovarov, M., Nahrendorf, M., Ntziachristos, V., & Weissleder, R. (2009). Born normalization for fluorescence optical projection tomography for whole heart imaging. *J Vis Exp (28)*.

von Wallbrunn, A., Höltke, C., Zühlsdorf, M., Heindel, W., Schäfers, M., & Bremer, C. (2007). In vivo imaging of integrin alpha v beta 3 expression using fluorescence-mediated tomography. *Eur J Nucl Med Mol Imaging 34(5)*, 745-754.

Wall, A., Persigehl, T., Hauff, P., Licha, K., Schirner, M., Muller, S., von Wallbrunn, A., Matuszewski, L., Heindel, W., & Bremer, C. (2008). Differentiation of angiogenic burden in human cancer xenografts using a perfusion-type optical contrast agent (SIDAG). *Breast Cancer Res 10(2)*, R23.

Wang, K., Li, W., Huang, T., Li, R., Wang, D., Shen, B., & Chen, X. (2009). Characterizing breast cancer xenograft epidermal growth factor receptor expression by using near-infrared optical imaging. *Acta Radiol 50(10)*, 1095-1103.

Wang, W., Ke, S., Wu, Q., Charnsangavej, C., Gurfinkel, M., Gelovani, J.G., Abbruzzese, J.L., Sevick-Muraca, E.M., & Li, C. (2004). Near-infrared optical imaging of integrin alphavbeta3 in human tumor xenografts. *Mol Imaging 3(4)*, 343-351.

Watmough, D.J. (1982a). Diaphanography: mechanism responsible for the images. *Acta Radiol Oncol 21(1)*, 11-15.

Watmough, D.J. (1982b). A light torch for the transillumination of female breast tissues. *Br J Radiol 55(650)*, 142-146.

Weissleder, R., Tung, C.H., Mahmood, U., & Bogdanov, A., Jr. (1999). In vivo imaging of tumors with protease-activated near-infrared fluorescent probes. *Nat Biotechnol 17(4)*, 375-378.

Weissleder, R., & Ntziachristos, V. (2003). Shedding light onto live molecular targets. *Nat Med 9(1)*, 123-128.

Winter, P.M., Morawski, A.M., Caruthers, S.D., Fuhrhop, R.W., Zhang, H., Williams, T.A., Allen, J.S., Lacy, E.K., Robertson, J.D., Lanza, G.M., & Wickline, S.A. (2003). Molecular imaging of angiogenesis in early-stage atherosclerosis with alpha(v)beta3-integrin-targeted nanoparticles. *Circulation 108(18)*, 2270-2274.

Winter, P.M., Neubauer, A.M., Caruthers, S.D., Harris, T.D., Robertson, J.D., Williams, T.A., Schmieder, A.H., Hu, G., Allen, J.S., Lacy, E.K., Zhang, H., Wickline, S.A., & Lanza, G.M. (2006). Endothelial alpha(v)beta3 integrin-targeted fumagillin nanoparticles inhibit angiogenesis in atherosclerosis. *Arterioscler Thromb Vasc Biol 26(9)*, 2103-2109.

Xie, J., Chen, K., Lee, H.Y., Xu, C., Hsu, A.R., Peng, S., Chen, X., & Sun, S. (2008). Ultrasmall c(RGDyK)-coated Fe3O4 nanoparticles and their specific targeting to integrin alpha(v)beta3-rich tumor cells. *J Am Chem Soc 130(24)*, 7542-7543.

Yanagisawa, M., Kurihara, H., Kimura, S., Tomobe, Y., Kobayashi, M., Mitsui, Y., Yazaki, Y., Goto, K., & Masaki, T. (1988). A novel potent vasoconstrictor peptide produced by vascular endothelial cells. *Nature 332(6163)*, 411-415.

Ye, Y., Bloch, S., Xu, B., & Achilefu, S. (2006). Design, synthesis, and evaluation of near infrared fluorescent multimeric RGD peptides for targeting tumors. *J Med Chem 49(7)*, 2268-2275.

Ye, Y., & Chen, X. (2011). Integrin Targeting for Tumor Optical Imaging *Theranostics 1*, 102-126.

Yuan, B., & Liu, Y. (2010). Ultrasound-modulated fluorescence from rhodamine B aqueous solution. *J Biomed Opt 15(2)*, 021321.

13

Intraductal Breast Cytology and Biopsy to the Detection and Treatment of Intraductal Lesions of the Breast

Tadaharu Matsunaga
Nagumo Clinic
Japan

1. Introduction

Detection of breast cancer at an early stage is the most effective approach to decrease mortality, and bloody nipple discharge is an important clue to detect ductal cancer. In case of bloody nipple discharge the intraductal approach is a minimally invasive method to detect intraductal lesions. The intraductal approach does not destroy the ductal structure and does not cause needle tract dissemination. Though bloody nipple discharge is a significant clue in the detection of ductal carcinoma of the breast that do not display any tumor images and calcifications, the sensitivity of discharge cytology is not sufficiently high. Mammary duct endoscopy (MS) has been employed to detect intraductal lesions and MS yields both an optical image and biopsy. Intraductal breast biopsy (IDBB) and direct ductal lavage cytology were used to obtain pathological and cytological diagnoses in intraductal lesions with nipple discharge. The usefulness of MS, IDBB and direct ductal lavage cytology for intraductal lesions, with particular regard to differential diagnosis of ductal carcinoma and intraductal papilloma.

2. Materials and methods

Four hundred and sixty two MS procedures were performed in 348 patients who had nipple discharge but no overt mass between October 1993 and September 2009 at Tokyo Metropolitan Cancer Detection Center (October 1993 to December 2002), Minamiaoyama Breastopia Clinic (April 2003 to June 2006), and Tokyo Medical University Hachioji Medical Center (November 2006 to Sep 2009). In these 348 cases, nipple discharge was the primary diagnostic finding and there were no specific findings on mammography or sonography. Of these 348 patients, 81 patients with breast cancer and 163 patients of intraductal papilloma (IDP) were diagnosed pathologically. The other 104 patients were diagnosed as benign with cytology and followed clinically for more than 5 years.

In these 348 patients, mammography, ultrasound and cytology of nipple discharge were performed routinely. Nipple discharge was examined with a glass slide touching the nipple directly and immediately immersed into 90% alcohol as a routine cytology method (touch method). The presence of a cluster of ductal cells was taken to indicate the presence of an intraductal papillary lesion. Nipple discharge was collected in a narrow vessel containing cell fixation liquid three times a day for three days at home in 70 breast cancer patients (collection method). This collection method was performed to obtain much cytologic specimen. Galactography was done if a papillary lesion was suggested by cytology or if there was an obvious bloody background. MS was indicated based on the galactographic findings and the cytological findings

2.1 Intraductal approach to the detection of intraductal lesions

At the time of the MS procedure, 4 % procaine was sprayed on the nipple. After injecting 1% procaine into the duct, the nipple orifice and ductal sphincter were dilated with a tear duct bougie. MS measuring 0.72 mm in outer diameter (Fiber Tech Company, Tokyo, Japan) were used. Intraductal breast biopsy (IDBB) under mammoscopic observation was performed in 226 intraductal papillomas (in a total of 128 patients) and in 38 ductal carcinomas (in a total of 35 patients). In most cases, IDBB was performed using a metallic tube with a side aperture near the tip (JN Biopsy Needle, Hakko Company, Tokyo, Japan). In directed ductal lavage cytolology, an epidural tube was used. After MS, the tube was inserted and advanced into the ductal branch where the papillary lesion was observed. When the lesion could not be observed by MS, emanation of bloody discharge from periphery suggested the direction of the lesion.We usually insufflated air to observe the ductal lumen by MS. Since after MS the lumen of the duct was enlarged, making it easy to selectively advance an epidural tube into an abnormal branch. When the lesion could not be observed by MS, emanation of bloody discharge from periphery suggested the direction of the lesion. An epidural tube, a 1 ml syringe of saline, and a 20 ml syringe were connected with a three-way valve. First the valve was turned to a 1-ml saline syringe and negative pressure was applied using a 20-ml syringe. Then the valve was turned to a-20 ml syringe and saline was sucked into the duct using the negative intraductal pressure. Then the valve was turned to a 1-ml syringe and intraductal fluid was collected into a 20-ml syringe. These procedures were repeated several times while changing the saline solution. Directed ductal lavage cytology was performed in this way in 38 patients. The cytologic findings were assessed by both cytology technician and a pathologist. These MS, IDBB and lavage procedures were performed in outpatient clinics..

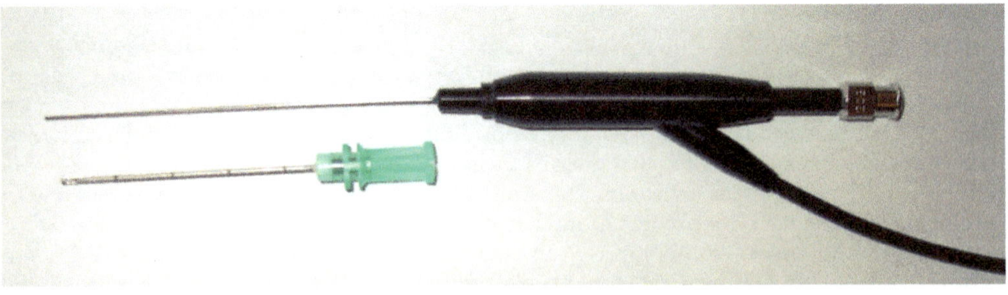

Fig. 1. Mammary duct endscopy (MS) and biopsy needle

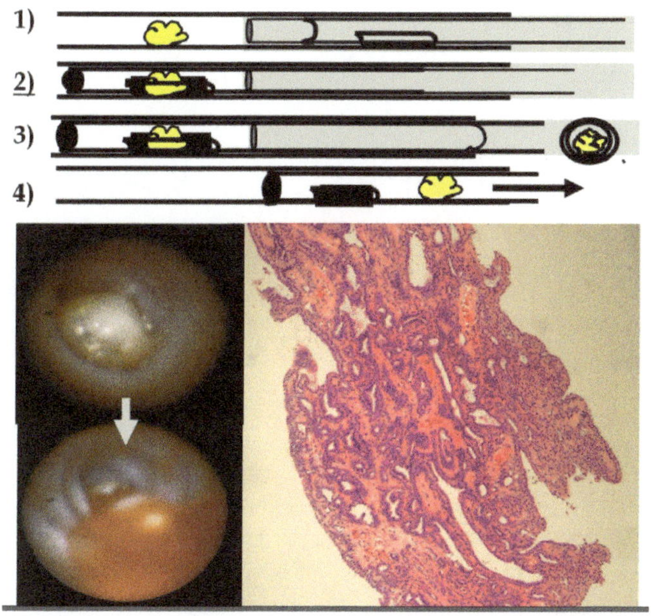

Fig. 2. Method of intraductal breast biopsy (IDBB) 1)The MS is covered with a metalic tube with a side aperture near the tip and the MS with a metalic tube is inserted into the mammary duct. 2) The metallic tube is advanced along the outside of the mammoscope to the intraductal mass and the mass is entrapped in the tube through a side aperture under observation by the MS. 3)Then the metallic tube was turned to cut off the intraductal mass. 4) Afterwards, the MS is removed and then the tissue piece within a metallic tube is collected by manually applied negative pressure. The specimen was diagnosed as IDP.

2.2 Assessment of ductal cytology and IDBB

The cytologic findings were classified into 4 categories; cancer, suspected cancer, suspected benign papillary lesion with the presence of a ductal cells cluster without atypia, and considered normal without any cluster. Cancer and suspected cancer categories were defined as positive findings. The diagnostic accuracy of these three methods , i.e. touch, collection, and directed ductal lavage were compared to IDBB in detecting malignancy. The therapeutic effect of IDBB for intraductal papillomas was also studied in 73 patients followed for more than 5 years (consisting of a total of 78 ducts).

3. Result

3.1.1 Visualization of intraductal lesions with MS

The normal mammary duct wall is white or light pink in color. The wall is smooth and lustrous with discharge and capillary veins might be observed. Of 81 breast cancer lesions, intraductal lesions were observed in 50 (61.7%) by MS. Then feature of MS were classified into three types; hemispheric, papillary and flat, irregular ductal wall. The hemispheric and papillary shape were most common in intraductal papilloma and the flat irregular pattern was most common in ductal carcinoma. In the other 26 lesions, bloody secretion emanating from the periphery suggested the presence of ductal carcinoma were observed. So the lesional ductal brunches were recognized in 76/81 cases (93.8%). Five carcinoma lesions could not be recognized by MS because the MS could not be advanced into the peripheral duct.

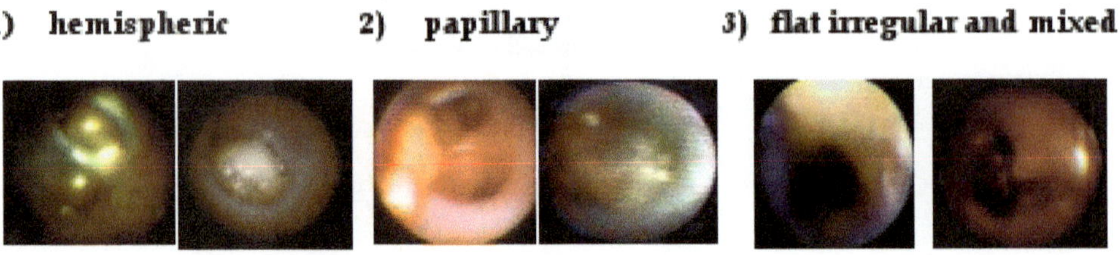

Fig. 3. Shape of intraductal lesions observed with MS. 1) Left; carcinoma, Right; IDP 2) Left; IDP, Right; cancer 3) Both cancer

Shape	total	solitary	multiple
hemispheric	6	4	2
papillary	6	4	2
flat irregular and mixed	38	16	22

Table 1. Recognition of intraductal lesions of cancer with MS

3.1.2 Ability of IDBB in obtaining specimen

IDBB was performed 38 times in 35 of 47 cancer cases in which intraductal lesions were observed. Of the 35 cases, IDBB yielded diagnostic specimens in 29 cases (82.9%) but in the remaining 6 there was insufficient material for diagnosis. With IDBB it was difficult to collect diagnostic specimens in some carcinoma cases because the lesion located periphery and low tissue cohesiveness compared with intraductal papilloma. IDBB provided a definite diagnosis of carcinoma in 15 of the 35 (42.9%), while 9 lesions were in the carcinoma suspected category (atypical papillary lesion; 25.7%) and 5 were diagnosed as intraductal papilloma (14.3%). In 4 of 5 cases which were misdiagnosed as intraductal papilloma, coexistence of intraductal papilloma and carcinoma were confirmed on the resected specimen. In these 35 cases, the sensitivity of IDBB was 68.6% (24/35), directed ductal lavage cytology was 82.8% (29/35), and conventional touch cytology was 37.1% (13/35). The sensitivity of IDBB was 82.8% limited in successful IDBB cases (24/29) and it was equal to directed ductal lavage cytology. IDBB was performed in 226 IDP lesions from 128 patients. The diagnostic specimen was obtained in 197 of 226 IDBB (87.1%) and the successful IDBB yielded IDP in all 197 cases.

3.1.3 Comparison in detecting cells cluster between each method of cytology with regard to diagnostic cell cluster

Touch cytology yielded no false positive result among the 348 patients. Twenty eight of 81 cancer cases were diagnosed as cancer or cancer suspected category. The sensitivity of touch cytology was 34.6% (28/81) and specificity was 100%. The presence of a cluster of ductal cells was the clue to take diagnostic procedure to detect intraductal papillary lesions and the method to obtain a lot of cells must be considered. Collection method and direct ductal lavage method were performed to obtain much cytologic specimen.

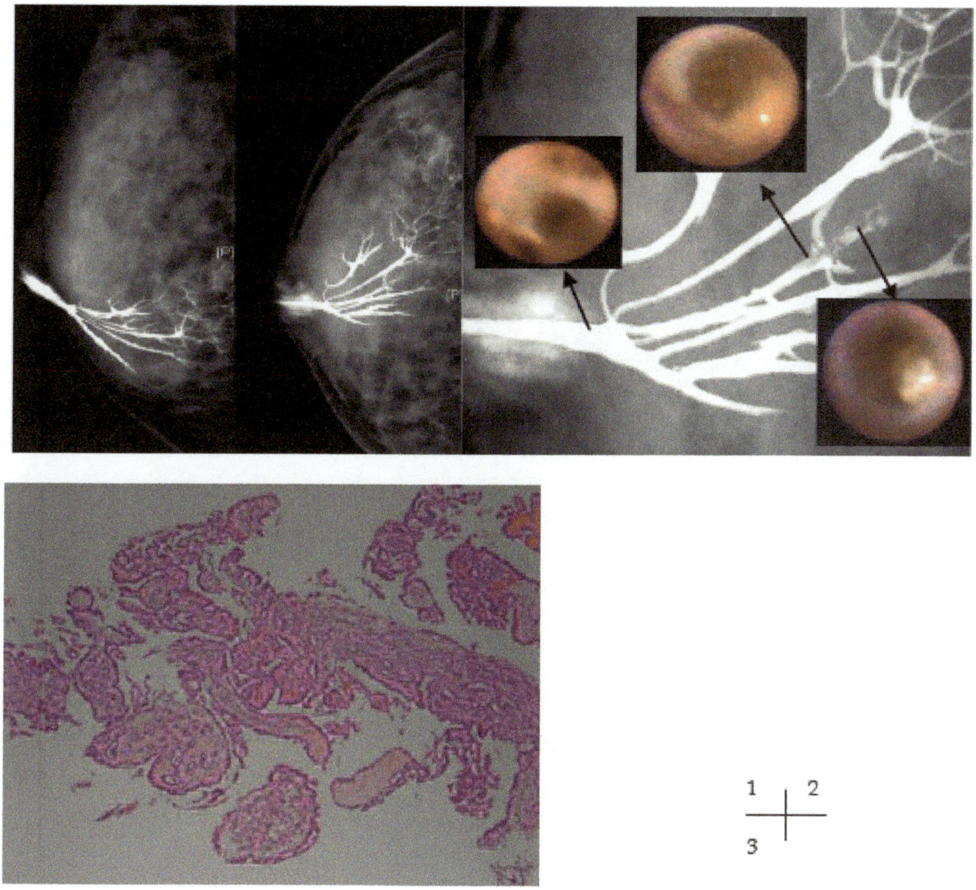

Fig. 4. A 27 years old woman with right bloody nipple discharge. 1) Galactography showed multiple filling defects in proximal brunches. 2) MS views corresponding to galactography were shown. There was intraductal papillary masses at the third bifurcation. 3) IDBB was performed to the papillary lesion at the third bifurcation and presence of large stalks and biphasic structure with mioepithelial cells were revealed. These character indicated IDP.

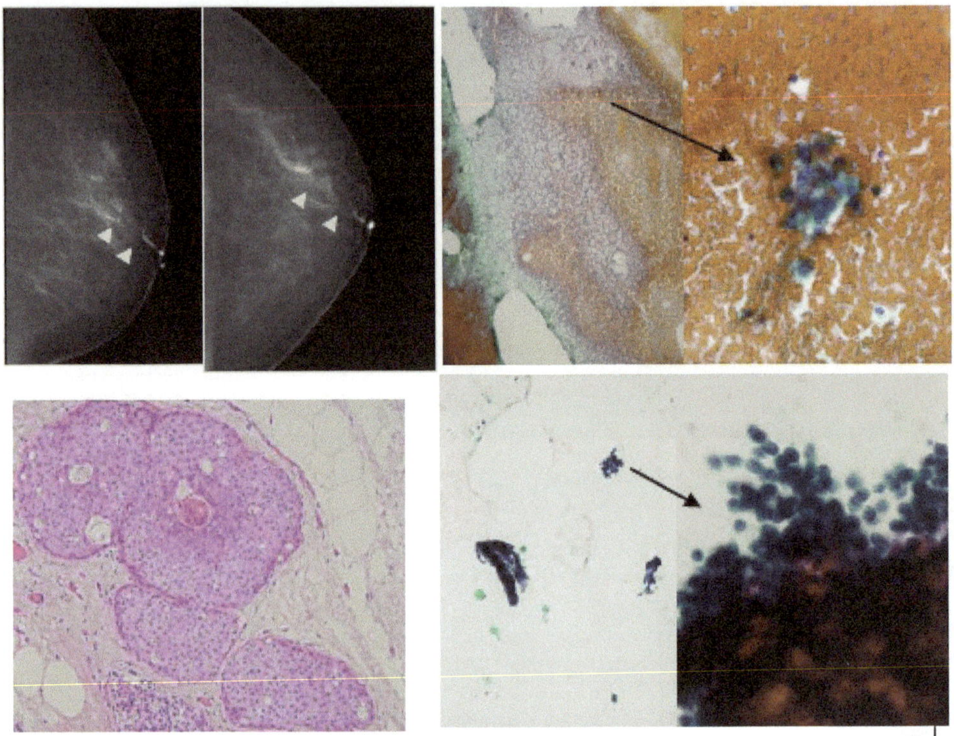

Fig. 5. A 78 years old woman with left bloody nipple discharge. 1) Galactography showed irregularity and defect of duct (arrow heads). 2) Excisional biopsy revealed DCIS, extended 8 mm in maxumum dimater with comedo~solid intraductal component. 3) Only a few cells clusters without atypia were recognized in touch cytology and diagnosed as benign. 4) MS could not be advanced into the lesion because of the narrow ductal caliber and directed ductal lavage cytology was performed. A diagnostic large papillary cells clusters were obtained by directed ductal lavage cytology and could be diagnosed as cancer.

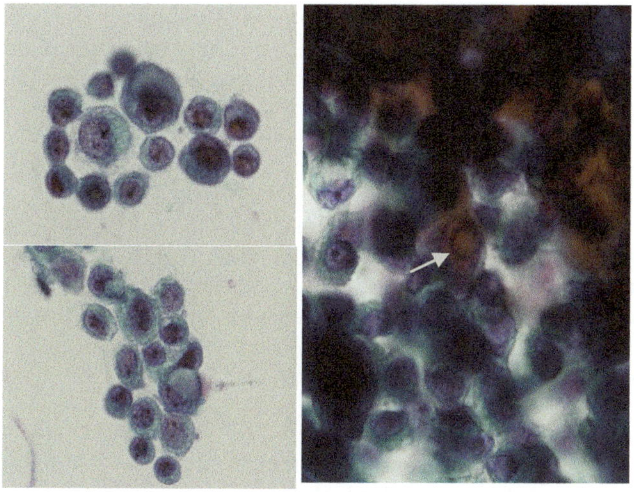

Fig. 6. Magnified view of directed lavage cytology. High NC ratio atypical cells, uneven distribution of nucleus, intranuclear enclosed body (arrow), and lack of cohesiveness were recognized.

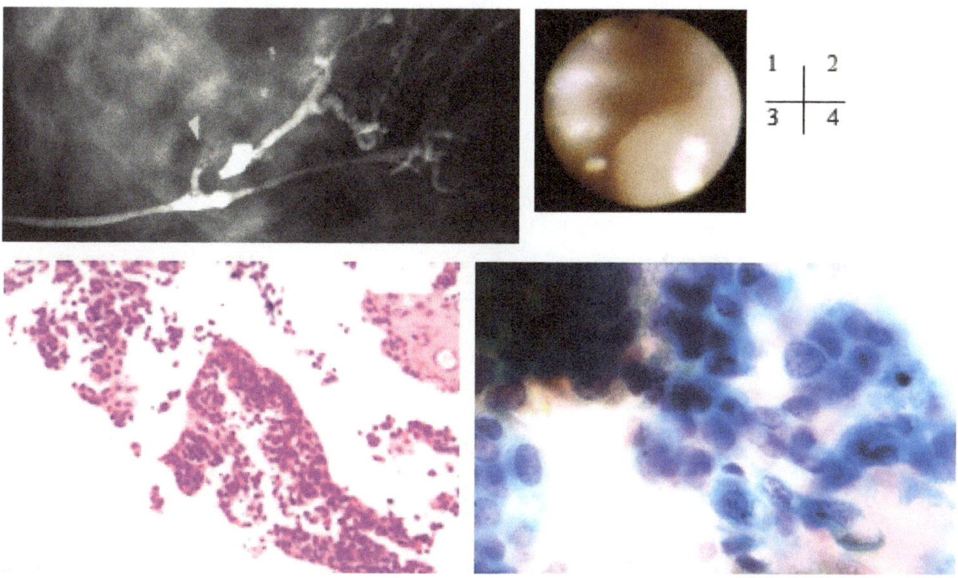

Fig. 7. A 35 years old woman with right bloody nipple discharge. 1) Galactography showed irregularity and defect at second branch (arrowhesd). 2) Hemispheric intraductal mass and flat irregulariry were observed with MS. 3) IDBB suggested atypical papillary lesion. 4) Ductal lavage cytology suggested atypical papillary lesion. Excisional biopsy was recommended for definite diagnosis but was denied. After 3 years, breast lump occurred at this area and it was proven to be cancer.

3.2.1 Comparison of the accuracy in detecting malignancy

The sensitivities of the cytologic methods differed somewhat. The collection method was applied in 243 benign cases and only one case was converted from the benign category on touch cytology to the cancer suspected category by the collection method. The rate of atypia (involving the suspicious category) increased from 35.0% in touch cytology to 37.1% in collection cytology and 84.2% in directed ductal lavage cytology. Collection and directed ductal lavage cytology were not performed when cancer was already diagnosed by a prior modality. The presence of a cluster of ductal cells indicated the presence of papillary lesion. Of 38 cases of cancer lesions, papillary clusters were detected in 37 by directed ductal lavage, (sensitivity in 97.4%). The remaining case had a mucinous intraductal component and the lesion was located beyond second bifurcation and about 4 cm length from nipple (Table2). In 35 cases who underwent IDBB, the rate of atypia was 68.6% (24/35) in IDBB, 82.8% (29/35) in directed ductal lavage cytology, and 37.1% (13/35) in conventional touch cytology.

Method	n	carcinoma	Suspicious atypical papillary	benign benign papillary	normal
Touch	81	16	12	37	16
		19.8%	14.8%	45.7%	12.3%
Collecting	70	16	10	24	20
		22.8%	14.2%	34.3%	28.6%
Lavage	38	21	11	5	1
		55.3%	28.9%	13.2%	2.6%
IDBB	35	15	9	5	insufficient; 6
		42.9%	31.4%	14.3%	

Table 2. Sensitivity of cytology and IDBB in detecting cancer

3.2.2 Sensitivity of cytology and localization of the lesions

The locations of the lesions were described as in the thoraco-bronchial tree, as the number of divergences of ductal branches approached from the nipple orifice. When cancer was recognized in a major duct (nondivergent), sensitivity of touch cytology was 73.3% (11/15). The sensitivity was 35.0% (7/20) in the first divergent branch, 35.3% in the second branch and 35.8% in the third branch and beyond. The sensitivity was extremely high only when cancer was present in a major duct (Table 3). The sensitivity of directed ductal lavage cytology was also studied in relation to the location of intraductal cancer. The sensitivity rates were 85.7% for lesions in a major duct, 75.0% for those in the first bifurcation, 72.7% beyond the second bifurcation, and 100% for those beyond the third bifurcation . The sensitivity of directed ductal lavage cytology did not depend on the location at the number of divergences of ductal branches (Table 4).

There were 15 cases in which coexistence of benign and malignant papillary lesions in the same duct-lobular unit was confirmed pathologically by sequential section slices at 3 mm of the surgically resected specimen. In these 15 cases, papillary lesions in which severe atypia was not recognized and myoepithelial cells remained in the side of proximal to the nipple orifice and ductal cancer was present in a more internal location. Coexistence of intraductal papilloma in a major duct and ductal cancers separately in a peripheral duct were recognized in 4 cases. In these 4 cases, IDBB revealed IDP in a major duct. Multiple foci of benign and malignant papillary lesions beyond the first bifurcation were recognized in 11 cases. In these 15 cases, 3 cases were positive by touch cytology (20.0%). Collection cytology was performed in 14 cases and 5 cases were positive (35.7%). Directed ductal lavage cytology was performed in 11 cases and 5 cases were positive (45.5%). IDBB was performed in 14 of these 15 cases. The coexistence of papilloma and carcinoma was confirmed by the first IDBB in a case (Fig. 9). Of these cases, the diagnosis obtained by IDBB was definitely cancer in 2, atypical papillary lesions in 4, intraductal papilloma in 5, and insufficient material in 3. In a case of a 31-year-old woman, IDBB was performed 4 times during 8 months and finally atypia was diagnosed (Fig. 10,11).

	diagnosis of cytology			
	cancer	atypia	benign	
Bifurcation			cluster+	cluster-
0	5	6	3	1
1	4	3	9	4
2	3	3	9	2
3~	4	0	16	9
Total	16	12	37	16

Table 3. Localization of intraductal lesions and sensitivity of touch cytology

	diagnosis of cytology			
	cancer	atypia	benign	
Bifurcation			cluster+	cluster-
0	3	3	1	0
1	4	2	2	0
2	4	4	2	1
3~	10	2	0	0
Total number	21	11	5	1

Table 4. Localization of intraductal lesions and sensitivity of ductal lavage cytology

3.2.3 Therapeutic effect of IDBB

Of 218 IDBB for 128 IDP patients, 197 specimens were diagnostic materials. There were 73 patients with IDP (composing a combined total of 78 lesions) who were followed for more than 5 years. Of these 73 patients, 39 experienced cessation of nipple discharge after the first IDBB and another 13 experienced cessation of nipple discharge after a subsequent IDBB. Thus the nipple discharge was halted in a total of 52 patients (71.2%). In another 5 patients, the bloody background and papillary clusters of ductal cells were not recognized after IDBB and intraductal masses could not be detected on either ductography or MS. Thus the therapeutic effectiveness of IDBB was recognized in 57 of 73 intraductal papilloma patients (78.1%). There was a tendency for lesions in the effective IDBB to be located in a major duct and hemispheric or papillary shape. There was less therapeutic efficacy of IDBB in flat lesions and in multiple nipple discharge orifices and intraductal lesions.

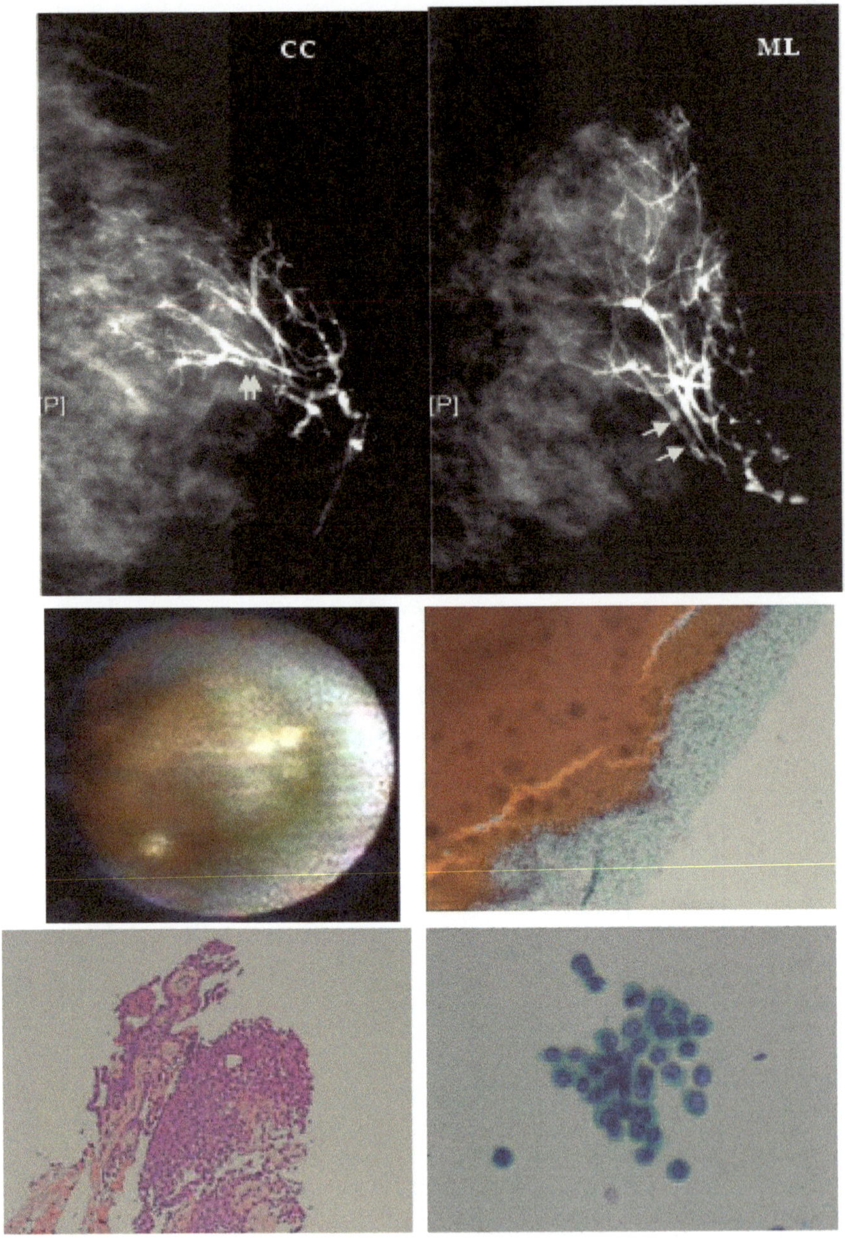

Fig. 8. A case of ductal cacer; Ductography showed defect beyond third bifurcation of the duct (upper, arrows). The hemispheric intraductal mass was detected by MS (middle, left). There was no atypical cell obtained by touch cytology (middle, right) but carcinoma was indicated by direct ductal lavage cytology and IDBB (lower left; IDBB and right; lavage cytology).

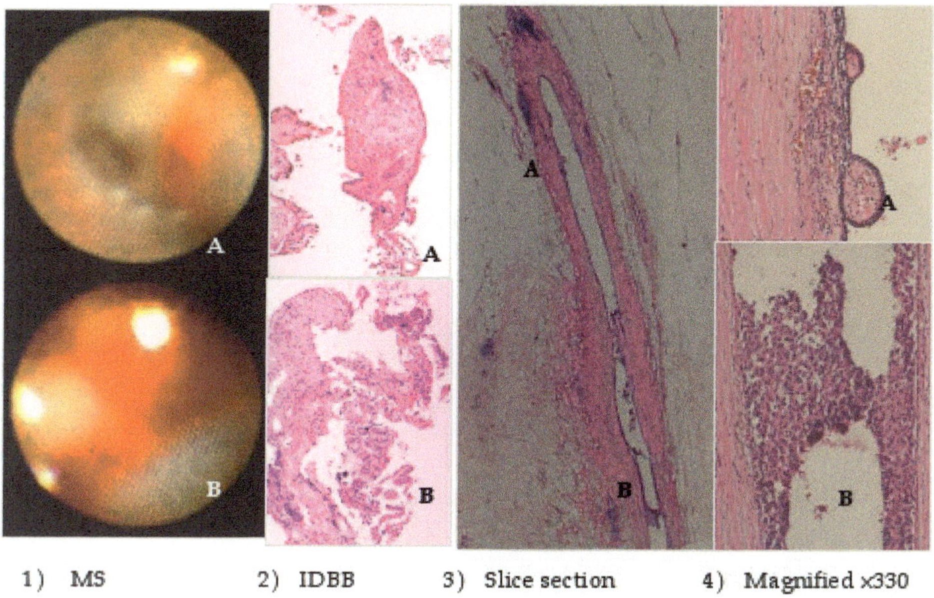

Fig. 9. 1&2) Yellow hemispherical and red papillary intraductal masses (A) were recognized in a proximal duct and were diagnosed as IDP by IDBB. A whitish-yellow flat mass coated with bloody discharge (B) was recognized distal to the site shown in A. This was diagnosed as ductal carcinoma by IDBB. 3) The slice section just on the line of the major duct in the direction of the nipple showed intraductal papilloma in the proximal duct (A; side central to the nipple) and ductal carcinoma in the disal duct (B). 4) The epithelium of the intraductal papilloma was abraded and was mechanically exfoliated by IDBB (A; HE stain, X330). Ductal cancer was recognized in the distal duct (B; HE stain, X330). In this case, the IDP was located at the proximal portion and the breast cancer was located at the distal portion to the IDP. Cancer was overlooked by discharge cytology alone. The value of MS lay in observation of the peripheral lesion by inserting the MS to the periphery beyond the proximal lesion after removing the proximal mass and biopsying the distal lesion and sampling with directed ductal lavage cytology.

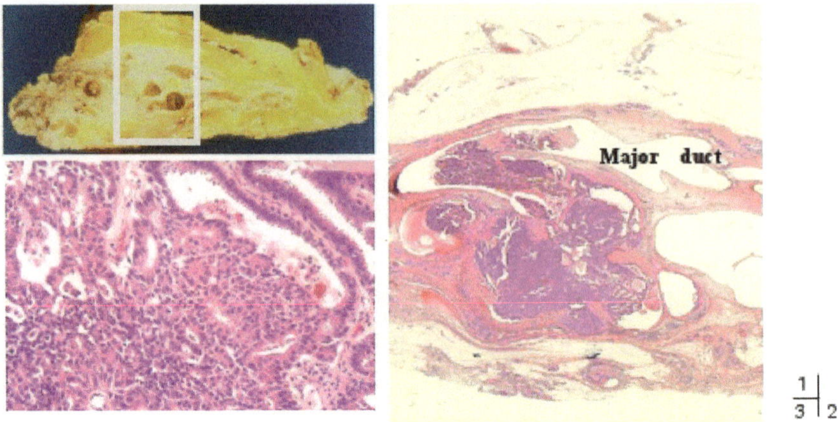

Fig. 10. 1) Section slice of intraductal lesion. The square surrounded part was the lesion concerned. 2) The slice section of major duct to the pariphery where the intraductal papillary lesion exsisted. 3) Magnification of the area of intraductal lesions in which coexsistenced biphasic (upper area) and lack of biphasic structure (lower area).

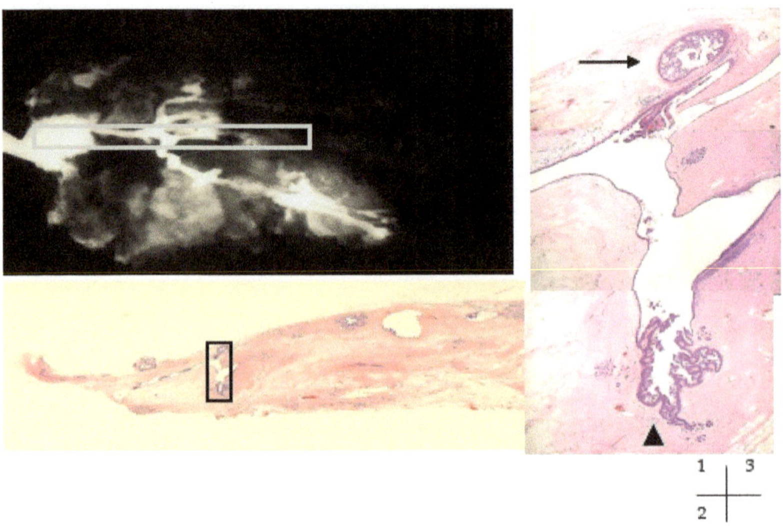

Fig. 11. 1) Specimen galactography. A 24 gage cannula was inserted into nipple orifice and the dye (methylene blue) was injected during excisional biosy (microdochectom). After excision, specimen galactography was performed. 2) The slice section just on the line of the major duct in the derection from specimen galactography (; the square surrounded part of the specimen 1). There were multiple intraductal lesions in periphery (; the square surrounded part). 3) Magnification of the area of intraductal papillary lesions. The myoepithelial cells were seen in the lesion showned with arrow head but were few in the lesion showned with arrow. The structural and cellular atypia were observed in the latter lesion. There was coexsistenced biphasic (arrow head) and lack of biphasic structure (arrow) and diagnosed as ductal cancer.

4. Discussion

Surgical excision previously was the only method available for pathological diagnosis and treatment for nipple discharge. MS contributes not only to the diagnosis of cases of nipple discharge, but also is of benefit in the treatment of IDP. The development of the MS has opened a new era in the diagnosis and treatment of secreting IDP by IDBB under direct observation. The MS helps to eliminate unnecessary surgical excision for benign lesions. Surgical excision has now been superseded by IDBB under endoscopic observation for the treatment of solitary IDP. In the previous report, neither the amount of specimen collected nor the amount of residual lesion after IDBB had a significant influence on the effect of treatment for nipple discharge. Some morphological changes after MS were also reported. It was speculated that the necrosis of IDP could be caused by the biopsy procedure. One factor related to the poor therapeutic effects of IDBB for IDP is lesion multiplicity. It was suggested that there was a tendency towards multifocal generation of intraductal papillary lesions in cases with multiple nipple orifices. Duct-lobular unit distribution patterns are infinite and all mammary ductal braches could not always be visualized by galactography. When IDP was located in a branch diverging at a sharp angle, only the proximal margin in a major duct could be detected by MS.

MS was also effective in cases of coexisting intraductal papilloma and carcinoma in the same duct-lobular unit. In these cases, the IDP is usually located at the proximal portion of the duct-lobular unit, and the breast cancer could be overlooked by discharge cytology and galactography. The value of MS in such cases lay in observation of the peripheral lesion by inserting the MS to the periphery beyond the proximal lesion or removing the proximal mass and biopsying the peripheral lesion. Thus MS finally contributed to the pathological diagnosis of intraductal masses with limited invasiveness compared with excisional biopsy.

Although IDBB is a definitive method for cancer diagnosis but the drawback of IDBB is the difficulty of obtaining diagnostic specimen. In addition, pathological diagnosis of intraductal papillary lesions was difficult in IDBB even with sufficient materials. Because of these technical defects of IDBB, the most reliable method in detecting ductal cancer was turned out to be directed ductal lavage cytology. The usefulness of cytologic specimens of nipple aspirate fluid has been reported in the evaluation of prognostic and predictive factors of breast cancer. Fluorescence in situ hybridization of ductal lavage samples was reported to be more effective in identifying malignancy. Ductal lavage was reported to detect intraductal breast cells 3.2 times more frequently than nipple aspiration but the actual cytological materials are very similar to those obtained by nipple aspiration devices. Directed ductal lavage cytology was complementary and helps to obtain most sensitive results, detecting intraductal papillary lesions in 97.4%. In only one case of mucinous intraductal component, was mucous fluid thought to be a negative factor for collecting peripheral ductal cells by lavage.

At present, the terminal duct-lobular unit from which carcinoma originates cannot be observed with MS. But MS contributes to the diagnosis of intraductal lesions through observation of the proximal portion of intraductal carcinoma and to in obtaining specimens. MS contribute the high sensitivity in cancer detection by directed ductal lavage cytology by selecting the abnormal branch to which the tube is advanced. The MS can be an important adjunct in breast-conservation management. Multiple intraductal lesions in peripheral ducts suggest cancer development. Surgical excision should be performed in patients with atypical papillary lesions revealed by IDBB or directed ductal lavage cytology. There were 2 patients in whom carcinoma was detected 3 years after IDBB showed no malignancy. Follow-up at a 6-month interval with ultrasound, checking for nipple discharge by palpation and annual mammography is considered appropriate instead of excision in patients with multiple lesions in peripheral ducts, when ductal lavage cytology showed benign result. The patients without surgical resection after IDBB showed no malignancy should be followed up as long as possible in principle (mean follow-up interval was 74.2 months; 36 to 204 months in our survey).

Cancer arises more frequently in the duct-lobular unit with bloody nipple discharge and bloody nipple discharge is thought to be an independent risk factor. Even in cases of nipple discharge with no atypia the associated relative risks for breast cancer increased compared with women who have no nipple discharge. Clinical follow-up was thought to be important to the patients with bloody nipple discharge. In previous study, carcinoma was detected in 3 patients during follow-up among 89 patients with negative MS and cytology. In these 3 patients, nipple discharge ceased after MS and carcinomas were detected at the different areas from previous galactography.

5. Conclusion

Directed ductal lavage cytology was the most sensitive method in detecting malignancy. MS and IDBB were benefit in the treatment of intraductal papilloma.

6. Acknowledgment

The author owe this work to all those who supported me. The author is indebted to Prof. Masahiko Fujii of the Department of Pathology of Kyorin University School of Health Science, Dr. Hutoshi Akiyama of the Department of Pathology of Cancer Institute Hospital, Dr. Hiromi Serizawa of the Department of Pathology of Tokyo medical University Hachioji Medical Center for pathological diagnosis and the author is grateful to the chairman of the board of directors Dr Yoshinori Nagumo for his understanding to continue this work.

7. References

Teboul, M. A new concept in breast investigation: echo-histological acino-ductal analysis or analytic echography. *Biomed & Pharmacother* 42, 1988, 282-296.

Namba, K, et al. Intraductal biopsy of the breast (IDBB) for intraductal lesions: a case of breast cancer diagnosed by IDBB. *Jpn J Breast Cancer* 4, 1989, 253-258

Makita, M, et al. Duct endoscopy and endoscopic biopsy in the evaluation of nipple discharge. *Breast Cancer Res Treat* 18, 1991, 179-188, DOI:10.1007/BF01990034

Okazaki, A, et al. Fiberoptic Ductoscopy of the Breast: a new diagnostic procedure for nipple discharge. *Jpn J Clin Oncol* 21, 1991. 188-193

Berna J, Garcia-Medina V, Kuni C: Ductoscopy: a new technique ductal exploration. *Eur J Radiol* 12, 1991. 127-129, DOI:10.1016/0720-48X(91)90112-9

Nagase, J & Endo, M. Endoscopic biopsy in the intraductal lesions of the breast for the mammary duct fiberscope. *Jpn J Breast Cancer* 10, 1995, 405-409

Love, SM & Barsky, SH. Breast-duct endoscopy to study stages of cancerous breast disease *Lancet* 348, 1996, 997-999, DOI 10.1016/S0140−6736(96)04145-1

Shen, KW, et al. Fiberoptic ductoscopy for patients with nipple discharge. *Cancer* 89, 2000, 1512-1519, DOI:10.1002/1097-0142(2000010001)89:7<1512::AID-CNCR14>3.0CO;2-L

Yamamoto, D, et al. A utility of ductography and fiberoptic ductoscopy for patients with nipple discharge. *Breast Cancer Res Treat* 70, 2001 103-108, DOI:10.1023/A:10129*90809466

Matsunaga, T, et al. Mammary ductoscopy for diagnosis and treatment of intraductal lesions of the breast. *Breast Cancer* 8, 2001, 213-221, DOI: 10.1007/BF02967511

Matsunaga, T, et al. Intraductal biopsy for diagnosis and treatment of intraductal lesions of the breast. *Cancer* 101, 2004, 2164-2169, DOI:10.1002/cncr.20657

Mtsunaga, T et al. Intraductal approach to the detection of intraductal lesions of the breast. *Breast Cancer Res Treat,* 2008118(1), 9-13, DOI:10.1007/s10549-008-0203-2

Matsunaga, T, et al. Breast cancer screening for nipple discharge: diagnostic procedure for cancer detection. *J Jpn. Assoc. Breast Cancer Screen.* 11 , 2002, 281-288

Sarakbi, WA, et al. Does mammary ductoscopy have a role in clinical practice? *Int Semin Surg Oncol.* 2006, 2006, 3-16

Danforth, DN, et al. Combined breast ductal lavage and ductal endoscopy for the evaluation of the high-risk breast: a feasibility study. *J Surg Oncol.* , 2006, 94:, 555-564

Escobar, PF, et al. The clinical applications of mammary ductoscopy. *Am J. Surg.* 191, 2006, 211-215

Ling H, et al. Fiberoptic ductoscopy-guided intraductal biopsy improve the diagnosis of nipple discharge. Breast J 15(2), 2009,168-75

Mokbel, K, et al. Mammary ductoscopy: current status and future prospects. *Eur. J Surg Oncol.* 331, 2005, 3-8

Zhi-Ming, S & Mai, N. Nipple Aspiration in diagnosis of breast cancer. *Seminars in Surgical Oncology* 20, 2001, 175-180

Dooley, WC, et al. Ductal lavage for detection of cellular atypia in woman at high risk for breast cancer. *J Natl Cancer Inst* 93, 2001, 1624-1632

Ljung, BM, et.al. Cytology of ductal lavage fluid of the breast. *Diagn. Cytopathol.* 30, 2004, 143-150

Wrensch, MR, et al. Breast cancer incidence in women with abnormal cytology in nipple aspirates of breast fluid. *Am J Epidemiol* 135, 1992 130-141

Wrensch, MR, et al. Breast cancer risk in women with abnormal cytology in nipple aspirates of breast fluid. *J Natl Cancer Inst* 93, 2001, 1791-1798

Dooley, WC. Routine operative breast endoscopy for bloody nipple discharge. *Ann Surg Oncol.* 9, 2002, 920-923

Dooley, WC. Routine operative breast endoscopy during lumpectomy. *Ann Surg Oncol.* 10, 2003 38-42

Dietz, JR, et al. Directed duct excision by using mammary ductoscopy in patients with pathologic nipple discharge. *Surgery* 132, 2002, 582-7. Doi:10.1067/msy.2002.127672

Tresserra, F, et al. Morphologic changes in breast biopsies after duct endoscopy. Breast. 10, 2001, 149-54

Wong, L, et al. Microdochectomy for single-duct nipple discharge. *Ann Acad Med Singapore* 29, 2000, 198-200

Babcock, WW. A simple operation for the discharge nipple. *Surgery* 4, 1938, 914-916

Urban, JA & Egeli, RA. Non-lactational nipple discharge. *CA Cancer J Clin* 28, 1978, 130-140

Van Zee, KJ, et al. Preoperative galactography increased the diagnostic yield of major duct excision for nipple discharge. *Cancer* 82, 1997, 1874-1880

Locker, AP, et al: Microdochectomy for single-duct discharge from the nipple. *Br J Surg* 75, 1988, 700-701

Florio MG, Manganaro T, Pollicino A, et al: Surgical approach to nipple discharge: A ten-year experience. *J Surg Oncol* 71, 1999, 235-238

Bauer, RL, et al. Ductal carcinoma in situ-associated nipple discharge: A clinical marker for locally extensive disease. *Ann Surg Oncol* 5, 1998, 452-455

Ling H, et al. Fiberoptic ductoscopy-guided intraductal biopsy improve the diagnosis of nipple discharge. *Breast J* 15(2); 2009, 168-75

14

Radiotracers for Molecular Imaging of Breast Cancer

Fan-Lin Kong and David J. Yang
Department of Experimental Diagnostic Imaging,
University of Texas MD Anderson Cancer Center, Houston, Texas
USA

1. Introduction

Breast cancer is the most prevailing malignancy among women in the world. 207,090 new cases of invasive breast cancer, along with 54,010 new cases of non-invasive types are expected to be diagnosed in women in the United States in 2010. Moreover, about 39,840 women are projected to die from this disease in the U.S in 2010. According to National Cancer Institute, the 5-year survival rate of breast cancer ranges from 23.4% in patients with stage IV to 98% in patients with stage I, highlighting the importance of early detection and diagnosis of this disease(American Cancer Society, 2010).

Molecular imaging does not only serve as an essential tool in breast cancer diagnosis and staging, but also provides significant amount of information for surgical management, radiation planning, chemotherapeutic assessment, and follow-up evaluation of patients. Currently, positron emission tomography (PET), single photon emission computed tomography (SPECT), and their combinations with CT, are major functional molecular imaging modalities used in clinic. Both PET and SPECT are based on the detection of radiolabeled ligands, termed "radiotracers", which are assumed to target tumor-specific characteristics at molecular levels. The accumulating understanding of the breast cancer molecular biology has highlighted pivotal factors that are critical for breast cancer progression, which allows researchers to select suitable targets for developing tumor-specific radiotracers. For instance, given that sustained tumor growth demands elevated glucose consumption for energy production in the lesion regions, PET radiotracer ^{18}F-labeled glucose analog ^{18}F-FDG has commonly been used to visualize the glucose metabolism of breast cancer cells(Buerkle & Weber, 2008). And yet, ^{18}F-Fluoroestradiol is used to image estrogen receptor, which is highly overexpressed in a large proportion of breast tumor tissues(Jonson & Welch, 1998). Many other radiotracers have been designed to image cell proliferation, cell apoptosis, angiogenesis and hypoxia of breast tumors. Since breast cancer treatment has become more individualized in compliance with the distinct biological characteristics of tumors from each patient, the more target-specific molecular imaging radiotracers may play a key role to guide treatment selection and evaluate treatment response in the early stages.

This chapter has firstly been focused on two major molecular imaging modalities, PET and SPECT, their principles, limitations, as well as the typical radionuclides applied for those modalities. The most commonly-used radiotracers, ^{18}F-FDG for PET and ^{99m}Tc-sestamibi for γ-imaging, have then been reviewed, respectively. In the following sections, we have discussed the radiotracers currently applied for breast cancer imaging other than ^{18}F-FDG and ^{99m}Tc-sestamibi, such as radiolabeled trastuzumab targeting HER2 receptor and ^{18}F-fluorothymidine imaging cell proliferation. Those radiotracers have been described according to the categories of the tumor-specific targets.

2. Molecular imaging modalities and radionuclides

2.1 Positron emission tomography (PET) and its radionuclides

Positron emission tomography (PET) is a 3-D nuclear medicine imaging technique, which is based on detection of the annihilation radiation emitted from a certain positron-emitting radionuclide(Buerkle & Weber, 2008). When the radionuclide decays, the positron will annihilate with an electron nearby, thus create two 511 keV photons emitted opposite to each other (180 degree). This process is called "coincidence event", which can be observed by PET detectors arranged in an array of full or partial ring around the patient body axis. Data are then reconstructed using standard algorithm. By using this coincidence-detection method, the traditional collimator of the SPECT scanner can be removed, therefore, the spatial resolution and sensitivity can be highly improved.

Commonly used PET imaging radionuclides are listed in Table 1. In order to monitor a small bioactive molecule *in vivo* without changing its chemical structure, ^{11}C is often labeled as a substitute for the stable carbon atom ^{12}C in that molecule. Given that ^{11}C has only 20 min half-life, ^{18}F can then be an alternative. In fact, ^{18}F is currently the most frequently used/developed PET radionuclide. The best example of ^{18}F-based radiotracers, ^{18}F-labeled glucose analogue ^{18}F-FDG, has been discussed in the next section. In addition to ^{11}C- and ^{18}F-labeled biomarkers, there are some other "non-targeted" radiotracers such as ^{15}O-labeled water and ^{13}N-labeled ammonia that measure blood flow in the patient body(Wijns & Camici, 1997). Moreover, copper-64 (^{64}Cu) and zirconium-89 (^{89}Zr), because of their long half-life (12.7 h and 78.4 h, respectively), have been increasingly recognized in the past decade for labeling nanoparticles or slowly localizing antibodies(DeNardo, 2005). Other than those cyclotron-produced PET radionuclides mentioned above, generator-produced gallium-68 (^{68}Ga) and rubidium-82 (^{82}Rb) have also shown high potentials in PET imaging. The advantage of in-house generator produced radionuclide is that generator itself serves as a top-of-the-bench source for short half-life radionuclides in the places that are located far from the cyclotron facility. Besides, it is quite simple to obtain radionuclides from the generator, and less expensive compared to cyclotron-produced radionuclides.

2.2 Single photon emission computed tomography (SPECT) and its radionuclides

Single photon emission computed tomography (SPECT) is a widely used nuclear medicine imaging modality, which utilizes radiotracers emitting gamma-ray photons directly from the labeling radionuclide. The energy of the radionuclide is generally from 70 to 364 keV (Table 2). A typical SPECT system consists of one or more rotating gamma camera(s) to obtain multiple projection images from different views around the patient, and a computer algorithm for 3D image reconstruction. A collimator is required to collect the γ-ray photons that only are emitted from the patient body in a particular direction(Benard & Turcotte, 2005).

Radionuclide	Half-life	Production
^{11}C	20.4 min	Cyclotron
^{13}N	9.97 min	Cyclotron
^{15}O	2.03 min	Cyclotron
^{18}F	109.7 min	Cyclotron
^{64}Cu	12.8 h	Cyclotron
^{89}Zr	78.4 h	Cyclotron
^{68}Ga	68 min	Generator
^{82}Rb	1.25 min	Generator

Table 1. Radionuclides commonly used in PET imaging.

Radionuclide	Decay Mode	Half-life	Emitted Photon Energy [keV]
^{99m}Tc	IT	6.01 h	140 (87.7%)
^{201}Tl	EC	73.0 h	71 (47%), 135 (3%), 167 (10%)
^{123}I	EC	13.2 h	159 (83.3%)
^{131}I	B^-	8.02 d	364 (81.2%)
^{111}In	EC	67.4 h	171(90.3%), 245 (94%)
^{67}Ga	EC	78.3 h	93 (37%), 184 (20.4%), 300 (16.6%)

Table 2. Radionuclides commonly used in SPECT imaging (IT: isomeric transition, EC: electron capture).

Technetium-99m (^{99m}Tc, $t_{1/2}$=6.02 h) is the most common radionuclide for SPECT imaging. It emits a 140 keV gamma ray in 89% abundance, which can be detected by NaI detectors. In addition, it is produced with in-house generator that contains the parent nuclide molybdenum-99 (^{99}Mo), and does not require the cyclotron. Since the chemistry of diagnostic radionuclide ^{99m}Tc is very similar to that of the therapeutic radioisotope rhenium-188 (^{188}Re), they could be labeled to the same ligand, which leads to the diagnostic/therapeutic matched pair(Schechter et al., 2007).

Although the resolution and sensitivity of SPECT is not as good as PET scan due to its physical nature, SPECT and SPECT/CT still play important and irreplaceable roles in nuclear imaging area. First of all, SPECT radiopharmaceuticals are comparatively easier and less costly to produce. In addition, given that most SPECT radionuclides have longer half-life than PET radionuclides, SPECT offers more possibility to broaden the observational time window that allows the doctors to monitor biological processes *in vivo* several hours or even days after radiopharmaceutical administration. Furthermore, only limited facilities around the world can afford complete armamentarium of PET instruments and cyclotron for the local production of short-lived positron-emitters. Clinical data have shown that 15.9 million SPECT procedures were performed in 2007, while only 1.6 million of PET procedures were performed, in comparison(Mariani et al., 2008).

3. The most common radiotracers for breast cancer imaging in clinic

3.1 ^{18}F-FDG for PET/CT and PEM (positron emission mammography)

In recent years, ^{18}F-fluoro-deoxy-glucose (^{18}F-FDG), which is an ^{18}F-labeled analog of glucose, has become the most common and attractive radiotracer for PET scans. Both ^{18}F-FDG and glucose are transported across the cell membrane by glucose transporters. ^{18}F-FDG is phosphorylated by hexokinase to ^{18}F-FDG-6-phosphate while glucose is phosphorylated to glucose-6-phosphate. Unlike glucose-6-phosphate, ^{18}F-FDG-6-phosphate cannot be further metabolized, and therefore, is trapped and accumulates steadily in the tumor cells(Buerkle & Weber, 2008). Hence, ^{18}F-FDG is able to provide high sensitivity and specificity for detecting, staging, and restaging tumors by imaging high glucose metabolic rates in tumor cells. For breast cancer cells, increased glucose utilization is caused by the overexpression of glucose transporters Glut-1/3 and increased hexokinase activity. The rate-limiting step in the uptake of ^{18}F-FDG in breast cancer appears to be the phosphorylation process by hexokinase, particularly hexokinase I(Buck et al., 2004).

Although ^{18}F-FDG-PET generally has high sensitivity and specificity in detecting malignancies, whole-body ^{18}F-FDG-PET is not quite suitable for primary breast cancer diagnosis, especially for the low grade tumors and tumors with a size less than 1 cm in diameter(Lim et al., 2007). In addition, it is not appropriate for breast cancer screening as well. Therefore, ^{18}F-FDG with positron emission mammography (PEM) has been introduced as an alternative. In comparison with PET, PEM has a much higher spatial resolution by putting two opposite detector heads on each side of the breast and thus minimizing the distance between radiation source and the detectors. Schilling *et al.* have reported that PEM can detect tumor as small as 1.5 mm in diameter, with much less breast compression compared to traditional mammography(Schilling et al., 2011). They have also indicated that PEM is not affected by breast density and it has good sensitivity (90%) in detecting ductal carcinoma *in situ* (DCIS), which cannot be detected by PET very well.

For breast cancer logoregional staging, ^{18}F-FDG-PET has shown high sensitivity in axillary staging of late-stage cancer patients, but not sensitive enough in detecting the early-stage micrometastases and small tumor-infiltrated axillary lymph nodes(Aukema et al., 2010). Therefore, ^{18}F-FDG-PET is not sufficient to replace the sentinel lymph node (SLN) biopsy in this case. Instead, ^{18}F-FDG-PET appears to be suitable for distant (systemic) staging, as well as for staging locally advanced breast cancer (LABC) because LABC usually has large primary tumor (> 5 cm in diameter) or advanced axillary disease without clinically apparent distant metastases(Mahner et al., 2008). Moreover, several studies have demonstrated that

^{18}F-FDG-PET is superior to traditional bone scintigraphy in the detection of osteolytic and intramedullary metastases but inferior in the detection of primary osteoblastic lesions(Schirrmeister, 2007).

An increasing number of studies have been performed to evaluate treatment response using ^{18}F-FDG-PET. Although ^{18}F-FDG has not been recommended as a routine assessment agent yet, it has been proven to be an accurate early predictor of poor response to therapy. Patients with a high ^{18}F-FDG uptake associated with low blood flow/perfusion rate in their tumors were more likely to have poor response and early relapse(Tseng et al., 2004).

3.2 ^{99m}Tc-sestamibi for scintimammography and BSGI (breast-specific γ-imaging)

^{99m}Tc-methoxyisobutylisonitrile (^{99m}Tc-MIBI or ^{99m}Tc-sestamibi) scintimammography has been increasingly used to assess the suspicious lesions of patients with a negative or indeterminate mammography in the clinic(Filippi et al., 2006). This small lipophilic cation was originally developed as a myocardial perfusion agent. The first report of its application in breast cancer detection was by Aktolun *et al.* in 1992(Aktolun et al., 1992). The cellular uptake mechanisms of ^{99m}Tc-sestamibi still remain unclear; however, its uptake is driven by a negative transmembrane potential and most of the radioactivity is found in the mitochondria(Scopinaro et al., 1994). ^{99m}Tc-sestamibi scintimammography shows higher sensitivity (85%) and specificity (87%) than the traditional mammography, and its sensitivity is independent of breast density(Liberman et al., 2003). In addition, ^{99m}Tc-sestamibi is a substrate of the transmembrane P-glycoprotein (Pgp), which is a member of the MDR/TAP subfamily that is involved in the multidrug resistance. Therefore, the uptake, clearance, and retention of ^{99m}Tc-sestamibi have been investigated as predictors of response to chemotherapy in human breast cancer(Kim et al., 2006). In a study of 45 patients with primary breast cancer, Cayre *et al* concluded that a negative ^{99m}Tc-sestamibi scintimammography predicted chemoresistance with a specificity of 100%. Besides, ^{99m}Tc-sestamibi uptake was inversely correlated to the expression of multidrug resistance protein MDR1 ($P<0.05$) in invasive ductal carcinomas(Cayre et al., 2002).

Nevertheless, ^{99m}Tc-sestamibi scintimammography demonstrates relatively low sensitivity in detecting the nonpalpable lesions or tumors smaller than 1 cm. Therefore, the high resolution small field-of-view breast-specific γ-imaging (BSGI) has been developed as an alternative. Similar to PEM, the single-head detector used in BSGI is mounted opposite to a compression plate, so the patient's breast is compressed between detector and plate. According to a 6-year BSGI study performed by Hruska *et al.* at Mayo Clinic, the sensitivity of BSGI for tumors larger than 1 cm was 97%, while that for tumors smaller than 1 cm was 74%(Hruska et al., 2008). When compare BSGI with PEM, although the average sensitivity of PEM (93%) is slightly higher than that of BSGI (89%), BSGI has a much higher negative predictive value (100%) than that of PEM (88%)(Ferrara, 2010). Thus, both of the imaging modalities have great detection ability in existing studies, and there is no proven clinically significant advantage to either modality over the other so far.

4. Other radiotracers imaging breast cancer molecular biomarkers

4.1 Radiotracer targeting hormone receptors

^{18}F-Fluoroestradiol (^{18}F-FES) targets Estrogen receptor (ER)

More than 70% of the breast tumors are positive for hormone receptors such as estrogen receptor (ER+), and ER-directed breast cancer therapeutic agents such as tamoxifen and aromatase inhibitors are highly effective to these patients with fewer side effects, while compared to the traditional chemotherapy(Oude Munnink et al., 2009). To date, ^{18}F-16α-17β-fluoroestradiol (^{18}F-FES) has been proven to be the most successful PET radiotracer in determining ER status and prognosis of ER-directed hormonal therapy in breast cancer patients(Jonson & Welch, 1998).

For clinical use, an automated synthesis of ^{18}F-FES can be achieved in a decay-corrected yield of 30% at 60 minutes after end of bombardment with high radiochemical purity (>99%)(Romer et al., 2001). ^{18}F-FES has a high binding affinity to ER, especially the ERα subtype(Yoo et al., 2005). In both human and rodents, ^{18}F-FES is rapidly taken up and metabolized by the liver. By 20 min after injection, 80% of the ^{18}F-FES is converted to radiolabeled glucuronide and sulfate conjugates in blood. The recommended injection dose and imaging time of ^{18}F-FES is 6mCi at 30 min after injection(Sundararajan et al., 2007). Peterson *et al* demonstrated excellent agreement (r=0.99) between ^{18}F-FES-PET and ER expression assayed by immunohistochemistry (IHC) in 17 patients. In addition, their study indicated that ER- tumors in those patients had partial-volume-corrected SUV of less than 1.0, while that of ER+ tumors were above 1.1(Peterson et al., 2008).

4.2 Radiotracers imaging HER 2

Radiolabled trastuzumab

Human epidermal growth factor receptor 2 (HER2) is a transmembrane glycoprotein that forms heterodimers with other EGFR family members to activate distinct signaling pathways, which are involved in cell growth, survival, differentiation, adhesion, and migration. HER2 has been found to be overexpressed in many types of cancers. For breast cancer patients, about 25-30% of breast tumors have HER2/*neu* gene amplification and/or HER2 protein overexpression(Moasser, 2007). Therefore, HER2 has become an attractive target for breast cancer imaging and treatment. The humanized monoclonal antibody trastuzumab has been successfully used for HER2-positive breast cancer treatment. By labeling trastuzumab with different radionuclides, we can assess the HER2 expression and localization in breast cancer patients non-invasively, and thus, select the patients with HER2-positive tumors that are qualified for trastuzumab treatment(Capala & Bouchelouche, 2010).

Zirconium-89 (^{89}Zr; $t_{1/2}$= 78.41 h) has been chosen for trastuzumab labeling because it has the longest half-life among the positron-emitting radionuclides, which allows PET imaging up to 7 days after injection(Holland et al., 2009). The antibodies like trastuzumab often have high molecular weight, thus slow metabolism and clearance. Hence, longer half-life radionuclides are more suitable to obtain better tumor-to-blood ratios even several days post injection. Dijkers *et al* have performed their first clinical trial of ^{89}Zr-trastuzumab PET in 14 patients with HER2-positive metastatic breast cancer. They have determined the optimal imaging time and dose as 4-5 days post injection and 50 mg dose for trastuzumab-naïve patients or 10 mg dose for patients already on trastuzumab treatment, respectively(Dijkers et al., 2010). Other than ^{89}Zr, trastuzumab has also been labeled with ^{124}I, ^{86}Y, and ^{76}Br for PET(Orlova et al., 2009; Winberg et al., 2004; Xu et al., 2007). In addition, the antibody has been labeled with ^{111}In for SPECT imaging(Sampath et al., 2007). To date, only ^{89}Zr and ^{111}In-labeled trastuzumab have been applied to human in the clinical trials. Although the tumor uptake levels of ^{89}Zr-trastuzumab and ^{111}In-trastuzumab were similar, ^{89}Zr-labled counterpart demonstrated better image quality due to higher spatial resolution and sensitivity of PET.

4.3 Radiotracer imaging cell proliferation

^{18}F-fluorothymidine (18F-FLT)

^{18}F-fluoro-3′-deoxy-3′-L-fluorothymidine (^{18}F-FLT) is a nucleoside-based radiotracer that was developed to target DNA replication and cell proliferation in tumors in 1998(Shields et al., 1998). ^{18}F-FLT enters the tumor cells mainly by Na^+-dependent active nucleoside transporters, which are generally upregulated in tumor cells(Reske & Deisenhofer, 2006). The same as thymidine, ^{18}F-FLT follows the salvage pathway of DNA synthesis and undergoes phosphorylation by thymidine kinase 1 (TK1). Since the 3′-hydroxyl group is converted to 3′-fluorine, ^{18}F-FLT cannot be incorporated into DNA and is trapped in cytosol(Seitz et al., 2002). Therefore, the rate-limiting step for ^{18}F-FLT-PET imaging is phosphorylation by TK1. TK1 has little activity in the quiescent cells but increased activity in proliferating cells, especially in the cells in S-phase(Munch-Petersen et al., 1995).

In clinical studies, ^{18}F-FLT-PET is commonly used in detecting brain tumor given its low uptake in the normal brain tissue(Spence et al., 2009). The high uptake in bone marrow and liver limits its diagnostic application especially in the assessment of liver and bone matastases. Besides, ^{18}F-FLT-PET is not superior to ^{18}F-FDG for cancer staging due to its low tumor-to-background ratios. Therefore, the imaging potential of ^{18}F-FLT in breast cancer has been evaluated more often in the prediction and assessment of tumor response to a certain treatment. For instance, Pio *et al* scanned 14 breast cancer patients before and two weeks after the first cycle of the treatment, and found out that ^{18}F-FLT uptake was strongly correlated with percentage change in CA27.29 tumor marker levels ($r = 0.79$; $p = 0.001$). In addition, the ^{18}F-FLT uptake change after the chemotherapy course was predictive of late change in tumor size ($r = 0.74$; $p = 0.01$) as measured by CT scans(Pio et al., 2006). In a more recent study, Kenny *et al* assessed ^{18}F-FLT response to a combined chemotherapy using 5-fluorouracil, epirubicin, and cyclophosphamide in 13 breast cancer patients with 17 discrete lesions. Their observations indicated a significant difference in ^{18}F-FLT uptake change between the responders and non-responders. The average decrease in responding lesions at 90 min were 41.3% for SUV and 52.9% for Ki (net irreversible plasma to tumor transfer constant), while those of non-responding lesions were 3.1% and 1.9%, respectively(Kenny et al., 2007).

To meet the clinical application needs, however, significant improvements are required in^{18}F-FLT radiosynthesis. So far, there are two synthesis methods using different precursors, but neither could achieve an optimal radiochemical yield within a short preparation time. By using precursor 3′-O-nosyl thymidine with its pyrimidine ring protected with N-BOC, Yun *et al* achieved a high radiochemical yield of 42±5.4% within 60 min in a radiochemical purity >97%(Yun et al., 2003). On the other hand, Machulla *et al* used 5′-O-(4,4′-dimethoxytriphenylmethyl)-2,3′-anhydrothymidine (DMTThy) as the precursor to achieve the preparation time within 10 min at 160°C, however, the radiochemical yield was only 14.3±3.3%(Machulla et al., 2000).

4.4 Radiotracers imaging amino acid transporters and protein synthesis

^{11}C/^{99m}Tc-methionine

Amino acid-based radiotracers are developed for tumor imaging based on the fact that tumor cells uptake and consume more amino acids to sustain their uncontrolled growth compared with the normal cells. Most of those radiotracers are reported to enter the tumor cells via amino acid transporters, such as Na^+-independent L-type amino acid transporter system LAT, and Na^+-dependent transport systems A and B^0(Jager et al., 2001).

^{11}C-methionine (^{11}C-MET) can be synthesized with an automation module within 20 min after the bombardment in a radiochemical yield of >30%. The specific activity was 3.3 Ci/mmol, and the radiochemical purity was >96%(Davis et al., 1982). ^{11}C-MET has recently been evaluated by Lindholm *et al* for its potential in assessing early response to therapy in advanced breast cancer. Twenty-five out of 26 metastatic sites from 13 patients could be detected by ^{11}C-MET-PET. The standard uptake value (SUV) in all six responding metastatic sites decreased by 30-54% ($P < 0.05$), while that of non-responding sites did not decrease significantly (11-13%; P =NS)(Lindholm et al., 2009).

On the other hand, ^{99m}Tc-labeld methionine has also been successfully used to detect breast cancer in a recent clinical trial performed by Sharma *et al.* ^{99m}Tc-methionine is proven to have the same biological properties as ^{11}C-methionine, but the longer half-life of in-house generator-produced radioisotope ^{99m}Tc ($t_{1/2}$ =6 h) provides a more simple and affordable way to image breast tumor using conventional scintimammography. ^{99m}Tc-methionine was synthesized by conjugating methionine with diethylene triamine pentaacetic acid and ^{99m}Tc, and the radiochemical yield was >95%. The sensitivity, specificity, and positive predictive value of ^{99m}Tc-methionine in this clinical trial with 47 patients were 87.8%, 92.8%, and 96.6%, respectively(Sharma et al., 2009).

4.5 Radiotracers imaging angiogenesis

Radiolabeled RGD peptides

Angiogenesis, which stands for the formation of new blood vessels, is required for solid tumor to obtain essential oxygen and nutrients for growth. Integrins, one kind of glycoproteins located on the cell surface, are extremely important in angiogenesis to mediate cell-cell or cell-extracellular matrix interactions(Takada et al., 2007). There are 24 integrins being reported up to date; among these, integrin $\alpha_V\beta3$ is the best-studied subtype as the molecular marker for targeting angiogenic cascade. A small peptide sequence consists of arginine-glycine-aspartic acid (RGD) has been identified as the motif of integrins for binding to their α_V subunit, including $\alpha_V\beta3$(Ruoslahti & Pierschbacher, 1987). Several radiolabled RGD peptides have been developed to image breast tumors in human. Here, two major radiotracers are introduced, ^{99m}Tc-NC100692 for SPECT imaging and ^{18}F-galacto-RGD for PET imaging.

NC100692 is a cyclic synthetic ligand containing RGD binding site with high affinity to $\alpha_V\beta3$ and $\alpha_V\beta5$, which are upregulated during angiogenesis. ^{99m}Tc-NC100692 is currently under Phase II clinical trial by GE healthcare. In the study performed by Bach-Gansmo *et al*, 19 out of 22 malignant lesions from 20 breast cancer patients were detected by ^{99m}Tc-NC100692 scintigraphy (86%)(Bach-Gansmo et al., 2006). In the Phase 2a study performed by Axelsson *et al*, ^{99m}Tc-NC100692 scintigraphy detected 1 out of 7 liver, 4 out of 5 lung, 8 out of 17 bone, and 1 out of 1 brain metastases in 10 patients with breast cancer(Axelsson et al., 2010).

^{18}F-galacto-RGD was first developed by Haubner *et al* in 2001(Haubner et al., 2001). By adding a sugar amino acid to the RGD peptide, the lipophilicity of the tracer could be reduced, which resulted in less uptake in liver and increased uptake in tumor. The overall radiochemical yield of ^{18}F-galacto-RGD was 29±5%, and the purity was >98%(Haubner et al., 2004). Beer *et al* performed ^{18}F-galacto-RGD-PET in 16 patients with invasive ductal breast cancer in 2007. All of the invasive carcinomas could be identified (SUV = 3.6±1.8, tumor-to-muscle ratios = 6.2±2.2), however, only 3 out of 8 lymph node metastases were detected(Beer et al., 2008). In addition, ^{18}F-galacto-RGD images were found to represent the mixture of $\alpha_V\beta3$ expressed in both tumor cells and endothelial cells, so the agent was not tumor specific. According to several preclinical and clinical studies, ^{18}F-galacto-RGD-PET may not be suitable to differentiate tumor from inflammation, because $\alpha_V\beta3$ is also highly expressed in the macrophages and other inflammatory lesions(Gaertner et al., 2010).

4.6 Radiotracers for bone scan

^{99m}Tc-methylene diphosphonate (^{99m}Tc-MDP)

The most common site of breast cancer metastases is bone, mainly spine and pelvis. The distribution of bone metastases is a prognostic factor of breast cancer(Hamaoka et al., 2004). Bone scintigraphy using ^{99m}Tc-methylene diphosphonate (^{99m}Tc-MDP) is the standard initial imaging technique to assess bone metastases. The uptake mechanism of ^{99m}Tc-MDP in bone is the chemical absorption onto the surface of hydroxyapatite and then incorporation into the crystalline structure of hydroxyapatite(Kanishi, 1993). The specificity and sensitivity of ^{99m}Tc-MDP bone scintigraphy for breast cancer bone metastases are 78-100% and 62-100%, respectively(Hamaoka et al., 2004). Since its detection rate in early stages breast cancer patient is very low (0.82% for stage I disease), the routine screening is only recommended to patients in advanced stages(Yeh et al., 1995). In addition, ^{99m}Tc-MDP bone scintigraphy may not be suitable to monitor hormonal therapy response because of the increased ^{99m}Tc-MDP uptake caused by new bone formation during the repair process after the therapy ("flare phenomenon")(Mortimer et al., 2001). In summary, given its high availability and affordability, as well as its rapid generation of whole-body images, the advantage of bone scintigraphy is rather for screening the patient with late stage (III and IV) breast cancer, than diagnosis. Instead of bone scintigraphy, ^{99m}Tc-MDP using SPECT or SPECT/CT is more suitable for the diagnosis of breast cancer bone metastases given its higher resolution and accuracy. The specificity and sensitivity of ^{99m}Tc-MDP-SPECT are 91-93% and 87-92%, respectively(Han et al., 1998).

^{18}F-fluoride

^{18}F-labeled sodium fluoride (^{18}F-fluoride) is a non-specific PET radiotracer for whole-body bone metastases imaging. Its uptake is via the exchange of hydroxyl ions in the hydroxyapatite crystal, mainly at the surface of the skeleton(Hawkins et al., 1992). ^{18}F-fluoride PET has higher resolution, sensitivity (99%) and specificity (97%) than ^{99m}Tc-MDP-SPECT(Even-Sapir et al., 2004). Besides, the absolute uptake of ^{18}F-fluoride in normal bone was twice as high as that of ^{99m}Tc-MDP. Although ^{18}F-fluoride is not tumor-specific, it can differentiate tumor from benign tissues better than ^{99m}Tc-MDP bone scintigraphy thanks to the superior spatial resolution of PET scanner. Among all the benign abnormalities detected by ^{18}F-fluoride PET, 80% are caused by endplate factures and arthritis of the articular facets, both of which have a typical uptake pattern of ^{18}F-fluoride(Schirrmeister et al., 1998). In ^{18}F-fluoride PET images, lesions that are not located at joint surfaces are suspicious for metastases. In addition, the lesions that do not show the typical pattern of endplate fracture, osteophytes, or serial rib fractures are suspicious for metastases as well.

5. Conclusion

Molecular imaging such as PET and SPECT plays an important role in non-invasive breast cancer diagnosis, staging, and treatment response evaluation. In this chapter, we have focused on introducing the radiotracers commonly used in molecular imaging of breast cancer, according to the classification of the tumor-specific characteristics to which they are targeting. To date, ^{18}F-FDG and ^{99m}Tc-sestamibi are still the two most extensively used radiopharmaceuticals in breast cancer for PET and γ-imaging, respectively. The advances in molecular cancer biology have led to an increased understanding of the cancer biomarkers that contribute to cancer progression, and thus led to the rapid development of more personalized and specifically tumor-targeted treatments. There is an increasing demand on molecular imaging and tracer development to help direct and assess the treatment response in an early stage.

6. References

Aktolun, C., Bayhan, H. & Kir, M. (1992). "Clinical experience with Tc-99m MIBI imaging in patients with malignant tumors. Preliminary results and comparison with Tl-201." *Clin Nucl Med* 17(3): 171-176

American Cancer Society. (2010, n.d.). "Breast Cancer Facts & Figures 2009-2010." from http://www.cancer.org/acs/groups/content/@nho/documents/document/f861009final90809pdf.pdf.

Aukema, T. S., Rutgers, E. J., Vogel, W. V., Teertstra, H. J., Oldenburg, H. S., Vrancken Peeters, M. T., Wesseling, J., Russell, N. S. & Valdes Olmos, R. A. (2010). "The role of FDG PET/CT in patients with locoregional breast cancer recurrence: a comparison to conventional imaging techniques." *Eur J Surg Oncol* 36(4): 387-392

Axelsson, R., Bach-Gansmo, T., Castell-Conesa, J. & McParland, B. J. (2010). "An open-label, multicenter, phase 2a study to assess the feasibility of imaging metastases in late-stage cancer patients with the alpha v beta 3-selective angiogenesis imaging agent 99mTc-NC100692." *Acta Radiol* 51(1): 40-46

Bach-Gansmo, T., Danielsson, R., Saracco, A., Wilczek, B., Bogsrud, T. V., Fangberget, A., Tangerud, A. & Tobin, D. (2006). "Integrin receptor imaging of breast cancer: a proof-of-concept study to evaluate 99mTc-NC100692." *J Nucl Med* 47(9): 1434-1439

Beer, A. J., Niemeyer, M., Carlsen, J., Sarbia, M., Nahrig, J., Watzlowik, P., Wester, H. J., Harbeck, N. & Schwaiger, M. (2008). "Patterns of alphavbeta3 expression in primary and metastatic human breast cancer as shown by 18F-Galacto-RGD PET." *J Nucl Med* 49(2): 255-259

Benard, F. & Turcotte, E. (2005). "Imaging in breast cancer: Single-photon computed tomography and positron-emission tomography." *Breast Cancer Res* 7(4): 153-162

Buck, A. K., Schirrmeister, H., Mattfeldt, T. & Reske, S. N. (2004). "Biological characterisation of breast cancer by means of PET." *Eur J Nucl Med Mol Imaging* 31 Suppl 1: S80-87

Buerkle, A. & Weber, W. A. (2008). "Imaging of tumor glucose utilization with positron emission tomography." *Cancer Metastasis Rev* 27(4): 545-554

Capala, J. & Bouchelouche, K. (2010). "Molecular imaging of HER2-positive breast cancer: a step toward an individualized 'image and treat' strategy." *Curr Opin Oncol* 22(6): 559-566

Cayre, A., Cachin, F., Maublant, J., Mestas, D., Feillel, V., Ferriere, J. P., Kwiaktowski, F., Chevillard, S., Finat-Duclos, F., Verrelle, P. & Penault-Llorca, F. (2002). "Single static view 99mTc-sestamibi scintimammography predicts response to neoadjuvant chemotherapy and is related to MDR expression." *Int J Oncol* 20(5): 1049-1055

Davis, J., Yano, Y., Cahoon, J. & Budinger, T. F. (1982). "Preparation of 11C-methyl iodide and L-[S-methyl-11C]methionine by an automated continuous flow process." *Int J Appl Radiat Isot* 33(5): 363-369

DeNardo, S. J. (2005). "Radioimmunodetection and therapy of breast cancer." *Semin Nucl Med* 35(2): 143-151

Dijkers, E. C., Oude Munnink, T. H., Kosterink, J. G., Brouwers, A. H., Jager, P. L., de Jong, J. R., van Dongen, G. A., Schroder, C. P., Lub-de Hooge, M. N. & de Vries, E. G. (2010). "Biodistribution of 89Zr-trastuzumab and PET imaging of HER2-positive lesions in patients with metastatic breast cancer." *Clin Pharmacol Ther* 87(5): 586-592

Even-Sapir, E., Metser, U., Flusser, G., Zuriel, L., Kollender, Y., Lerman, H., Lievshitz, G., Ron, I. & Mishani, E. (2004). "Assessment of malignant skeletal disease: initial experience with 18F-fluoride PET/CT and comparison between 18F-fluoride PET and 18F-fluoride PET/CT." *J Nucl Med* 45(2): 272-278

Ferrara, A. (2010). "Nuclear imaging in breast cancer." *Radiol Technol* 81(3): 233-246

Filippi, L., Pulcini, A., Remediani, S., Masci, E., Redler, A., Scopinaro, F. & De Vincentis, G. (2006). "Usefulness of scintimammography with tc-99m MIBI in clinical practice." *Clin Nucl Med* 31(12): 761-763

Gaertner, F. C., Schwaiger, M. & Beer, A. J. (2010). "Molecular imaging of avb3 expression in cancer patients." *Q J Nucl Med Mol Imaging*

Hamaoka, T., Madewell, J. E., Podoloff, D. A., Hortobagyi, G. N. & Ueno, N. T. (2004). "Bone imaging in metastatic breast cancer." *J Clin Oncol* 22(14): 2942-2953

Han, L. J., Au-Yong, T. K., Tong, W. C., Chu, K. S., Szeto, L. T. & Wong, C. P. (1998). "Comparison of bone single-photon emission tomography and planar imaging in the detection of vertebral metastases in patients with back pain." *Eur J Nucl Med* 25(6): 635-638

Haubner, R., Kuhnast, B., Mang, C., Weber, W. A., Kessler, H., Wester, H. J. & Schwaiger, M. (2004). "[18F]Galacto-RGD: synthesis, radiolabeling, metabolic stability, and radiation dose estimates." *Bioconjug Chem* 15(1): 61-69

Haubner, R., Wester, H. J., Weber, W. A., Mang, C., Ziegler, S. I., Goodman, S. L., Senekowitsch-Schmidtke, R., Kessler, H. & Schwaiger, M. (2001). "Noninvasive imaging of alpha(v)beta3 integrin expression using 18F-labeled RGD-containing glycopeptide and positron emission tomography." *Cancer Res* 61(5): 1781-1785

Hawkins, R. A., Choi, Y., Huang, S. C., Hoh, C. K., Dahlbom, M., Schiepers, C., Satyamurthy, N., Barrio, J. R. & Phelps, M. E. (1992). "Evaluation of the skeletal kinetics of fluorine-18-fluoride ion with PET." *J Nucl Med* 33(5): 633-642

Holland, J. P., Sheh, Y. & Lewis, J. S. (2009). "Standardized methods for the production of high specific-activity zirconium-89." *Nucl Med Biol* 36(7): 729-739

Hruska, C. B., Boughey, J. C., Phillips, S. W., Rhodes, D. J., Wahner-Roedler, D. L., Whaley, D. H., Degnim, A. C. & O'Connor, M. K. (2008). "Scientific Impact Recognition Award: Molecular breast imaging: a review of the Mayo Clinic experience." *Am J Surg* 196(4): 470-476

Jager, P. L., Vaalburg, W., Pruim, J., de Vries, E. G., Langen, K. J. & Piers, D. A. (2001). "Radiolabeled amino acids: basic aspects and clinical applications in oncology." *J Nucl Med* 42(3): 432-445

Jonson, S. D. & Welch, M. J. (1998). "PET imaging of breast cancer with fluorine-18 radiolabeled estrogens and progestins." *Q J Nucl Med* 42(1): 8-17

Kanishi, D. (1993). "99mTc-MDP accumulation mechanisms in bone." *Oral Surg Oral Med Oral Pathol* 75(2): 239-246

Kenny, L., Coombes, R. C., Vigushin, D. M., Al-Nahhas, A., Shousha, S. & Aboagye, E. O. (2007). "Imaging early changes in proliferation at 1 week post chemotherapy: a pilot study in breast cancer patients with 3'-deoxy-3'-[18F]fluorothymidine positron emission tomography." *Eur J Nucl Med Mol Imaging* 34(9): 1339-1347

Kim, I. J., Bae, Y. T., Kim, S. J., Kim, Y. K., Kim, D. S. & Lee, J. S. (2006). "Determination and prediction of P-glycoprotein and multidrug-resistance-related protein expression in breast cancer with double-phase technetium-99m sestamibi scintimammography. Visual and quantitative analyses." *Oncology* 70(6): 403-410

Liberman, M., Sampalis, F., Mulder, D. S. & Sampalis, J. S. (2003). "Breast cancer diagnosis by scintimammography: a meta-analysis and review of the literature." *Breast Cancer Res Treat* 80(1): 115-126

Lim, H. S., Yoon, W., Chung, T. W., Kim, J. K., Park, J. G., Kang, H. K., Bom, H. S. & Yoon, J. H. (2007). "FDG PET/CT for the detection and evaluation of breast diseases: usefulness and limitations." *Radiographics* 27 Suppl 1: S197-213

Lindholm, P., Lapela, M., Nagren, K., Lehikoinen, P., Minn, H. & Jyrkkio, S. (2009). "Preliminary study of carbon-11 methionine PET in the evaluation of early response to therapy in advanced breast cancer." *Nucl Med Commun* 30(1): 30-36

Machulla, H. J., Blocher, A., Kuntzsch, M., Piert, M., Wei, R. & Grierson, J. R. (2000). "Simplified labeling approach for synthesizing 3 '-deoxy-3 '-[F-18]fluorothymidine ([F-18]FLT)." *Journal of Radioanalytical and Nuclear Chemistry* 243(3): 843-846

Mahner, S., Schirrmacher, S., Brenner, W., Jenicke, L., Habermann, C. R., Avril, N. & Dose-Schwarz, J. (2008). "Comparison between positron emission tomography using 2-[fluorine-18]fluoro-2-deoxy-D-glucose, conventional imaging and computed tomography for staging of breast cancer." *Ann Oncol* 19(7): 1249-1254

Mariani, G., Bruselli, L. & Duatti, A. (2008). "Is PET always an advantage versus planar and SPECT imaging?" *Eur J Nucl Med Mol Imaging* 35(8): 1560-1565

Moasser, M. M. (2007). "The oncogene HER2: its signaling and transforming functions and its role in human cancer pathogenesis." *Oncogene* 26(45): 6469-6487

Mortimer, J. E., Dehdashti, F., Siegel, B. A., Trinkaus, K., Katzenellenbogen, J. A. & Welch, M. J. (2001). "Metabolic flare: indicator of hormone responsiveness in advanced breast cancer." *J Clin Oncol* 19(11): 2797-2803

Munch-Petersen, B., Cloos, L., Jensen, H. K. & Tyrsted, G. (1995). "Human thymidine kinase 1. Regulation in normal and malignant cells." *Adv Enzyme Regul* 35: 69-89

Orlova, A., Wallberg, H., Stone-Elander, S. & Tolmachev, V. (2009). "On the selection of a tracer for PET imaging of HER2-expressing tumors: direct comparison of a 124I-labeled affibody molecule and trastuzumab in a murine xenograft model." *J Nucl Med* 50(3): 417-425

Oude Munnink, T. H., Nagengast, W. B., Brouwers, A. H., Schroder, C. P., Hospers, G. A., Lub-de Hooge, M. N., van der Wall, E., van Diest, P. J. & de Vries, E. G. (2009). "Molecular imaging of breast cancer." *Breast* 18 Suppl 3: S66-73

Peterson, L. M., Mankoff, D. A., Lawton, T., Yagle, K., Schubert, E. K., Stekhova, S., Gown, A., Link, J. M., Tewson, T. & Krohn, K. A. (2008). "Quantitative imaging of estrogen receptor expression in breast cancer with PET and 18F-fluoroestradiol." *J Nucl Med* 49(3): 367-374

Pio, B. S., Park, C. K., Pietras, R., Hsueh, W. A., Satyamurthy, N., Pegram, M. D., Czernin, J., Phelps, M. E. & Silverman, D. H. (2006). "Usefulness of 3'-[F-18]fluoro-3'-deoxythymidine with positron emission tomography in predicting breast cancer response to therapy." *Mol Imaging Biol* 8(1): 36-42

Reske, S. N. & Deisenhofer, S. (2006). "Is 3'-deoxy-3'-(18)F-fluorothymidine a better marker for tumour response than (18)F-fluorodeoxyglucose?" *Eur J Nucl Med Mol Imaging* 33 Suppl 1: 38-43

Romer, J., Fuchtner, F., Steinbach, J. & Kasch, H. (2001). "Automated synthesis of 16alpha-[18F]fluoroestradiol-3,17beta-disulphamate." *Appl Radiat Isot* 55(5): 631-639

Ruoslahti, E. & Pierschbacher, M. D. (1987). "New perspectives in cell adhesion: RGD and integrins." *Science* 238(4826): 491-497

Sampath, L., Kwon, S., Ke, S., Wang, W., Schiff, R., Mawad, M. E. & Sevick-Muraca, E. M. (2007). "Dual-labeled trastuzumab-based imaging agent for the detection of human epidermal growth factor receptor 2 overexpression in breast cancer." *J Nucl Med* 48(9): 1501-1510

Schechter, N. R., Yang, D. J., Azhdarinia, A. & Chanda, M. (2007). "Technologies for translational imaging using generators in oncology." *Recent Pat Anticancer Drug Discov* 2(3): 251-258

Schilling, K., Narayanan, D., Kalinyak, J. E., The, J., Velasquez, M. V., Kahn, S., Saady, M., Mahal, R. & Chrystal, L. (2011). "Positron emission mammography in breast cancer presurgical planning: comparisons with magnetic resonance imaging." *Eur J Nucl Med Mol Imaging* 38(1): 23-36

Schirrmeister, H. (2007). "Detection of bone metastases in breast cancer by positron emission tomography." *Radiol Clin North Am* 45(4): 669-676, vi

Schirrmeister, H., Rentschler, M., Kotzerke, J., Diederichs, C. G. & Reske, S. N. (1998). "Skeletal imaging with (FNa)-F-18-PET and comparison with planar skeletal scintigraphy." *Rofo-Fortschritte Auf Dem Gebiet Der Rontgenstrahlen Und Der Bildgebenden Verfahren* 168(5): 451-456

Scopinaro, F., Schillaci, O., Scarpini, M., Mingazzini, P. L., Di Macio, L., Banci, M., Danieli, R., Zerilli, M., Limiti, M. R. & Centi Colella, A. (1994). "Technetium-99m sestamibi: an indicator of breast cancer invasiveness." *Eur J Nucl Med* 21(9): 984-987

Seitz, U., Wagner, M., Neumaier, B., Wawra, E., Glatting, G., Leder, G., Schmid, R. M. & Reske, S. N. (2002). "Evaluation of pyrimidine metabolising enzymes and in vitro uptake of 3'-[(18)F]fluoro-3'-deoxythymidine ([(18)F]FLT) in pancreatic cancer cell lines." *Eur J Nucl Med Mol Imaging* 29(9): 1174-1181

Sharma, R., Tripathi, M., Panwar, P., Chuttani, K., Jaimini, A., Maitra, S., Chopra, M. K., Sawroop, K., Shukla, G., Mondal, A. & Mishra, A. (2009). "99mTc-methionine scintimammography in the evaluation of breast cancer." *Nucl Med Commun* 30(5): 338-342

Shields, A. F., Grierson, J. R., Dohmen, B. M., Machulla, H. J., Stayanoff, J. C., Lawhorn-Crews, J. M., Obradovich, J. E., Muzik, O. & Mangner, T. J. (1998). "Imaging proliferation in vivo with [F-18]FLT and positron emission tomography." *Nat Med* 4(11): 1334-1336

Spence, A. M., Muzi, M., Link, J. M., O'Sullivan, F., Eary, J. F., Hoffman, J. M., Shankar, L. K. & Krohn, K. A. (2009). "NCI-sponsored trial for the evaluation of safety and preliminary efficacy of 3'-deoxy-3'-[18F]fluorothymidine (FLT) as a marker of proliferation in patients with recurrent gliomas: preliminary efficacy studies." *Mol Imaging Biol* 11(5): 343-355

Sundararajan, L., Linden, H. M., Link, J. M., Krohn, K. A. & Mankoff, D. A. (2007). "18F-Fluoroestradiol." *Semin Nucl Med* 37(6): 470-476

Takada, Y., Ye, X. & Simon, S. (2007). "The integrins." *Genome Biol* 8(5): 215

Tseng, J., Dunnwald, L. K., Schubert, E. K., Link, J. M., Minoshima, S., Muzi, M. & Mankoff, D. A. (2004). "18F-FDG kinetics in locally advanced breast cancer: correlation with tumor blood flow and changes in response to neoadjuvant chemotherapy." *J Nucl Med* 45(11): 1829-1837

Wijns, W. & Camici, P. G. (1997). "The value of quantitative myocardial perfusion imaging with positron emission tomography in coronary artery disease." *Herz* 22(2): 87-95

Winberg, K. J., Persson, M., Malmstrom, P. U., Sjoberg, S. & Tolmachev, V. (2004). "Radiobromination of anti-HER2/neu/ErbB-2 monoclonal antibody using the p-isothiocyanatobenzene derivative of the [76Br]undecahydro-bromo-7,8-dicarba-nido-undecaborate(1-) ion." *Nucl Med Biol* 31(4): 425-433

Xu, H., Baidoo, K., Gunn, A. J., Boswell, C. A., Milenic, D. E., Choyke, P. L. & Brechbiel, M. W. (2007). "Design, synthesis, and characterization of a dual modality positron emission tomography and fluorescence imaging agent for monoclonal antibody tumor-targeted imaging." *J Med Chem* 50(19): 4759-4765

Yeh, K. A., Fortunato, L., Ridge, J. A., Hoffman, J. P., Eisenberg, B. L. & Sigurdson, E. R. (1995). "Routine bone scanning in patients with T1 and T2 breast cancer: a waste of money." *Ann Surg Oncol* 2(4): 319-324

Yoo, J., Dence, C. S., Sharp, T. L., Katzenellenbogen, J. A. & Welch, M. J. (2005). "Synthesis of an estrogen receptor beta-selective radioligand: 5-[18F]fluoro-(2R,3S)-2,3-bis(4-hydroxyphenyl)pentanenitrile and comparison of in vivo distribution with 16alpha-[18F]fluoro-17beta-estradiol." *J Med Chem* 48(20): 6366-6378

Yun, M., Oh, S. J., Ha, H. J., Ryu, J. S. & Moon, D. H. (2003). "High radiochemical yield synthesis of 3'-deoxy-3'-[18F]fluorothymidine using (5'-O-dimethoxytrityl-2'-deoxy-3'-O-nosyl-beta-D-threo pentofuranosyl)thymine and its 3-N-BOC-protected analogue as a labeling precursor." *Nucl Med Biol* 30(2): 151-157

15

Molecular Imaging of Breast Cancer Tissue *via* Site-Directed Radiopharmaceuticals

Andrew B. Jackson, Lauren B. Retzloff,
Prasant K. Nanda and C. Jeffrey Smith
University of Missouri Department of Radiology, Columbia, MO
United States of America

1. Introduction

The American Cancer Society reports that ~261,100 new cases of invasive and in situ breast cancer were diagnosed in 2010, and nearly 40,000 fatalities were attributed to this disease (American Cancer Society, 2010). Although death rates have steadily decreased since 1990, breast cancer currently ranks second in cancer deaths among women. Improvements in detection, treatment, and prevention education contribute to slow the incidence rate, and rapidly evolving nuclear medicine techniques have emerged as a formidable opponent to female breast cancer. The involvement of nuclear medicine imaging modalities in both the detection and diagnosis of breast cancer has increased in recent years (Gopalan et al., 2002). In contrast to earlier imaging methods, in which the transmission of various forms of energy through tissue is employed to generate an image, nuclear medicine imaging techniques are based on detection of the energy emitted from radioactive tracers that are injected into the body and subsequently accumulate locally in specific tissues (Nass et al., 2001). The classification of these techniques as either positron emission tomography (PET) or single photon emission computed tomography (SPECT) imaging modalities is determined by the radionuclide that is utilized to synthesize a given radiotracer.

The theory behind nuclear medicine imaging techniques to detect and diagnose breast cancer is founded on preferential radiopharmaceutical uptake by cancerous cells as a result of alterations in metabolic rate, vascularity, or receptor expression which are associated with malignancy. Although both PET and SPECT are commonly employed to detect a variety of malignancies, neither imaging technique has achieved clinical acceptance as a method of imaging breast cancer due to the lack of sensitivity and specificity demonstrated by available radiotracers (Gopalan et al., 2002; Nass et al., 2001; Rosen et al., 2008).

Presently, there is only one radiopharmaceutical, the SPECT imaging agent technetium-99m methoxy-isobutyl-isonitrile (^{99m}Tc-sestamibi, Miraluma®), that has received FDA approval for use as a diagnostic adjunct to mammography (Gopalan et al., 2002; Nass et al., 2001; Rosen et al., 2008). Although the mechanism governing the concentration of ^{99m}Tc-sestamibi in cancer cells is not fully understood, it may be related to the degree of cellular proliferation and vascular permeability (Nass et al., 2001). Once inside malignant cells, ^{99m}Tc-sestamibi is sequestered within the cytoplasm as a result of the strong electrostatic attraction between the positively charged lipophilic ^{99m}Tc-sestamibi and the negatively charged mitochondria. This sequestration allows for the accumulation of ^{99m}Tc-sestamibi in cancer cells over time, presenting with high contrast on the resulting SPECT image (Gopalan et al., 2002). Despite the relatively high overall sensitivity (75-95%), specificity (71-100%), positive predictive value (67-100%), and accuracy (67-92%) demonstrated in numerous trials, ^{99m}Tc-sestamibi has proven unsuitable for the diagnosis of lesions smaller than 12 millimeters due to a significant decrease in both sensitivity (30-50%) and specificity (50%) (Gopalan et al., 2002).

2. Current research: Toward receptor-targeted radiopharmaceuticals

The continued interest in the development of radiopharmaceuticals for the detection and diagnosis of breast cancer is based on the fact that current methods fail to both detect and accurately diagnose early stage lesions in a large percentage of patients (Berghammer et al., 2001; Gopalan et al., 2002; Olsen & Gotzsche 2001). Nuclear medicine imaging techniques are well suited to address this situation given their ability to noninvasively detect a variety of physiological alterations associated with malignancy. The potential clinical applications of scintigraphic evaluation of breast cancer patients fall into five categories: 1) the early detection of breast cancer, 2) the differentiation between benign and malignant masses, 3) the staging of newly discovered breast cancer, 4) the detection of distant metastatic sites, and 5) the evaluation of tumor response to therapy (Berghammer et al., 2001; Rosen et al., 2008).

2.1 Early radiopharmaceuticals

While radiolabeled small molecules have accounted for the vast majority of imaging agents initially investigated for breast cancer detection and diagnosis, their non-specificity has resulted in low accumulation in target tissues, high levels of background radioactivity, and poor image resolution (Anderson & Welch, 1999). As a consequence of these findings, research efforts have shifted towards the utilization of monoclonal antibodies, which have been designed to target specific antigens that are over-expressed on tumor cells (Signore et al., 2001).

However, radiolabeled monoclonal antibodies have had limited clinical success due to several factors including the immunogenicity of the murine antibodies frequently employed in radiotracer preparation, the predominately hepatobiliary route of excretion, and the reduced ability to extravasate and access the target antigen as a result of the large size of intact monoclonal antibodies (Blok et al., 1999).Although the introduction of Fab´ and $F(ab)_2$´ fragments, chimeric, and humanized antibodies have diminished these effects, accumulation of monoclonal antibodies in tumor tissue continues to be insufficient, generating unfavorable target to background ratios.The advent of radiolabeled biologically active peptides in the early 1990s provided a means to overcome the limitations associated with these early radiopharmaceuticals (Table 1) (Fischman et al., 1993).The unique over-expression of specific receptors on malignant cells allows for their selective targeting using radiolabeled peptides that are designed to act as ligands for these receptors (Katzenellenbogen et al., 1995). A number of these receptor targets that are described herein have been identified on breast cancer cells, including those for somatostatin, vasoactive intestinal peptide, neuropeptide Y, and gastrin releasing peptide.

	Small Molecules	Monoclonal Antibodies	Peptides
Synthesis	Facile	Lengthy	Facile
Size	Less than 1,500Da	MAb: ~160kDa, Fab′ and F(ab)$_2$′ Fragments: 10-100kDa	Less than 10,000Da
Specificity	Moderate	High, Inflammation Sites: Nonspecific IgG uptake	High
Binding Affinity	Perfusion Agents: N/A, Others: Moderate	High	High
***In Vivo* Binding**	Perfusion Agents: N/A, Others: Moderate	Limited by size	High
Target to Background Ratio	Moderate	Moderate	Moderate to High
Blood Clearance	Variable	Slow	Rapid
Immunogenicity	No	Potential for HAMA response	No

Table 1. Comparison of Early Radiopharmaceuticals (Blok et al., 1999; Fischman et al., 1993; Signore et al., 2001)

2.2 Somatostatin receptor scintigraphy

Somatostatin (SST) is a peptide hormone with two endogenous forms, SST-14 and SST-28, which are the cleavage products of the SST prohormone. SST may be found in several organ systems, including the central nervous system, the hypothalamopituitary system, the gastrointestinal tract, the exocrine and endocrine pancreas, and the immune system. This widespread distribution highlights the varied actions of SST throughout the body, ranging from inhibition of peptide hormone secretion to modulation of neurotransmission to inhibition of cellular proliferation. These effects are mediated *via* interaction with G protein-coupled SST receptors, which may lead to a number of intracellular actions including the inhibition of the adenylyl cyclase-cAMP-protein kinase A and MAP kinase (MAPK) pathways, modulation of potassium channels, stimulation of phopholipase A2, and activation of phosphotyrosine phosphatases. To date, five SST receptor subtypes have been identified ($SSTR_1$, $SSTR_2$, $SSTR_3$, $SSTR_4$, $SSTR_5$), which differ in both their expression pattern and their affinity for structural analogs of SST (Pomper & Gelovani, 2008; Reubi, 2008).

The observation that the administration of SST inhibits the growth of various tumor cell lines as a result of their over-expression of the SST receptor led to the development of OctreoScan® (^{111}In-diethylenetriaminepentaacetic acid (DTPA)-octreotide), a radiolabeled synthetic SST analog that became the first peptide-based radiopharmaceutical to receive FDA approval for the scintigraphic localization of SST receptor-positive neuroendocrine tumors. Due to the fact that endogenous SST exhibits a short *in vivo* half-life as a result of rapid degradation by both aminopeptidases and endopeptidases, OctreoScan® incorporates modified amino acids into the Phe-(D)Trp-Lys-Thr receptor binding motif of octreotide to inhibit its metabolism and allow for increased tumor uptake.

The discovery that SST receptors are expressed on a multitude of tumor types, including those of the breast (50-75%), coupled with the diagnostic and therapeutic success of OctreoScan® in patients with neuroendocrine carcinomas, generated interest in the potential expansion of OctreoScan®'s clinical use. While the successful scintigraphic detection of both primary and metastatic breast cancer has been reported with OctreoScan® in 50 to 94% of breast cancer cases, these figures may represent an overestimation as nonspecific uptake by nonmalignant breast tissue is observed in 15% of patients (Bajc et al., 1996; Reubi, 2008; Wang et al., 2008). In addition to the nonspecific uptake observed with OctreoScan®, the low density of SST receptors ($SSTR_{2A}$ and $SSTR_5$) present in carcinomas of the breast combined with their heterogeneous expression pattern have prevented the acceptance of this agent for the routine diagnosis of breast cancer.

2.3 Vasoactive intestinal peptide scintigraphy

Vasoactive intestinal peptide (VIP) is a neuropeptide composed of 28 amino acids that belongs to the glucagon secretion family of peptides. VIP, and the closely related pituitary adenylate cyclase-activating polypeptide (PACAP), are among the most important neurotransmitters employed in the digestive system. In addition to its actions in the gut, VIP has a modulatory role in both the central nervous and immune systems. These actions are mediated by binding to G protein-coupled VIP receptors ($VPAC_1$, $VPAC_2$), which may be internalized after ligand binding, resulting in various intracellular effects including stimulation of adenylyl cyclase activity (Pomper & Gelovani, 2008; Reubi, 2008). The $VPAC_1$ and $VPAC_2$ receptors exhibit distinct distribution patterns, with preferential expression of the $VPAC_1$ receptor in a number of tissues including hepatocytes, gastrointestinal mucosa, pancreatic ducts, lung acini, thyroid follicles, prostatic glands, bladder and ureter urothelium, and breast lobules and ducts and of the $VPAC_2$ receptor in smooth muscle. In addition to its ubiquitous *in vivo* biodistribution pattern, the $VPAC_1$ receptor has been reported to be expressed in up to 93% of all primary tumors and metastatic sites of lung and breast cancer, generating interest in the development of $VPAC_1$-targeted radiotracers that may be employed in the detection and diagnosis of various neoplasms (Moody & Gozes, 2007; Pomper & Gelovani, 2008; Reubi, 2008).

Radiopharmacological targeting of the $VPAC_1$ receptor in colon cancer tumors was initially accomplished by radiolabeling native VIP with iodine-123 (^{123}I). While promising scintigraphic images have been obtained using this agent, the rapid *in vivo* degradation of endogenous VIP, combined with both the cost and the difficulty associated with ^{123}I-VIP conjugate synthesis, have hindered widespread clinical use of this compound. In an effort to address these issues, investigators have constructed a variety of VIP analogs that are suitable for labeling with a number of radioisotopes including technetium-99m (^{99m}Tc), copper-64 (^{64}Cu), and fluorine-18 (^{18}F) (Moody & Gozes, 2007; Pomper & Gelovani, 2008; Thakur et al., 2004). Although these radiotracers have proven capable of *in vivo* targeting of $VPAC_1$ receptor-bearing tumors, the significant background radioactivity that is present as a result of ubiquitous $VPAC_1$ receptor expression and the rapid *in vivo* degradation of these VIP analogs reduces the resolution of the images obtained. These results, coupled with the fact that $VPAC_1$ receptors are found in high (>2,000 dpm/mg tissue) density in only 37% of breast tumors, suggest that radiolabeled VIP conjugates are unlikely to gain widespread clinical acceptance for use in routine breast cancer detection and diagnosis.

2.4 Neuropeptide Y receptor scintigraphy

Neuropeptide Y (NPY) is a neurotransmitter that belongs to a family of 36 amino-acid-long peptides that also includes peptide YY and pancreatic polypeptide. In the central nervous system, the actions of NPY consist of stimulation of feeding behavior and inhibition of anxiety, while in the peripheral nervous system NPY regulates a variety of functions such as vasoconstriction, gastrointestinal motility and secretion, insulin release, and renal function (Koglin & Beck-Sickinger, 2004; Reubi, 2008). These effects are mediated by interaction with various metabotropic G protein-coupled NPY receptor subtypes (Y_1, Y_2, Y_3, Y_4, Y_5, Y_6), among which Y_1, Y_2, Y_4, and Y_5 have been well characterized.

In contrast to other regulatory peptides, NPY has not often been associated with human cancer. However, a recent *in vitro* study, which included over 100 human breast cancer samples, reported that the NPY receptor, predominantly the Y_1 subtype, was expressed in 85% of primary carcinomas and 100% of lymph node metastases of receptor-positive primary tumors. These results are higher than those reported in a subsequent trial, in which the NPY(Y_1) receptor was observed in only 69% of the primary breast tumor samples analyzed and at high density (>2,000 dpm/mg tissue) in only 66% of those samples.

The recent development of receptor subtype selective NPY analogs, combined with novel strategies for the synthesis and radiolabeling of these analogs, has enabled progress in the construction of NPY receptor targeted radiopharmaceuticals that may be employed for breast cancer detection and diagnosis. Radiolabeling of NPY(Y_1)-selective conjugates was initially achieved by exploiting the high tyrosine content of these derivatives which allowed for the oxidative incorporation of iodine-125 (^{125}I). Although this represents a rapid and facile radiosynthetic method, it is also non-selective, allowing for the potential incorporation of ^{125}I into residues that are involved in receptor binding. In order to address this limitation, subsequent radiolabeling techniques have employed photolabile protecting groups and bifunctional chelating agents (BFCA) (Zwanziger et al., 2008).

Despite these advances in the field of NPY(Y_1) receptor imaging, proof of principle remains to be established. In fact, in a recent study which utilized NMRI nu/nu mice bearing MCF-7 tumors to analyze the biodistribution of the NPY(Y_1)-selective peptide DOTA-[Phe_7, Pro_{34}] NPY radiolabeled with indium-111 (^{111}In), tumor uptake of the conjugate was relatively low at all time points (30 minutes post-injection (p.i.) = 1.7 ± 0.5% injected dose per gram (%ID/g)). In addition, although the NPY(Y_1) receptor is found in high density in 66% of *in situ*, invasive, and metastatic breast cancers, it is also present in both the lobules and ducts of normal breast tissue, which decreases the tumor-to-background ratio and degrades the overall image resolution. Thus, the suitability of radiolabeled NPY(Y_1) receptors for the routine detection and diagnosis of breast cancer remains in question.

2.5 Gastrin releasing peptide receptor (GRPr) sScintigraphy

Gastrin releasing peptide (GRP) is a peptide hormone composed of 27 amino acids that, along with neuromedin C, are the cleavage products of a 148 amino acid preproprotein. GRP belongs to the bombesin-like (bombesin = BBN) family of peptides that regulates numerous functions in the enteric and the central nervous systems, including circadian rhythm, immune function, thermoregulation, satiety, gastrointestinal hormone release, smooth muscle contraction, and epithelial cell proliferation (Knigge et al., 1984). These actions are mediated by binding to $G_{q/11}$ protein-coupled receptors of the bombesin family (BB_1- Neuromedin B receptor, BB_2- GRPr, BB_3- Orphan receptor, BB_4- BBN receptor) expressed in the pancreas, stomach, adrenal cortex, and brain, which activates the intracellular phospholipase C signal transduction cascade leading to inositol triphosphate (IP_3) and diacylglycerol (DAG) generation, and subsequent intracellular calcium elevation (Gugger & Reubi, 1999; Smith et al., 2005).

Of all the physiological effects of GRP, the most studied is the one related to cancer. Investigation into the role of GRP in cancer progression began with the observation in 1981 that both cancer cell lines and primary human tumors can synthesize GRP as well as its amphibian analog BBN (Moody et al., 1981). Four years later, Cuttitta et al. demonstrated that GRP and BBN stimulate the growth of small cell lung cancer, and that this ability is part of an autocrine feedback mechanism that involves the interaction of these peptides with their receptors, which are expressed on the surface of tumor cells (Cuttitta et al., 1985). The mitogenic role of GRP and BBN in other cancers has since been established, including those of the lung, pancreas, prostate, central nervous system, and breast (Reubi, 2008). While the mechanism of growth stimulation does not appear to be constant for all carcinomas, it generally involves the transactivation and up-regulation of epidermal growth factor (EGF) receptors (Van de Wiele et al., 2000).

Although GRPrs have been readily detected in various tumor cell lines, identification of these receptors in primary human tumors has proven to be more difficult. While the presence of GRPr proteins has not been conclusively established in either gastrointestinal or exocrine pancreatic carcinomas, both GRP mRNA and receptor proteins have been detected in neoplasms of the prostate and breast (Reubi, 2008). Expression of GRPrs in neoplastic epithelial mammary cells have been reported in approximately two thirds (62-71%) of all breast carcinomas, and in high density (>2,000 dpm/mg tissue) in 65% of these cases. In addition, all of the lymph node metastases from GRPr-positive primary breast carcinomas were positive for this receptor, whereas the surrounding lymphoreticular tissue was GRPr-negative. Although GRPrs are present in both the ducts and lobules of nonneoplastic breast tissue, their heterogeneous distribution, coupled with the strong GRPr expression by primary breast carcinomas as well as metastatic sites, indicates that breast cancer may be effectively imaged using GRP and BBN analogs (Gugger & Reubi, 1999; Reubi, 2008).

For over a decade, the feasibility of using radiolabeled BBN analogs to detect and diagnose GRPr-positive breast cancer has been investigated. The translation of these efforts into human subjects first occurred in 2000, with the publication of the results from the first human trial (Van de Wiele et al., 2000). In order to evaluate the diagnostic utility of ^{99m}Tc-RP527, Van de Wiele et al. administered this agent to six patients with metastatic breast cancer prior to image acquisition (planar, SPECT). While low physiological uptake of ^{99m}Tc-RP527 was observed in normal breast tissue, it did not affect the visualization of either the primary tumor or metastatic sites, which were successfully imaged in 4 out of 6 patients with tumor-to-background ratios of 1.7 to 3.4 and 2.6 to 7.2 at 1 and 6 hours p.i., respectively. Similar results were obtained by Scopinaro et al. in a 2002 trial which compared the diagnostic capacity of a ^{99m}Tc-labeled BBN analog with that of ^{99m}Tc-sestamibi in five patients with infiltrating ductal carcinoma (Scopinaro et al., 2002). Although the identification of metastatic sites was achieved with both agents, detection of the primary tumor was higher for ^{99m}Tc-BBN (100%) than for ^{99m}Tc-sestamibi (80%). This may be related to the higher affinity of BBN analogs for malignant breast tissue which often over-express the GRPr, allowing for improved tumor-to-background ratios when compared with ^{99m}Tc-sestamibi (1.4-2.3 vs. 1.0-1.8 at 5 minutes) (Scopinaro et al., 2002). While the results of these trials indicate that the detection/diagnosis of both primary breast cancer and metastatic sites can be achieved using radiolabeled BBN derivatives, the disadvantages demonstrated by these agents (moderate tumor-to-background ratios, hepatobiliary excretion) need to be addressed in order to recognize their full potential.

2.6 GRPr-expressing T-47D human bBreast cancer cells

The ability of radiolabeled BBN analogs to detect and diagnose both primary breast carcinomas and metastatic sites which express the GRPr, coupled with the expression of this receptor in 62-71% of breast cancer cases, has fueled continued interest in the development of BBN-based tumor targeting agents. In order to produce high quality SPECT images, radiotracer accumulation and residualization in GRPr-expressing cells must be maximized to optimize the contrast and hence the resolution of the resulting image. While there are other cell lines that express the GRPr in relative high numbers, our group and many others have used the T-47D human breast cancer cell line in a variety of studies to evaluate the therapeutic and diagnostic efficacy of potential radiopharmaceuticals. This differentiated cell line, with breast epithelial morphology, was derived from a metastatic pleural effusion originating from an infiltrating ductal carcinoma in a 54 year-old Caucasian patient (Lacroix & Leclercq, 2004; Engel & Young, 1978). The cell line is described as "luminal epithelial-like" with markers indicating its pre-metastatic state according to the EMT (epithelial-mesenchymal transition) hypothesis for metastatic transformation. It has been shown that the GRPR is over-expressed on the surface of T-47D breast carcinoma cells while being absent from normal breast tissues (Giacchetti et al., 1990). This receptor has served as a target for a number of diagnostic and therapeutic strategies (Prasanphanich et al., 2007; Garrison et al., 2007; Parry et al., 2007; Biddlecombe et al., 2007; Guojun et al., 2008; Zhou et al., 2003; Ma et al., 2007). T-47D xenografts in mice have been used in preclinical investigations of a variety of diagnostic modalities (Giblin et al., 2006; Aliaga et al., 2004).

T-47D Cell Line	
Cell Line Origin	Female patient. Age = 54. Pleural effusion from an invasive ductal carcinoma.
Acquisition Data	Dr. Keydar, 1974
In Vitro Invasion	Positive (low)
Estrogen Receptor	Positive
Progesterone Receptor	Positive
GRPr	Positive (36,000 sites/cell)
^{125}I-Tyr^{4}-BBN(7-14)NH_2: Binding Capacity and Affinity	$9.7x10^{-13}$M/mg K_D = 1 nM

Table 2. T-47D Cell line characteristics (Giacchetti et al., 1990)

3. Site-directed radiopharmaceutical composition

The use of peptide-based bioconjugates in molecular investigations is common. Typically, a peptide is covalently modified with a bifunctional chelating agent (BFCA) capable of complexing and stabilizing a radionuclide. Pharmacokinetic modifiers can be introduced between the peptide and the BFCA to fine-tune the biodistribution of the bioconjugate. The potential of using peptide-based site-directed radiopharmaceuticals for *in vivo* single-photon emission computed topography (SPECT) and PET imaging has recently become apparent (Sprague et al., 2007; Weiner & Thakur, 2005).

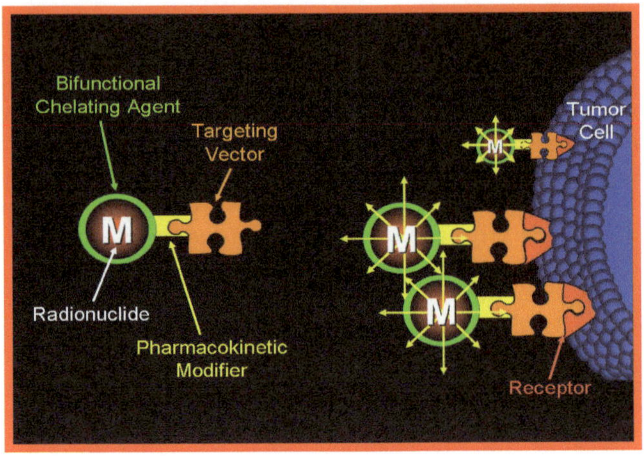

Fig. 1. Schematic representation of a radiolabeled targeting vector for treatment of human disease.

3.1 Bombesin targeting vectors

Radiopharmaceuticals designed to target the GRPr employ modified analogs of bombesin, a tetradecapeptide initially isolated from the skin of the fire-bellied toad *Bombina bombina* in 1971 (Reubi, 2008; Smith et al., 2003; Zhang et al., 2004). The amidated C-terminus sequence of seven amino acids (**Trp-Ala-Val-Gly-His-Leu-Met-NH$_2$**), which is homologous to that of GRP (Table 3), is utilized for conjugate synthesis as a result of the fact that this sequence is sufficient for specific high affinity binding to the GRPr.

GRP	Val-Pro-Leu-Pro-Ala-Gly-Gly-Gly-Thr-Val-Leu-Thr-Lys-Met-Tyr-Pro-Arg-Gly-Asn-His-**Trp-Ala-Val-Gly-His-Leu-Met-NH$_2$**
BBN*	Pyr-Gln-Arg-Leu-Gly-Asn-Gln-**Trp-Val-Gly-His-Leu-Met-NH$_2$** Pyr-Gln-Arg-Leu-Gly-Asn-Gln-**Trp-Ala-Val-Gly-His-Phe-Met-NH$_2$**

*Two distinct forms of BBN have been identified for the BB_4 receptor subtype.

Table 3. Amino Acid Sequence Comparison, GRP versus BBN (Smith et al., 2003)

The utilization of radiolabeled receptor agonists for cancer detection, diagnosis, and treatment has traditionally been accepted due to the fact that agonists often undergo rapid internalization upon receptor binding and are subsequently residualized within the tumor cell for an extended period of time. The internalization mechanism for BBN-based agonists involves the endocytosis of the agonist/GRPr complex into clathrin-coated vesicles and endosomes. This is followed by migration to the perinuclear space where lysosomal entrapment of the agonist occurs, prolonging the residence time of agonist-bound radioactivity in the target tissue. This allows for the accumulation of radioactivity in GRPr-positive tissues, thereby facilitating breast cancer diagnosis and treatment (Van de Wiele et al., 2000). While a number of BBN-based agonists have been developed, in order to maintain a high binding affinity for the GRPr subtype, these analogs all contain the seven amino acid GRPr binding motif with limited substitution (Coy et al., 1988; Pomper & Gelovani, 2008). The production of radiopharmaceutial agents from these BBN(7-14)NH_2 based compounds may be readily achieved using a variety of radiometal chelates. The resulting radiotracers have been demonstrated to retain high specific binding to the GRPr in a variety of human cancer cell lines, including those of the prostate, pancreas, and breast (Inhibitory Concentration at 50% (IC_{50}) = 1-10 nM).

3.2 Pharmacokinetic modification—"Linking groups"

An important aspect in the design of new radiopharmaceuticals is the adjustment of the pharmacokinetic properties of an agent, which influence its biodistribution and clearance. These factors have a significant impact on the tumor-to-background ratio, and hence the diagnostic and therapeutic utility that will be exhibited by a radiotracer. While the GRPr binding motif is not generally modified during conjugate production, amendments to this basic sequence are commonly employed for a number of reasons including augmentation of conjugate resistance to degradation by plasma peptidases, alteration of the pharmacokinetic properties of the derivative, and facilitation of the radiolabeling procedure (Blok et al., 1999; Signore et al., 2001).

Incorporation of an inert spacer group into a BBN-based radiopharmaceutical is an effective method of modifying both the physiochemical properties and the metabolic fate of the bioconjugate, improving both the residualization of radioactivity by GRPr-positive malignant cells and clearance of the radiotracer from the blood and non-target tissues (Pomper & Gelovani, 2008). Both length and charge of the spacer group influence the pharmacokinetic properties, GRPr binding affinity, and tumor uptake of the BBN analog. Addition of a peptide sequence such as polyglycine or polyserine can be used to augment the hydrophilicity of a conjugate, thereby enhancing renal clearance, while the incorporation of a simple hydrocarbon chain may be employed to increase its lipophilicity in order to prolong its residence time in the bloodstream. An alternative approach to reduce the circulatory clearance rate of an analog is the insertion of a polyethyleneglycol (Peg) linker, which slows the extraction of the conjugate by hepatocytes (Krause, 2002). In the case of BBN(8-14)NH_2 based analogs, the incorporation of a tethering moiety between the receptor binding sequence and the radiometal complex influences not only the pharmacokinetic properties and renal retention of the resulting conjugate, but also the binding affinity and the degree of receptor-mediated analog uptake that is observed in GRPr rich tissues. In order to maintain a GRPr binding affinity that is similar to native BBN, the receptor binding sequence and the radiometal chelate must be separated by a distance of five or more atoms and the spacer sequence employed to serve this purpose must not introduce an extra negative charge at the N-terminus (Hoffman et al., 2001; Zhang et al., 2004).

Additionally, a spacer group creates distance between the appended radiometal chelate and the receptor binding sequence, which promotes the biological integrity of the radiotracer (Pomper & Gelovani, 2008). As both the receptor binding sequence and the C-terminus are essential to the *in vivo* interaction between BBN-based conjugates and the GRPr, attachment of the tethering moiety occurs at the N-terminal tryptophan in position 8 (Trp^8). Spacer group selection is critical because the effect of side chain conjugation to the Trp^8 residue is unpredictable. The attachment of some amino acid chains or other groups has been demonstrated to dramatically decrease the binding affinity of the BBN analog (Coy, et al., 1988). To avoid this issue, glutamine is frequently appended to the Trp^8 residue prior to the addition of the linker as its inclusion is not only compatible with maintaining high GRPr binding affinity, but also with reducing the renal retention of the resulting BBN(7-14)NH_2 conjugate (Hoffman et al., 2001).

3.3 Radiolabeling techniques and bifunctional chelating agents (BFCAs)

Radiolabeling may result in substantial alterations to both the lipophilicity and the charge of the radiopharmaceutical and has important consequences for both the biodistribution and the kinetic properties of the resulting agent (Blok et al., 1999; Signore et al., 2001). For instance, the introduction of a negative charge at the N-terminus of a BBN analog leads to a loss of binding affinity, while a positive charge augments it, resulting in the potential for increased accumulation in GRPr rich tissues. Radioisotope complexation to biologically active peptide based targeting vectors may be accomplished *via* either direct or indirect radiolabeling approaches (Stigbrand et al., 2008). While there are distinct advantages and disadvantages associated with each of these methods, the production of high specific activity products is essential to the generation of high resolution scintigraphic images.

Direct radiolabeling is a relatively rapid, facile synthetic method that utilizes functional groups, such as sulfhydryls or thioethers, which are present within the peptide to complex the radioisotope. However, this technique often suffers from a lack of specificity as the location of radioisotope incorporation into the resulting radiopharmaceutical may involve functional groups within or near the receptor binding sequence. This can decrease the affinity of the conjugate for its receptor, resulting in diminished accumulation in target tissues, which reduces the resolution, and hence the diagnostic utility of the scintigraphic image that is produced.

Indirect radiolabeling overcomes many of these difficulties by employing a bifunctional chelating agent (BFCA) to complex the radioisotope, providing distance between the metal chelate and the receptor binding sequence in order to preserve the biological activity of the radiopharmaceutical. BFCAs are designed not only to form stable, high yield complexes with metallic radionuclides, but also to covalently link these radioisotopes to the targeting vector. The BFCA may be conjugated to the targeting vector either prior to or subsequent to the radiolabeling procedure. In the pre-conjugation technique, synthesis of the BFCA-radiometal complex occurs in advance of conjugation to the targeting vector. This method is employed when the BFCA-radionuclide complex can only be generated under harsh reaction conditions, such as extreme temperature or pH, which may destroy the receptor binding region of the molecule (Stigbrand et al., 2008). The preferred method of indirect radiolabeling is the post-conjugation approach as it represents an effective, one-step method of radiopharmaceutical synthesis in which the BFCA is directly conjugated to the targeting vector prior to radioisotope complexation. Ideally, only specific donor atoms of the BFCA will coordinate the radiometal to produce a high yield conjugate with both high receptor affinity and *in vivo* stability. In order to achieve a high degree of *in vivo* stability, the BFCA must impart both thermodynamic and kinetic inertness to the resulting radiometal complex. This serves to decrease not only the *in vivo* metabolism of the radiopharmaceutical but also the subsequent retention of these metabolites by non-target tissues such as the stomach, liver, and kidneys, thereby increasing the tumor-to-background ratio.

4. microSPECT imaging using technetium-99m-BBN agents

Although a multitude of radioisotopes have been utilized in the development of diagnostic radiopharmaceuticals, ^{99m}Tc remains the most widely employed radionuclide in diagnostic nuclear medicine, accounting for approximately 85% of all nuclear medicine procedures performed (Smith et al., 2003). Technetium-99m is well suited for use as a radionuclide due to its ready availability *via* on site $^{99}Mo/^{99m}Tc$ generator systems, ideal nuclear characteristics (half-life ($t_{1/2}$) = 6.04 hours, gamma energy = 140.5 keV (89%), high specific activity), favorable dosimetry, and well-established labeling chemistries using a variety of BFCAs (Fischman et al., 1993; Smith et al., 2003 and 2005; Varvarigou et al., 2004). In addition, the chemistry of ^{99m}Tc is parallel to that of the therapeutic radioisotopes $^{186/188}Re$, allowing for the development of diagnostic/therapeutic radiopharmaceutical pairs. As such, the diagnostic agent may be employed in prescreening patients prior to therapy, which would provide valuable individual information regarding drug pharmacokinetics, receptor density, and dosimetry, potentially reducing or even eliminating unsuccessful radiotherapeutic regimens.

While ^{99m}Tc can exist in a variety of oxidation states ranging from +7 to -1, it is most stable in the +7 state (i.e. TcO_4^-, pertechnetate). Lower oxidation states may be stabilized by complexation with numerous ligands, resulting in radiometal chelates that have coordination numbers between 4 and 9. While oxidation states below +4 are easily oxidized to the +4 state, ^{99m}Tc in the +5 and +6 states frequently undergoes disproportionation into the +4 and +7 states, respectively. However, the type of complex formed and its stability are highly dependent on labeling conditions, which include pH, BFCA, reducing agent, and concentration. Initially, ^{99m}Tc chemistry focused on the +5 oxidation state as it may be complexed using a broad range of thiol-, isonitrile-, or phosphine-containing chelates to produce compounds that are highly stable in aqueous media (Blok et al., 1999). However, it is often difficult to produce well-defined conjugates with high specific activity *via* direct or indirect radiolabeling techniques, due to the fact that the reduction of the disulfide bonds in the targeting vector or the ligand framework may occur as a consequence of the presence of excess reducing agent (Sn^{2+}) in the labeling cocktail (Schibli & Schubiger, 2002). In addition, the resulting derivatives frequently suffer from significant *in vivo* hydrophobicity, prolonging their residence time in both the circulatory system and non-target tissues, which decreases the target-to-background ratio, and hence the resolution, of the resulting scintigraphic image, while simultaneously increasing the radiation exposure to the patient (Smith et al., 2003).

Both of these issues have been addressed utilizing the organometallic tricarbonyl core, *fac*-$^{99m}Tc(CO)_3$, formulated in the late 1990s (Alberto et al., 1998). Although initially the *fac*-$[^{99m}Tc\text{-}(H_2O)_3(CO)_3]^+$ precursor was obtained by direct carbonylation of the permetallate salt ($Na[TcO_4]$) using sodium borohydride under atmospheric carbon monoxide pressure, a method was subsequently devised for the fully aqueous, normal pressure preparation by employing potassium boranocarbonate ($K_2[H_3BCO_2]$) as both the reducing agent and the source of carbon monoxide (Alberto et al., 2001; Schibli & Schubiger, 2002). This method eliminates undesired disulfide bond reduction in the conjugates because excess reducing agent is destroyed prior to the radiolabeling procedure. The synthetic ease, high yield, excellent radiochemical purity, reproducibility, and improved safety associated with this new method of radiolabeling using the tricarbonyl core spurred the development of a commercial kit (Isolink®) for $[^{99m}Tc\text{-}(H_2O)_3(CO)_3]^+$ preparation (Biersack & Freeman, 2007).

The remarkable kinetic and thermodynamic stability demonstrated by the $[^{99m}Tc-(H_2O)_3(CO)_3]^+$ aqua ion in aerobic, aqueous solutions over a wide range of pH values is derived from two factors: 1) the shape of the ^{99m}Tc-labeled precursor, and 2) the oxidation state of ^{99m}Tc. The $^{99m}Tc(CO)_3$ metal core is compact, with an almost spherical shape, which if "closed" with an appropriate ligand system will form an octahedral coordination sphere that effectively protects the metal center against further ligand attack or reoxidation. Conversely, $^{99m}Tc(V)$-complexes possess an "open" quadratic pyramidal structure, which is prone to ligand attack and/or protonation often resulting in decomposition of the original complex (Schibli & Schubiger, 2002). In addition, $^{99m}Tc(I)$ has a low spin d^6 electron configuration that is responsible for the octahedral shape of these complexes, endowing them with large crystal field stabilization energies in the presence of strong field ligands such as CO, further contributing to the kinetic and the thermodynamic stability of these compounds. Unlike the CO ligands in the aqua ion, the water ligands are not π-electron acceptors and as a result their binding to the metal center is not stabilized by synergic bonding. This accounts for the substitution lability of these ligands which can undergo facile exchange reactions with a number of donor groups including amines, thioethers, phosphines, and thiols (Jones & Thornback, 2007). The ease of these reactions contributes to the excellent labeling efficiencies exhibited by the $[^{99m}Tc-(H_2O)_3(CO)_3]^+$ precursor, which results in the production of metallated conjugates with remarkable *in vitro* and *in vivo* stability against serum-based proteins and superior uptake and retention when compared with $^{99m}Tc(V)$- agents.

In recent studies, we have evaluated conjugates of the type DPR-Y-BBN(7-14)NH_2 where DPR = 2,3-diaminopropionic acid (DPR), and Y= GSG or SSS (Retzloff et al., 2010) that when radiolabeled with *fac*-$[^{99m}Tc-(H_2O)_3(CO)_3]^+$ produced metallated conjugates $^{99m}Tc-(CO)_3$-DPR-Y-BBN(7-14)NH_2 in very high yield (~90%) (Figure 2) These products demonstrated *in vitro* stability in excess of 24 hours as monitored by reverse phase-high performance liquid chromatography (RP-HPLC), with no observable degradation or transchelation to inherent functional donor atoms present in either histidine solution (1 mM) or human serum albumin.

In competitive radioligand binding assays against ^{125}I-[Tyr^4]-BBN(7-14)NH_2, the standard for the evaluation of GRPr specific binding, these derivatives demonstrated very high affinities for the GRPr, with IC_{50} values of 8.1 ± 1.3 nM for Y = GSG, and 5.9 ± 0.8 nM for Y = SSS in the T-47D cell line (Retzloff et al., 2010). The internalization and externalization (trapping) of the $^{99m}Tc-(CO)_3$-DPR-Y-BBN(7-14)NH_2 derivatives, when assessed in T-47D cell lines showed that the apex of internalization occurred between 45 and 120 minutes, when uptake levels reached 80-88% of all cell-associated radioactivity in the T-47D cell line. This level of internalization remained relatively constant for subsequent time points, with no significant efflux of radiotracer observed over a 90-minute period.

Results obtained from biodistribution studies in SCID mice bearing human T-47D xenografted tumors suggested that analog size and lipophilicity strongly influence *in vivo* pharmacokinetic behavior. While the $^{99m}Tc-(CO)_3$-DPR-Y-BBN(7-14)NH_2 derivatives were eliminated primarily *via* the renal-urinary system, both the rate and the extent of clearance was affected by the DPR BFCA and the amino acid spacer sequence of the derivative. The prompt elimination of the DPR analogs from the body, where Y = GSG or SSS, can be attributed to the small size and hydrophilic nature of both the DPR BFCA and the amino acid linkers which served to mitigate the lipophilic character of the $^{99m}Tc(CO)_3$ metal core. As a result of this clearance pattern, these $^{99m}Tc-(H_2O)(CO)_3$-DPR-Y-BBN(7-14)NH_2 analogs demonstrated consistently lower levels of background radioactivity in non-target tissues, such as the liver and the gastrointestinal tract. In addition to aiding in their prompt elimination *via* the renal-urinary pathway, the small size and hydrophilic nature of the DPR derivatives containing amino acid linkers allowed for the rapid penetration of these conjugates into GRPr-positive target tissues, as evidenced by their comparatively high levels of uptake by both GRPr-expressing pancreatic and tumor tissues. Tumor uptake and retention in T-47D xenografted breast cancer tumors were 2.3-2.4 ± 0.4-0.8% ID/g (Y = GSG) and from 2.4-3.7 ± 0.7-1.8% ID/g (Y = SSS) at 1 hour p.i., respectively.

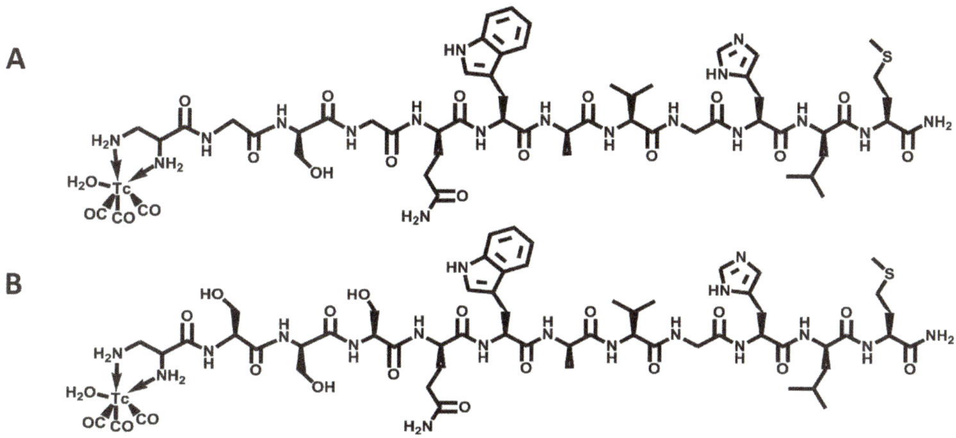

Fig. 2. $^{99m}Tc-(CO)_3-(H_2O)$-DPR-GSG-BBN(7-14)NH_2 (A) and $^{99m}Tc-(CO)_3-(H_2O)$-DPR-SSS-BBN(7-14)NH_2 (B) conjugates.

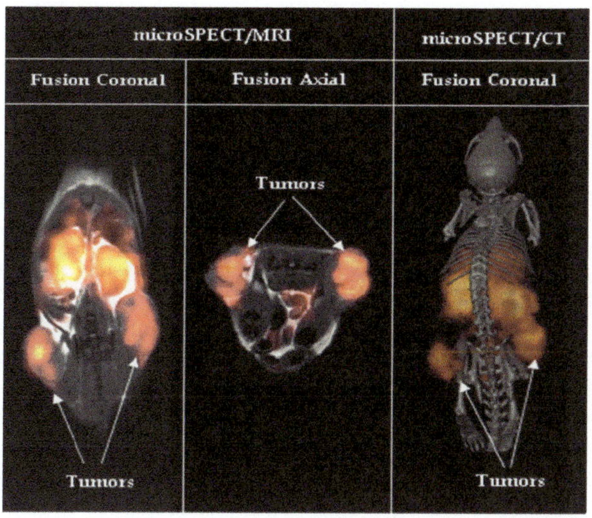

Fig. 3. microSPECT/MRI/CT imaging of $^{99m}Tc-(H_2O)_3(CO)_3$-DPR-SSS-BBN(7-14)NH_2 after 24 h p.i.

Due to each rapid elimination from non-target tissues *via* the renal-urinary excretion pathway and moderate accumulation and retention in tumor tissue, $^{99m}Tc-(H_2O)(CO)_3$-DPR-Y-BBN(7-14)NH_2 conjugates were evaluated for microSPECT imaging in T-47D tumor-bearing SCID mice at 24 hours p.i.(Figure 3). These conjugates produced favorable tumor-to-background ratios, which allowed for clear visualization of tumor tissue, despite some level of background radioactivity. Although the location and intensity of this background radioactivity fluctuated slightly among these conjugates, the kidneys and the gastrointestinal tract were consistently the predominant sources of radioactivity at the time of imaging. Despite these subtle differences in biodistribution, clear identification of tumor tissue was readily achieved with both derivates, supporting the hypothesis that radiolabeled $^{99m}Tc(I)$-BBN conjugates may be employed to diagnose GRPr-expressing breast cancers.

5. microPET imaging with copper-64-BBN conjugates

While a variety of diagnostic imaging techniques exist for identifying breast cancer, low-dose mammography is still considered to be the most accurate and dependable procedure (Prasad & Houserkova, 2007). Still, digital mammography is most accurate in women under 50, with low-density breast, who have either not entered or recently passed through menopause (Pisano et al., 2005). PET imaging using FDG (^{18}F-fluorodeoxyglucose) has been an effective technique for diagnosis of primary breast cancer and benefited from PET imaging devices designed specifically for breast imaging. While FDG-PET was able to identify tumors in the breast, a high false-positive rate, 87%, limits its wide-spread use. (Kaida et al., 2008). Thus there is a need to develop diagnostic modalities with increased specificity for malignant breast tissues and capable of overcoming these limitations. Targeting a unique physiological manifestation of breast malignancy, such as over-expression of an extracellular receptor with a diagnostic radionuclide, might be a procedure capable of imaging tumors of the breast with higher resolution and lower false-positive rates.

Copper-64 is one of few radionuclides possessing physical properties that allow for medical imaging and therapy (Nijsen et al., 2007). The utility of ^{64}Cu ($t_{1/2}$ = 12.7 h, cyclotron generated as $^{64}CuCl_2$) results from its diverse decay profile. Electron capture, with corresponding gamma emission at 1346 keV, accounts for 41% of the decay profile for ^{64}Cu. This is accompanied by emission of a β^- particle (40%, 190 keV) and a positron (β^+, 19%, 278 keV). The degree of β^+ decay is sufficient for PET imaging *in vivo* and has been extensively investigated. Moreover, ^{67}Cu-containing radiopharmaceuticals possess therapeutic potential and provide *in vivo* pharmacokinetic profiles nearly identical to ^{64}Cu-containing drugs (Blower et al., 1996). ^{67}Cu has ideal physical characteristics that are well-suited for radionuclide therapy (β^-, 100%, 121 keV, $t_{1/2}$ = 62 h) (Voss, et al., 2007). As such, ^{64}Cu can be used as a dose-determinant indicator in ^{67}Cu-based therapeutic regimens.

While the physical properties of copper are well-suited for use in radiopharmaceuticals, the metabolism and physiological properties of copper in the human body present a challenge to the development and wide-spread use of copper-containing radiopharmaceuticals. Ideally, site-directed radiopharmaceuticals accumulate at the target site quickly with little accumulation in non-target tissues and rapidly clear non-target tissues after administration. Hence, hepatobiliary clearance of radiopharmaceuticals is much less desirable to renal/urinary clearance. Since the liver is the anatomical location of copper metabolism, the stability of the copper chelate in a ^{64}Cu-containing radiopharmaceutical under physiological conditions is very important (Wadas et al., 2007). Increasing the stability of copper complexes *in vivo* has been a major focus in the field of nuclear medicine for some time (Di Bartolo et al., 2001 and 2006; Gasser et al., 2008; Kukis et al., 1993; Voss et al., 2007; Pippin et al., 1991; Geraldes et al., 2000; Wieghardt et al., 1982; van der Merwe et al., 1985; Prasanphanich et al., 2007; Soluri et al., 2003; Maina et al., 2005; Monstein et al., 2006; Sun & Chen, 2007) as the development of stable copper complexes will allow for a variety of copper-based diagnostic and therapeutic strategies.

Recent work in the field of copper radiochemistry has produced very promising results. A majority of the work has focused on synthesis of new ligand frameworks to chelate copper in a multi-dentate fashion to prevent loss of the Cu^{2+} ion under *in vivo* conditions. Cross-bridged TETA (1,4,8,11-tetraazacyclotetradecane-1,4,8,11-tetracetic acid) derivatives, such as 4,11-bis(carboxymethyl)-1,4,8,11-tetraazabicyclo[6.6.2]hexadecane (CB-TE2A) and 1-N-(4-aminobenzyl)-3,6,10,13,16,19-hexa-aza-bicyclo-[6.6.6]eichosane-1,8-diamine (SarAr), have shown increased copper-complex stability *in vivo* versus the TETA and DOTA (1,4,7,10-tetraazacyclododecane-1,4,7,10-tetraacetic acid) chelators (Garrison et al., 2007; Di Bartolo et al., 2001 and 2006). Additionally, derivatives of the triazacyclononane macrocycle have produced improved stability of copper complexes (Prasanphanich et al., 2007). Pippin et al., have shown that complexes of Cu(II) with NOTA (1,4,7-triazacyclononane-1,4,7-triacetic acid) are more inert towards isotopic exchange with ^{67}Cu than DOTA or TETA (Pippin et al., 1991). Recent work by Gasser, et al., demonstrated a 2-[4,7-bis(2-pyridylmethyl)-1,4,7-triazacyclononan-1-yl] acetic acid (PMCN) bifunctional chelator containing the ^{64}Cu radionuclide (Gasser et al., 2008). Recently, we have reported on the superior microPET imaging quality of NOTA bifunctional chelator over that of the DOTA using ^{64}Cu in a GRPR-positive human prostate cancer mouse model (Prasanphanich et al., 2007). Previous investigations have reported a highly stable complex consisting of NOTA and divalent copper (Kukis et al., 1993; Geraldes et al., 2000; Wieghardt et al., 1982). Also reported are biomolecules conjugated with NOTA and chelating ^{64}Cu. Interestingly, one investigation reported a crystal structure of [CuCl(TACNTA)$^-$], or [CuCl(NOTA)$^-$], with a pentadentate NOTA in which one carboxylate arm of the triazacyclononane macrocycle is not involved in the coordination of copper(II) (van der Merwe et al., 1985). This implies that occupation of this non-chelating carboxylate of NOTA, as in our bifunctional NO2A, may not alter the native structure of the Cu-NOTA complex.

We have recently evaluated ^{64}Cu-NO2A-8-Aoc-BBN(7-14)NH_2 radiopharmaceutical (Figure 4) to be used as a PET targeting agent for primary or metastatic breast cancer disease (Prasanphanich et al., 2009). In this study, we were able to prepare high specific activity ^{64}Cu-NO2A-8-Aoc-BBN(7-14)NH_2 conjugate in very high radiochemical yield and to evaluate the 1) targeting capacity of ^{64}Cu-NO2A-8-Aoc-BBN(7-14)NH_2 for GRPr-positive tissues *in vivo*; 2) particular routes of clearance; and 3) extent of retention of radiopharmaceutical in radiosensitive tissues.

A number of *in vitro* assays were used to evaluate the uptake and affinity of ^{64}Cu-NO2A-8-Aoc-BBN(7-14)NH_2 for the GRPr in T-47D human breast cancer cells. Competitive binding displacement assays using ^{125}I-[Tyr^4]-BBN(7-14)NH_2, as the radioligand were used to quantify the relative binding affinity of Cu-NO2A-8-Aoc-BBN(7-14)NH_2 for GRPrs located on the surface of T-47D cells. The concentration of Cu-NO2A-8-Aoc-BBN(7-14)NH_2 needed to inhibit ^{125}I-[Tyr^4]-BBN(7-14)NH_2 binding by 50% was determined to be 7.56 ± 2.23 nM. The rate at which cell-associated radioactivity was internalized within the T-47D cells was also measured. After incubating T-47D cells in media containing ^{64}Cu-NO2A-8-Aoc-BBN(7-

14)NH_2 for 45 min, nearly 90% of all cell-associated radioactivity had internalized. This remained nearly constant for subsequent time points. The externalizaton of ^{64}Cu-NO2A-8-Aoc-BBN(7-14)NH_2 from T-47D cells was measured by removing cells from conjugate-containing media after 45 min and washing them to remove all surface-bound radioactivity. No significant efflux of radiotracer was observed over the 90 min period.

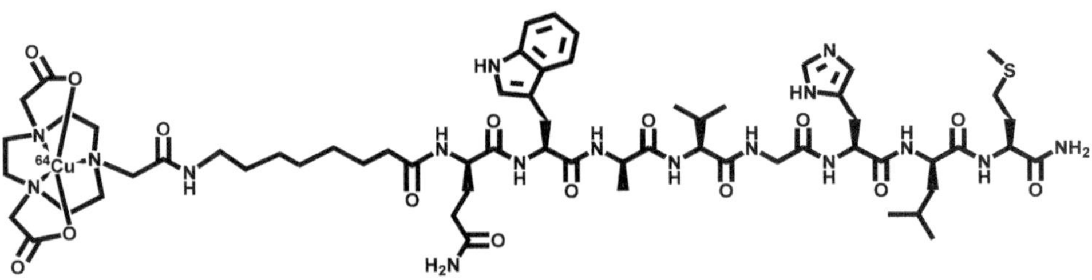

Fig. 4. ^{64}Cu-NO2A-8-Aoc-BBN(7-14)NH_2 conjugate.

Results obtained from biodistribution studies in SCID mice bearing human T-47D xenografted tumors suggested uptake in GRPr expressing tissues was receptor mediated. The average uptake and retention of conjugate in T-47D xenografted tumors at 1, 4, and 24 h p.i. were 2.27 ± 0.08, 1.35 ± 0.14, and 0.28 ± 0.07% ID/g. The primary mode of excretion for this conjugate was the renal-urinary excretion pathway. A receptor blocking assay in which BBN(1-14)NH_2 was administered 15 min prior to targeting vector in T-47D tumor-bearing mice showed a significant decrease in the accumulation of ^{64}Cu-NO2A-8-Aoc-BBN(7-14)NH_2 in tumor tissue. For example, uptake/accumulation of ^{64}Cu-NO2A-8-Aoc-BBN(7-14)NH_2 conjugate was reduced to 0.58±0.10% ID/g (1 h p.i.) with the addition of the blocking agent to the study. Furthermore, in the blocking assay, the degree of urinary excretion increased to 82 ± 18% ID and suggests that the radioactivity detected in the intestines were at least partially the result of a receptor-mediated process located along the lower gastrointestinal tract and not solely a function of hepatobiliary excretion. Additionally, accumulation of radiotracer in pancreatic tissue and tumors was significantly decreased in this blocking experiment, suggesting that the ^{64}Cu-NO2A-8-Aoc-BBN(7-14)NH_2 conjugate is intact and that GRPr-mediated binding is facilitating uptake in the tissues.

As a result of optimal uptake and retention of ^{64}Cu-NO2A-8-Aoc-BBN(7-14)NH_2 in T-47D xenografted tumor, microPET/MicroCT/microMRI multimodal imaging experiments were conducted in tumor-bearing mice (Figure 5). A SCID mouse bearing T-47D xenografted tumors on the left and right hind flanks underwent microMR and microPET/CT imaging 24 h following injection with 5.1 mCi of ^{64}Cu-NO2A-8-Aoc-BBN(7-14)NH_2. Anatomical structures observed *via* microPET imaging were consistent with pharmacokinetic data obtained from *in vivo* experiments. For example, tumors, pancreas, liver and kidneys, to a lesser extent, were clearly identifiable *via* microPET imaging analysis. Analysis of MRI data indicated small necrotic regions in the xenografted tumors as evident by increased water diffusivity. Observable in the microPET data were regions of reduced intensity that correlated well to these necrotic regions of the tumors. Additionally, the liver is observed to lack a uniform intensity. The drop in intensity correlates to the separation between the median and left lobes of the liver. The identification of such fine structures in the microPET data is a goal of diagnostic nuclear medicine. High-resolution imaging may aid in identifying structural boundaries as well as possible malignant sites.

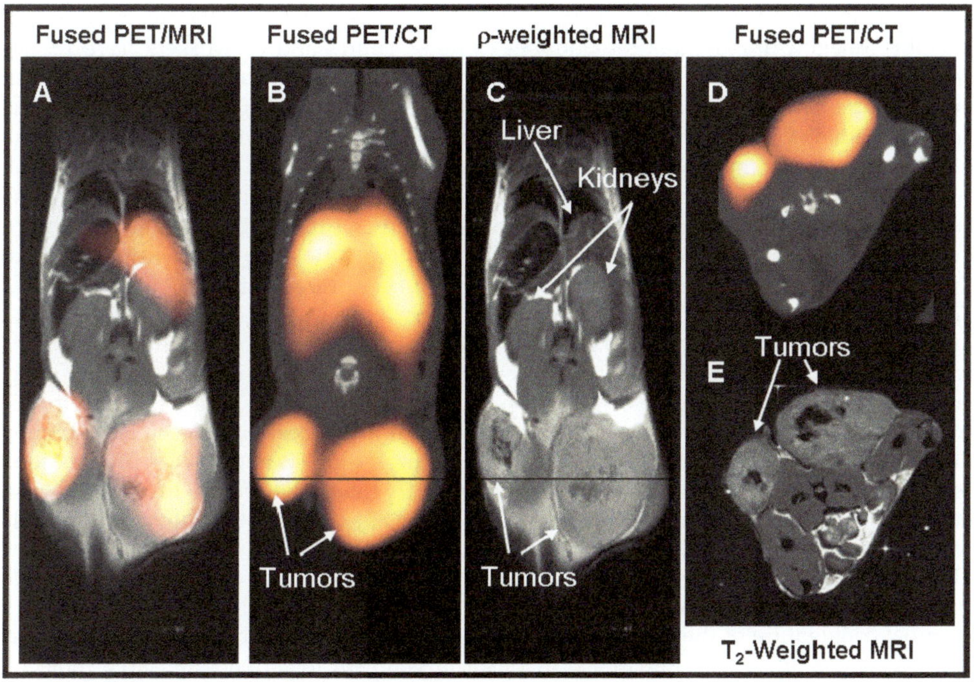

Fig. 5. *In vivo* microPET/CT and microMRI images of a T-47D tumor-bering mouse 24 h after 5.1 mCi tail vein injection of ^{64}Cu-NO2A-8-Aoc-BBN(7-14)NH_2 conjugate. (A) MicroPET/MRI fusion coronal image. (B) MicroPET/CT fused coronal image showing specific uptake of ^{64}Cu-NO2A-8-Aoc-BBN(7-14)NH_2 conjugate. (C) Proton density-weghted microMRI coronal image. (D) An axial cross section of microPET/CT images showing functional image of tumor uptake. (E) The corresponding high-resolution T2-weighted microMRI axial image correlating anatomical features of the xenografted tumors to (D).

6. Fluorescence molecular imaging using alexa fluor 680-BBN conjugates

Alternative optical imaging technologies such as fluorescence molecular tomography are emerging as new and exciting molecular imaging tools for diagnosis of human disease (Montet et al., 2006; Young & Rozengurt, 2005; Pu et al., 2005). Studies show that the high-throughput signal afforded by fluorescence imaging might offer an alternative to traditional tomographic imaging by alleviating many of the imaging artifacts seen in imaging systems of this general type (Weissleder & Ntziachristos, 2003; Zacharakis et al., 2005; Kwon et al., 2005). Therefore, design and development of new site-directed, fluorescent, targeting vectors for dynamic optical imaging of human cancers holds some significance.

Monet and co-workers have described a new peptide-nanoparticle conjugate based upon bombesin that may be potentially useful for imaging pancreatic ductal adenocarcinoma. They reported the ability of this new conjugate to specifically target GRPrs expressed on normal pancreatic tissue with minimal accumulation in normal and surrounding tissues. Furthermore, the utility of this new conjugate to be used as a dual modality MRI contrast agent was shown *in vivo* in T2 weighted MR images of rodents bearing MIA-PaCa2 pancreatic tumors (Montet et al., 2006). This study well demonstrates the potential of dual-modality imaging for diagnosis of human cancers. Young and co-workers have recently described the use of quantum dots conjugated to bombesin to successfully image living mouse Swiss 3T3 and Rat-1 cells *in vitro* (Young & Rozengurt, 2005) and Pu et al., have described a new Cypate-bombesin Peptide Analogue Conjugate (Cybesin) that has potential use as a prostate tumor receptor-mediated contrast agent (Pu et al., 2005). All of these studies provide either *in vivo* or *in vitro* evidence for production of fluorescence-based targeting vectors of bombesin for early detection of human cancers. In addition, fluorescence molecular tomography shows advantages as a relatively low cost, noninvasive procedure that utilizes highly sensitive, non-ionizing probes for tissue targeting.

To complement our work using technetium-99m and copper-64 tagged bombesin tracers to image T-47D breast cancer cells, we developed a new non-radioactive, fluorescent probe based upon BBN having high tumor uptake and optimal pharmacokinetics for specific targeting and optical imaging of the same cell line. In this study, we have developed a conjugate of bombesin having very high affinity for the GRP-receptor holding an N-terminal fluorescent tag that might be useful in determining the diagnosis and disease progression of estrogen receptor positive (ER+) breast cancer. Targeting ER+ breast cancer cells *via* a targeting vector bearing a fluorescent label is a viable alternative to traditional radiolabeled conjugates of this general type.

The new Alexa Fluor 680-GGG-BBN(7-14)NH_2 conjugate (Figure 6) was conveniently synthesized by solid phase peptide synthesis of the parent BBN ligand followed by N-terminal conjugation of the active succinimidyl ester of the Alexa Fluor molecule (Ma et al., 2007). This conjugation technology provides a mechanism for appending large molecular weight molecules having inherent fluorescent properties to either the N-terminal primary amine or the epsilon primary amines of lysine-containing peptides or antibodies to produce stable conjugates for dynamic *in vivo* optical imaging. Less-reactive amidated C-termini, however, do not readily react with succinimidyl esters, making this a very selective conjugation method. In our hands, AF 680-GGG-BBN(7-14)NH_2 conjugate was stable at temperatures of -80 °C for periods extending 6 months. Other Alexa Fluor® 680 compounds of this general type designed and developed in our laboratory have demonstrated similar stability profiles.

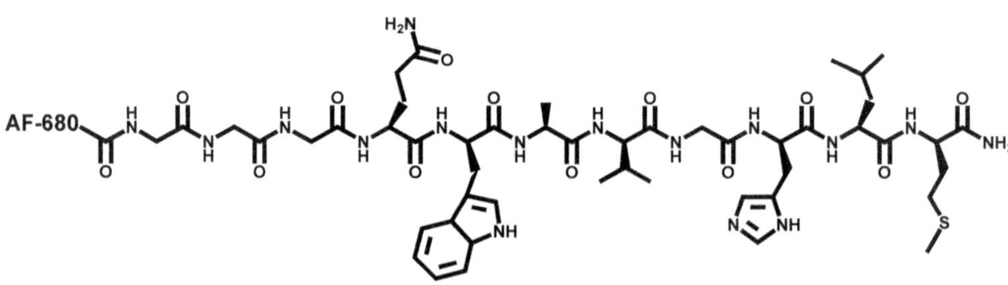

Fig. 6. AF 680-GGG-BBN(7-14)NH_2 conjugate.

In order to assess the binding affinity of the Alexa Fluor 680-GGG-BBN(7-14)NH_2 conjugate for the GRPr, *in vitro* competitive cell-binding assays were performed on T-47D breast cancer cells using ^{125}I-[Tyr^4]-BBN(7-14)NH_2 as the displacement radioligand. This new peptide conjugate demonstrated very high affinity for the GRPr in T-47D breast cancer cells, exhibiting an IC_{50} value of 7.7 ± 1.4 nM.

Figure 7 summarizes the results of studies to assess the degree of uptake, internalization, and blocking of the Alexa Fluor-GGG-BBN(7-14)NH_2 conjugate in T-47D breast cancer cells *via* confocal fluorescence microscopy. Assessment of the degree of AF 680-GGG-BBN(7-14)NH_2 conjugate associated with the cells after a 40 min incubation period was evaluated following a cell wash with pH 7.4 incubation media. Results of these studies clearly indicate the effectiveness of AF 680-GGG-BBN(7-14)NH_2 to specifically target the GRPr. To assess receptor-mediated internalization of AF 680-GGG-BBN(7-14)NH_2 conjugate, surface-bound conjugate was removed using pH 2.5 (0.2 M acetic acid and 0.5 M NaCl) buffer. After the acid wash, much of the conjugate remained internalized within the cells. *In vitro* blocking studies, in which high levels of BBN(1-14) were administered to the cells prior to the AF 680-GGG-BBN(7-14)NH_2 conjugate, reduced the uptake/retention in normal GRPr-expressing T-47D cells. This illustrates the high affinity and selectivity of this conjugate for GRPrs over-expressed on T-47D breast cancer cells. In fact, there is little or no indication of fluorescent signal associated with the cells following the blocking experiment.

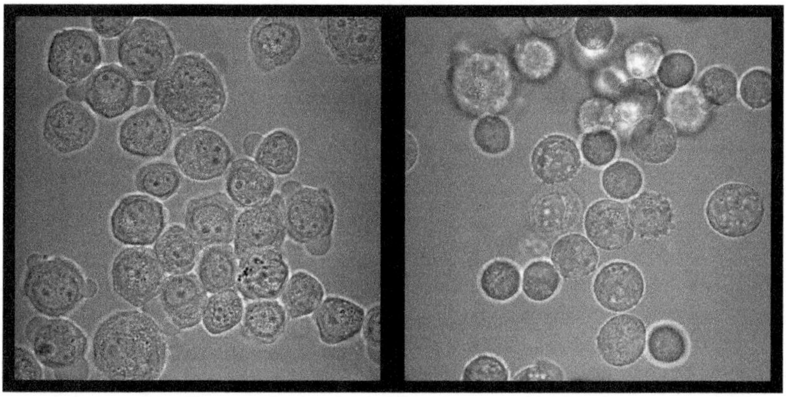

Fig. 7. Confocal fluorescence photomicrograph of internalized uptake of Alexa Fluor 680-GGG-BBN(7-14)NH_2 in human T-47D breast cancer cells (left). Confocal fluorescence photomicrograph of blocked uptake of Alexa Fluor 680-G-G-G-BBN(7-14)NH_2 in human T-47D breast cancer cells by wild-type BBN(1-14).

To assess the *in vivo* uptake of the Alexa Fluor conjugate, we have evaluated AF 680-GGG-BBN(7-14)NH_2 in rodents bearing human T-47D cancer cell xenografted tumors. In this study, dynamic optical imaging studies of T-47D breast cancer tumor xenografts in rodent models demonstrated the effectiveness of AF 680-GGG-BBN(7-14)NH_2 to specifically target GRPr-expressing cells *in vivo*. Montet and co-workers have demonstrated the effectiveness of fluorescent bombesin conjugates to effectively target implanted tumors of the pancreas (Montet et al., 2006). However, the effectiveness of imaging was only demonstrated using excised pancreatic/tumor tissue. Our more recent investigations have indicated specific uptake of conjugate in human tumor tissue (Figure 8a) in xenografted rodent models. Some degree of uptake was also observed in collateral tissue of the abdomen. This, however, is not entirely unexpected due to the hydrophobic nature of the high molecular weight targeting vector. Blocking investigations (Figure 8b), in which BBN(1-14) was used to saturate the GRPr prior to administration of AF 680-GGG-BBN(7-14)NH_2, showed little or no fluorescent signal associated with tumor tissue. To complement and verify the presence of GRPr-expressing tumors, magnetic resonance imaging was performed (Figure 8c and 8d). These studies further demonstrate the high degree of selectivity and affinity of AF 680-GGG-BBN(7-14)NH_2 conjugate for the GRPr.

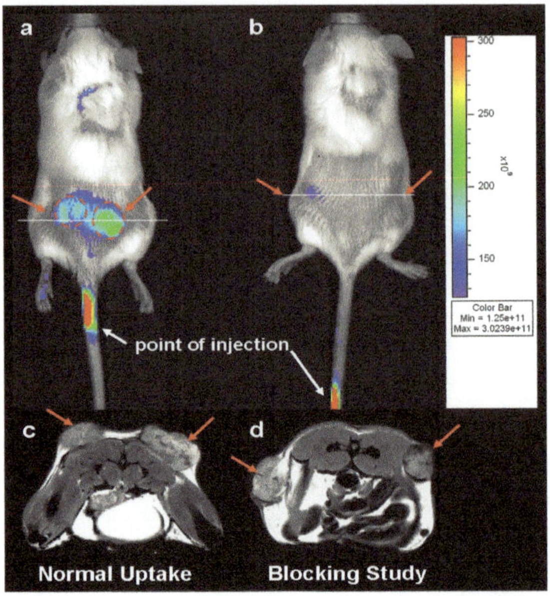

Fig. 8. *In vivo* uptake and blocking experiment of Alexa Fluor 680-GGG-BBN(7-14)NH_2 in SCID mice bearing human T-47D breast cancer cell xenografts. Xenogen fluorescence images of mice with (A) normal uptake and (B) blocking assay. Magnetic resonance images of cross sections through tumors for (C) normal uptake and (D) blocking assay.

7. Conclusion

The clinical successes of Octreoscan® have paved the way for exploration and radiolabeling of biologically-active peptides for targeted molecular imaging and peptide receptor scintigraphy of receptors that are highly expressed on specific human tumors. This book chapter has focused primarily upon those peptides that are potentially useful for molecular imaging of human breast cancer. Specifically, our research investigations have focused primarily upon targeting GRPrs with truncated analogues of BBN peptide, as these receptors tend to be expressed in very high numbers on the surface of breast cancer cells. However, there are other cancer types that also express regulatory peptide receptors in very high numbers, making possible early diagnosis and staging of primary and metastatic disease for these cancers as well. More importantly, continued research efforts toward development of thermodynamically stable, kinetically inert radiolabeled peptides for specific targeting of receptors that are highly expressed on the surfaces of human cancer cells creates the opportunity to use peptide receptor targeted radiotherapy as a highly selective treatment strategy for tumor targeting of breast cancer and many others, or as a mechanism for this treatment strategy to complement traditional, clinically-useful chemotherapeutic regimens of treatment.

8. Future work

Until now, the molecular basis for GRPr-targeted diagnosis or therapy of receptor-positive neoplastic disease has primarily focused upon targeting receptor over-expression using radiolabeled agonist ligands with inherent internalizing capability. However, recent reports by Nock et al., show compelling evidence that radiopharmaceutical design and development based upon antagonist-type ligand frameworks bear reexamination (Nock et al., 2003 and 2005). Antagonist ligands are presumably not internalized, and therefore are not expected to residualize as effectively in tumor tissue when compared to agonist-based ligand frameworks. Studies using ^{99m}Tc-Demobesin1 ([^{99m}Tc-N_4^{0-1},bzlg^0,D-Phe^6,Leu-NHEt^{13},des-Met^{14}]BBN(6-14)) demonstrated very high affinity and selectivity for the GRPR with pronounced accumulation and retention of radioactivity in human tumor xenografts in rodents (Nock et al., 2003 and 2005). In addition, Maecke and co-workers have begun investigating another antagonist-like targeting vector, [DOTA-4-amino-1-carboxymethyl-piperidine-D-Phe-Gln-Trp-Ala-Val-Gly-His-Sta-Leu-NH_2], having high selectivity for the GRPr (Mansi et al., 2009 and 2011). Therefore, selective targeting of specific receptor subtypes expressed on the surfaces of primary or metastatic breast cancer tissues with new and improved radiolabeled antagonists might provide a new avenue for earlier diagnosis and staging of patients presenting with disease.

In addition, we should point out that discussions herein have only considered monomeric peptide targeting vectors for molecular imaging of breast cancer tissue. It is important to note that the clinical utility of monomeric radiolabeled peptides can be limited by a number of factors including receptor density, binding affinity, and pharmacokinetics. For example, high-quality, high tumor-to-background PET or SPECT images require a high degree of receptor expression on tumor cells as compared to normal, collateral tissue. For these reasons, multimeric or multivalent peptide probes have recently become a new avenue for diagnostic molecular imaging tumors expressing either singly- or multi-targetable receptors. Continued design and development of multimeric or multivalent peptides capable of targeting multiple receptor subtypes highly expressed on human cancers could do much to improve image resolution and contrast, all but eliminating the high false-positive rates and non-target uptake that oftentimes limits some of the clinically-approved radiopharmaceuticals from widespread usage for diagnosis of malignant tissues.

9. Acknowledgment

This material is the result of work supported with resources and the use of facilities at the Harry S. Truman Memorial Veterans' Hospital and the University of Missouri School of Medicine. This work was funded in part by grants from the National Institutes of Health and the United States Department of Veterans' Affairs VA Merit Award.

10. References

American Cancer Society. *Cancer Facts and Figures 2010, Detailed Guide: Breast Cancer.* The American Cancer Society, Atlanta: 2010. Available at www.cancer.org/acs/groups /content/@epidemiologysurveilance/documents/document/acspc-026210.pdf

Abd-Elgaliel WR, Gallazzi F, Garrison JC, et al. (2008). Design, Synthesis, and Biological Evaluation of an Antagonist-Bombesin Analogue as Targeting Vector. *Bioconj. Chem.*, Vol. 19: pp. 2040-2048.

Alberto R, Ortner K, Wheatley N, et al. (2001). Synthesis and properties of boranocarbonate: a convenient in situ CO source for the aqueous preparation of $[^{99m}Tc(OH_2)_3(CO)_3]^+$. *J. Am. Chem. Soc.*, Vol. 123, pp. 3135-3136.

Alberto R, Schibli R, Egli A, et al. (1998). A novel organometallic aqua complex of technetium for the labeling of biomolecules: synthesis of $[^{99m}Tc(OH_2)_3(CO)_3]^+$ from $[^{99m}TcO_4]^-$ in aqueous solution and its reaction with a bifunctional ligand. *J. Am. Chem. Soc.*, Vol. 120, pp. 7987-7988.

Aliaga A, Rousseau JA, Ouellette R, et al. (2004). Breast cancer models to study the expression of estrogen receptors with small animal PET imaging. *Nucl. Med. Biol.*, Vol. 31, pp. 761-770.

Anderson CJ & Welch MJ. (1999). Radiometal-Labeled Agents (Non-Technetium) for Diagnostic Imaging. *Chem. Rev.*, Vol. 99, pp. 2219-2234.

Bajc M, Ingvar C. & Palmer J. (1996). Dynamic Indium-111-Pentetreotide Scintigraphy in Breast Cancer. *J. Nuc. Med.*, Vol. 37, pp. 622-626.

Berghammer P, Obwegeser R, & Sinzinger H. (2001). Nuclear medicine and breast cancer: a review of current strategies and novel therapies. *The Breast*, Vol. 10, pp. 184-197.

Biddlecombe GB, Rogers BE, de Visser M, et al. (2007) Molecular imaging of GRP receptor positive tumors in mice using ^{64}Cu- and ^{86}Y-DOTA-(Pro1,Tyr4)-BBN(1-14). *Bioconj. Chem.*, Vol. 18, pp. 724-730.

Biersack HJ & Freeman LM (eds). (2007). *Clinical Nuclear Medicine*, Springer, New York.

Blok D, Feitsma RIJ, Vermeij P, et al. (1999). Peptide radiopharmaceuticals in nuclear medicine. *Eur. J. Nucl. Med.*, Vol. 26, pp. 1511-1519.

Blower PJ, Lewis JS, & Zweit J. (1996). Copper radionuclides and radiopharmaceuticals in nuclear medicine. *Nucl. Med. Biol.*, Vol. 23, pp. 957-980.

Coy DH, Heinz-Erian P, Jiang NY, et al. (1988). Probing peptide backbone function in bombesin. A reduced peptide bond analogue with potent and specific receptor antagonist activity. *Bioconj. Chem.*, Vol. 263, pp. 5056-5060.

Cuttitta F, Carney DN, Mulshine J, et al. (1985). BBN-like peptides can function as autocrine growth factors in human small-cell lung cancer. *Nature*, Vol. 316, pp. 823-825.

Di Bartolo NM, Sargeson AM, Donlevy TM, et al. (2001). Synthesis of a new cage ligand, SarAr, and its complexation with selected transition metal ions for potential use in radioimaging. *J Chem. Soc., Dalton Trans*, pp. 2303-2309.

Di Bartolo NM, Sargeson AM & Smith SV. (2006). New ^{64}Cu PET imaging agents for personalized medicine and drug development using the hexa-aza cage, SarAr. *Org. Biomol. Chem.*, Vol. 4, pp. 3350-3357.

Engel LW & Young NA. (1978). Human breast carcinoma cells in continuous culture: a review. *Can. Res.*, Vol. 38, pp. 4327-4339.

Fischman AJ, Babich JW, & Strauss HW. (1993). A Ticket to Ride: Peptide Radiopharmaceuticals. *J. Nucl. Med.*, Vol. 34, pp. 2253-2263.

Garrison JC, Rold TL, Sieckman GL, et al. (2007). *In vivo* evaluation and small-animal PET/CT of a prostate cancer mouse model using ^{64}Cu BBN analogs: side-by-side comparison of the CB-TE2A and DOTA chelation systems. *J. Nucl. Med.*, Vol. 48, pp. 1327-1337.

Gasser G, Tjioe L, Graham B, et al. (2008). Synthesis, copper(II) complexation, ^{64}Cu-labeling, and bioconjugation of a new bis(2-pyridylmethyl) derivative of 1,4,7-triazacyclononane. *Bioconj. Chem.*, Vol. 19, pp. 719-730.

Geraldes CFGC, Marques MP, de Castro B, et al. (2000). Study of copper(II) polyazamacrocyclic complexes by electronic absorption spectrophotometry and EPR spectroscopy. *Eur. J. Inorg. Chem.*, pp. 559-565.

Giacchetti S, Gauville C, De Cremoux P, et al. (1990). Characterization, In Some Human Breast Cancer Cell Lines, of Gastrin-Releasing Peptide-Like Receptors Which are Absent in Normal Breast Epithelial Cells. *Int. J. Can.*, Vol. 46, pp. 293-298.

Giblin MF, Gali H, Sieckman GL, et al. (2006). *In vitro* and *in vivo* evaluation of ^{111}In-labeled E. coli heat-stable enterotoxin analogs for specific targeting of human breast cancers. *Breast Can. Res. Treat.*, Vol. 98, pp. 7-15.

Gopalan D, Bomanji JB, Costa DC, et al. (2002). Nuclear Medicine in Primary Breast Cancer Imaging. *Clin. Radiol.*, Vol. 57, pp. 565-574.

Gugger M & Reubi JC. (1999). Gastrin-Releasing Peptide Receptors in Non-Neoplastic and Neoplastic Human Breast. *Am. J. Path.*, Vol. 155, pp. 2067-2076.

Guojun W, Wei G, Kedong O, et al. (2008). A novel vaccine targeting pastrin-releasing peptide: efficient inhibition of breast cancer growth *in vivo*. *Endocrine-Related Cancer*, Vol. 15, pp. 149-159.

Hoffman TJ, Quinn TP, & Volkert WA. (2001). Radiometallated receptor-avid peptide conjugates for specific *in vivo* targeting of cancer cells. *Nucl. Med. Biol.*, Vol. 28, pp. 527-539.

Jones CJ and Thornback JR. (2007). *Medical Applications of Coordination Chemistry*, RSC Publishing, Cambridge, UK.

Kaida H, Ishibashi M, Fujii T, et al. (2008). Improved detection of breast cancer on FDG-PET cancer screening using breast positioning device. *Ann. Nucl. Med.*, Vol. 22, pp. 95-101.

Katzenellenbogen JA, Coleman RE, Hawkins RA, et al. (1995). Tumor Receptor Imaging: Proceedings of the National Cancer Institute Workshop, Review of Current Work, and Prospective for Further Investigations. *Clin. Can. Res.*, Vol. 1, 921-932.

Knigge U, Holst JJ, Knuhtsen S, et al. (1984). Gastrin-Releasing Peptide: Pharmacokinetics and Effects on Gastroentero-Pancreatic Hormones and Gastric Secretion in Normal Men. *J. Clin. Endocrin. Metab.*, Vol. 59, pp. 310-315.

Koglin N & Beck-Sickinger AG. (2004). Novel modified and radiolabelled neuropeptide Y analogues to study Y-receptor subtypes. *Neuropeptides*, Vol. 38, pp. 153-161.

Krause W. (ed.) (2002). *Contrast Agents II: Optical, Ultrasound, X-Ray, and Radiopharmaceutical Imaging*, Springer, New York.

Kukis DL, Li M, & Meares CF. (1993). Selectivity of antibody-chelate conjuates for binding copper in the presence of competing metals. *Inorg. Chem.*, Vol. 32, pp. 3981-3982.

Kwon S, Ke S, Houston JP, et al. (2005). Imaging dose-dependent pharmacokinetics of an RGD-fluorescent dye conjugate targeted to avb3 receptor expressed in Kaposi's sarcoma. *Mol. Imaging*, Vol. 4, No. 2, pp. 75-87.

Lacroix M & Leclercq G. (2004). Relevance of breast cancer cell lines as models for breast tumors: an update. *Breast Can. Res. Treat.*, Vol. 83, pp. 249-289.

Lixin M, Yu P, Veerendra B, et al. (2007). *In vitro* and *In vivo* Evaluation of AF 680-BBN[7-14]NH_2 Peptide Conjugate, a High-Affinity Fluorescent Probe with High Selectivity for the GRP Receptor. *Mol. Imaging*, Vol. 6, pp. 171-180.

Maina T, Nock BA, Zhang H, et al. (2005). Species differences of bombesin analog interactions with GRP-R define the choice of animal models in the development of GRP-R-targeting drugs. *J. Nucl. Med.*, Vol. 46, pp. 823-830.

Mansi, R., Wang X, Forrer F et al. (2009). Evaluation of a 1,4,7,10-tetraazacyclododecane-1,4,7,10-tetraacetic acid-conjugated BBN-based radioantagonist for the labeling with single-photon emission computed tomography, positron emission tomography, and therapeutic radionuclides. *Clin. Can. Res.*, Vol. 15, No. 16, pp. 5240-5249.

Mansi, R., Wang X, Forrer F, et al. (2011). Development of a potent DOTA-conjugated BBN antagonist for targeting GRPr-positive tumours. *Eur. J. Nucl. Med. Mol. Imag.*, Vol. 38, No. 1, pp. 97-107.

Monstein HJ, Grahn N, Truedsson M, et al. (2006). Progastrin-releasing peptide and gastrin-releasing peptide receptor mRNA expression in non-tumor tissues of the human gastrointestinal tract. *World J. Gastroenterol.*, Vol. 12, pp. 2574-2578.

Montet X, Weissleder R & Josephson L (2006). Imaging pancreatic cancer with a peptide-nanoparticle conjugate targeted to normal pancreas. *Bioconj. Chem.*, Vol. 27, pp. 905-911.

Moody TW & Gozes I. (2007). Vasoactive Intestinal Peptide Receptors: A Molecular Target in Breast and Lung Cancer. *Cur. Pharmaceutical Des.*, Vol. 13, pp. 1099-1104.

Moody TW, Pert CB, Gazdar AF, et al. (1981). High levels of intracellular BBN characterize human small cell lung carcinoma. *Science*, Vol. 214, pp. 1246-1248.

Nass SJ, Henderson IC, & Lashof JC (eds). (2001). *Mammography and Beyond: Developing Technologies for the Early Detection of Breast Cancer.* Natl. Acad. Press, Washington.

Nijsen JFW, Krijer GC, & van het Schip AD. (2007). The bright future of radionuclides for cancer therapy. *Anti Canc. Agents Med. Chem.*, Vol. 7, pp. 271-290.

Nock B, Nikolopoulou A, Chiotellis E, et al. (2003). [^{99m}Tc] Demobesin 1, a novel potent bombesin analogue for GRPr-targeted tumour imaging. *Eur. J. Nucl. Med. Mol. Imag.*, Vol. 30, pp. 247-258.

Nock B, Nikolopoulou A, Galanis A, et al. (2005). Potent bombesin-like peptides for GRP-receptor targeting of tumors with ^{99m}Tc: A preclinical study. *J. Med. Chem.*, Vol. 48, No. 1, pp. 100-110.

Olsen, O & Gotzsche PC. (2001). Cochrane Review on Screening for Breast Cancer with Mammography. *Lancet.* Vol. 358, pp. 1340-1342.

Parry JJ, Andrews R, & Rogers BE. (2007). MicroPET imaging of breast cancer using radiolabeled bombesin analogs targeting the gastrin-releasing peptide receptor. *Breast Can. Res. Treat.*, Vol. 101, pp. 175-183.

Pippin CG, Kumar K, Mirzadeh S, et al. (1991). Kinetics of the isotopic exchange between copper(II) and copper(II) 1,4,7-triazacyclononane-*N,N',N''* triacetate. *J. Labeled Comp. Rad.*, Vol. 30, p. 221.

Pisano ED, Gatsonis C, Hendrick E, et al. (2005). Diagnostic performance of digital versus film mammography for breast-cancer screening. *New Engl. J. Med.*, Vol. 353, pp. 1773-1783.

Pomper MG & Gelovani JG (eds). (2008). *Molecular Imaging in Oncology.* Informa Healthcare, New York.

Prasad NS, & Houserkova D. (2007). The roles of various modalities in breast imaging. *Biomed Pap Fac Univ Palacky Olomouc Czech Republic*, Vol. 151, pp. 209-218.

Prasanphanich AF, Lane SR, Figueroa SD, et al. (2007). The effects of linking substituents on the *in vivo* behavior of site-directed, peptide-based, diagnostic radiopharmaceuticals. *In Vivo*, Vol. 21, pp. 1-16.

Prasanphanich AF, Nanda PK, Rold TL, et al. (2007). [^{64}Cu-NO2A-8-Aoc-BBN(7-14)NH_2] targeting vector for PET imaging of gastrin-releasing peptide receptor-expressing tissues. *Proc. Natl. Acad. Sci. USA*, Vol. 104, pp. 12462-12467.

Prasanphanich AF, Retzloff L, Lane SR, et al. (2009). *In vitro* and *in vivo* analysis of [^{64}Cu-NO2A-8-Aoc-BBN(7-14)NH_2]: a site-directed radiopharmaceutical for positron emission tomography imaging of T-47D human breast cancer tumors. *Nucl. Med. and Biol.*, Vol. 36, pp. 171-181.

Pu Y, Wang WB, Tang GC, et al. (2005). Spectral polarization imaging of human prostate cancer tissue using a near-infrared receptor-targeted contrast agent. *Tech. Canc. Res. Treat.* Vol. 4, No. 4, pp. 429-436.

Retzloff, LB, Heinzke, L, Figureoa, SD et al. (2010). Evaluation of [^{99m}Tc-$(CO)_3$-X-Y-Bombesin(7-14)NH_2] Conjugates for Targeting Gastrin-releasing Peptide Receptors Over-expressed on Breast Carcinoma. *Antican. Res.*, Vol. 30, pp.19-30.

Reubi, JC. (2008). Peptide Receptors as Molecular Targets for Cancer Diagnosis and Therapy. *Endocrine Rev.*, Vol. 124, pp. 389-427.

Rosen ST, Blake MA, & Kalra MK (eds). (2008). *Cancer Treatment and Research, Volume 143: Imaging in Oncology.* Springer, New York.

Schibli R & Schubiger PA. (2002). Current use and future potential of organometallic radiopharmaceuticals. *Eur. J. Nucl. Med.*, Vol. 29, pp. 1529-1542.

Scopinaro F, Varvarigou AD, Ussof W, et al. (2002). Technetium Labeled Bombesin-like Peptide: Preliminary Report on Breast Cancer Uptake in Patients. *Canc. Biother. Rad.*, Vol. 17, pp. 327-335.

Signore A, Annovazzi A, Chianelli M, et al. (2001). Peptide radiopharmaceuticals for diagnosis and therapy. *Eur. J. Nucl. Med.*, Vol. 28, pp. 1555-1565.

Smith CJ, Gali H, Sieckman GL, et al. (2003). Radiochemical Investigations of ^{99m}Tc-N_3S-X-BBN[7-14]NH_2: An *in vitro/in vivo* Structure-Activity Relationship Study Where X = 0-, 3-, 5-, 8-, and 11-Carbon Tethering Moieties. *Bioconj.Chem.*, Vol. 14, pp. 93-102.

Smith CJ, Volkert WA, & Hoffman TJ. (2003). Gastrin releasing peptide receptor targeted radiopharmaceuticals: A concise update. *Nucl. Med. Biol.*, Vol. 30, pp. 861-868.

Smith CJ, Volkert WA, & Hoffman TJ. (2005). Radiolabeled peptide conjugates for targeting of the BBN receptor superfamily subtypes. *Nucl. Med. Biol.*, Vol. 32, pp. 733-740.

Soluri A, Scopinaro F, de Vincentis G, et al. (2003). ^{99m}Tc [13Leu] bombesin and a new gamma camera, the probe, are able to guide mammotome breast biopsy. *Antican. Res.*, Vol. 23, pp. 2139-2142.

Sprague JE, Peng Y, Fiamengo AL, et al. (2007). Synthesis, characterization and *in vivo* studies of Cu(II)-64-labeled cross-bridged tetraazamacrocycle-amide complexes as models of peptide conjugate Imaging Agents. *J. Med. Chem.*, Vol. 50, pp. 2527-2535.

Stigbrand T, Carlsson J, & Adams GP (eds). (2008). *Targeted Radionuclide Tumor Therapy: Biological Aspects.* Springer, New York.

Sun YG, & Chen ZF. (2007). A gastrin-releasing peptide receptor mediates the itch sensation in the spinal cord. *Nature*, Vol. 488, pp. 700-703.

Thakur ML, Aruva MR, Gariepy J, et al. (2004). PET Imaging of Oncogene Over-expression Using: ^{64}Cu-Vasoactive Intestinal Peptide (VIP) Analog: Comparison with ^{99m}Tc-VIP Analog. *J. Nucl. Med.*, Vol. 45, pp. 1381-1389.

Van de Wiele C, Dumont F, Broecke RV, et al. (2000). Technetium-99m RP527, a GRP analogue for visualisation of GRPr-expressing malignancies: a feasibility study. *Eur. J. Nucl. Med.*, Vol. 27, pp. 1694-1699.

van der Merwe MJ, Boeyens JCA, & Hancock RD. (1985). Crystallographic and thermodynamic study of metal ion size selectivity in the ligand 1,4,7-triazacyclononane-*N,N′,N″*-triacetate. *Inorg. Chem.*, Vol. 24, pp. 1208-1213.

Varvarigou A, Bouziotis P, Zikos C, et al. (2004). Gastrin-Releasing Peptide (GRP) Analogues for Cancer Imaging. *Canc. Biother. Rad.*, Vol. 19, pp. 219-229.

Voss SD, Smith SV, Di Bartolo NM, et al. (2007). Positron emission tomography (PET) imaging of neuroblastoma and melanoma with ^{64}Cu-SarAr immunoconjugates. *Proc. Natl. Acad. Sci. USA*, Vol. 104, pp. 17489-17493.

Wadas TJ, Wong EH, Weisman GR, et al. (2007). Copper chelation chemistry and its role in copper radiopharmaceuticals. *Cur. Pharmaceutical Des.*, Vol. 13, pp. 3-16.

Wang F, Wang Z, Wu J, et al. (2008). The role of technetium-99m-labeled octreotide acetate scintigraphy in suspected breast cancer and correlates with expression of SSTR. *Nucl. Med. Biol.*, Vol. 35, pp. 665-671.

Weiner RE, & Thakur ML. (2005). Radiolabeled peptides in oncology. *Biodrugs*, Vol. 19, pp. 145-163.

Weissleder R, & Ntziachristos, V (2003). Shedding light onto live molecular targets. *Nat. Med.*, Vol. 9, pp. 123-128.

Wieghardt K, Bossek U, Chaudhuri P, et al. (1982). 1,4,7-Triazacyclononane-*N,N′,N″*-triacetate (TCTA), a hexadentate ligand for divalent and trivalent metal ions. Crystal structures of [Cr^{III}(TCTA)], [Fe^{III}(TCTA)], and Na[Cu^{II}(TCTA)]•2NaBr•$8H_2O$. *Inorg. Chem.*, Vol. 21, pp. 4308-4314.

Young SH, & Rozengurt E (2006). Quantum dots conjugated to bombesin or angiotensin II label the cognate G protein-coupled receptor in living cells. *Am. J. Physiol. Cell Physiol.*, Vol. 290, No. 3, pp. 728-732.

Zacharakis, G, Ripoll, J, & Ntziachristos, V (2005). Fluorescent protein tomography scanner for small animal imaging. *IEEE Trans. Med. Imag.*, Vol. 24, pp. 878-885.

Zhang H, Chen J, Waldherr C, et al. (2004). Synthesis and Evaluation of Bombesin Derivatives on the Basis of Pan-Bombesin Peptides Labeled with Indium-111, Lutetium-177, and Yttrium-90 for Targeting Bombesin Receptor-Expressing Tumors. *Can. Res.*, Vol. 64, pp. 6707-6715.

Zhou J, Chen J, Mokotoff M, et al. (2003). Bombesin/gastrin-releasing peptide receptor: a potent target for antibody-mediated therapy of small cell lung cancer. *Clin. Can. Res.*, Vol. 9, pp. 4953-4960.

Zwanziger D, Khan IU, Neundorf I, et al. (2008). Novel Chemically Modified Analogues of Neuropeptide Y for Tumor Targeting. *Bioconj. Chem.*, Vol. 19, pp. 1430-1438.

16

Computer Aided System for Nuclear Stained Breast Cancer Cell Counting

Pornchai Phukpattaranont, Somchai Limsiroratana, Kanita Kayasut and Pleumjit Boonyaphiphat
Prince of Songkla University
Thailand

1. Introduction

1.1 Image characteristics

Immunohistochemistry is a technique used for detecting *in situ* a tissue antigen by a specific antibody. An antigen-antibody reaction is visualized by the color development of specific dye and can be seen by light microscope. The tissue antigen is presented at any part of the cell, i.e., cell membrane, cytoplasm or nucleus. Therefore, it is a useful technique to demonstrate the protein markers including cancer cell. Estrogen receptor (ER) and progesterone receptor (PR) are prognostic markers for breast cancer detected by this method. Evaluation of ER and PR positive cells are useful for hormonal therapy.

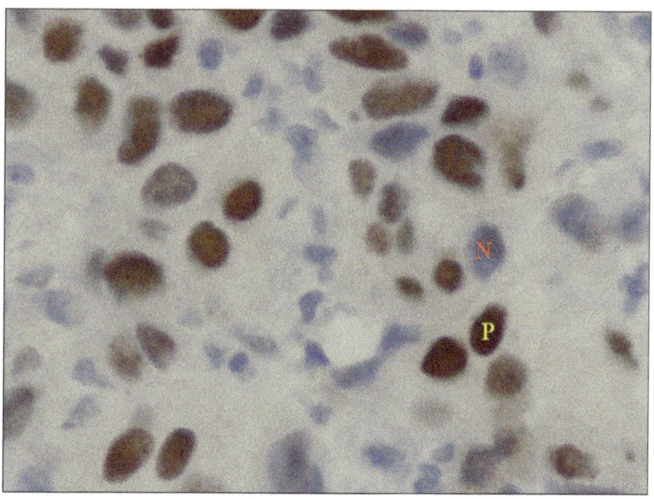

Fig. 1. An example of a stained cancer cell image. The brown and blue nuclei with the added labels are representative samples of positive and negative staining of estrogen receptor of breast cancer cells, respectively.

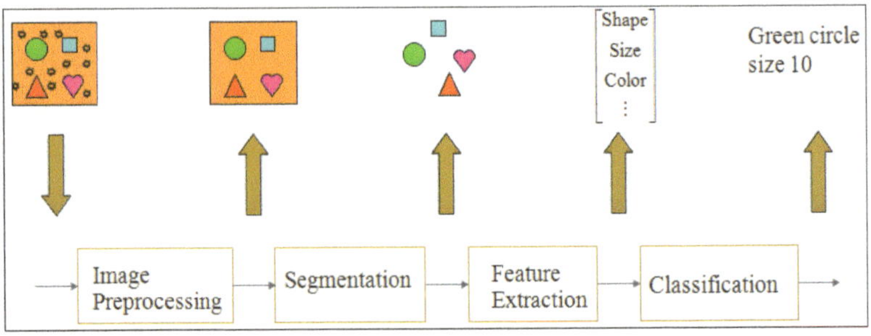

Fig. 2. The principle of image analysis in computer aided system for cancer cell classification.

Figure 1 shows an example of stained cancer cell image from microscope with a magnification of 40x. This staining procedure is utilized to demonstrate the existing of estrogen or progesterone receptors in the breast cancer cells. In other words, stained cancer cells are classified into two categories according to their nuclear color contents, i.e. brown and blue. The brown color indicates a positive (P) staining while the blue one demonstrates a negative (N) result. The brown and blue cells with the added labels shown in Figure 1 are representative samples of positive and negative staining of estrogen receptor of cancer cells, respectively. The ratio of the total number of positive cancer cells to the total number of cancer cells in the whole image is used by a doctor for medical planning and treatment.

Traditionally, the percentage of positive cells of those markers is semi-quantitatively counted. However, it is time consuming, costly, subjective and tedious. To overcome these problems, image analysis that previously requires manual operations is performed on the basis of the developments in computer capabilities and image processing algorithms (Fang et al., 2003; Petushi et al., 2004; Thiran & Macq, 1996). There are a number of benefits that result from image analysis with computer aided system. These include an acceleration of the process, a reduction in cost for image analysis, as well as a decrement in a false inspection due to fatigue. Additionally, the computer aided analysis provides a quantitative description. Based on this quantitative measurement, the analysis result is objective. Furthermore, the correlation of the quantitative categorization with patient symptoms may allow for an automated diagnostic system (O'Gorman et al., 1985). However, it is not expected that computer aided image analysis will replace pathologist's experience. It is only an aid to the pathologist for the repeated routine work and yields quantitative results that complement and enhance interpretations by pathologists. Visual examination by the pathologist is still required where the objects that the method is not trained to deal with are encountered.

1.2 Image analysis

The principle of image analysis in computer aided system for classifying cancer cells is composed of four stages as shown in Figure 2. After the preprocessing stage, the image is segmented in order to keep the interesting parts and remove the undesirable components. Next, the feature extraction process is applied in order to extract the useful information from the segmented objects. Finally, the classification is performed using the characteristics extracted from the previous stage. The ultimate goal of our research project is to develop an automatic algorithm for counting positive and negative cancer cells on immunohistological stained slides from breast cancer tissue.

One of the most important stages for the image analysis is cell image segmentation, which is the main focus of this work. Cell image segmentation methods for pathology are largely relied on two image processing techniques: thresholding and region growing. Thresholding identifies each pixel in the image into either object or background based on its intensity. Image thresholding is a simple yet often effective means for obtaining a segmentation of images in which cells of interest situate in uniform background intensity across the image. Consequently, it is often used as a part in a sequence of image processing operations. For example, thresholding is one of important steps in segmenting live cell image (Wu et al., 1995). For the image with uneven background, local adaptive thresholding method is an effective technique because the threshold value can be adapted to the background intensity variations. In other words, the threshold value is derived in each subregion, which is considered to be composed of both background and objects. Examples of medical image analysis that contain the local adaptive thresholding algorithm are as follows: (1) Segmentation of fluorescence tumor cells from tissue sections (Fang et al., 2003), (2) Segmentation of cell nuclei from the stroma and fat like regions (Petushi et al., 2004), (3) Segmentation of tissue components in liver tissue (O'Gorman et al., 1985), (4) Segmentation of dead and live hepatocytes (liver cells) in cultures from microscopic images (Refai et al., 2003), and (5) Segmentation of nuclei from a breast tissue image (Zhao & Ong, 1998). One of disadvantages of the thresholding technique is that it does not take into account the spatial characteristics of the image. This causes it to be sensitive to noise and intensity heterogeneity. Therefore, further image processing algorithms that consider spatial modeling of the image need to be incorporated (Li et al., 1995).
Region growing separates objects of interest from background in the image based on some predetermined criteria, i.e. intensity and/or edges (Haralik & Shapiro, 1985). While edge-based methods are sensitive to noise and artifacts, the intensity-based algorithms are usually more computationally expensive. Additionally, one of main disadvantage of region growing is the requirement of manual interaction to obtain the seed point (Adams & Bischof, 1994). Similar to thresholding, region growing is partially used in a set of image processing operations (Beveridge & et al., 1989; Wani & Batchelor, 1994). An example of region growing used in medical image analysis includes the extraction of noisy cell contour as appear in (Wu & Barba, 1994). In addition to thresholding and region growing, other techniques are the segmentation of white blood cells based on morphological granulometries (Theera-Umpon & Gader, 2000) and the segmentation of white blood cells based on the principle of least commitment (Park & Keller, 1997).
We propose two image segmentation methods for breast cancer cell counting. Firstly, we present the segmentation algorithm for breast cancer cell image based on local adaptive thresholding (Phukpattaranont & Boonyaphiphat, 2006). The method is appropriate for microscopic images with low histological noise, i.e., low variations on background color and intensity. However, the degree of histological noise in breast cancer images varies. For the image with high histological noise, the local adaptive thresholding approach is sensitive to noise and intensity heterogeneity. In addition, the computational time for the approach is quite lengthy. To address these problems, we propose a strategy for segmenting cancer cells in a microscopic image of immunohistological nuclear staining of breast cancer tissue based on the color of pixel(Phukpattaranont & Boonyaphiphat, 2007; Phukpattaranont et al., 2009). This is motivated from the way that a pathologist determines the positive and negative of tumor cells by using their color contents manually. As a result, we propose the use of pixel color partitioning based on a neural network classifier for segmenting cancer cells microscopically as the second algorithm. The remainder of this chapter is organized as

follows: Section 2 describes the cell counting technique based on local adaptive thresholding; Section 3 presents the cell counting technique based on neural network; and Section 4 gives conclusions and recommendations for future work.

2. Cell counting based on local adaptive thresholding

2.1 Method

In this section, we present an approach on segmenting cancer cells from a microscopic tissue image of breast cancer. Color space changing and anisotropic diffusion filtering for noise removal are performed in the preprocessing stage. Subsequently, the preprocessing result is segmented using local adaptive thresholding, morphological operations, and cell size considerations. Finally, cell types are classified based on their color content.

2.1.1 Image preprocessing

Two processes are performed in the preprocessing stage. Firstly, we transform the red-green-blue (RGB) color space to CIELab space. The CIELab space is chosen due to the close correlation between its Euclidean distances and human perception of colors. The CIELab space can be defined by (Trussell et al., 2005)

$$L^* = 116\left(\frac{Y}{Y_n}\right)^{\frac{1}{3}} - 16 \tag{1}$$

$$a^* = 500\left[\left(\frac{X}{X_n}\right)^{\frac{1}{3}} - \left(\frac{Y}{Y_n}\right)^{\frac{1}{3}}\right] \tag{2}$$

$$b^* = 200\left[\left(\frac{Y}{Y_n}\right)^{\frac{1}{3}} - \left(\frac{Z}{Z_n}\right)^{\frac{1}{3}}\right] \tag{3}$$

for $\frac{X}{X_n}, \frac{Y}{Y_n}, \frac{Z}{Z_n} > 0.01$. The values X_n, Y_n, Z_n are the CIE (Commission Internationale de l'eclairage) tristimulus values of the reference white under the reference illumination, and X, Y, Z are the tristimulus values, which are mapped to the CIE color space. While the L^* component represents intensity, the a^* and b^* components are proportional to red-green and yellow-blue color contents, respectively.

Secondly, we apply the anisotropic diffusion with the L^* component from the first step. The objective of this operation is to smooth regions inside cancer cells while still preserve the edge and contrast at sharp intensity gradients. The image resulting from this step significantly facilitates the segmentation algorithm in the next stage. The anisotropic diffusion equation can be expressed as (Perona & Malik, 1990)

$$I_t = div(c(x, y, t)\nabla I), \tag{4}$$

where div is the divergence operator, $c(x, y, t)$ is the diffusion coefficient, and ∇I is the gradient operator. In order to smooth the area within an object of interest and simultaneously preserve high gradient boundaries, the diffusion coefficient is given by

$$c(x, y, t) = g(\|\nabla I(x, y, t))\|) = e^{-(\|\nabla I(x,y,t))\|/\kappa)^2}, \tag{5}$$

where κ is a constant that controls conduction. We implement the numerical solution of Equation (4) using the algorithm provided in (Perona & Malik, 1990), which is given by

$$I_{i,j}^{t+1} = I_{i,j}^{t} + \lambda[c_N \cdot \nabla_N I + c_S \cdot \nabla_S I + c_E \cdot \nabla_E I + c_W \cdot \nabla_W I], \tag{6}$$

where $0 \leq \lambda \leq 1/4$ for numerical scheme to be stable. Please see (Perona & Malik, 1990) for more details.

2.1.2 Segmentation

We use the combination of local adaptive thresholding, morphological operations, and cell prior knowledge in our segmentation algorithm. For local adaptive thresholding, we apply M-by-M sliding blocks with the output image from the anisotropic diffusion. The threshold of each local block is determined using Otsu's method (Otsu, 1979). After finishing adaptive thresholding for all local blocks, we process the black and white image using morphological opening in combination with a cell size consideration. These two operations are successively used to eliminate spike noise, fill holes, and separate touching cancer cells.

2.1.3 Feature extraction and cell classification

In this step, we use the features based on color components to classify cancer cells. The average values of L^*, a^* and b^* from the representative regions of light brown (P1), brown (P2), dark brown (P3), and blue (N) cells are selected to serve as the reference markers. All segmented cancer cells are categorized using the following two steps. First, we classify each N cancer cell from the others, i.e. P1, P2, and P3, in the image. The Euclidean distances between the average values of a^* and b^* of the considering cell and those of all reference markers are compared. The smallest distance will tell us that the cell most closely matches that reference marker. For example, if the distance between the considering cell and the N reference marker is the smallest, then it would be labeled as the N cancer cell. Second, we separate the remaining P1, P2, and P3 cancer cells using the average value of L^* component. Also similar to the first step, the minimum Euclidean distance is used to determine the class of cancer cells.

2.2 Results and discussion

2.2.1 Image preprocessing

Figure 3(a) shows the original color image used in demonstrating the proposed algorithm. Figure 3(b) shows the intensity image resulting from the L^* component of CIELab color space of stained cancer cell image. We can see that most of cancer cells stay separately and have the round shape. Figure 3 (c) shows output images from anisotropic diffusion. Parameters used for the numerical solution of anisotropic diffusion are as follows: speed of diffusion (λ) = 0.2, conduction coefficient (κ) = 20, and number of iterations = 50. It can be seen from the image that the anisotropic diffusion filtering successfully removes undesirable noise while still preserving sharp edges of cancer cells.

2.2.2 Segmentation

Segmented images resulting from the local adaptive thresholding with block sizes 7, 11, 15, and 19 are investigated. Results show that the pixel elements of cells from the output image with block size 7 is not uniform and not well connected. Cells from the output image with increasing block sizes, i.e. 11, 15 and 19, show more homogenous and completed shapes. However, cell sizes also appear larger and any two cells that stay closely may merge together. As a result, the local adaptive thresholding that operates with block size 11 is the most appropriate for image segmentation. When the 11-by-11 sliding block is used for local adaptive thresholding in the demonstrating image, the output image is shown in Figure 3(d). In order to eliminate spike noise, the binary image is processed using

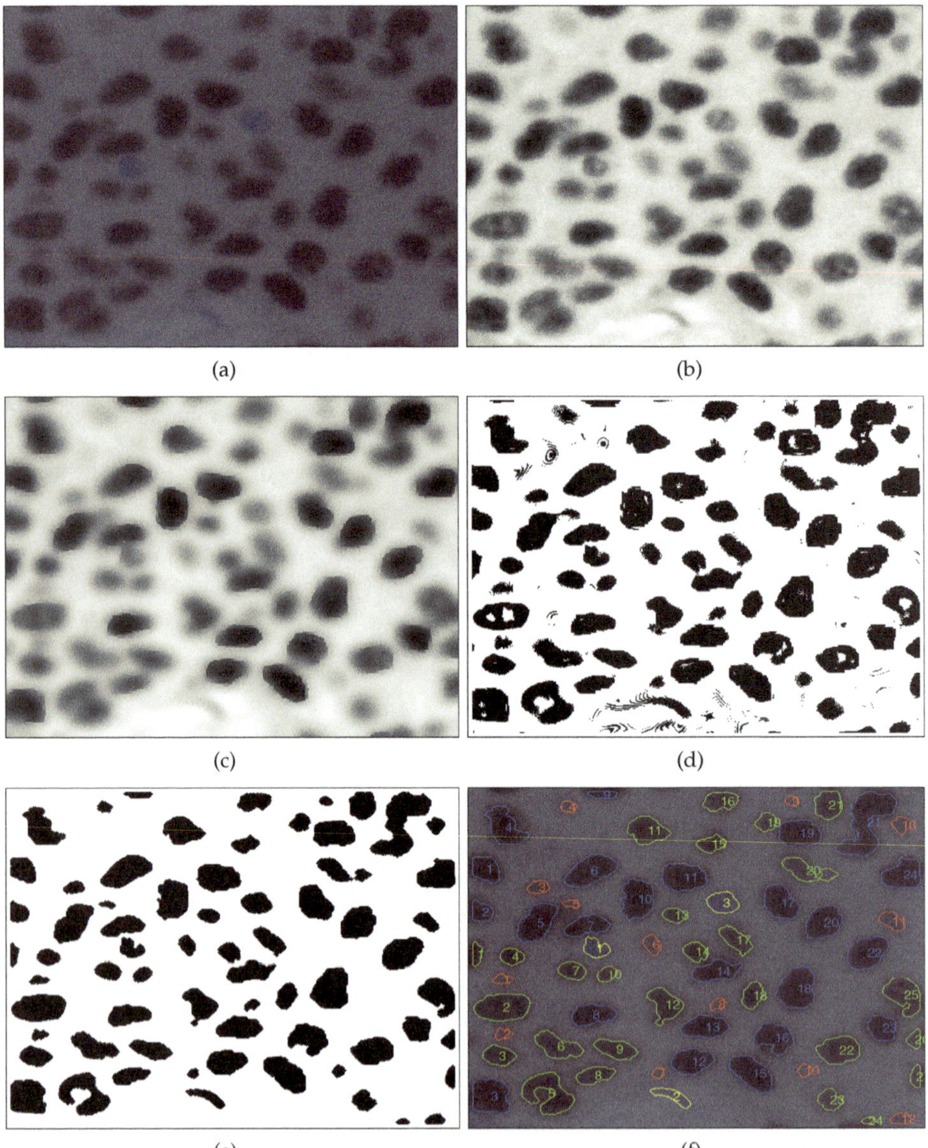

Fig. 3. Images resulting from the algorithm based on local adaptive thresholding. (a) Original color image. (b) Intensity image of stained cancer cell image. (c) Image from the anisotropic diffusion filtering. (d) Image from local adaptive thresholding. (e) Image from morphological operations. (f) Cell classification results.

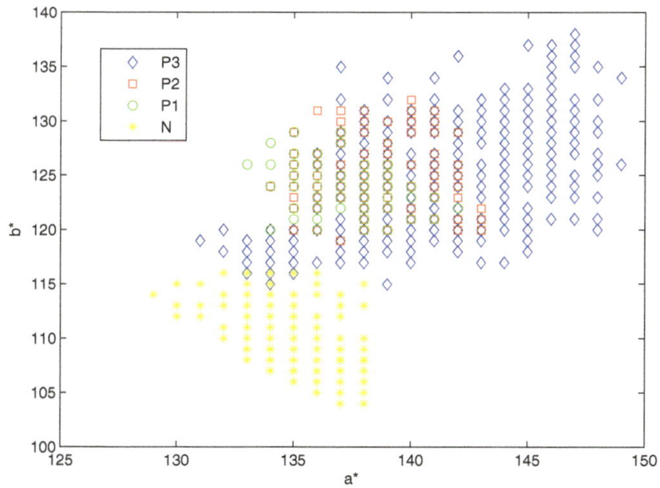

Fig. 4. Scatter plot between the a^* and b^* components of pixels from four different classes of reference cancer cells. Diamond: Light brown (P1). Square: Brown (P2). Circle: Dark brown (P3). Point: Light blue (N).

morphological opening with the disk-shaped structuring element. The algorithm based on morphological reconstruction is subsequently used to fill holes in the image. Additionally, the size of cancer cells under consideration must be greater than 140. A segmentation result after morphological operations is shown in Figure 3(e). We can clearly see that the boundaries of segmented cancer cells are in agreement with those of their original images shown in Figure 3(a).

2.2.3 Feature extraction and cell classification

The scatter plot between the a^* and b^* components of pixels from four different classes of reference cancer cells in demonstrating image is displayed in Figure 4. Color components of pixels from P1, P2, P3, and N cancer cells are shown using diamond, square, circle, and point markers, respectively. The scatter plot shows a good separation of the a^* and b^* components of N cancer cells from those of P1, P2, and P3.

Cell type	L^*	a^*	b^*
P1	102± 4	137± 2	124± 2
P2	87± 5	138± 2	125± 2
P3	42± 8	139± 3	121± 3
N	95± 5	134± 2	110± 2

Table 1. Average values ± standard deviation (SD) of color components from reference cancer cells.

Table I reports the average values and corresponding standard deviation (SD) of the L^*, a^* and b^* components of P1, P2, P3, and N reference cancer cells. The average values shown in the table are used as the reference markers for classifying all cancer cells in the image. We can clearly see from Table I that the separation degree of average values of a^* and b^* agrees with the scatter plots shown in Figure 4. Moreover, values of L^* component from CIELab color space in Table I suggest that we can use intensity of pixels to classify P1, P2, and P3 cancer cells due to their degree of separation.

Classification result of the cancer cell image using minimum Euclidean distances of color components is shown in Figure 3(f). While N cancer cells are shown using yellow contour plots, P1, P2, and P3 cancer cells are shown in red, green, and blue contour plots, respectively. A total number of cancer cells in the image are 67. The number of P1, P2, P3, and N cancer cells are 13, 27, 24, and 3, respectively. This classification result is consistent with the manual result from a specialist. However, we need to develop an additional segmentation algorithm for overlapping and irregular-shaped cancer cells such as the cells shown in the bottom left and top right corners of Figure 3(a).

2.2.4 Image with high histological noise

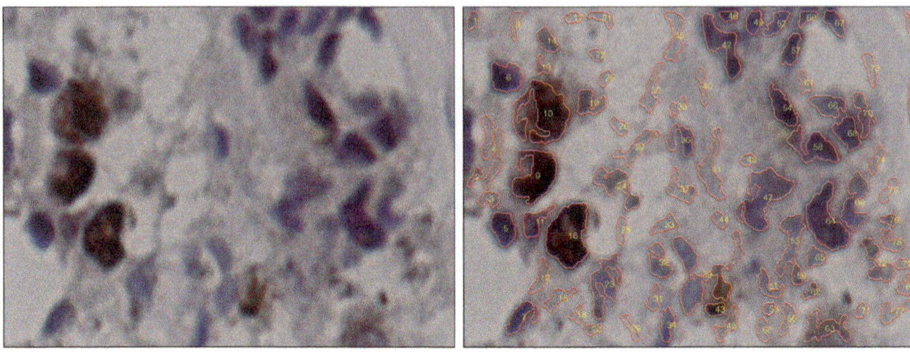

(a) (b)

Fig. 5. (a) Breast cancer cell image with high histological noises. (b) Results of image analysis based on local adaptive thresholding.

The cell counting based on local adaptive thresholding is appropriate for microscopic images with low histological noise, i.e., low variations on background color and background intensity. However, the degree of histological noise in breast cancer images is varied image by image. Figure 5(a) shows an example of breast cancer cell with high histological noise, i.e., high variations on background color and background intensity. When the image is applied with the local adaptive thresholding algorithm, the result is shown in Figure 5(b). Not only the cancer cells but also other artifacts are detected. This causes the so called over-segmentation problem. In addition, the computational time for the approach is quite lengthy. To address these problems, we propose a strategy for segmenting cancer cells in a microscopic image of immunohistological nuclear staining of breast cancer tissue based on the color of pixel in the next section.

3. Cell counting based on neural network

3.1 Method

The originally acquired image is in the red-green-blue (RGB) color space. That is, the color image is formed by the combination of red, green, and blue monochrome images. In the first step, we classify color pixels in the image into one of three categories, i.e. background, positive (P), or negative (N), based on their RGB components. There are many classifiers that can be used for partitioning color of a pixel. However, a neural network is chosen due to its well known as a successful classifier for many applications (Gelenbe et al., 1996; Heermann & Khazenie, 1992; Reddick et al., 1997). Subsequently, morphology operations are used for addressing the spatial characteristics of cells. Finally, in order to obtain accurate cell counting results, the marker-controlled watershed, a classical method for separating overlapping objects, is applied for separating attached multiple cells into distinct single cells. An algorithm for segmenting cancer cells based on their colors and sizes is as follows.

An algorithm for cancer cell segmentation

```
Read image file
Classify pixels using neural network
Do threshoding
Do morphology opening
Fill holes
Label objects in the image
Classify each object using its size
IF size < 400 THEN
   Ignore object
ELSE IF 400 ≤ size ≤ 1000 THEN
   Object is a distinct single cell
   Apply morphology closing (1)
ELSE size > 1000 THEN
   Object is attached multiple cells
   Apply morphology opening
   Apply marker-controlled watershed (2)
ENDIF
Combine the results from (1) and (2)
```

Details of the algorithm are given below.

3.1.1 Neural network

We use backpropagation neural network to classify pixels in the microscopic image according to their color contents. Backpropagation is created by generalizing the Widrow-Hoff learning rule to multiple-layer networks and nonlinear differentiable transfer functions. Input vectors and the corresponding target vectors are used to train the network until it can classify the defined pattern. The training algorithms use the gradient of the performance function to determine how to adjust the weights to maximize performance. The gradient is determined by a technique called backpropagation, which involves performing computations backwards through the network. The backpropagation computation is derived using the chain rule of calculus (Hagan et al., 1996).

Based on our experiences, the number of neural network layer between two and three is appropriate for classifying color of pixels in cancer cell images. Therefore, a backpropagation

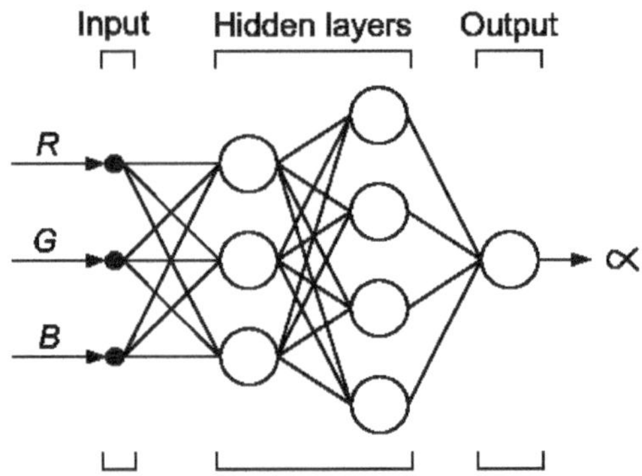

Fig. 6. Diagram of backpropagation neural network.

neural network of three layers shown in Figure 6 is chosen to classify image pixels whether they are from background, P, or N regions. The input vector is composed of 3 elements corresponding to the RGB color vector of pixel. Two hidden layers are determined empirically to be 3 and 4 neurons and the output layer consists of one neuron. In addition, the transfer functions of hidden and output layers are tan-sigmoid and linear, respectively. For the training of neural network, the target is assigned to be -1, 0, and 1, which are corresponding to RGB components from background, P, and N regions, respectively. The networks are trained using the Levenberg-Marquardt (LM) algorithm. The training stops when the maximum number of epochs reaches 100 or the mean square error is less than 1×10^{-12}. The number of pixels used for training neural network from each reference region is 1600.

3.1.2 Morphology operations

Mathematical morphology is a nonlinear operator based on set theory operating on object shape. It is a powerful tool to numerous image processing problems, for example, image preprocessing, segmentation using object shape, and quantitative description objects (Gonzalez & Woods, 2002). We utilize mathematical morphology as a tool for noise filtering and shape simplification in our work. Note that the disk-shaped structuring element (SE) with a radius of R is used for all morphological operations. As a result, the size of SE matrix is $2R + 1$ by $2R + 1$. In addition, all mathematical morphology operations are applied once for each stage.

After finishing color partition for all pixels, the output image from neural network is transformed to a black and white image by thresholding. That is, while the pixels in background region are transformed to zero, the pixels in P and N regions, i.e., objects of interest, are transformed to one. In order to eliminate spike noise, the binary image is processed using morphological opening. The disk-shaped SE with a radius of 1 is used in this stage. The algorithm based on morphological reconstruction is subsequently used to fill holes in the image before performing size consideration.

In the next step, we classify each object in the image into one of three categories according to its size: small, medium, and large. The value of sizes used for cell classification is predetermined from guidance by a specialist. The small object is regarded as noise and is ignored. The medium object is considered to be a distinct single cell. For the large object, it is determined as attached multiple cells. All distinct single cells are processed further with mathematical closing to complete their shape. It is used as spatial compensation for an uneven distribution of color in the cell. The SE used in this stage has a radius of 4. On the other hand, all attached multiple cells are applied with morphological opening. The radius of the SE in this stage is 4. There are two explanations for doing this performing. First, the multiple cells with small degree of attachment can be kept apart. Second, it can be used as a preparation step before marker-controlled watershed processing.

3.1.3 Marker-controlled watershed

In order to separate attached cancer cells into individual objects, we further process the result from last step with marker-controlled watershed. The watershed algorithm is shown to be a powerful tool for dividing attached objects (Vincent, 1993). The marker computation is used as an additional processing because the direct use of watershed transform usually yields the over-segmented result (Fang et al., 2003). The computational procedures for marker-controlled watershed are as follows.

Step 1. Use the Sobel edge marks to compute the gradient magnitude of all attached cells,

Step 2. Determine the marker, which is connected blobs of pixels inside each cell, based on the distant transform.

Step 3. Combine the results of Step 1 and Step 2,

Step 4. Compute the watershed transform of the result from Step 3.

Finally, to obtain whole cancer cells, we combine the image of attached multiple cells with the image of distinct single cells using a logical operator OR.

3.2 Results and discussion

3.2.1 Neural network

Figure 7(a) shows an original RGB image of cancer cells. Most of cancer cells are located separately, but some of them attach with their neighborhood. We also see an uneven distribution of color and intensity in the background region surrounding cancer cells. It is considered as histological noise. The R-, G- and B-components of pixel values from background, P, and N reference regions (Boxes **B1**, **B2**, and **B3**) shown in Figure 7(a) are used as the input vectors for training neural network. After the backpropagation neural network is trained, network responses of pixel values throughout the image are calculated.
Figure 7(b) shows the output image from neural network. Pixels from background, P, and N regions are shown in white, gray, and black colors, respectively. Results demonstrate that the neural network can classify color pixels very well. That is, pixel values are appropriately categorized into a connected region corresponding to the cancer cells shown in Figure 7(a). Additionally, the results from neural network show that color contents of pixel values for each cancer cell are unevenly distributed. For example, we can notice the mixture appearance of positive and negative colors of the cell situating at the left hand side of box **B1**. This is in agreement with the original RGB image.

3.2.2 Morphology operations

Figure 8(a) shows the binary image after thresholding and morphological opening for spike noise removal. Subsequently, hole filling is performed using the algorithm based on morphological reconstruction. Each object in the image is classified into three categories

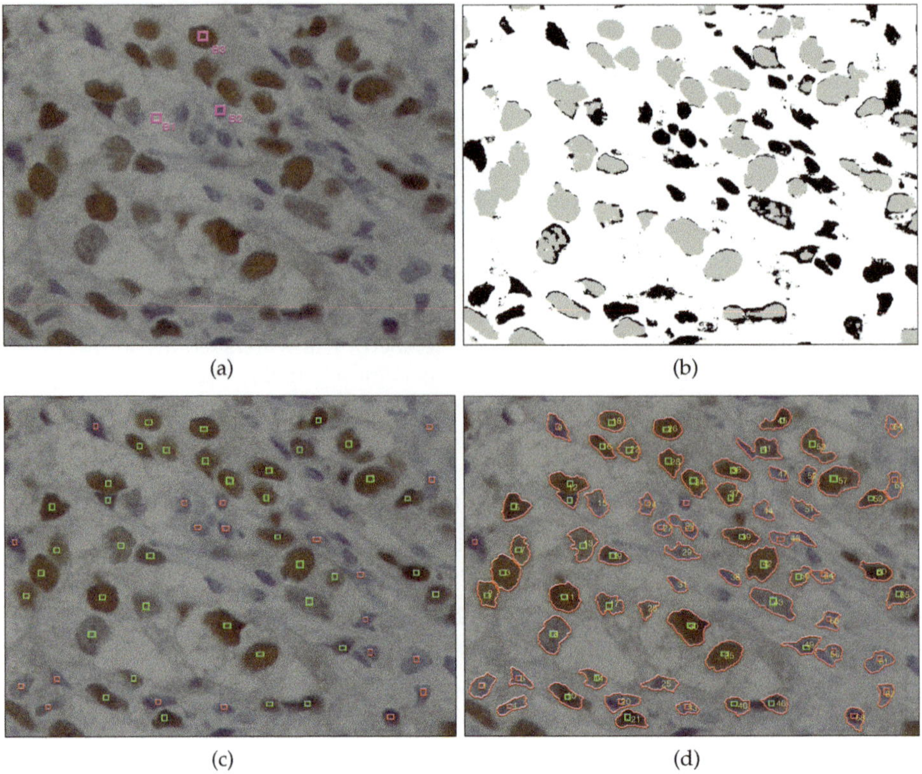

Fig. 7. (a) Original RGB image of stained cancer cells. Boxes **B1**, **B2**, and **B3** indicate reference regions from background, P, and N, respectively. Pixel values in the box regions are used for training neural network. (b) Output image from neural network. Pixels from background, P, and N regions are shown in white, gray, and black colors, respectively. (c) Positive and negative cancer cells marked by an expert. (d) Segmented image superimposed on the original RGB image compared with the result from the expert.

according to its size. Figure 8(b) shows the binary image of distinct single cells after size consideration. One can notice that some cells do not have the complete shape due to an uneven distribution of color and intensity. To compensate for this shortcoming, we perform mathematical closing and show result in Figure 8(c). It is shown that distinct single cells with perfect round shape are obtained after mathematical closing.

Figure 8(d) shows the binary image of attached multiple cells after size consideration. The size of cancer cells in this image is large in terms of area compared with the size of distinct single cell. Figure 8(e) shows the binary image of attached multiple cells after morphological opening. One can see that a slightly attached multiple cell is separated into two distinct single cells as we expect. In addition, the shape of each cell is smoothed and simplified, which make it appropriate for marker-controlled watershed processing.

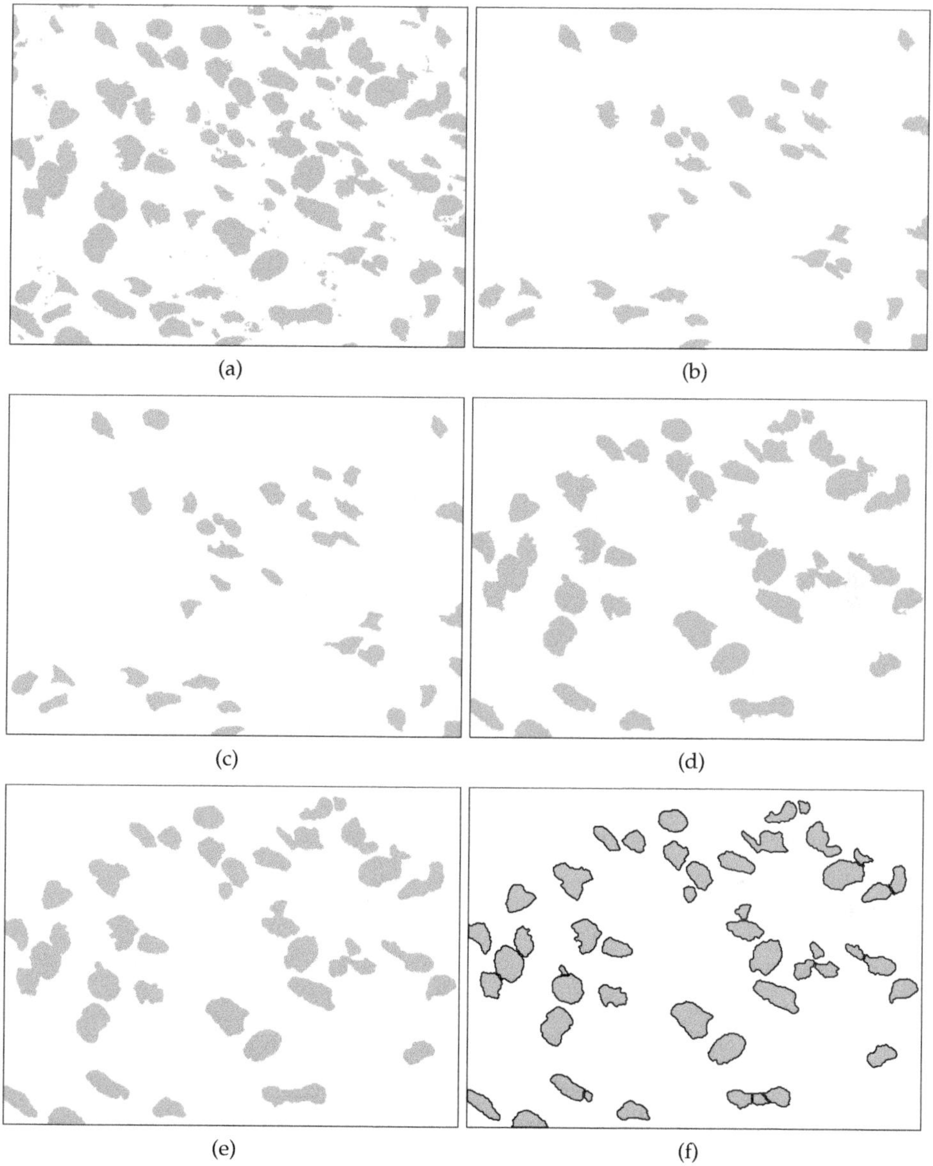

Fig. 8. (a) Binary image after thresholding and morphological operations of the image from neural network. (b) Binary image of distinct single cells before morphological closing. (c) Binary image of distinct single cells after morphological closing. (d) Binary image of attached multiple cells before morphological opening. (e) Binary image of attached multiple cells after morphological opening. (f) Binary image of attached multiple cells after marker-controlled watershed.

3.2.3 Marker-controlled watershed

Figure 8(f) shows the segmented image after the application of marker-controlled watershed. A more accurate segmented result is achieved. That is, the attached multiple cells are appropriately separated into the distinct single cells. Figure 7(c) shows positive and negative cancer cells marked by an expert. While the positive nuclei marked by the expert are shown with green rectangular windows, the negative nuclei are shown with red rectangular windows. To compare the results from the proposed algorithm with those from the expert, we superimpose the segmented image on the original RGB image and demonstrate the result in Figure 7(d). The number of segmented cancer cells is 65. It can be clearly seen that the perception of segmented cancer cells is in agreement with their original visualization.

4. Conclusions

We present two segmentation methods for nuclear stained breast cancer cell counting. While one is based on a local adaptive thresholding, another is based on the separation of pixel color using neural network. The segmenting results of cancer cells from the background are used as a preliminary step before extracting cell features and classifying cell types. The excellent segmentation results from the proposed algorithm are demonstrated with microscopic images under various histological noise conditions. Quantitative evaluations of the neural network approach compared with the counting results from the expert provide similar agreement to image visualization(Phukpattaranont et al., 2009). In other words, sensitivity and positive predictive value of cell segmentation are 88% and 82%, respectively. Moreover, sensitivity, positive predictive value, specificity, and negative predictive value of color classification are 94%, 99%, 91%, and 78%, respectively. However, to make the method automatic and gain higher accuracy, the following issues have to be addressed:

- The algorithm that can compensate for the selection of training data by a specialist need to be incorporated.
- The more sophisticated algorithm for the separation of overlapping cells is needed.
- More features are necessary such as the texture of cell and its neighborhood and the shape of each cell.

They are ongoing research. Results will be reported in the near future.

5. Acknowledgments

This research was supported by Department of Electrical Engineering, Department of Computer Engineering, Faculty of Engineering through contract no. ENG-51-2-7-02-0018-S and Department of Pathology, Faculty of Medicine, Prince of Songkla University.

6. References

Adams, R. & Bischof, L. (1994). Seeded region growing, *IEEE Trans. Pattern Anal. Mach. Intell.* 16: 641–647.

Beveridge, J. R. & et al. (1989). Segmenting images using localized histograms and region merging, *International Journal of Computer Vision* 2: 311–347.

Fang, B., Hsu, W. & Lee, M. L. (2003). On the accurate counting of tumor cells, *IEEE Trans. Nanobiosci.* 2(2): 94–103.

Gelenbe, E., Feng, Y. & Krishnan, K. R. R. (1996). Neural network methods for volumetric magnetic resonance imaging of the human brain, *Proc. IEEE* 84(10): 1488–1496.

Gonzalez, R. C. & Woods, R. E. (2002). *Digital Image Processing*, Prentice-Hall, Inc.

Hagan, M. T., Demuth, H. B. & Beale, M. H. (1996). *Neural Network Design*, PWS Publishing Company, Boston, MA.

Haralik, R. M. & Shapiro, L. G. (1985). Image segmentation techniques, *Comput. Vis. Graph. Image Proc.* 29: 100–132.

Heermann, P. D. & Khazenie, N. (1992). Classifiation of multispectral remote sensing data using a back-propagation neural network, *IEEE Trans. Geosci. Remote Sensing* 30(1): 81–88.

Li, H. D., Kallergi, M., Clarke, L. P., Jain, V. K. & Clark, R. A. (1995). Markov random field for tumor detection in digital mammography, *IEEE Trans. Med. Imag.* 14(3): 565–576.

O'Gorman, L., Sanderson, A. C. & Jr., K. P. (1985). A system for automated liver tissue image analysis: Methods and results, *IEEE Trans. Biomed. Eng.* 32(9): 696–706.

Otsu, N. (1979). A threshold selection method from gray-level histograms, *IEEE Trans. Syst., Man, Cybern.* 9(1): 62–66.

Park, J. & Keller, J. (1997). Fuzzy patch label relaxation in bone marrow cell segmentation, *Proc. IEEE Int. Conf. Syst. Man. Cybern.*, Vol. 2, pp. 1133–1138.

Perona, P. & Malik, J. (1990). Scale-space and edge detection using anisotropic diffusion, *IEEE Trans. Pattern Anal. Mach. Intell.* 12(7): 629–639.

Petushi, S., Katsinis, C., Coward, C., Garcia, F. & Tozeren, A. (2004). Automated identification of microstructures on histology slides, *IEEE International Symposium on Biomedical Imaging: Macro to Nano*, Vol. 1, pp. 424–427.

Phukpattaranont, P. & Boonyaphiphat, P. (2006). Automatic classification of cancer cells in microscopic images: Preliminary results, *The 2006 ITC-CSCC International Conference*, Vol. 1, pp. 113–116.

Phukpattaranont, P. & Boonyaphiphat, P. (2007). Color based segmentation of nuclear stained breast cancer cell images, *ECTI Transactions on Electrical Eng. Electronics and Communications* 5(2): 158–164.

Phukpattaranont, P., Limsiroratana, S. & Boonyaphiphat, P. (2009). Computer-aided system for microscopic images: Application to breast cancer nuclei counting, *International Journal of Applied Biomedical Engineering* 2(1): 69–74.

Reddick, W. E., Glass, G. O., Cook, E. N., Elkin, T. D. & Deaton, R. J. (1997). Automated segmentation and classification of multispectral magnetic resonance images of brain using artificial neural network, *IEEE Trans. Med. Imag.* 16: 911–918.

Refai, H., Li, L. & Teague, T. K. (2003). Automatic count of hepatocytes in microscopic images, *International Conference on Image Processing*, Vol. 2, pp. 1101–1104.

Theera-Umpon, N. & Gader, P. D. (2000). Counting white blood cells using morphological granulometries, *Journal of Electronic Imaging* 9(2): 170–177.

Thiran, J. P. & Macq, B. (1996). Morphological feature extraction for the classification of digital images of cancerous tissues, *IEEE Trans. Biomed. Eng.* 43(10): 1011–1020.

Trussell, H. J., Saber, E. & Vrhel, M. (2005). Color image processing (basics and special issue overview), *IEEE Signal Process. Mag.* 22(1): 14–22.

Vincent, L. (1993). Morphological grayscale reconstruction in image analysis: applications and efficient algorithms, *IEEE Trans. Image Process.* 2(2): 176–201.

Wani, M. A. & Batchelor, B. G. (1994). Edged-region-based segmentation of range images, *IEEE Trans. Pattern Anal. Mach. Intell.* 16: 314–319–647.

Wu, H. S. & Barba, J. (1994). An algorithm for noisy cell contour extraction via area merging, *J. Imag. Sci. Technol.* 38: 604–607.

Wu, K., Gauthier, D. & Levine, M. D. (1995). Live cell image segmentation, *IEEE Trans. Biomed. Eng.* 42(1): 1–12.

Zhao, X. & Ong, S. H. (1998). Adaptive local thresholding with fuzzy-validity-guided spatial partitioning, *International Conference on Pattern Recognition*, Vol. 2, pp. 988–990.

17

Imaging the Sigma-2 Receptor for Diagnosis and Prediction of Therapeutic Response

Chenbo Zeng[1], Jinbin Xu[1] and Robert H. Mach[1,2,3]
[1]*Department of Radiology,*
[2]*Department of Cell Biology and Physiology,*
[3]*Department of Biochemistry and Molecular Biophysics,*
Washington University School of Medicine, St. Louis, MO,
USA

1. Introduction

Sigma (σ) receptors represent a class of proteins that were initially classified as a subtype of the opiate receptors. Subsequent studies revealed that σ binding sites are a distinct class of receptors that are located in the central nervous system as well as in a variety of tissues and organs [1, 2]. Two σ binding site subtypes were distinguished based on differences in their drug-binding profiles and molecular weight. The two binding sites are known as σ_1 and σ_2 receptors. σ_1 receptors have a molecular weight of ~25 kDa, whereas σ_2 receptors have a molecular weight of ~21.5 kDa [3]. The σ_1 receptor has been cloned and displays a 30% sequence homology with the enzyme, yeast C8-C7 sterol isomerase [4, 5], but this receptor lacks C8-C7 isomerase activity. Recent studies have shown that neuroactive steroids bind with moderate affinity to σ_1 sites, and suggest that σ_1 receptors may modulate the activity of GABA and NMDA receptors in the CNS [6-8]. The σ_2 receptor has not been cloned, and most of what is known regarding the σ_2 receptor has been obtained through the use of in vitro receptor binding studies aimed at the pharmacological characterization of this receptor.

2. Characterization of the σ_2 receptor as a biomarker of the proliferative status of solid tumors

The first report suggesting that there is an overexpression of σ receptors in tumors cells was by Bem et al. in 1991[9]. In this study, σ binding in tumors was found to be greater than or equal to 2-fold higher than that of control nonmalignant tissue. Later, Vilner et al.[10] demonstrated that many murine and human tumor cells possess a high density of σ_2 receptors when grown under cell culture conditions. These studies clearly indicate that σ_2 receptors may serve as a biomarker for differentiating solid tumors from the surrounding normal tissues. The proliferative status of a solid tumor, which is defined as the ratio of proliferating (P) cells in a solid tumor to those driven into a quiescent (Q) state by nutrient deprivation and/or hypoxia (the P:Q ratio), is an important parameter in determining how to treat a tumor with either radiation or chemotherapy[11]. Tumors having a high proliferative status (i.e., high P:Q ratio) typically respond better to hyperfractionated radiation therapy versus conventional radiation therapy. Similarly, tumors having a high P:Q ratio will respond better to cell cycle specific agents such as Ara-C and gemcitabine, whereas tumors having a lower proliferative status will respond better to non-cell cycle specific agents such as cisplatin and BCNU [11]. Also, a change in the proliferative status of a tumor during or after treatment has the potential to serve as a predictor of response and allow further tailoring of therapy.

In order to investigate the relationship between the density of σ_2 receptors and the proliferative status of tumors, Wheeler and colleagues used the mouse mammary adenocarcinoma cell line 66[12, 13] to determine if there was a difference in the density of σ_2 receptors in proliferating (66P) and quiescent (66Q) tumor cells in cell culture or in solid tumor xenografts. This group demonstrated that the density of σ_2 receptors in 66P cells was about 10 times greater than the density observed in 66Q cells (Figure 1A)[14]. The density of σ_2 receptors in the 66P cells was found to be quite high, ~900,000 copies/cell versus ~90,000 receptors/cell in the 66Q cells. This group also reported that the expression kinetics of σ_2 receptors follows the growth kinetics of the 66 cells (Figure 1B)[15]. A subsequent study in solid tumor xenografts of the same tumor cell lines demonstrated the identical P:Q ratio to that measured in the cell culture condition[16]. The agreement between the solid tumor and tissue culture data indicates that the σ_2 receptor is a receptor-based biomarker of cell proliferation in breast tumors. Thus the σ_2 receptor possesses properties similar to Ki-67, a marker of proliferation [17]. Ki-67 expression level is determined by immunohistochemistry using Ki-67 antibody. This method requires biopsy or surgical specimens of tumor. In contrast, radiotracers having a high affinity and high selectivity for σ_2 receptors have the potential to assess the proliferative status of human breast tumors using noninvasive imaging techniques such as Positron Emission Tomography (PET) and Single Photon Emission Computed Tomography (SPECT). In addition, it is likely that this approach can be extended to assess the proliferative status of other human tumors, such as head and neck, melanoma, and lung tumors, which are known to express a high density of σ_2 receptors[10]. Imaging the proliferative status with σ_2 receptors radiotracers can provide useful information regarding the prognosis and aggressiveness of tumors, and this information can be used to guide treatment of cancer in clinical practice. Rapidly proliferating tumors requires aggressive initial treatment. A reduction in the proliferative status of a tumor can serve as a predictor of the tumor's response to therapy.

3. Development of σ_2 receptor selective ligands

A number of structurally-diverse compounds have been shown to possess a high affinity to σ receptors [2]. However, most of these compounds bind selectively to σ_1 receptor or have similar affinities to both σ_1 and σ_2 receptors. One of the first σ_2 selective ligands reported was the benzomorphan-7-one analog, **CB-64D** [18]. This compound was identified as part of a structure-activity relationship (SAR) study aimed at refining the affinity of (−)-2-methyl-5-(3-hydroxyphenyl)morphan-7-one for μ versus κ opioid receptors [19]. A second series of compounds having a high affinity for σ_2 receptors are the 3-(ω-aminoalkyl)-1H-indole analogs [20, 21]. SAR studies with compounds that were originally designed to be serotonin 5-HT_{1A} agonists, resulted in the synthesis of **Lu 28-179** [22], also known as siramesine, which has a subnanomolar affinity for σ_2 receptors and a 140-fold selectivity for σ_2 versus σ_1

receptors. Other compounds that were found to have a higher affinity for σ_2 versus σ_1 receptors are: 1) the hallucinogen, ibogaine [23, 24]; 2) the mixed serotonin 5-HT_3 antagonist/5-HT_4 agonist **BIMU-1**[25]; 3) the tropane analog **SM-21**, an acetylcholine releaser that has been utilized as an antinociceptive agent [26, 27]; 4) the trishomocubane analog **ANSTO-19** [28]; and 5) the piperazine analog **PB28** [29].

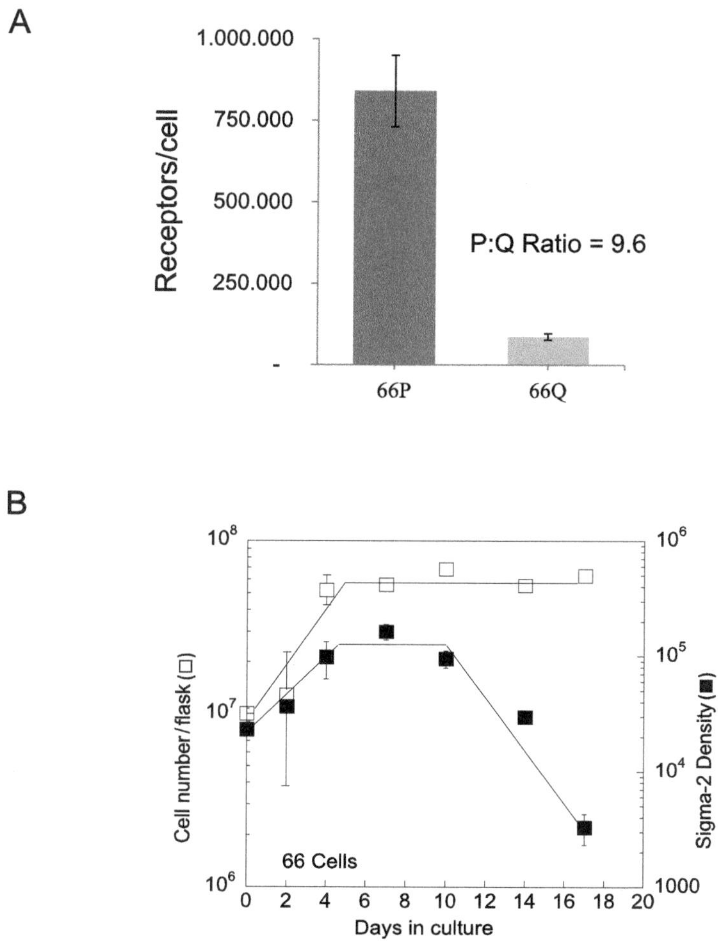

Fig. 1. The σ_2 receptor densities in proliferating and quiescent cells. A: Differences of the σ_2 receptor densities in 66P and 66Q cells. B: The σ_2 receptor expression kinetics in 66 cells during the Q to P transition and the downregulation of the σ_2 receptor densities during the P to Q transition.

A number of SAR studies using **BIMU-1** as the lead compound have identified high affinity, high selectivity σ_2 receptor ligands [30-32]. **BIMU-1** is an ideal lead compound for SAR studies since it provides a variety of regions where structural modifications can be made to optimize the σ_2 receptor affinity and reduce the affinity for serotonin 5-HT_3 and 5-HT_4 receptors (Figure 2). The structures of **BIMU-1** were altered in three different regions: 1) replacement of the urea linkage with a comformationally-flexible carbamate moiety; 2) replacement of the N-methyl group with an N-benzyl group to diminish serotonin receptor affinity; and 3) preparation of both tropane (i.e., [3.2.1]azabicyclonoctane) and granatane (i.e., [3.3.1]azabicyclononane) ring systems. The most interesting analog from this initial SAR study was the compound **ABN-1**, which had a σ_2 receptor affinity of ~ 3 nM and a σ_2: σ_1 selectivity of ~30 (Figure 2)[31]. Compound **ABN-1** was used as a secondary lead compound for a series of subsequent SAR studies aimed at producing second-generation granatane analogs having an improved σ_2 receptor affinity and high σ_2: σ_1 selectivity ratio. Consequently, this led to the development of a number of fluorescent probes, **K05-138, SW120, SW107 and SW116**, that have proven useful in two photon and confocal microscopy studies of σ_2 receptors in tumor cells growing under cell culture conditions[33, 34].

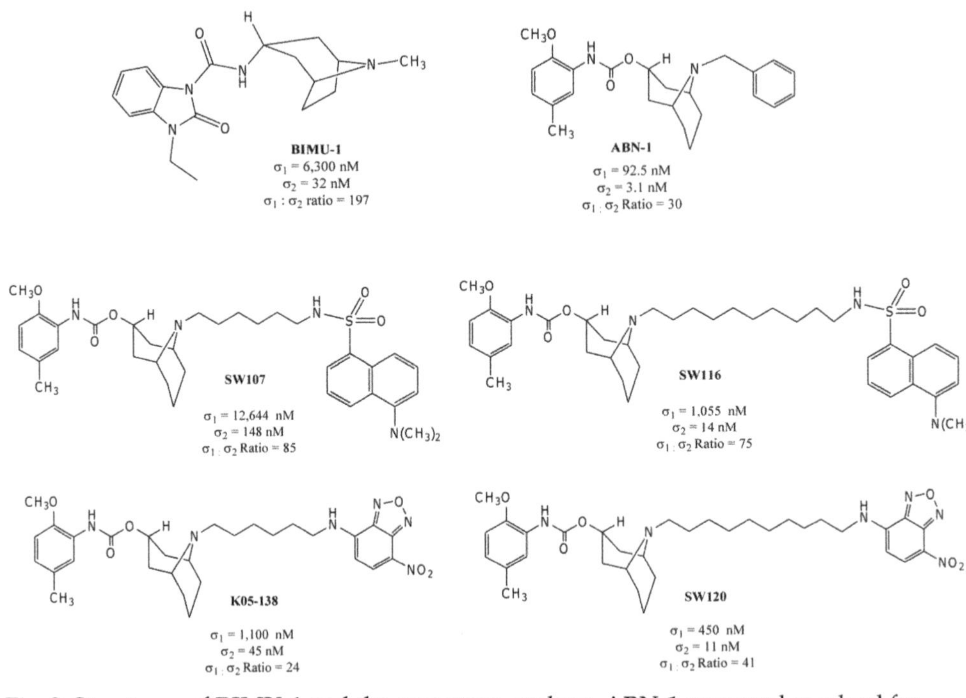

Fig. 2. Structures of **BIMU-1** and the granatane analogs. **ABN-1** was used as a lead for producing second-generation granatane-based σ_2 receptor ligands, which led to the development of a number of fluorescent probes, **K05-138, SW120, SW107 and SW116,** for two photon and confocal microscopy studies of σ_2 receptors in tumor cells.

A second class of compounds having a high affinity for σ_2 receptors and excellent σ_1 : σ_2 selectivity ratios are the conformationally-flexible benzamide analogs. These compounds were identified in an SAR study of the benzamide analog, **YUN250,** that was developed as a dopamine D_3-selective ligand (Figure 3A) [35]. The relatively high lipophilicity of **YUN250** (log P = 5.76) suggests that it is not capable of readily crossing the blood-brain barrier and being active in behavioral studies. In order to reduce the lipophilicity of **YUN250,** the 4-(2,3-dichlorophenyl) piperazine moiety of **YUN250** was replaced with other aromatic amine groups. Although this strategy resulted in a number of useful dopamine D_3 receptor ligands [36], it was also observed that replacement of the 4-phenylpiperazine moiety with a 6,7-dimethoxy-1,2,3,4-tetrahydroisoqinoline ring resulted in compounds having a high affinity and excellent selectivity for σ_2 versus σ_1 receptors, and a dramatic reduction in affinity for dopamine receptors [35]. As discussed in greater detail below, the conformationally-flexible benzamide analogs have proven to be an important class of σ_2-selective compounds for the preparation of radiolabeled probes to image this receptor in vitro and in vivo.

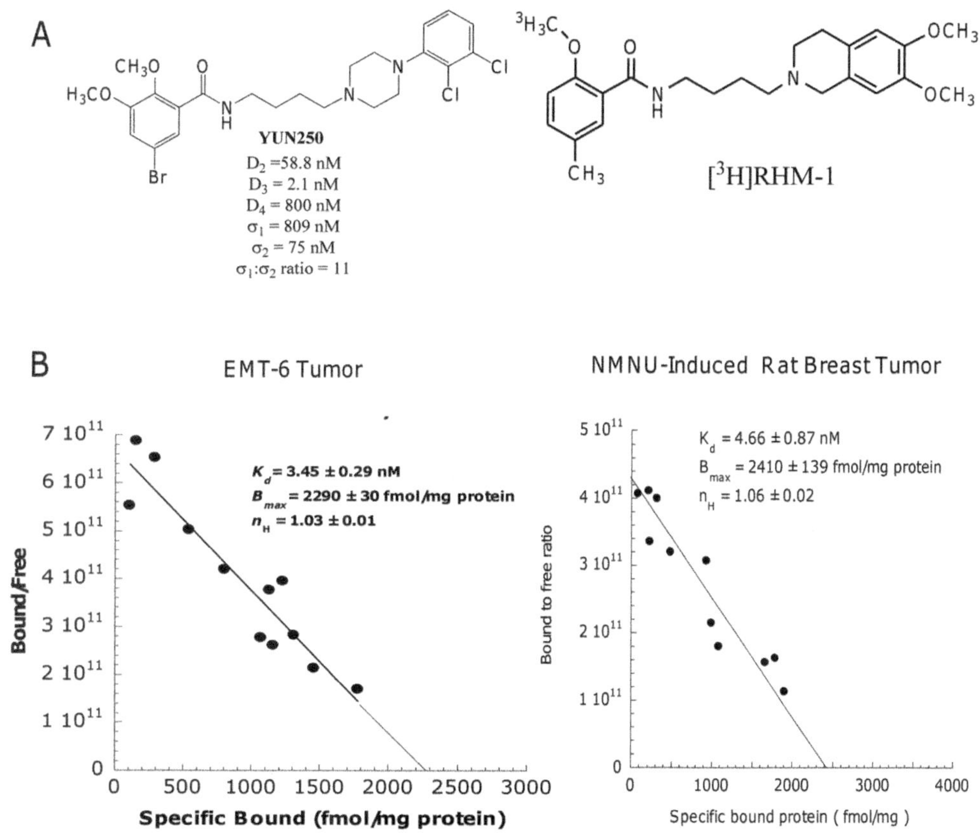

Fig. 3. The conformationally-flexible benzamide-based σ_2 receptor ligands for in vitro studies of the σ_2 receptor. **A**: **YUN250** was a lead for generating the conformationally-flexible benzamide analogues which are selective for σ_2 receptors. The tritium labeled ligand, [^{3}H]**RHM-1** , has been used to conduct the receptor binding assay. **B**: Scatchard studies of σ_2 receptors in EMT-6 mouse breast tumors and NMNU-induced rat breast tumors with **[^{3}H]RHM-1.** This probe has high affinity to the σ_2 receptors in the rodent breast tumors and is useful for in vitro binding studies.

4. In vitro binding and in vivo imaging studies of σ_2 receptors

The conformationally-flexible benzamide analogs have been used to develop the σ_2 radioligands for in vitro binding studies. The tritium labeled σ_2 selective ligand, [^{3}H]**RHM-1**, has been used to conduct Scatchard studies of σ_2 receptors in tumors and normal tissues (Figure 3A)[37, 38]. The in vitro receptor binding studies indicate that **[^{3}H]RHM-1** binds with a high affinity to both EMT-6 mouse breast tumors (K_d=3.45 nM) and chemically-induced rat breast tumors (K_d=4.66 nM). The σ2 receptor densities of both tumors are found to be high (B_{max} =2290 fmol/mg of protein for EMT-6 mouse breast tumors and B_{max}=2410 fmol/mg of protein for *N*-methyl-*N*-nitrosourea (NMNU)-induced rat breast tumors) (Figure 3B). The pharmacologic profile of **[^{3}H]RHM-1** is in agreement with that of [^{3}H]di-o-tolylguanidine ([^{3}H]DTG), a most commonly used radioligand for the σ_2 receptor binding assay. These results indicate that **[^{3}H]RHM-1** is a useful radioligand for studying σ_2 receptors in vitro.

The high correlation between the density of σ_2 receptors and the proliferative status of solid tumors indicates that σ_2 selective radiotracers can be used for imaging the proliferative status of solid tumors with PET and SPECT. The conformationally-flexible benzamide analogs have been used for the development of PET radiotracers for imaging the σ_2 receptor status of solid tumors. The first PET radiotracers prepared were [^{11}C]**1-4** (Figure 4A), which involves labeling the corresponding ortho-hydroxy group with [^{11}C]methyl iodide [38]. MicroPET and tumor uptake studies were conducted with [^{11}C]**1-4**; the most promising analog proved to be [^{11}C]**4**. Although all four analogs had a high affinity for σ_2 receptors, the optimal lipophilicity of [^{11}C]**4** was responsible for the high tumor uptake and suitable signal: normal tissue ratios for imaging. These data indicate that both receptor affinity and lipophilicity are important properties for successful receptor-based tumor imaging agents. MicroPET and MicroCT imaging studies in a murine solid breast tumor EMT-6 clearly show the potential of [^{11}C]**4** as a radiotracer for imaging the σ_2 receptor status of breast tumors with PET.

Although [^{11}C]**4** provides a clear image of breast tumors in microPET imaging studies, the short half life of carbon 11 ($t_{1/2}$ = 20.4 min) is not ideal for the development of radiotracers which can be used in clinical PET imaging studies. The longer half-life of ^{18}F ($t_{1/2}$ =109.8 min) compared to ^{11}C places fewer time constraints on tracer synthesis, allows imaging studies to be conducted up to 2 h after injection of the radiotracers, and usually results in higher tumor: normal tissue ratios. A number of ^{18}F-labeled radiotracers [^{18}F]**5-8** (Figure 4B) based on the conformationally-flexible benzamide analogs have been generated and evaluated in murine breast tumor models[39]. The strategy involved replacement of the 2-methoxy group in the benzamide ring with a 2-fluoroethoxy group. The 2-fluoroethoxy- for methoxy-substitution is a common strategy used in the development of ^{18}F-labeled radiotracers. Biodistribution studies in female Balb/c mice bearing EMT-6 tumor allografts demonstrated that all four ^{18}F -labeled compounds had a high tumor uptake (2.5-3.7% ID/g) and acceptable tumor/normal tissue ratios at 1 and 2 h post-i.v. injection (Figure 4C). The moderate to high tumor/normal tissue ratios and the rapid clearance from the blood for [^{18}F]**5** and [^{18}F]**8** suggests that these radiotracers are likely the best candidates for imaging of solid tumors with PET. MicroPET imaging studies indicate that [^{18}F]**5** and [^{18}F]**8** are suitable probes for imaging the σ_2 receptor status of solid tumors with PET (Figure 4D). Clinical studies of [^{18}F]**8** are currently in progress in the US.

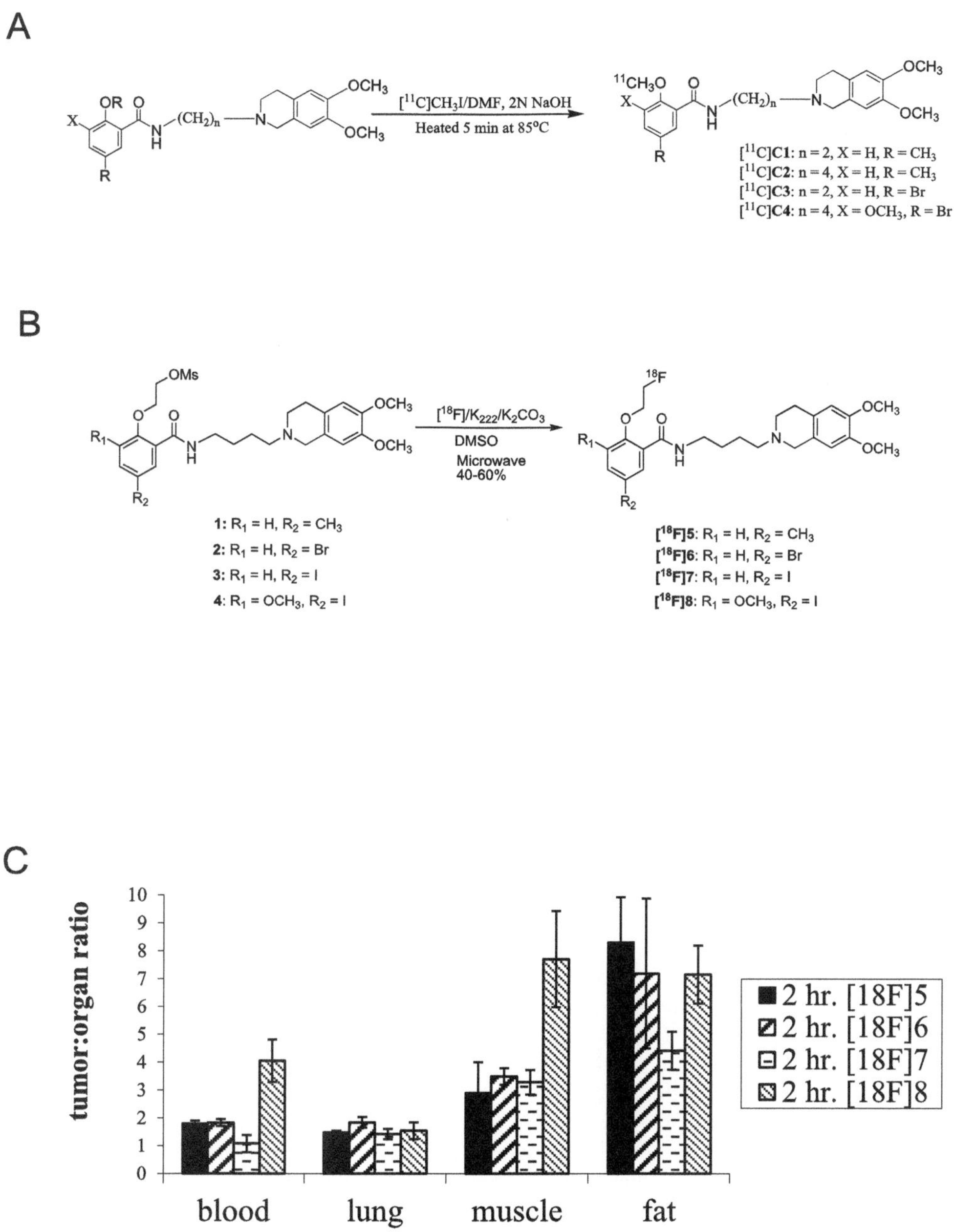
A
[11C]CH3I/DMF, 2N NaOH
Heated 5 min at 85°C
[11C]C1: n = 2, X = H, R = CH3
[11C]C2: n = 4, X = H, R = CH3
[11C]C3: n = 2, X = H, R = Br
[11C]C4: n = 4, X = OCH3, R = Br
B
[18F]/K222/K2CO3
DMSO
Microwave
40-60%
1: R1 = H, R2 = CH3
2: R1 = H, R2 = Br
3: R1 = H, R2 = I
4: R1 = OCH3, R2 = I
[18F]5: R1 = H, R2 = CH3
[18F]6: R1 = H, R2 = Br
[18F]7: R1 = H, R2 = I
[18F]8: R1 = OCH3, R2 = I
C
tumor:organ ratio
blood
lung
muscle
fat
2 hr. [18F]5
2 hr. [18F]6
2 hr. [18F]7
2 hr. [18F]8

D

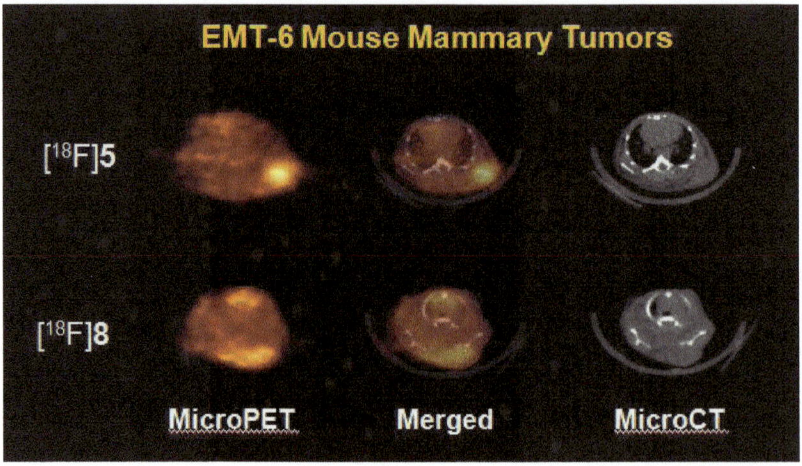

Fig. 4. The synthetic schemes for generating conformationally-flexible benzamide-based PET radiotracers. A: A number of ^{11}C-labeled radiotracers, [^{11}C]**1-4,** are prepared by labeling the corresponding ortho-hydroxy group with [^{11}C]methyl iodide. B: A number of ^{18}F-labeled radiotracers, [^{18}F]**5-8,** are generated by replacing of the 2-methoxy group in the benzamide ring with a 2-fluoroethoxy group. C: Biodistribution studies in female Balb/c mice bearing EMT-6 tumor allografts demonstrating that all four ^{18}F -labeled compounds had a high tumor uptake (2.5-3.7% ID/g) and acceptable tumor/normal tissue ratios at 2 h post-i.v. injection. D: MicroPET imaging studies indicate that [^{18}F]**5** and [^{18}F]**8** are suitable probes for imaging the σ_2 receptor status of solid tumors with PET.

5. Confocal and two photon microscopy studies of σ_2 receptors in tumor cells

Since the σ_2 receptor protein has not been cloned, current knowledge of this receptor is based predominantly on receptor binding studies with radiolabeled probes such as [^{3}H]DTG. The function of the σ_2 receptors has also been investigated by studying their effects on the biochemical and physiological properties of tumor cells. Several studies have shown that σ_2 ligands induced cell death. The proposed mechanisms of cell death include caspase-independent apoptosis [40], lysosomal leakage [41], Ca^{2+} release [42, 43], oxidative stress [41], ceramide production [44] and autophagy [45]. However, the subcellular localizations where the σ_2 ligands bind and function were not known. Using the fluorescent probes shown in Figure 2, Zeng and colleagues[33, 34] recently conducted a series of confocal and two photon microscopy studies that have provided the information regarding the localization of σ_2 receptors in breast tumor cells.

MDA-MB-435 cells were incubated with 30 nM **SW120** and each of the five subcellular organelle markers: the mitochondria tracker, MitoTracker Red CMXRos (20 nM), the endoplasmic reticulum tracker, ER-Tracker™ Red (500 nM), the lysosome tracker, LysoTracker Red DND-99 (50 nM), the nuclear marker, DAPI (300 nM), or the plasma membrane tracker, FM 4-64FX (5 μg/mL). The results showed that **SW120** partially co-localized with MitoTracker, ER-Tracker, LysoTracker and the plasma membrane tracker, suggesting that σ_2 receptors may localize in mitochondria, endoplasmic reticulum, lysosomes and the plasma membrane (Figure 5). The data also showed that **SW120** did not co-localize with the nuclear marker, DAPI, suggesting that either the σ_2 receptor does not exist in the nucleus or **SW120** does not enter the nucleus. The similar results were obtained for the other σ_2 fluorescent probes (**SW116, K05-138** and **SW107**)[33, 34].

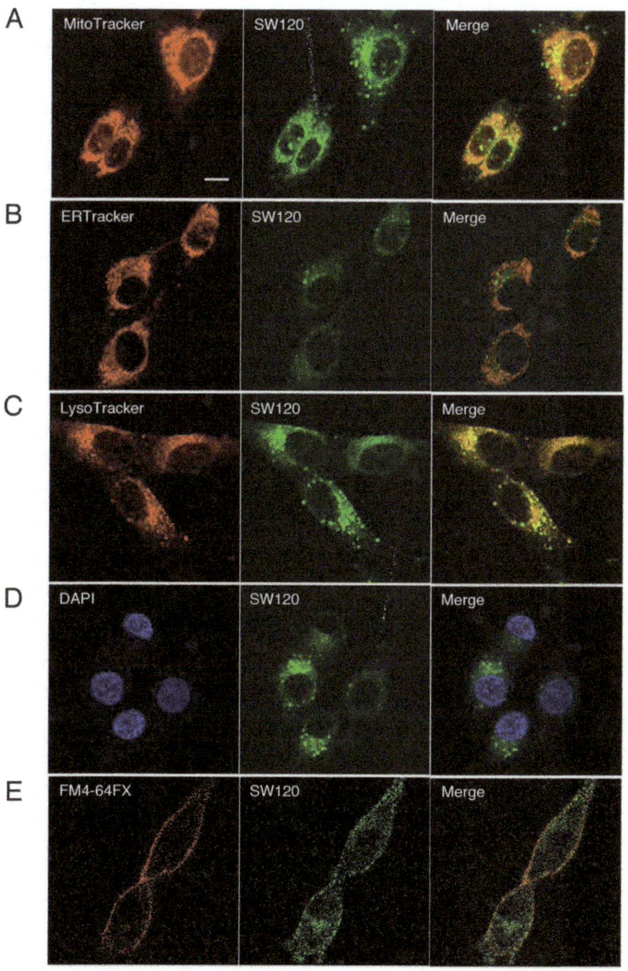

Fig. 5. Determination of the intracellular distribution of **SW120** in MDA-MB-435 cells with and without MitoTracker (A), ER-Tracker (B), LysoTracker (C), a nuclear marker, DAPI (D), or a membrane tracker, FM®4-64FX (E), using confocal microscopy. MDA-MB-435 cells were incubated with 30 nM **SW120** and either 20 nM MitoTracker, 500 nM ER-Tracker, 50 nM LysoTracker, or 300 nM DAPI. After incubating for 2 h at 37°C, live cells were imaged by confocal microscopy. MDA-MB-435 cells were also incubated with 50 nM **SW120** and 5 μg/mL of the membrane tracker, FM®4-64FX, for 15 min at 0°C. The live cells were imaged by confocal microscopy. Scale bar = 10 μm.

The kinetic studies of internalization of σ_2 fluorescent probes in MDA-MB-435 cells were conducted using confocal microscopy[33, 34]. σ_2 fluorescent probes enter tumor cells rapidly. For example, **K05-138** and **SW120** reach 50% of the maximal fluorescent intensity ($T_{1/2}$) in 16 seconds and 11 minutes, respectively (Figure 6A). The internalization of **SW120** can be blocked by the σ_2 selective ligands, **SW43** and siramesine, by 52% and 44%, respectively (Figure 6B). This internalization can not be blocked by the σ_1 selective ligand, (+)-pentazocine. The data suggest that the internalization of the σ_2 selective ligand is partially mediated by σ_2 receptor. In order to study whether the internalization of the σ_2 ligand is mediated by endocytosis, Zeng et al examined the effect of phenylarsine oxide (PAO), a well-characterized endocytosis inhibitor [46], on the internalization of **SW120**. MDA-MB-435 cells were pretreated with 5 or 10 μM PAO for 30 min, and then treated with 10 nM **SW120** in the absence or presence of PAO for an additional 30 min. Flow cytometric analysis (Figure 6C) showed that 10 μM PAO significantly blocked internalization of **SW120** by 30%. These data demonstrate that 30% of the σ_2 receptor ligand was internalized by an endocytosis-mediated mechanism, while the remaining 70 % was internalized by other mechanisms such as passive diffusion. The rapid internalization of σ_2 receptors via endocytosis suggests that σ_2 selective ligands may potentially serve as receptor-mediated probes for delivering cytotoxic agents to solid tumors.

The two photon and confocal microscopy studies conducted by Zeng et al.[33, 34] have provided useful information for the interpretation of studies demonstrating that σ_2 receptor ligands may have a role as cancer chemotherapeutic agents. Mitochondria are a key organelle to regulate the intrinsic apoptotic pathway. Apoptotic signals such as UV irradiation or treatment with chemotherapeutic agents cause the release of cytochrome C from the mitochondria and the subsequent activation of caspase-3 leading to an apoptotic cell death[47]. The subcellular localization of σ_2 ligands in mitochondria is consistent with the previous studies that σ_2 ligands trigger apoptosis in tumor cells by acting on mitochondria [48]. The data are also consistent with our observation by transmission electron microscopy that the σ_2 ligand siramesine induces distortion of mitochondria (unpublished data). The endoplasmic reticulum (ER) serves as a dynamic Ca^{2+} storage pool [49]. σ_2 selective ligands have been reported to induce transient Ca^{2+} release from the ER, which may be responsible for σ_2 ligand-induced cell death [42]. The presence of the σ_2 fluorescent probes in the ER is consistent with these results. Additional research will be required to determine how σ_2 receptors regulate the Ca^{2+} release channels in the ER. Lysosomal proteases, such as cathepsins, calpains and granzymes, have been reported to contribute to apoptosis [50]. Under physiological conditions, these proteases are found within the lysosomes but are released into the cytoplasm upon exposure to cell damaging agents, thereby triggering a cascade of intracellular events leading to cell death. The σ_2 selective ligand siramesine has been reported to cause lysosomal leakage and induce cell death by caspase-independent mechanisms [41, 45]. The localization of fluorescent σ_2 receptor probes in the lysosomes is consistent with the hypothesis that siramesine induces cell death partially by targeting lysosomes to cause lysosomal damage, the release of proteases, and eventually cell death. Evidence has also been reported that σ_2 receptors exist in lipid rafts which are mainly found in the plasma membrane [51]. Lipid rafts play an important role in the signaling associated with a variety of cellular events including adhesion, motility, and membrane trafficking [52, 53]. The observation that σ_2 fluorescent ligands are co-localized with cytoplasmic membrane markers, and undergo receptor mediated endocytosis, is consistent with their localization in lipid rafts. How the σ_2 receptor is involved in lipid raft function deserves further investigation.

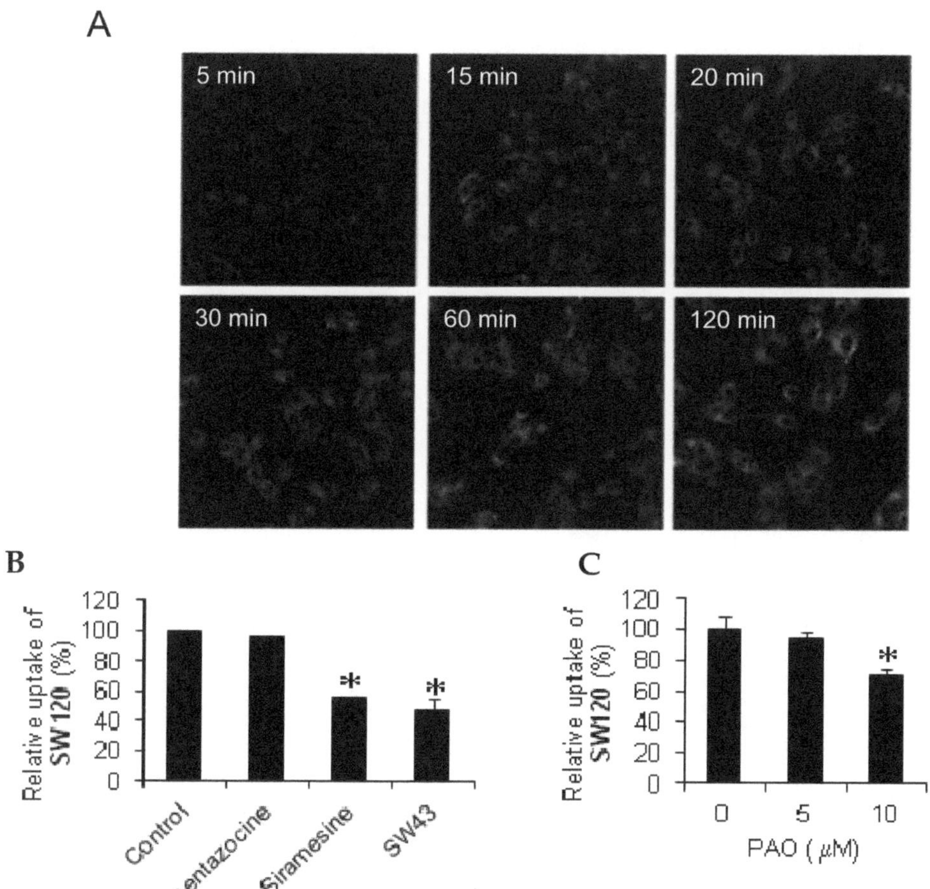

Fig. 6. Characterization of σ_2 fluorescent probes. A: The internalization kinetics of **SW120** in MDA-MB-435 cells by confocal microscopy studies show that **SW120** enters tumor cells rapidly. B: The internalization of **SW120** in MDA-MB-435 cells are partially blocked by σ_2 selective ligands, **SW43** and siramesine, but not by a σ_1 selective ligand, (+)-pentazocine. C: The inhibition of **SW120** internalization by phenylarsine oxide (PAO). MDA-MB-435 cells were preincubated with 5 or 10 μM PAO for 30 min at 37°C, and then incubated with 10 nM **SW120** for an additional 30 min. The cells were analyzed by flow cytometry. The internalization of **SW120** was significantly reduced by 10 μM PAO (* $P < 0.05$).

The σ_2 receptor has been validated as a proliferation marker in cell culture and in solid tumors. Therefore it is possible that σ_2 fluorescent probes could preferentially label proliferating cells versus non-proliferating cells and serve as agents to image cell proliferation in vivo. This hypothesis was tested in nude mice implanted with murine mammary adenocarcinoma 66 cells and BALB/C mice implanted with mouse mammary carcinoma cell line EMT6[34]. The mice were treated with **SW120** (50 μg in 100 μL PBS) for one hour. The peripheral blood mononuclear cells (PBMC), which are commonly used as controls for non-proliferative cells, and tumor cells were prepared. These cells were analyzed by flow cytometry for **SW120** uptake and for Ki67 expression, a commonly-used proliferation marker. Our data showed that PBMC were Ki67 negative, whereas a large portion of the tumor cells were Ki-67 positive (Figure 7). The data also showed that PBMC were not labeled by **SW120**, whereas a portion of the tumor cells were labeled with **SW120**. The trend of the positive correlation between Ki67 expression and **SW120** labeling implies that the fluorescent may possess in vivo selectivity toward proliferating cells versus non-proliferative cells. These data suggest that σ_2 fluorescent probes could be used as imaging agents for monitoring cell proliferation in mice. The data also suggest that σ_2 selective ligands hold a potential to serve as therapeutic agents to selectively target tumor cells in vivo.

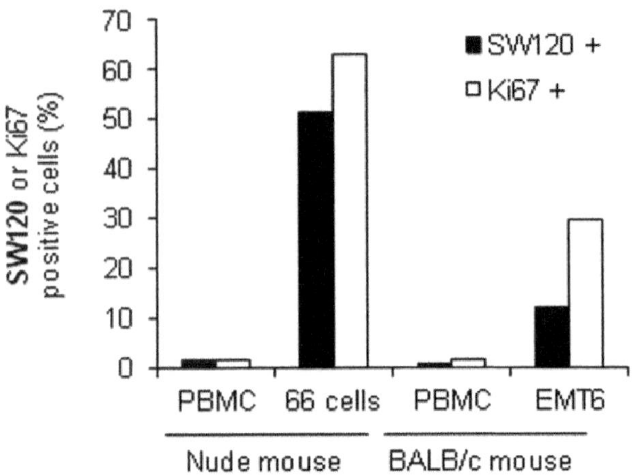

Fig. 7. Ki67 expression and **SW120** fluorescent intensity in solid mouse breast tumors and peripheral blood mononuclear cells (PBMC) of mice by flow cytometric analysis. The female nude mice were implanted with murine mammary adenocarcinoma 66 cells. BALB/C mice were implanted with mouse mammary carcinoma cell line EMT6. The mice were i.v. injected with **SW120** (50 µg/ mouse) and tissues harvested after 1 hour. The 66 cells and EMT6 cells were dissociated from the solid tumors. PBMC were prepared from the blood of mice. The cells were analyzed for the fluorescent intensity of **SW120** and the Ki67 expression determined by Ki67 immunostaining using a flow cytometer. The data indicate the trend of the positive correlation between Ki67 expression and **SW120** labeling.

6. Conclusions

The σ_2 receptor continues to be an important molecular target in the field of tumor biology. The high expression of this receptor in proliferating versus quiescent breast tumors indicates that the σ_2 receptor is an important clinical biomarker for determining the proliferative status of solid tumors using the functional imaging techniques PET and SPECT. The σ_2 receptor fluorescent probes are useful to study the subcellular localization and the function of σ_2 receptors using confocal and two photon microscopy techniques, and may be used to image tumor proliferation in mice using optical imaging techniques. The full utility of the σ_2

receptor in the diagnosis and prediction of therapeutic response will rely on the cloning of the σ_2 receptor and elucidation of its functional role in normal and tumor cell biology.

Note: While this article is accepted, a paper from our group is published in Nature Communication[54]. In this paper we have identified progesterone receptor membrane component 1(PGRMC1) as the putative σ_2 receptor. This finding will greatly facilitate investigations of the functions of the σ_2 receptor in normal and tumor cells.

7. Acknowledgement

This research was supported by grants CA80452, CA81825, and CA102869 awarded by the National Cancer Institute, and grant DAMD17-01-1-0446 awarded by the Department of Defense Breast Cancer Research Program of the US Army Medical Research and Materiel Command Office.

8. References

[1] Hellewell, S.B., et al., Rat liver and kidney contain high densities of sigma 1 and sigma 2 receptors: characterization by ligand binding and photoaffinity labeling. Eur J Pharmacol, 1994. 268(1): p. 9-18.

[2] Walker, J.M., et al., Sigma receptors: biology and function. Pharmacol Rev, 1990. 42(4): p. 355-402.

[3] Rothman, R.B., et al., Labeling by [3H]1,3-di(2-tolyl)guanidine of two high affinity binding sites in guinea pig brain: evidence for allosteric regulation by calcium channel antagonists and pseudoallosteric modulation by sigma ligands. Mol Pharmacol, 1991. 39(2): p. 222-32.

[4] Seth, P., F.H. Leibach, and V. Ganapathy, Cloning and structural analysis of the cDNA and the gene encoding the murine type 1 sigma receptor. Biochem Biophys Res Commun, 1997. 241(2): p. 535-40.

[5] Hanner, M., et al., Purification, molecular cloning, and expression of the mammalian sigma1-binding site. Proc Natl Acad Sci U S A, 1996. 93(15): p. 8072-7.

[6] Maurice, T., F.J. Roman, and A. Privat, Modulation by neurosteroids of the in vivo (+)-[3H]SKF-10,047 binding to sigma 1 receptors in the mouse forebrain. J Neurosci Res, 1996. 46(6): p. 734-43.

[7] Maurice, T., J.L. Junien, and A. Privat, Dehydroepiandrosterone sulfate attenuates dizocilpine-induced learning impairment in mice via sigma 1-receptors. Behav Brain Res, 1997. 83(1-2): p. 159-64.

[8] Romieu, P., et al., Sigma 1 receptor-related neuroactive steroids modulate cocaine-induced reward. J Neurosci, 2003. 23(9): p. 3572-6.

[9] Bem, W.T., et al., Overexpression of sigma receptors in nonneural human tumors. Cancer Res, 1991. 51(24): p. 6558-62.

[10] Vilner, B.J., C.S. John, and W.D. Bowen, Sigma-1 and sigma-2 receptors are expressed in a wide variety of human and rodent tumor cell lines. Cancer Res, 1995. 55(2): p. 408-13.

[11] Mach, R.H., F. Dehdashti, and K.T. Wheeler, PET Radiotracers for Imaging the Proliferative Status of Solid Tumors. PET Clin, 2009. 4(1): p. 1-15.

[12] Wallen, C.A., R. Higashikubo, and L.A. Dethlefsen, Murine mammary tumour cells in vitro. II. Recruitment of quiescent cells. Cell Tissue Kinet, 1984. 17(1): p. 79-89.

[13] Wallen, C.A., R. Higashikubo, and L.A. Dethlefsen, Murine mammary tumour cells in vitro. I. The development of a quiescent state. Cell Tissue Kinet, 1984. 17(1): p. 65-77.

[14] Mach, R.H., et al., Sigma 2 receptors as potential biomarkers of proliferation in breast cancer. Cancer Res, 1997. 57(1): p. 156-61.

[15] Al-Nabulsi, I., et al., Effect of ploidy, recruitment, environmental factors, and tamoxifen treatment on the expression of sigma-2 receptors in proliferating and quiescent tumour cells. Br J Cancer, 1999. 81(6): p. 925-33.

[16] Wheeler, K.T., et al., Sigma-2 receptors as a biomarker of proliferation in solid tumours. Br J Cancer, 2000. 82(6): p. 1223-32.

[17] Weigel, M.T. and M. Dowsett, Current and emerging biomarkers in breast cancer: prognosis and prediction. Endocr Relat Cancer, 2010. 17(4): p. R245-62.

[18] Bowen, W.D., et al., CB-64D and CB-184: ligands with high sigma 2 receptor affinity and subtype selectivity. Eur J Pharmacol, 1995. 278(3): p. 257-60.

[19] Bertha, C.M., et al., A marked change of receptor affinity of the 2-methyl-5-(3-hydroxyphenyl)morphans upon attachment of an (E)-8-benzylidene moiety: synthesis and evaluation of a new class of sigma receptor ligands. J Med Chem, 1994. 37(19): p. 3163-70.

[20] Perregaard, J., et al., Sigma ligands with subnanomolar affinity and preference for the sigma 2 binding site. 1. 3-(omega-aminoalkyl)-1H-indoles. J Med Chem, 1995. 38(11): p. 1998-2008.

[21] Moltzen, E.K., J. Perregaard, and E. Meier, Sigma ligands with subnanomolar affinity and preference for the sigma 2 binding site. 2. Spiro-joined benzofuran, isobenzofuran, and benzopyran piperidines. J Med Chem, 1995. 38(11): p. 2009-17.

[22] Soby, K.K., et al., Lu 28-179 labels a sigma(2)-site in rat and human brain. Neuropharmacology, 2002. 43(1): p. 95-100.

[23] Bowen, W.D., et al., Ibogaine and its congeners are sigma 2 receptor-selective ligands with moderate affinity. Eur J Pharmacol, 1995. 279(1): p. R1-3.

[24] Mach, R.H., C.R. Smith, and S.R. Childers, Ibogaine possesses a selective affinity for sigma 2 receptors. Life Sci, 1995. 57(4): p. PL57-62.

[25] Bonhaus, D.W., et al., [3H]BIMU-1, a 5-hydroxytryptamine3 receptor ligand in NG-108 cells, selectively labels sigma-2 binding sites in guinea pig hippocampus. J Pharmacol Exp Ther, 1993. 267(2): p. 961-70.

[26] Mach, R.H., et al., The analgesic tropane analogue (+/-)-SM 21 has a high affinity for sigma2 receptors. Life Sci, 1999. 64(10): p. PL131-7.

[27] Ghelardini, C., N. Galeotti, and A. Bartolini, Pharmacological identification of SM-21, the novel sigma(2) antagonist. Pharmacol Biochem Behav, 2000. 67(3): p. 659-62.

[28] Nguyen, V.H., et al., Comparison of binding parameters of sigma 1 and sigma 2 binding sites in rat and guinea pig brain membranes: novel subtype-selective trishomocubanes. Eur J Pharmacol, 1996. 311(2-3): p. 233-40.

[29] Azzariti, A., et al., Cyclohexylpiperazine derivative PB28, a sigma2 agonist and sigma1 antagonist receptor, inhibits cell growth, modulates P-glycoprotein, and synergizes with anthracyclines in breast cancer. Mol Cancer Ther, 2006. 5(7): p. 1807-16.

[30] Vangveravong, S., et al., Synthesis of N-substituted 9-azabicyclo[3.3.1]nonan-3alpha-yl carbamate analogs as sigma2 receptor ligands. Bioorg Med Chem, 2006. 14(20): p. 6988-97.

[31] Ariazi, E.A., et al., Estrogen receptors as therapeutic targets in breast cancer. Curr Top Med Chem, 2006. 6(3): p. 181-202.

[32] Arttamangkul, S., et al., Binding and internalization of fluorescent opioid peptide conjugates in living cells. Mol Pharmacol, 2000. 58(6): p. 1570-80.

[33] Zeng, C., et al., Subcellular localization of sigma-2 receptors in breast cancer cells using two-photon and confocal microscopy. Cancer Res, 2007. 67(14): p. 6708-16.

[34] Zeng, C., et al., Characterization and Evaluation of Two Novel Fluorescent Sigma-2 Receptor Ligands as Proliferation Probes. Mol Imaging, 2011 (in press)

[35] Mach, R.H., et al., Conformationally-flexible benzamide analogues as dopamine D3 and sigma 2 receptor ligands. Bioorg Med Chem Lett, 2004. 14(1): p. 195-202.

[36] Chu, W., et al., Synthesis and in vitro binding of N-phenyl piperazine analogs as potential dopamine D3 receptor ligands. Bioorg Med Chem, 2005. 13(1): p. 77-87.

[37] Xu, J., et al., [3H]N-[4-(3,4-dihydro-6,7-dimethoxyisoquinolin-2(1H)-yl)butyl]-2-methoxy-5 -methylbenzamide: a novel sigma-2 receptor probe. Eur J Pharmacol, 2005. 525(1-3): p. 8-17.

[38] Tu, Z., et al., Carbon-11 labeled sigma2 receptor ligands for imaging breast cancer. Nucl Med Biol, 2005. 32(5): p. 423-30.

[39] Tu, Z., et al., Fluorine-18-labeled benzamide analogues for imaging the sigma2 receptor status of solid tumors with positron emission tomography. J Med Chem, 2007. 50(14): p. 3194-204.

[40] Crawford, K.W. and W.D. Bowen, Sigma-2 receptor agonists activate a novel apoptotic pathway and potentiate antineoplastic drugs in breast tumor cell lines. Cancer Res, 2002. 62(1): p. 313-22.

[41] Ostenfeld, M.S., et al., Effective tumor cell death by sigma-2 receptor ligand siramesine involves lysosomal leakage and oxidative stress. Cancer Res, 2005. 65(19): p. 8975-83.

[42] Vilner, B.J. and W.D. Bowen, Modulation of cellular calcium by sigma-2 receptors: release from intracellular stores in human SK-N-SH neuroblastoma cells. J Pharmacol Exp Ther, 2000. 292(3): p. 900-11.

[43] Cassano, G., et al., F281, synthetic agonist of the sigma-2 receptor, induces Ca2+ efflux from the endoplasmic reticulum and mitochondria in SK-N-SH cells. Cell Calcium, 2009. 45(4): p. 340-5.

[44] Crawford, K.W., A. Coop, and W.D. Bowen, sigma(2) Receptors regulate changes in sphingolipid levels in breast tumor cells. Eur J Pharmacol, 2002. 443(1-3): p. 207-9.

[45] Ostenfeld, M.S., et al., Anti-cancer agent siramesine is a lysosomotropic detergent that induces cytoprotective autophagosome accumulation. Autophagy, 2008. 4(4): p. 487-99.

[46] Hertel, C., S.J. Coulter, and J.P. Perkins, A comparison of catecholamine-induced internalization of beta-adrenergic receptors and receptor-mediated endocytosis of epidermal growth factor in human astrocytoma cells. Inhibition by phenylarsine oxide. J Biol Chem, 1985. 260(23): p. 12547-53.

[47] Jiang, X. and X. Wang, Cytochrome C-mediated apoptosis. Annu Rev Biochem, 2004. 73: p. 87-106.

[48] Balakumaran, B.S., et al., MYC activity mitigates response to rapamycin in prostate cancer through eukaryotic initiation factor 4E-binding protein 1-mediated inhibition of autophagy. Cancer Res, 2009. 69(19): p. 7803-10.

[49] Berridge, M.J., The endoplasmic reticulum: a multifunctional signaling organelle. Cell Calcium, 2002. 32(5-6): p. 235-49.
[50] Chwieralski, C.E., T. Welte, and F. Buhling, Cathepsin-regulated apoptosis. Apoptosis, 2006. 11(2): p. 143-9.
[51] Gebreselassie, D. and W.D. Bowen, Sigma-2 receptors are specifically localized to lipid rafts in rat liver membranes. Eur J Pharmacol, 2004. 493(1-3): p. 19-28.
[52] Brown, D.A. and E. London, Functions of lipid rafts in biological membranes. Annu Rev Cell Dev Biol, 1998. 14: p. 111-36.
[53] Simons, K. and D. Toomre, Lipid rafts and signal transduction. Nat Rev Mol Cell Biol, 2000. 1(1): p. 31-9.
[54] Xu, J., et al., Identification of the PGRMC1 protein complex as the putative sigma-2 receptor binding site. Nat Commun, 2011. 2: p. 380.

Part 4

Therapeutics

18

Translational Research on Breast Cancer: miRNA, siRNA and Immunoconjugates in Conjugation with Nanotechnology for Clinical Studies

Arutselvan Natarajan[1] and Senthil Kumar Venugopal[2]
[1]Department of Radiology, Stanford University, California,
[2]Institute of Liver and Biliary Sciences, New Delhi,
[1]USA
[2]India

1. Introduction

Currently, breast cancer is a global public health issue. However, recent progress in phenotyping and expression profiling of human cancers have greatly enhanced the diagnosis and biological classification of several tumors, in particular breast cancers. Despite significant advances in cytotoxic chemotherapy, endocrine therapy and novel targeted agents, metastatic breast cancer remains an incurable disease (Ocana et al., 2006; Ocana & Pandiella, 2008). The lack of curative potential is partially explained by the heterogeneous biology of this disease which exhibits both *de novo* and acquired resistance to many treatment modalities (Ocana & Pandiella, 2008).

Breast cancers are classified into distinct subtypes using microarray-based gene expression signatures identification; these are largely based on their (Estrogen) ER, progesterone (PR), and HER2 receptor status (Perou et al., 2000; Sorlie et al., 2001; Sorlie et al., 2006). Subtypes were designated *Luminal A*, which strongly expressed ER and/or PR, but not HER2; *Luminal B*, which were ER, PR and HER2 positive; *Basal* tumors which were ER, PR, and HER negative, preferentially affecting young women and women of African origin, usually of high histological grade and more aggressive clinical behavior (Yehiely et al., 2006) .

Genomic tumor profiling has provided us with important insights to mechanisms of tumorigenesis and translational data for clinical advances (Bauer et al.). Relative to some cancer types, there is tremendous genomic information available for breast cancers, which includes tumor DNA copy number (Adelaide et al., 2007; Bergamaschi et al., 2006; Chin et al., 2006; Han et al., 2008; Neve et al., 2006) DNA sequence and mutations (Leary et al., 2008; Nikolsky et al., 2008; Shah et al., 2009; Sjoblom et al., 2006; Stephens et al., 2009; Wood et al., 2007), gene expression and protein profiles(Boyd et al., 2008; Hennessy et al., 2009), as well as epigenetics (Andrews et al.; Ruike et al.) and microRNAs (Iorio et al., 2005a; Mattie et al., 2006a).

Promising new targeted agents, such as small molecule tyrosine kinase inhibitors and monoclonal antibodies such as trastuzumab, which targets breast cancer cells overexpressing her2neu, are rapidly making their way into general oncology practice in high-resource countries. These "smart bombs" of the oncologywill, no doubt, have increasing utility either as stand-alone or adjunct drugs in the armamentarium of anti-neoplastics. However, given the experience to date with cost of these agents, and the likelihood that any of these drugs will be off-patent and "genericized" in the coming decade, it is presently entirely beyond the reach of low and middle-resource countries to even consider their use.

According to the WHO, a drug may be considered cost-effective if the annual cost per quality-adjusted life year saved, or QALY, is no greater than a country's per capita GDP (gross domestic product) ("https://www.cia.gov/library/publications/the-world-factbook/,"). Although major share of drug development budgets are focused on targeted agents, which escalates the cost of the drug. Hence to decrease drug cost, drug activity should be improved, and treatment failures need to avoided, to achieve this identification of common 'drugable' oncogenic mechanisms is an important area to focus research.

Many strategies have been developed to treat cancer by targeting the cancer cells without affecting normal cells. Recent research on gene delivery such as, siRNAs, miRNAs which have been proven to control breast cancer tumors can be introduced into breast tissue through the use of nanoparticle technology and breast cancer targeting immunoconjugates. Hence, in this chapter we will focus mainly translational research on novel formulation that contains miRNA or siRNA or immunoconjugate modified to nanoparticles for specific delivery to breast cancer tissues. Thus this chapter will divides into four sub sections, first three will be briefing current updates on miRNA, siRNA, immunoconjugates, relevant to breast cancer research ;and the fourth one is clinical applications on nanoparticles modified with targeting agents to deliver into breast cancer cells. Hence this book chapter will be an unique one to all breast cancer researchers with the following expertise; gene delivery, nanotechnology, immunologists, clinicians, and clinical translational scientists.

2. MicroRNAs

MicroRNAs (miRNAs) are a family of endogenous, noncoding, small single stranded RNAs (21-25 nucleotides) that regulate the gene expression at post-transcriptional levels (Venugopal et al., 2009; Yoon et al., 2010). miRNAs bind to the target sequences by partial or complete binding to the 3′ untranslated region (UTR) of their target mRNAs, and thereby mediate mRNA degradation or translational inhibition, which depends on the degree of complementarity between miRNAs and their targets (Carthew, 2006). They appear to function via several mechanisms in repressing gene expression and regulating cellular activities, such as development (Ambros, 2004), cell proliferation (Zhang et al., 2006), differentiation (Esau et al., 2004), apoptosis (Cimmino et al., 2005), glucose metabolism (Poy et al., 2004), stress resistance (Dresios et al., 2005), and cancer (Calin et al., 2002). One of the miRNAs, which is abundantly expressed in the liver, and appears to affect hepatic function, is microRNA-122a (miR-122a)(Krutzfeldt et al., 2005). Using antagomiR-122a, when miR-122a expression was silenced, there was a 44% decrease in cholesterol synthesis in hepatocytes (Krutzfeldt et al., 2005). The mechanism of this effect appears to be that inhibition of miR-122a caused the activation of a transcriptional repressor protein involved in cholesterol biosynthesis (Krutzfeldt et al., 2005). Another study reported that inhibition of miR-122a in the liver caused a marked loss of hepatitis C viral RNAs, and that miR-122a may represent a target for antiviral intervention (Jopling et al., 2005). Several miRNAs have

been implicated in the process of apoptosis and cell proliferation in non-liver systems (Cimmino et al., 2005; Xu et al., 2004). For example, miR-21 has been shown to inhibit caspase activation, thereby promoting anti-apoptosis (Chan et al., 2005). miR-15 and miR-16 were shown to promote apoptosis by interacting with Bcl-2 (Cimmino et al., 2005), and down-regulation of miR-27b caused apoptosis (Scott et al., 2006). Another study shows that miR-126 increased the growth and proliferation of megakaryocytes (Garzon et al., 2006), and that miR-451 enhanced the differentiation of erythroid cells (Rathjen et al., 2006). The miRNAs, which are secreted to the blood stream, can be detected and used as diagnostic markers, one such example is miR-21 released to the blood stream. It has shown by various investigators that several of these miRNAs including miR-21, miR-126 have been shown to be involved in the progression of breast cancer. Anti-cancer therapies are also focused in modulating the expression of miRNAs to inhibit cell growth, proliferation and invasion.
The biogenesis of miRNA occurs in nucleus, like other genes, **(Figure 1)** and a longer primary miRNA is transcribed by RNA polymerase II or III. The primary miRNA is processed by the RNAse III endonuclease Drosha and DGCR8 to form stem-loop structure

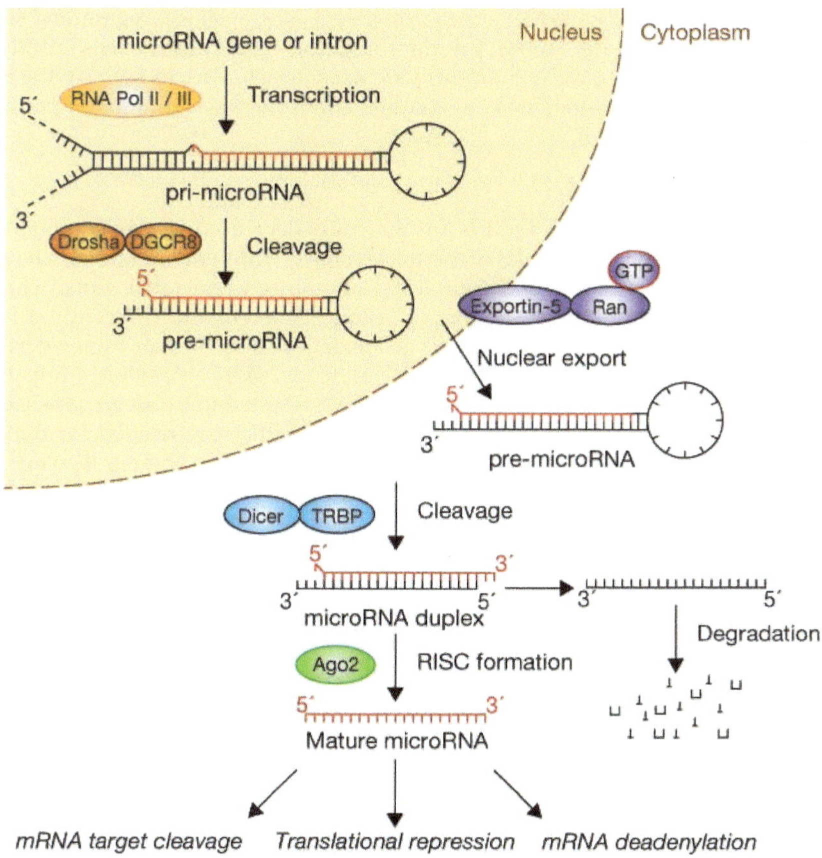

Fig. 1. Schematic diagram of the biogenesis of microRNA in eukaryotic cells. (Reproduced with permission from Nature Cell Biology, 2009)

of approximately 50 nculeotides long called "precursor miRNA" (pre-miRNA)(Borchert et al., 2006; Gregory et al., 2004; Han et al., 2004; Lee et al., 2004). The pre-miRNA is transported from the nucleus to the cytoplasm with the help of exportin 5, where this pre-miRNA will undergo further processing by another RNase III endonuclease, Dicer (Lee et al., 2003; Lund et al., 2004). Dicer removes the loop structure of the pre-miRNA to produce an imperfect duplex made up of the mature miRNA and a fragment of similar size (miRNA*), which is derived from the opposing arm of the pre-miRNA. The miRNA strand of the duplex is loaded onto the RNA-induced silencing complex (RISC); the miRNA* gets separated from the duplex and is degraded (Lee et al., 2002).

Regulation of gene expression by miRNAs occurs either by degrading the mRNA or by inhibiting the translation of the mRNA. The mechanisms by which the miRNAs inhibit the translation depends on the degree of complimentarity between the particular miRNA and the target mRNA. If there is a perfect complementarity, the target mRNA sequence is degraded and if there is an imperfect complementarity, the translation of the mRNA is blocked (Hutvagner & Zamore, 2002).

These miRNAs can bind to a seed sequence (about 6-8 bases) of the approximately 22 nucleotides aligns perfectly with the target mRNA's 3' untranslated region and can bind more than one target sequence. Hence, finding the target sequences for these miRNAs has been difficult for researchers. Using bioinformatic approaches, we can identify the putative targets of these miRNAs, but one needs to conduct confirmatory laboratory experiments to establish the target genes.

2.1 miRNA and cancer

In most of the cancers, expression of miRNA is generally decreased, as most of them may act as tumor suppressors (Lu et al., 2005). Furthermore, poorly differentiated tumors have lower miRNA levels compared to more differentiated tumors, indicating that global changes in miRNA expression may indicate the degree of cellular differentiation. Recently it has been shown that several miRNAs were expressed at lower levels in human tumor-derived cell lines compared to the corresponding tissue (Gaur et al., 2007). Another study has also shown that a loss in the expression of miRNA in cancer resulted in tumorigenesis (Kumar et al., 2007). When drosha and dicer were knocked down, which are needed for the miRNA biogenesis, there was a complete loss of miRNA expression. When these cells were injected in nude mice, they formed accelerated growth with increased invasive properties. These results suggest that the loss of miRNA expression enhances tumorigenesis.

2.2 miRNA in breast cancer

Several studies have been conducted in the recent past on profiling miRNAs and found that several of them were aberrantly expressed in breast cancer tissues. Although several of the functions of these miRNAs were studied, still an array of experiments needs to be conducted for utilizing them as diagnostic markers or therapeutic agents. In addition, tumor metastasis may be promoted by enhanced expression of prooncogenic/prometastatic and/or downregulation of antioncogenic/antimetastatic miRNAs.

Several miRNAs have shown to be deregulated in breast cancer, suggesting that these miRNAs may modulate oncogenesis (Iorio et al., 2005b; Lu et al., 2005; Yu et al., 2010). Lu et al. (Lu et al., 2005) had reported that miRNA expression is downregulated in tumors, including breast cancer. Several miRNAs, such as miR-10b, miR-125b and miR-145 were down regulated, while miR-21 and miR-155 were up regulated, suggesting that these miRNAs may play an important role as either tumor suppressor genes or oncogenes (Iorio et al., 2005b). A recent study has shown that miR-7, miR-128a, miR-210 and miR-51-3p were involved in breast cancer progression (Foekens et al., 2008). Upregulation of miR-373 and miR-520c promotes metastasis by inhibiting CD44 expression (Huang et al., 2008). Ma et al. (Ma et al., 2007) showed that a transcription factor, twist1, is involved in the upregulation of miR-10b. Suppression of miR-21 led to an increase in apoptosis and inhibition of bcl-2 (Si et al., 2007). miR-21 also has been shown to inhibit tropomyosin 1, which plays an important role in antioncogenic function including binding microfilaments and regulating cytosekleton miRNAs (Zhu et al., 2007). miR-27a is reported to inhibit the transcription factor ZBTB10/RINZF, which is a putative suppressor of specificity protein (Sp) (Mertens-Talcott et al., 2007). Overexpression of Sp by miR-27a contributes to the increased expression of Sp-dependent survival and angiogenic genes, including survivin, vascular endothelial growth factor (VEGF) and VEGF receptor 1. miR-175p is inhibited in breast cancer and it regulates AIB1 (Amplified in Breast Cancer-1 protein) (Hossain et al., 2006). AIB1 is a coactivator for nuclear receptors, such as estrogen receptor, and is overexpressed in breast cancer. Both miR-125a and miR-125b are down-regulated in breast cancer and these miRNAs suppress the HER2 and HER3, the two tyrosine kinase receptors frequently deregulated in breast cancer (Scott et al., 2007). miR-206 has been found to target the 3'UTR of the estrogen receptor-α protein, leading to an inverse correlation between miR-206 concentration and estrogen receptor-α status (Adams et al., 2007; Kondo et al., 2008). Some of the key miRNAs, which are shown to be involved in modulating tumor growth and metastasis, is described below.

2.3 Oncogenic miRNAs

miR-21

There have been several studies showing that miR-21 is consistently overexpressed in many tumors, including breast cancer (Iorio et al., 2005b; Volinia et al., 2006). It also has been shown that miR-21 was highly upregulated in breast tumors compared to the matched normal breast tissues among 157 human miRNAs analyzed by real-time RT-PCR arrays (Si et al., 2007), suggesting that miR-21 may function as an oncomiR. In the later study the authors have also shown that knocking down miR-21 resulted in a marginal decrease in cell survival (25% decrease), and the authors found that this growth inhibition increased when the transfected MCF-7 cells were treated with the anticancer drug topotecan, suggesting that suppression of miR-21 can sensitize tumor cells to anticancer agents. The target prediction using bioinformatics approaches followed by experimental validation showed that tropomyosin 1 (TPM1), which is known to be downregulated in breast cancer epithelial cell lines, was a target of miR-21 (Zhu et al., 2007). miR-21 has also been shown to inhibit the expression of the tumor suppressor PDCD4 (programmed cell death-4) (Frankel et al., 2008). Another important target of miR-21 is the tumor suppressor gene phosphatase and tensin homolog (*PTEN*) (Qi et al., 2009). These genes were shown to reduce invasiveness of a metastatic breast cancer cell line. These findings further establish miR-21 as an oncogenic miRNA and suggest that miR-21 has a role not only in tumor growth but also in invasion and tumor metastasis by targeting multiple anti-metastatic genes.

miR-155

MiRNA microarray has shown that miR-155 is over-expressed in a number of human malignancies, including breast cancer (Iorio et al., 2005b; Volinia et al., 2006). A recent study has shown that miR-155 is upregulated in normal mouse mammary gland epithelial cells (NMuMG cells) by the TGF-β/Smad4 pathway and mediates TGF-β-induced EMT and cell invasion (Kong et al., 2008). miR-155 directly inhibits the expression of *RhoA*, a gene that regulates many cellular processes, including cell adhesion, motility, and polarity, and is an important modulator of cell junction formation and stability. It also has been shown that miR-155 is highly expressed in invasive tumors but not in noninvasive cancer tissues.

miR-10b

miR-10b was found to influence the metastatsis of human cancer cells (Ma et al., 2007). Unlike miR-155, which is overexpressed in many breast tumors, miR-10b was highly expressed only in metastatic cancer cells and was found to promote cell migration and invasion *in vitro* and initiate tumor invasion and metastasis *in vivo*. miR-10b expression is shown to be regulated by a transcription factor Twist, and miR-10b inhibits the translation of the transcription factor homeobox D10 (HOXD10), resulting in a cascade of cellular alterations that include expression of the prometastatic gene *RHOC* (ras homologue gene family member C), a gene that promotes cancer cell migration and invasion.

miR-373/520c family

miRNAs of the miR-373/520c family were identified (Kato et al., 2009) as prometastatic using a forward genetic screen involving overexpression of almost 450 miRNAs in a nonmetastatic human breast cancer cell line (MCF-7 cells). MCF-7 cells were transduced with these miRNAs and subjected to a trans-well cell migration assay to identify miRNAs that stimulate cell migration. The authors found that miR-373 and miR-520c promoted cancer cell migration and invasion *in vitro* and *in vivo*. It has been shown that the downregulation of CD44 (a metastasis repressor) was found when miR-373 or miR-520c were overexpressed in MCF-7 cells.

2.4 Tumor suppressor miRNAs

miR-206

Using miRNA microarrays it was found that miR-206 is involved in suppressing breast cancer cells (Iorio et al., 2005b). miR-206 was upregulated in estrogen receptor (ER)α-negative breast cancers, suggesting a role of miR-206 in regulation of the estrogen receptor gene *ERa* (*ESR1*). Indeed, miR-206 was recently shown to inhibit the expression of *ESR1* mRNA through two binding sites in the *ESR1* 3' UTR (Kumar et al., 2007). The latter study also showed that miR-206 expression was strongly repressed by ERα agonists, but not by an ERβ agonist or progesterone, suggesting the existence of a feedback loop. Another study had shown that miR-206 expression decreased in ERα-positive human breast cancer tissues and that miR-206 suppresses ESR1 expression and inhibits growth of MCF7 breast cancer cells. In addition to miR-206, the authors found that *ESR1* mRNA was a direct target of miR-18a, miR-18b, miR-193b and miR-302c in breast cancer cells (Leivonen et al., 2009), most of which were shown to induce cell cycle arrest and to inhibit estrogen-induced proliferation. Bioinformatics approach had revealed that the direct targets of miR-335 are *PTPRN2*, *MERTK*, *TNC* and *SOX4*; among them, *TNC* (encoding an extracellular matrix component) and *SOX4* (encoding a transcription factor that is involved in tumorigenesis) were shown to be functional targets implicated in metastasis. Restoring miR-206 expression in metastatic cells did not influence their proliferation or sensitivity to apoptosis, but altered cellular morphology, possibly contributing to a decrease in cell motility that could limit the migration of metastatic cells (Tavazoie et al., 2008). These findings suggest that miR-206 could be a novel candidate for breast cancer therapy.

miR-17-5p

miR-17-5p, also known as miR-91, is located on chromosome 13q31, a genomic region that undergoes loss of heterozygosity in multiple cancers, including breast cancer (Eiriksdottir et al., 1998). The oncogene *AIB1* (amplified in breast cancer) is a direct target of miR-17-5p (Hossain et al., 2006). The protein encoded by the *AIB1* gene is a steroid receptor co-activator that enhances the transcriptional activity of *ERa, E2F1* (which is also directly regulated by miR-17-5p) and other transcription factor genes. Downregulation of AIB1 by miR-17-5p results in the suppression of estrogen-stimulated proliferation and estrogen/ER-independent breast cancer cell proliferation (Hossain et al., 2006). In breast cancer cells, the gene cyclin D1 (*CCND1*), which is overexpressed in approximately 50% of human cancers, was recently identified as a direct target of miR-17-5p (Yu et al., 2008). miR-17-5p inhibits the proliferation of breast cancer cells by suppressing cyclin D1 protein synthesis. *miR-125a and miR-125b*

miR-125a and miR-125b are downregulated in HER2-amplified and HER2-overexpressing breast cancers (Mattie et al., 2006b). These two miRNAs are potential tumor suppressors and their overexpression in SKBR3 cells (a HER2-dependent human breast cancer cell line) suppresses *HER2* and *HER3* mRNA and protein levels, leading to a reduction in anchorage-dependent growth, cell motility, and invasiveness (Scott et al., 2007). However, this influence was subtle in non-transformed HER2-independent breast cancer cells (MCF10A).

miR-200 family

Overexpression of miR-200 induced epithelial differentiation in undifferentiated breast cancer cells (MDA-MB231) whereas antagonizing it induced an EMT phenotype in the colorectal cancer cell line HCT116. *ZEB1* and *ZEB2* were again detected as targets of the miR-200 family members. These and other recent reports on the miR-200 family (Hurteau et al., 2009; Korpal et al., 2008) add important miRNAs to the growing list of tumor-associated miRNAs. Furthermore, a recent study showed that the expression of the miR-200 family was decreased by Akt2, suggesting that, in many cases, breast cancer metastasis may be under the control of the Akt-miR-200-E-cadherin pathway (Iliopoulos et al., 2009). Interestingly, a recent study showed that expression of miR-200 unexpectedly enhanced macroscopic metastases in mouse breast cancer cell lines (Dykxhoorn et al., 2009). Their results suggest that, for some tumors, tumor colonization at metastatic sites might be enhanced by mesenchymal-to-epithelial transition (MET). MET is a reversible biological process that involves the transition from motile, multipolar or spindle-shaped mesenchymal cells to planar arrays of polarized cells called epithelia. Thus the epithelial nature of a tumor would be difficult to predict metastatic outcome. Taken together, these studies suggest that miRNAs of the miR-200 family play important roles in regulating tumor progression and metastasis.

let-7 family

let-7 is poorly expressed or deleted in many human cancers. Recent data from both hematologic malignancies and solid tumors suggest that each includes minor populations of cells that are capable of tumor initiation (Clarke & Fuller, 2006). A recent study compared miRNA expression in self-renewing and differentiated cells from breast cancer lines and found that the expression of let-7 was strongly reduced in breast tumor initiating cells (BT-

ICs) and increased with differentiation (Yu et al., 2007). Introducing let-7 in BT-ICs reduced their proliferative capacity, their ability to form mammospheres and tumor formation and metastasis *in vivo*. Conversely, knocking down let-7 enhanced self-renewal of non-T-ICs *in vitro*. Known oncogenic targets of let-7, such as *H-RAS* and *HMGA2*, were downregulated by let-7 overexpression. Silencing *H-RAS* in a BT-IC-enriched cell line reduced self-renewal but had no effect on differentiation, while knocking down *HMGA2* enhanced differentiation but did not affect self-renewal. Their results suggest that let-7 regulates multiple BT-IC stem cell-like properties and that let-7 may offer a unique opportunity to attack tumor stem cells using therapeutic RNA. Delivery of the *let-7* miRNA to tumors could potentially deplete stem cells by inducing cellular differentiation.

miR-34a

miR-34a is one of several miRNAs that are downregulated in multiple cancers (Gaur et al., 2007) and has been shown to be transcriptionally regulated by p53. In the context of breast cancer, only one study (Kato et al., 2009) has shown that miR-34a levels were lower in triple negative and mesenchymal breast cancer cell lines compared with normal epithelial lines and HER-2+ lines. Increasing the levels of miR-34a protected the MDA-MB-231 cells from radiation-induced cell death, and downregulating it had the converse effect. These results show that miR-34a is necessary for the survival of MDA-MB-231 cells from non-apoptotic cell death and suggest that miR-34a may have therapeutic potential in breast cancers, since antagonizing miR-34a increases the sensitivity of breast cancer cells towards radiation.

miR-31

miR-31 was recently shown to prevent metastasis at multiple steps by inhibiting the expression of prometastatic genes (Valastyan et al., 2009). miR-31 is expressed in normal breast cells and its abundance was shown to be dependent on the metastatic state of the tumor. It is moderately decreased in non-metastatic breast cancer cell lines and is almost undetectable in metastatic mouse and human breast cancer cell lines. Importantly, the authors demonstrated that introducing miR-31 in metastatic breast cancer cells suppressed metastasis-related functions (motility, invasion and resistance to anoikis) *in vitro* and metastasis *in vivo*. Injecting miR-31 overexpressing cells directly into the circulation impeded the ability of the cells to survive and form secondary tumors in the lung, suggesting that miR-31 inhibits metastasis at multiple steps of the metastatic cascade. Conversely, inhibition of miR-31 function increased invasiveness and promoted metastasis *in vivo*. The targets have been identified for this miRNA is frizzled3 (*Fzd3*), integrin α-5 (*ITGA5*), myosin phosphatase-Rho-interacting protein (*M-RIP*), matrix metallopeptidase 16 (*MMP16*), radixin (*RDX*) and the ras homolog gene family member A (*RhoA*). Taken together, their findings demonstrate that miR-31 may also be an attractive therapeutic target for breast cancer as it exerts its antimetastatic effect by targeting multiple prometastatic genes of the metastasis cascade.

3. Nanoparticles in breast cancer translational research

Nanoparticles (NP) have been widely utilized in biomedical applications; such as drug delivery, transfection agents, molecular imaging, and as bioprobes. The size and surface area of NP provide unique features to modify various functions using organic/inorganic compounds. Thus NPs provide an excellent template for multimodality agents such as imaging, tracking, and sensitive detection of biomarkers specific to disease (Medarova et al.,

2007; Phillips et al., 2008; Sonnichsen et al., 2005; Yang et al., 2007). Several classes of NPs have been developed and utilized for various applications. For example, oligonucleotide-functionalized nanoparticles have been introduced as an effective bioassay tool, referred to as a bio-barcode assay, which allows for sensing small biomolecules such as β- amyloid related to Alzheimer's disease and small DNA fragments associated with various diseases such as human immunodeficiency virus (HIV) (Keating, 2005; Stoeva et al., 2006). Furthermore, NPs linked to antibodies have demonstrated selective binding of rare stem cells, immune cells and cancer cells presenting specific receptors on the cell surface (Pissuwan et al., 2007). Several study reports have been showed that antibodies linked to NP can detect or target cells with high specificity (Yang et al., 2007). In our recent study, we have used gold nanoparticles (AuNP) of a small size (10 nm) coated with streptavidin (SA) for conjugation of molecules to create a nanoimmunogene conjugate (Yoon et al., 2010). This conjugates includes an apoptosis-inducing miRNA (miRNA-491), breast cancer targeting MAb, and quantum dots to target breast cancer selectively and to induce apoptosis (Natarajan et al., 2009). This novel approach of making multifunctional nanoparticles, combining NP, miRNA and antibody, will target cell surface receptors, and subsequently nanoparticles will enhance the transfection of apoptosis-inducing miRNA into the cell to enhance the apoptosis **(Figure 2)**.

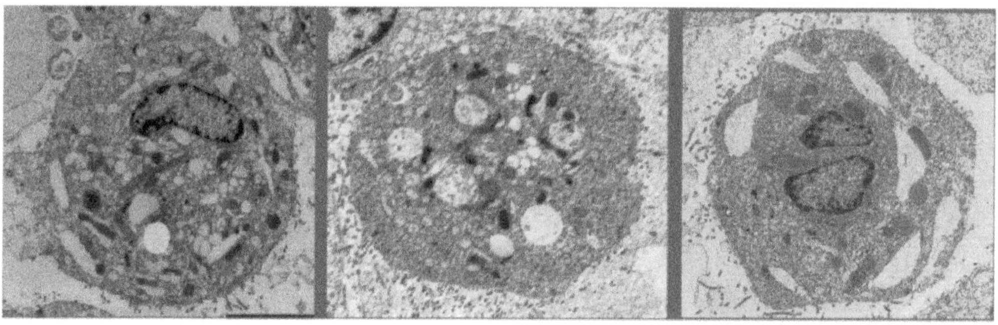

Fig. 2. Images left to right shows evidence of apoptosis in HBT3477 human breast cancer cells treated with miR-491-AuNP 10nm for 24h. The apoptotic effect was analyzed by Transmission Electron microscopy to confirm the morphological changes at a cellular level. Morphological changes show irregular nuclear contours, smudged chromatin (left panel), and focal breakdown of the nuclear membrane (center panel) as well as; marginated and clumped chromatin at the periphery (right panel).

3.1 Targeted nanoparticles

Nanomaterials or nanoparticles (NPs) are currently, synthesized by various polymers and lipids; iron, gold and silica particles. These particles are typically < 200 nm size used for drug delivery vehicles that can carry multiple drugs and/or imaging agents. Due to high surface-area-to-volume ratio, it is possible to achieve high ligand density on the surface for targeting purposes. Further, NPs can also be used to increase local drug concentration by carrying the drug within and control-releasing it when bound to the targets.

Targeted nanoparticles (NPs) conjugates are created by linking to targeting agents such as proteins (mainly antibodies and their fragments), nucleic acids (aptamers), or other receptor ligands (peptides, vitamins, and carbohydrates). These NPs that are chemically conjugated with drugs are often considered new chemical entities owing to a distinct pharmacokinetic profile from that of the parent drug.

In spite of variety of novel drug targets and sophisticated chemistries available, only four drugs (doxorubicin, camptothecin, paclitaxel, and platinate) and few polymers (N-(2-hydroxylpropyl)methacrylamide (HPMA) copolymer, poly-*L*-glutamic acid, poly(ethylene glycol) (PEG), and Dextran) have been reported quite often used to develop NP–drug conjugates(Duncan, 2006).

Many polymer based NP–drug conjugates have entered Phase I and II clinical trials and these are especially useful for targeting blood vessels in tumors. Examples include anti-endothelial immunoconjugates, fusion proteins (Arap et al., 1998; Halin et al., 2002; Schraa et al., 2002), and caplostatin, the first polymer-angiogenesis inhibitor conjugates (Satchi-Fainaro et al., 2004).

3.2 miRNA-NPs

The key to success of RNA-based therapeutics is to have effective strategies for the delivery of siRNA or miRNA in vivo (Hammond, 2006). For example, modification of antisense RNA with a cholesteryl functionality results in enhanced stability in the serum, improved cellular uptake and inhibition of target mRNA (Krutzfeldt et al., 2005). If the delivery of miRNAs through nanoparticles is proven to be an effective breast cancer therapeutic, this could revolutionize breast cancer treatment. In contrast to chemotherapy, targeted miRNA-nanoplatform is only the tumor would be targeted for treatment, preventing serious side-effects. Thus delivering siRNA and / or miRNA with nanoparticles simultaneously targeting several different oncogenic pathways is definitely an important advantage of the current approach.

Chen et al first developed an approach for co-delivery of siRNA and miRNA using liposome-polycation-hyaluronic acid particles with tumor targeting single-chain antibody fragment to target murine B16F10 melanoma (Chen et al., 2010). Targeted nanoparticles with miR-34a induced apoptosis inhibited survivin expression, in the metastatic tumor and reduced tumor load in the lung. This study clearly demonstrated this novel therapeutics enhanced the antitumor effect. Similarly in another study by Anand et al demonstrated mir-132 linked nanoparticles were able target $\alpha_v\beta_3$ integrins to manuplate miRNA levels in the endothelium to control pathological neovascularization (Anand et al., 2010).

Natarajan et al delivered miR491 to induce apoptosis in human breast cancer cells (HT3477) using quantum dots, gold nanoparticles, and HBT3477 targeting Mab. The transmission electron microscopy (Fig 2) clearly showed the apoptotic effect on cells due to delivery of Au-NP-miR491, compared to control cells which were not delivered miR-491.

3.3 SiRNA-NPs

Gene silencing using short interfering RNA (siRNA) is an attractive approach to probe gene function, and to silence cancer genes in mammalian cells. Recently some success in the delivery of siRNA using various methods; here we mainly discuss their delivery through non viral vectors using nanoparticles for breast cancer imaging and therapy. Kumar et al synthesized (Kumar et al., 2010) a tumor-targeting nanodrug of Iron oxide nanoparticles linked to peptide and small interfering RNA (siRNA), (MN-EPPT-siBIRC5) to specifically shuttle siRNA to human breast tumors. The nanodrug binds the tumor-specific antigen uMUC-1, which is found in >90% of human breast adenocarcinomas. MN-EPPT-siBIRC5 consists of superparamagnetic iron oxide nanoparticles [for magnetic resonance imaging (MRI)], the dye Cy 5.5 (for near-IR optical imaging), peptides (EPPT) that specifically target uMUC-1, and a synthetic siRNA that target the tumor-specific anti apoptotic gene BIRC5. Nanodrug uptake by human breast adeno carcinoma cells resulted in a significant down regulation of BIRC5. Following i.v. delivery into subcutaneous mouse models of breast cancer, the nanodrug showed a preferential tumor uptake, which could be visualized by MRI and near-IR optical imaging. Intravenous injection of the agent once a week over 2 weeks resulted in the induction of considerable levels of necrosis and apoptosis in the tumors, translating into a significant decrease in tumor growth rate. This strategy permits the simultaneous tumor-specific delivery of siRNA to tumors and the imaging of the delivery process.

Bouclier et al studied suppression (Bouclier et al., 2010) of oestrogen receptor alpha (ERalpha) functions by silencing RNAs in association with or not with anti-oestrogens (AEs) both in vitro and in breast cancer cell xenografts was assessed. In vitro, a prolonged decrease in ERalpha protein expression and an enhanced AE-induced inhibition of ERalpha-mediated transcription, together with antiproliferative activity, were observed. Incorporation of ERalpha-siRNAs in PEGylated nanocapsules (NC) was achieved; and their intravenous injections in MCF-7 xenografts, in contrast to scramble siRNA containing NCs, lead to decrease in ERalpha protein content and Ki67 labeling in tumour cells. In this study, co-injection of the two nanocarriers potentiated the decrease in ERalpha protein, concomitantly with decreasing tumour vasculature and glucose transporter-1. These data support that the targeted delivery of ERalpha-siRNA in breast tumors potentiates the inhibition of E(2)-induced proliferative activity by encapsulated AE through enhanced anti-vascular activity. The study findings suggest that the anti-oestrogen activity of RU as well as that of targeted ERalpha-siRNA leads to anti-angiogenic activity. Their delivery in "stealth" nanocarriers may constitute a new anti-cancer therapeutic strategy in solid tumors. For example to create "stealth" (sneaky) characteristics for nanoparticles the surface of the particles were coated with polyethylene glycol (PEG), a procedure called PEGylation to protect nanocarriers from the reticulo-endothelial system.

Tan et al (Tan et al., 2007) synthesized chitosan NPs with encapsulated quantum dots (QDs) to deliver HER2/neu siRNA. These constructs were tested for the delivery and track the siRNA by monitoring the presence of fluorescent QDs in the chitosan NPs. Chitosan is a linear polysaccharide compound composed of randomly distributed β-(1-4)-linked D-glucosamine (deacetylated unit) and N-acetyl-D-glucosamine (acetylated unit). It is a fiber isolated from shellfish. It has a unique property that allows it to bind with fat. Targeted delivery of HER2 siRNA to HER2-overexpressing SKBR3 breast cancer cells was shown to be specific with chitosan /QD NP surface labeled with HER2 antibody targeting the HER2 receptors on SKBR3 cells. In this study gene-silencing effects of the conjugated siRNA was established using the luciferase and HER2 ELISA assays. These self-tracking siRNA delivery NPs could be useful in the monitoring of future gene silencing studies both in vitro and in vivo.

3.4 Immunoconjugate linked NPs

DeNardo et al studied (DeNardo et al., 2005) radioisotope conjugated-chimeric L6 mAb-linked iron oxide nanoparticles (bioprobes) studied in athymic mice bearing human breast cancer HBT 3477 xenografts. These NP based bioprobes were given to i.v., escapes into the extravascular space and bind to cancer cell membrane antigen, later these bioprobes can be used in concert with externally applied alternating magnetic field (AMF) to deliver thermoablative cancer therapy. The pharmacokinetics, tumor uptake, and the therapeutic effect of inductively heating by bioprobes indicated these probes were capable of killing breast cancer cells selectively.

In another study Gao et al developed (Gao et al., 2009) PE38KDEL-loaded poly(lactic-co-glycolic acid) (PLGA) nanoparticles conjugated to Fab' fragments of a humanized anti-HER2 monoclonal antibody (rhuMAbHER2). The PE38KDEL-loaded nanoparticles-anti-HER2 Fab' bioconjugates (PE-NP-HER) were constructed modularly with Fab' fragments of rhuMAbHER2 covalently linked to PLGA nanoparticles containing PE38KDEL. Compared with nontargeted nanoparticles that lack anti-HER2 Fab', PE-NP-HER specifically bound to and were sequentially internalized into HER2 overexpressing breast cancer cells, which resulted in significant cytotoxicity in vitro.

Recently Chattopadhyay et al reported (Chattopadhyay et al., 2010) an immunoconjugate linked 30nm AuNPs for HER-2 targeting NPs. This nanotechnology-based radiosensitizer was tested on SK-BR-3 breast cancer cells *in vitro*. This newly designed trastuzumab-AuNPs described in this study could be useful to for breast cancer treatment.

4. Nanoparticles in clinical studies for breast cancer therapy

Ranson et al, published the treatment outcome of Caelyx (Doxil; Sequus Pharmaceuticals Inc, Menlo Park, CA), the PEGylated liposomal doxorubicin NP in advanced breast cancer (Ranson et al., 1997). In advanced breast cancer, standard therapy regimens yield infrequent complete responses, and continued therapy has been associated with an improved quality of life (Coates et al., 1987) and favorable time to progression (Muss et al., 1991) over intermittent therapy or observation, respectively. This study reported median survival of 7 months and the 9-month time to progression in the responding patients and it proposed if the majority of patients that completed six cycles had received additional Caelyx, the survival and time to progression might have been extended further.

Metastatic breast cancer is still incurable. Taxanes represent an important class of antitumor agents, which have proven to be fundamental in the treatment of advanced and early-stage breast cancer, but the clinical advances of taxanes have been limited by their highly hydrophobic molecular status. To overcome this poor water solubility, lipid-based solvents have been used as a vehicle, and new systemic formulations have been developed, mostly for paclitaxel, which are Cremophor-free and increase the circulation time of the drug. ABI-007 is a novel, albumin-bound, 130-nm particle formulation of paclitaxel, free from any kind of solvent. It has been demonstrated to be superior to an equitoxic dose of standard paclitaxel with a significantly lower incidence of toxicities in a large, international, randomized phase III trial. The availability of new drugs, such as Abraxane, in association with other traditional and non-traditional drugs (new antineoplastic agents and targeted molecules), will give the oncologist many different effective treatment options for patients in this setting (Miele et al., 2009).

In another study metastatic breast cancer (MBC) phase II study evaluated the efficacy and safety of weekly administration of nanoparticles with albumin-bound paclitaxel as a first-line treatment (Mirtsching et al.). The overall response rate (ORR) was 42.2% (95% CI, 30%-55%); 5 patients had a complete response (CR) and 22 patients had a partial response (PR). Additionally, 17 patients experienced stable disease (SD), providing an overall benefit (CR +

PR + SD) of 68.8%. These findings demonstrated that weekly NP- paclitaxel had a favorable safety profile and is well tolerated as a first-line treatment for MBC. An ORR of 42% and an overall benefit of 69% is extremely encouraging, particularly in the HER2-positive population where 52% of patients responded. Clinically approved NP-conjugates for breast cancer are listed in Table 1.

NP type /material (Brand Name)	Drug entrapped or linked	Current stage of development	References
PEG-liposomes (Doxil/Caelyx)	Doxorubicin	Phase I/II	(Coates et al., 1987; Ranson et al., 1997)
Albumin (Abraxane)	Paclitaxel	Phase II/III	(Lobo et al., 2007; Miele et al., 2009; Moreno-Aspitia & Perez, 2005)

Table 1. Nanoparticles and their current stage of development for use in breast cancer therapy

5. Summary

In conclusion, we envision that breast cancer targeting agents such as miRNAs, siRNAs, and immunoconjugates are already demonstrated that these agents could be potential molecules for molecular cancer therapy. Only few siRNAs are in clinical trials because of their off-target effects, and the efforts being made to develop miRNAs as either diagnostic or therapeutic markers, since these they are one of the natural mechanisms to control the gene expression. For example Rosetta Genomics, Israel-based microRNA Genomics Company is already actively planning for Investigational New drug (IND) study using miRNA for infectious disease and hepatocellular carcinoma the fifth most common cancer in the world. Similarly, the first in-human phase I clinical trial involving the systemic administration of siRNA to patients with solid cancers using a targeted, nanoparticle delivery system. Davis et al., (California Institute of Technology, Pasadena, California 91125, USA) study indicated the evidence of inducing an RNAi mechanism of action in a human from the delivered siRNA. Tumour biopsies from melanoma patients obtained after treatment show the presence of intracellularly localized nanoparticles in amounts that correlate with dose levels of the nanoparticles administered.

Several reports have shown that use of nanoparticles and nanotechnologies have been giving very encouraging results. One of the efficient ways to deliver these therapeutic molecules is through the use of nanoparticles. These novel technologies will help in achieving accurate early detection, prognosis, imaging and targeted therapy for breast cancer.

In spite of many positive reports on this area, very few nanoparticles linked with targeting agents are showed desired properties for clinical studies. Further studies are needed in translational research to incorporate these molecules into nanoparticles for the cancer treatment options. Therefore active research on nanotechnology warrants as answer for a number of questions prior to translational research: example specificity, toxicity, well defined characterization, stringent quality and in vivo clearance profile. Although active researches are ongoing in this area still we need to go a long way to achieve curable treatment outcome using these agents and technology.

6. References

Adams, B. D., et al. (2007). The micro-ribonucleic acid (miRNA) miR-206 targets the human estrogen receptor-alpha (ERalpha) and represses ERalpha messenger RNA and protein expression in breast cancer cell lines. *Mol Endocrinol, 21*(5), 1132-1147.

Adelaide, J., et al. (2007). Integrated profiling of basal and luminal breast cancers. *Cancer Res, 67*, 11565 - 11575.

Ambros, V. (2004). The functions of animal microRNAs. *Nature, 431*(7006), 350-355.

Anand, S., et al. (2010). MicroRNA-132-mediated loss of p120RasGAP activates the endothelium to facilitate pathological angiogenesis. *Nat Med, 16*(8), 909-914.

Andrews, J., et al. (2010). Multi-platform whole-genome microarray analyses refine the epigenetic signature of breast cancer metastasis with gene expression and copy number. *PLoS One, 5*, e8665.

Arap, W., et al. (1998). Cancer treatment by targeted drug delivery to tumor vasculature in a mouse model. *Science, 279*(5349), 377-380.

Bauer, J., et al. (2010). RNA interference (RNAi) screening approach identifies agents that enhance paclitaxel activity in breast cancer cells. *Breast Cancer Research, 12*(3), R41.

Bergamaschi, A., et al. (2006). Distinct patterns of DNA copy number alteration are associated with different clinicopathological features and gene-expression subtypes of breast cancer. *Genes Chromosomes Cancer, 45*, 1033 - 1040.

Borchert, G. M., et al. (2006). RNA polymerase III transcribes human microRNAs. *Nat Struct Mol Biol, 13*(12), 1097-1101.

Bouclier, C., et al. (2010). Coadministration of nanosystems of short silencing RNAs targeting oestrogen receptor alpha and anti-oestrogen synergistically induces tumour growth inhibition in human breast cancer xenografts. *Breast Cancer Res Treat, 122*(1), 145-158.

Boyd, Z., et al. (2008). Proteomic analysis of breast cancer molecular subtypes and biomarkers of response to targeted kinase inhibitors using reverse-phase protein microarrays. *Mol Cancer Ther, 7*, 3695 - 3706.

Calin, G. A., et al. (2002). Frequent deletions and down-regulation of micro- RNA genes miR15 and miR16 at 13q14 in chronic lymphocytic leukemia. *Proc Natl Acad Sci U S A, 99*(24), 15524-15529.

Carthew, R. W. (2006). Gene regulation by microRNAs. *Curr Opin Genet Dev, 16*(2), 203-208.

Chan, J. A., et al. (2005). MicroRNA-21 is an antiapoptotic factor in human glioblastoma cells. *Cancer Res, 65*(14), 6029-6033.

Chattopadhyay, N., et al. (2010). Design and characterization of HER-2-targeted gold nanoparticles for enhanced X-radiation treatment of locally advanced breast cancer. *Mol Pharm, 7*(6), 2194-2206.

Chen, Y., et al. (2010). Nanoparticles Modified With Tumor-targeting scFv Deliver siRNA and miRNA for Cancer Therapy. *Mol Ther, 18*(9), 1650-1656.

Chin, K., et al. (2006). Genomic and transcriptional aberrations linked to breast cancer pathophysiologies. *Cancer Cell, 10*, 529 - 541.

Cimmino, A., et al. (2005). miR-15 and miR-16 induce apoptosis by targeting BCL2. *Proc Natl Acad Sci U S A, 102*(39), 13944-13949.

Clarke, M. F.. & Fuller, M. (2006). Stem cells and cancer: two faces of eve. *Cell, 124*(6), 1111-1115.

Coates, A., et al. (1987). Improving the quality of life during chemotherapy for advanced breast cancer. A comparison of intermittent and continuous treatment strategies. *N Engl J Med, 317*(24), 1490-1495.

DeNardo, S. J., et al. (2005). Development of tumor targeting bioprobes ((111)In-chimeric L6 monoclonal antibody nanoparticles) for alternating magnetic field cancer therapy. *Clin Cancer Res, 11*(19 Pt 2), 7087s-7092s.

Dresios, J., et al. (2005). Cold stress-induced protein Rbm3 binds 60S ribosomal subunits, alters microRNA levels, and enhances global protein synthesis. *Proc Natl Acad Sci U S A, 102*(6), 1865-1870.

Duncan, R. (2006). Polymer conjugates as anticancer nanomedicines. *Nat Rev Cancer, 6*(9), 688-701.

Dykxhoorn, D. M., et al. (2009). miR-200 enhances mouse breast cancer cell colonization to form distant metastases. *PLoS One, 4*(9), e7181.

Eiriksdottir, G., et al. (1998). Mapping loss of heterozygosity at chromosome 13q: loss at 13q12-q13 is associated with breast tumour progression and poor prognosis. *Eur J Cancer, 34*(13), 2076-2081.

Esau, C., et al. (2004). MicroRNA-143 regulates adipocyte differentiation. *J Biol Chem, 279*(50), 52361-52365.

Foekens, J. A., et al. (2008). Four miRNAs associated with aggressiveness of lymph node-negative, estrogen receptor-positive human breast cancer. *Proc Natl Acad Sci U S A, 105*(35), 13021-13026.

Frankel, L. B., et al. (2008). Programmed cell death 4 (PDCD4) is an important functional target of the microRNA miR-21 in breast cancer cells. *J Biol Chem, 283*(2), 1026-1033.

Gao, J., et al. (2009). PE38KDEL-loaded anti-HER2 nanoparticles inhibit breast tumor progression with reduced toxicity and immunogenicity. *Breast Cancer Res Treat, 115*(1), 29-41.

Garzon, R., et al. (2006). MicroRNA fingerprints during human megakaryocytopoiesis. *Proc Natl Acad Sci U S A, 103*(13), 5078-5083.

Gaur, A., et al. (2007). Characterization of microRNA expression levels and their biological correlates in human cancer cell lines. *Cancer Res, 67*(6), 2456-2468.

Gregory, R. I., et al. (2004). The Microprocessor complex mediates the genesis of microRNAs. *Nature, 432*(7014), 235-240.

Halin, C., et al. (2002). Enhancement of the antitumor activity of interleukin-12 by targeted delivery to neovasculature. *Nat Biotechnol, 20*(3), 264-269.

Hammond, S. M. (2006). MicroRNA therapeutics: a new niche for antisense nucleic acids. *Trends Mol Med, 12*(3), 99-101.

Han, J., et al. (2004). The Drosha-DGCR8 complex in primary microRNA processing. *Genes Dev, 18*(24), 3016-3027.

Han, W., et al. (2008). DNA copy number alterations and expression of relevant genes in triple-negative breast cancer. *Genes Chromosomes Cancer, 47*, 490 - 499.

Hennessy, B., et al. (2009). Characterization of a naturally occurring breast cancer subset enriched in epithelial-to-mesenchymal transition and stem cell characteristics. *Cancer Res, 69*, 4116 - 4124.

Hossain, A., et al. (2006). Mir-17-5p regulates breast cancer cell proliferation by inhibiting translation of AIB1 mRNA. *Mol Cell Biol, 26*(21), 8191-8201.

https://www.cia.gov/library/publications/the-world-factbook/.

Huang, Q., et al. (2008). The microRNAs miR-373 and miR-520c promote tumour invasion and metastasis. *Nat Cell Biol, 10*(2), 202-210.

Hurteau, G. J., et al. (2009). Stable expression of miR-200c alone is sufficient to regulate TCF8 (ZEB1) and restore E-cadherin expression. *Cell Cycle, 8*(13), 2064-2069.

Hutvagner, G.. & Zamore, P. D. (2002). A microRNA in a multiple-turnover RNAi enzyme complex. *Science, 297*(5589), 2056-2060.

Iliopoulos, D., et al. (2009). MicroRNAs differentially regulated by Akt isoforms control EMT and stem cell renewal in cancer cells. *Sci Signal, 2*(92), ra62.

Iorio, M., et al. (2005a). MicroRNA gene expression deregulation in human breast cancer. *Cancer Res, 65*, 7065 - 7070.

Iorio, M. V., et al. (2005b). MicroRNA gene expression deregulation in human breast cancer. *Cancer Res, 65*(16), 7065-7070.

Jopling, C. L., et al. (2005). Modulation of hepatitis C virus RNA abundance by a liver-specific MicroRNA. *Science, 309*(5740), 1577-1581.

Kato, M., et al. (2009). The mir-34 microRNA is required for the DNA damage response in vivo in C. elegans and in vitro in human breast cancer cells. *Oncogene, 28*(25), 2419-2424.

Keating, C. D. (2005). Nanoscience enables ultrasensitive detection of Alzheimer's biomarker. *Proc Natl Acad Sci U S A, 102*(7), 2263-2264.

Kondo, N., et al. (2008). miR-206 Expression is down-regulated in estrogen receptor alpha-positive human breast cancer. *Cancer Res, 68*(13), 5004-5008.

Kong, W., et al. (2008). MicroRNA-155 is regulated by the transforming growth factor beta/Smad pathway and contributes to epithelial cell plasticity by targeting RhoA. *Mol Cell Biol, 28*(22), 6773-6784.

Korpal, M., et al. (2008). The miR-200 family inhibits epithelial-mesenchymal transition and cancer cell migration by direct targeting of E-cadherin transcriptional repressors ZEB1 and ZEB2. *J Biol Chem, 283*(22), 14910-14914.

Krutzfeldt, J., et al. (2005). Silencing of microRNAs in vivo with 'antagomirs'. *Nature, 438*(7068), 685-689.

Kumar, M., et al. (2010). Image-guided breast tumor therapy using a small interfering RNA nanodrug. *Cancer Res, 70*(19), 7553-7561.

Kumar, M. S., et al. (2007). Impaired microRNA processing enhances cellular transformation and tumorigenesis. *Nat Genet, 39*(5), 673-677.

Leary, R., et al. (2008). Integrated analysis of homozygous deletions, focal amplifications, and sequence alterations in breast and colorectal cancers. *Proc Natl Acad Sci USA, 105*, 16224 - 16229.

Lee, Y., et al. (2003). The nuclear RNase III Drosha initiates microRNA processing. *Nature, 425*(6956), 415-419.

Lee, Y., et al. (2002). MicroRNA maturation: stepwise processing and subcellular localization. *EMBO J, 21*(17), 4663-4670.

Lee, Y., et al. (2004). MicroRNA genes are transcribed by RNA polymerase II. *EMBO J, 23*(20), 4051-4060.

Leivonen, S. K., et al. (2009). Protein lysate microarray analysis to identify microRNAs regulating estrogen receptor signaling in breast cancer cell lines. *Oncogene, 28*(44), 3926-3936.

Lobo, C., et al. (2007). Paclitaxel albumin-bound particles (abraxane) in combination with bevacizumab with or without gemcitabine: early experience at the University of Miami/Braman Family Breast Cancer Institute. *Biomed Pharmacother, 61*(9), 531-533.

Lu, J., et al. (2005). MicroRNA expression profiles classify human cancers. *Nature, 435*(7043), 834-838.

Lund, E., et al. (2004). Nuclear export of microRNA precursors. *Science, 303*(5654), 95-98.

Ma, L., et al. (2007). Tumour invasion and metastasis initiated by microRNA-10b in breast cancer. *Nature, 449*(7163), 682-688.

Mattie, M., et al. (2006a). Optimized high-throughput microRNA expression profiling provides novel biomarker assessment of clinical prostate and breast cancer biopsies. *Mol Cancer, 5*, 24.

Mattie, M. D., et al. (2006b). Optimized high-throughput microRNA expression profiling provides novel biomarker assessment of clinical prostate and breast cancer biopsies. *Mol Cancer, 5*, 24.

Medarova, Z., et al. (2007). In vivo imaging of siRNA delivery and silencing in tumors. *Nat Med, 13*(3), 372-377.

Mertens-Talcott, S. U., et al. (2007). The oncogenic microRNA-27a targets genes that regulate specificity protein transcription factors and the G2-M checkpoint in MDA-MB-231 breast cancer cells. *Cancer Res, 67*(22), 11001-11011.

Miele, E., et al. (2009). Albumin-bound formulation of paclitaxel (Abraxane ABI-007) in the treatment of breast cancer. *Int J Nanomedicine, 4*, 99-105.

Mirtsching, B., et al. (2010). A Phase II Study of Weekly Nanoparticle Albumin-Bound Paclitaxel With or Without Trastuzumab in Metastatic Breast Cancer. *Clin Breast Cancer*, 1-8.

Moreno-Aspitia, A.. & Perez, E. A. (2005). North Central Cancer Treatment Group N0531: Phase II Trial of weekly albumin-bound paclitaxel (ABI-007; Abraxane) in combination with gemcitabine in patients with metastatic breast cancer. *Clin Breast Cancer, 6*(4), 361-364.

Muss, H. B., et al. (1991). Interrupted versus continuous chemotherapy in patients with metastatic breast cancer. The Piedmont Oncology Association. *N Engl J Med, 325*(19), 1342-1348.

Natarajan, A., et al. (2009). Breast Cancer Targeting Novel microRNA-Nanoparticles for Imaging. *Proc SPIE, 7171*(N), N1-N11.

Neve, R., et al. (2006). A collection of breast cancer cell lines for the study of functionally distinct cancer subtypes. *Cancer Cell, 10*, 515 - 527.

Nikolsky, Y., et al. (2008). Genome-wide functional synergy between amplified and mutated genes in human breast cancer. *Cancer Res, 68*, 9532 - 9540.

Ocana, A., et al. (2006). Concomitant versus sequential chemotherapy in the treatment of early-stage and metastatic breast cancer. *Clinical Breast Cancer, 6*(6), 495-504.

Ocana, A.. & Pandiella, A. (2008). Identifying breast cancer druggable oncogenic alterations: Lessons learned and future targeted options. *Clinical Cancer Research, 14*(4), 961-970.

Perou, C. M., et al. (2000). Molecular portraits of human breast tumours. *Nature, 406*(6797), 747-752.

Phillips, R. L., et al. (2008). Rapid and efficient identification of bacteria using gold-nanoparticle-poly(para-phenyleneethynylene) constructs. *Angew Chem Int Ed Engl, 47*(14), 2590-2594.

Pissuwan, D., et al. (2007). A golden bullet? Selective targeting of Toxoplasma gondii tachyzoites using antibody-functionalized gold nanorods. *Nano Lett, 7*(12), 3808-3812.

Poy, M. N., et al. (2004). A pancreatic islet-specific microRNA regulates insulin secretion. *Nature, 432*(7014), 226-230.

Qi, L., et al. (2009). Expression of miR-21 and its targets (PTEN, PDCD4, TM1) in flat epithelial atypia of the breast in relation to ductal carcinoma in situ and invasive carcinoma. *BMC Cancer, 9*, 163.

Ranson, M. R., et al. (1997). Treatment of advanced breast cancer with sterically stabilized liposomal doxorubicin: results of a multicenter phase II trial. *J Clin Oncol, 15*(10), 3185-3191.

Rathjen, T., et al. (2006). Analysis of short RNAs in the malaria parasite and its red blood cell host. *FEBS Lett, 580*(22), 5185-5188.

Ruike, Y., et al. (2010). Genome-wide analysis of aberrant methylation in human breast cancer cells using methyl-DNA immunoprecipitation combined with high-throughput sequencing. *BMC Genomics, 11*, 137.

Satchi-Fainaro, R., et al. (2004). Targeting angiogenesis with a conjugate of HPMA copolymer and TNP-470. *Nat Med, 10*(3), 255-261.

Schraa, A. J., et al. (2002). Targeting of RGD-modified proteins to tumor vasculature: a pharmacokinetic and cellular distribution study. *Int J Cancer, 102*(5), 469-475.

Scott, G. K., et al. (2007). Coordinate suppression of ERBB2 and ERBB3 by enforced expression of micro-RNA miR-125a or miR-125b. *J Biol Chem, 282*(2), 1479-1486.

Scott, G. K., et al. (2006). Rapid alteration of microRNA levels by histone deacetylase inhibition. *Cancer Res, 66*(3), 1277-1281.

Shah, S., et al. (2009). Mutational evolution in a lobular breast tumour profiled at single nucleotide resolution. *Nature, 461*, 809 - 813.

Si, M. L., et al. (2007). miR-21-mediated tumor growth. *Oncogene, 26*(19), 2799-2803.

Sjoblom, T., et al. (2006). The consensus coding sequences of human breast and colorectal cancers. *Science, 314*, 268 - 274.

Sonnichsen, C., et al. (2005). A molecular ruler based on plasmon coupling of single gold and silver nanoparticles. *Nat Biotechnol, 23*(6), 741-745.

Sorlie, T., et al. (2001). Gene expression patterns of breast carcinomas distinguish tumor subclasses with clinical implications. *Proc Natl Acad Sci U S A, 98*(19), 10869-10874.

Sorlie, T., et al. (2006). Distinct molecular mechanisms underlying clinically relevant subtypes of breast cancer: gene expression analyses across three different platforms. *BMC Genomics, 7*, 127.

Stephens, P., et al. (2009). Complex landscapes of somatic rearrangement in human breast cancer genomes. *Nature, 462*, 1005 - 1010.

Stoeva, S. I., et al. (2006). Multiplexed DNA detection with biobarcoded nanoparticle probes. *Angew Chem Int Ed Engl, 45*(20), 3303-3306.

Tan, W. B., et al. (2007). Quantum-dot based nanoparticles for targeted silencing of HER2/neu gene via RNA interference. *Biomaterials, 28*(8), 1565-1571.

Tavazoie, S. F., et al. (2008). Endogenous human microRNAs that suppress breast cancer metastasis. *Nature, 451*(7175), 147-152.

Valastyan, S., et al. (2009). A pleiotropically acting microRNA, miR-31, inhibits breast cancer metastasis. *Cell, 137*(6), 1032-1046.

Venugopal, S. K., et al. (2009). Liver fibrosis causes down-regulation of miRNA-150 and miRNA-194 in hepatic stellate cells and their over-expression causes decreased stellate cell activation. *Am J Physiol Gastrointest Liver Physiol.*

Volinia, S., et al. (2006). A microRNA expression signature of human solid tumors defines cancer gene targets. *Proc Natl Acad Sci U S A, 103*(7), 2257-2261.

Wood, L., et al. (2007). The genomic landscapes of human breast and colorectal cancers. *Science, 318*, 1108 - 1113.

Xu, P., et al. (2004). MicroRNAs and the regulation of cell death. *Trends Genet, 20*(12), 617-624.

Yang, J., et al. (2007). Multifunctional magneto-polymeric nanohybrids for targeted detection and synergistic therapeutic effects on breast cancer. *Angew Chem Int Ed Engl, 46*(46), 8836-8839.

Yehiely, F., et al. (2006). Deconstructing the molecular portrait of basal-like breast cancer. *Trends Mol Med, 12*(11), 537-544.

Yoon, S., et al. (2010). Acute liver injury upregulates microRNA-491-5p in mice, and its overexpression sensitizes Hep G2 cells for tumour necrosis factor-alpha-induced apoptosis. *Liver Int, 30*(3), 376-387.

Yu, F., et al. (2007). let-7 regulates self renewal and tumorigenicity of breast cancer cells. *Cell, 131*(6), 1109-1123.

Yu, Z., et al. (2010). microRNA, cell cycle, and human breast cancer. *Am J Pathol, 176*(3), 1058-1064.

Yu, Z., et al. (2008). A cyclin D1/microRNA 17/20 regulatory feedback loop in control of breast cancer cell proliferation. *J Cell Biol, 182*(3), 509-517.

Zhang, L., et al. (2006). microRNAs exhibit high frequency genomic alterations in human cancer. *Proc Natl Acad Sci U S A, 103*(24), 9136-9141.

Zhu, S., et al. (2007). MicroRNA-21 targets the tumor suppressor gene tropomyosin 1 (TPM1). *J Biol Chem, 282*(19), 14328-14336.

19

Preclinical and Clinical Developments in Molecular Targeting Therapeutic Strategies for Breast Cancer

Teruhiko Fujii[1,2,3], Hiroki Takahashi[1,2], Yuka Inoue[1], Masayoshi Kage[3,4], Hideaki Yamana[5] and Kazuo Shirouzu[2]

[1]*Breast Care Center, Clinical Research Institute, National Hospital Organization Kyushu Medical Cancer,*
[2]*Department of Surgery, Kurume University, Japan*
[3]*Center for Innovative Cancer Therapy, Kurume University,*
[4]*Department of Pathology, Kurume University,*
[5]*Multidisciplinary Treatment Center, Kurume University, Japan*

1. Introduction

The development of effective chemotherapy has greatly improved survival among patients with breast cancer, although molecular cancer therapeutics is also emerging as an important approach. Molecular-targeting therapy using agents such as trastuzumab has enhanced breast cancer treatment, while clinical trials have suggested that epidermal growth factor receptor (EGFR), vascular endothelial growth factor (VEGF), and mammalian target of rapamycin (mTOR) are potential targets. Our current efforts to identify molecular targets that might be useful for treatment are focused on two molecules: the putative metastasis-suppressor gene Cap43/NDRG1/Drg-1 (Cap43) protein and the Y-box binding protein-1 (YB-1). Here we describe the latest preclinical and clinical developments in molecular-targeting therapeutic strategies for breast cancer, including those using Cap43 and YB-1.

2. Current study of molecular-targeting agents

2.1 EGFR family signaling

The EGFR family of receptor tyrosine kinases is an attractive target for anticancer strategies. Members include EGFR, which is also known as human epidermal growth factor receptor 1 (HER1), HER2 (erbB2), HER3 (erbB3), and HER4 (erbB4). Through their interconnected cellular signaling network, EGFR family members regulate diverse biological processes including cell proliferation, differentiation, and survival. They also play key roles in the development and progression of breast cancer. High levels of EGFR and HER2 expression have been reported in 15–30% of breast cancers, and are correlated with poor prognosis (Schlotter et al., 2008; Witton et al., 2003). HER3 expression, observed in 18% of tumors, is correlated with reduced overall survival (OS) and it may provide a rout for resistance to agents targeting EGFE or HER2 (Koutras et al., 2010; Witton et al., 2003). By contrast, HER4 expression, observed in 12% of tumors, is associated with differentiation and growth inhibition, thus it is more consistently related with favorable prognosis in breast cancer (Koutras et al., 2010; Witton et al., 2003). EGFRs have an extracellular domain involved in ligand binding, a helical transmembrane segment, and an intracellular protein kinase domain. Upon ligand binding, the extracellular domain undergoes conformational changes that allow EGFR family members to form homodimers or heterodimers. Particularly, the combination of HER2 and HER3 receptors may be critical in breast cancer growth and progression. Ligand binding induces dimerization of the receptor and activation of the kinase through autophosphorylation, stimulating phosphoinositide 3-kinase (PI3K)/Akt and mitogen-activated protein kinase (MAPK) signaling. This is followed by proliferation, migration, adhesion, and angiogenesis (Atalay et al., 2003; Lin & Winer, 2004; Rosen et al., 2010; Russo & Ove, 2003; Schlotter, 2008).

2.2 EGFR family-targeted therapies

2.2.1 Trastuzumab

Targeting signaling has led to the development of therapies that reduce the activation of HER2 in breast cancer. Trastuzumab is a humanized monoclonal antibody that targets the extracellular domain of the transmembrane tyrosine kinase HER2, and is a key drug in the treatment strategy for HER2-positive breast cancer. National Comprehensive Cancer Network (NCCN) guidelines recommend both trastuzumab monotherapy and combined trastuzumab and chemotherapy as first-line treatments for metastatic breast cancer (MBC) (NCCN 2011), and these have both shown efficacy in HER2-positive MBC patients (Slamon et al., 2001; Vogel et al., 2002). Data from the National Surgical Adjuvant Breast and Bowel Project (NSABP) B-31 + North Central Cancer Treatment Group (NCCTG) N9831 trial, the HERceptin Adjuvant (HERA) trial, the Breast Cancer International Research Group (BCIRG) 006 trial, and the Finland Herceptin (FinHer) trial (Joensuu et al., 2006; Perez et al., 2007; Slamon et al., 2006; Smith et al., 2007) have suggested that adjuvant trastuzumab treatment improves both disease-free survival (DFS) and OS among early breast cancer patients. NCCN guidelines and the St Gallen consensus guidelines therefore recommend that adjuvant trastuzumab treatment should be used for node-positive and node-negative, high-risk early HER2-positive breast cancer patients (NCCN 2011; Goldhirsch et al., 2009). The efficacy of adjuvant trastuzumab therapy for HER2-positive breast cancer patients with a tumor size of less than 1 cm is unclear. Gonzalez-Angulo et al. reported that such patients who were HER2-positive had higher risks of recurrence and distant recurrence than those who were HER2-negative. These results suggest that patients with HER2-positive T1abN0M0 tumors have a significant risk of relapse and should be considered for trastuzumab adjuvant therapy (Gonzalez-Angulo et al., 2009). A retrospective analysis of the effect of adjuvant trastuzumab in patients with small, node-negative, HER2-positive breast cancer was reported at the 2010 American Society of Clinical Oncology (ASCO) meeting. This concluded that even small breast cancers probably derive significant benefit from adjuvant trastuzumab therapy (McArthur et al., 2010). The NeOAdjuvant Herceptin (NOAH) trial (Gianni et al., 2010a) was a randomized study that evaluated the addition of trastuzumab to anthracycline- and taxane-based chemotherapy for patients with HER2-positive locally advanced breast cancer in a neoadjuvant setting. Trastuzumab was well tolerated, and significantly improved the 3-year event-free survival (EFS) of patients with HER2-positive breast cancer (71% with trastuzumab vs 56% without trastuzumab, p=0.013). The addition of trastuzumab to neoadjuvant chemotherapy should therefore be considered for women with HER2-positive, locally advanced or inflammatory breast cancer in order to improve the EFS, survival, and clinical and pathological tumor responses.

2.2.2 Trastuzumab-DM1 (T-DM1)

T-DM1 is an antibody–drug conjugate that uses trastuzumab to deliver the maytansinoid antimicrotubule agent DM1 specifically to HER2-positive cells. T-DM1 was previously shown to be well tolerated with no dose-limiting cardiotoxicity, with an objective response rate by independent assessment of 25.9%, and a median progression-free survival (PFS) time of 4.6 months (Burris et al., 2011). These results suggest that T-DM1 monotherapy is useful in patients with heavily pretreated, HER2-positive MBC.

2.2.3 Pertuzumab

HER2-containing heterodimers elicit greater mitogenic responses than HER2 homodimers. The ligand-induced activation of either HER1 or HER3, and the subsequent formation of heterodimers with HER2, might therefore play an important role in resistance to conventional HER2 inhibitors. Pertuzumab is a humanized monoclonal antibody and a member of a new class of inhibitors, including EGFR family members such as HER3, that block HER2 dimerization, thereby inhibiting the downstream signaling processes associated with tumor growth and progression (Adams et al., 2006; Franklin et al., 2004). Clinical studies have indicated that pertuzumab monotherapy shows limited efficacy for HER2-positive or HER2-negative advanced breast cancer (Cortes et al., 2009; Gianni et al., 2010b). Trastuzumab and pertuzumab bind to distinct epitopes on the HER2 extracellular domain, and it has been hypothesized that a combination of the two agents might inhibit tumor growth more effectively than either agent alone (Franklin et al., 2004; Hubbard, 2005). Indeed, *in vivo* data showed that the combination had a strongly enhanced antitumor effect and induced tumor regression in breast cancer xenograft models, which was not achieved by either agent alone (Scheuer et al., 2009). In view of this synergistic effect, a phase II trial of pertuzumab and trastuzumab combination therapy in patients with HER2-positive MBC was performed. The objective response rate (ORR) was 24.2% and the clinical benefit rate (CBR) 50%. The combination was active and well tolerated in patients who had experienced progression during previous trastuzumab therapy (Baselga et al., 2010a). A phase Ib/II trial of T-DM1 with pertuzumab combination therapy for locally advanced or MBC was also reported, and nine partial responses (PRs) were observed among 23 patients (Miller et al., 2010). Due to the safety, tolerability, and efficacy of full-dose T-DM1 plus pertuzumab, this approach is a promising new treatment strategy for MBC. In addition, the ongoing, randomized, phase II Pertuzumab HERceptin Evaluation with XelodA (PHEREXA) study will evaluate the efficacy and safety of a combination of trastuzumab and capecitabine with or without pertuzumab in patients with HER2-positive MBC (ClinicalTrials.gov 1). Pertuzumab and trastuzumab combination therapy was also investigated in The Neoadjuvant Study of Pertuzumab and Herceptin in an Early Regimen Evaluation (NeoSphere) trial, which was a phase II clinical study of preoperative systemic therapy that ranked the antitumor activity and tolerability of the following combinations: trastuzumab+docetaxel, docetaxel+trastuzumab+pertuzumab, trastuzumab+pertuzumab, and docetaxel+pertuzumab. The clinical CR+PR rates were 80%, 88%, 68%, and 71%, respectively, while pathologic complete response (pCR) rates were 29%, 45.8%, 17.8%, and 24%, respectively (Gianni et al., 2010c). These data showed superior antitumor activity in the docetaxel+trastuzumab+pertuzumab group. Notably, the trastuzumab+pertuzumab group also showed excellent tolerability and effective antitumor activity, which is expected to lead to the establishment of molecular-targeting therapy that does not involve toxic chemotherapy.

2.3 Tyrosine kinase inhibitors

2.3.1 Lapatinib

Lapatinib is an oral small-molecule tyrosine kinase inhibitor that reversibly inhibits both EGFR and HER2 (Lackey, 2006). Binding of EGFR ligands to EGFR stimulates heterodimerization with HER2 and activation of downstream signaling pathways including PI3K, Akt protein kinase, and mTOR, resulting in an increase in cell proliferation. Phosphatase and tensin homolog (PTEN) has tumor-suppressor activity in this signaling pathway, and loss of PTEN, as well as up-regulation of insulin-like growth factor 1 receptor (IGF-1R) signaling, is associated with trastuzumab resistance. Lapatinib blocks the activation of the HER2 signaling pathway by inhibiting the intracellular tyrosine kinase of EGFR and HER2, and Lapatinib is believed to circumvent the trastuzumab resistance associated with the up-regulation of IGF-1R signaling. Lapatinib also binds to the p95 truncated variant of HER2 (p95 HER2) and inhibits cell proliferation in trastuzumab-resistant cells expressing p95 HER2. This suggests that lapatinib is a potential therapeutic for breast cancer patients who are resistant to trastuzumab (Vogel et al., 2010). In a phase II clinical trial (EGF20009), lapatinib monotherapy demonstrated clinical activity and was well tolerated as a first-line therapy in HER2-amplified locally advanced or MBC (Gomez et al., 2008). In a randomized phase III study, patients with HER2-positive MBC that had progressed after treatment with anthracycline, taxane, and trastuzumab were given combination therapy with lapatinib and capecitabine. The performance of this was superior to capecitabine alone, with no increase in serious toxic effects (Geyer et al., 2006). A phase III randomized study comparing lapatinib alone with lapatinib plus paclitaxel as first-line treatment for MBC also found that the combination therapy significantly improved clinical outcomes in HER2-positive patients (Di Leo et al., 2008). Preclinical studies have shown that lapatinib is active not only as a monotherapy but also in combination with trastuzumab (Konecny et al., 2006; Xia et al., 2002; Xia et al., 2005). A randomized phase III study (EGF104900) compared the activity of lapatinib alone and in combination with trastuzumab in patients with HER2-positive, trastuzumab-refractory MBC. The combination treatment performance was superior to lapatinib alone in terms of both the PFS and the CBR (Blackwell et al., 2010). This was also supported by the Neoadjuvant Lapatinib and/or Trastuzumab Treatment Optimization (NeoALTTO) phase III randomized neoadjuvant study which compared lapatinib and trastuzumab both alone and in combination with paclitaxel for the treatment of HER2-positive primary breast cancer. pCR rates for the three arms were 24.7% for lapatinib alone, 29.5% for trastuzumab alone, and 51.3% for the combination (Baselga et al., 2010b). These results suggested that combination therapy with lapatinib and trastuzumab is useful for both metastatic and primary breast cancers. Brain metastases are common among HER2-positive MCB patients, and usually imply poor prognosis and short survival. Because lapatinib is a small-molecule tyrosine kinase inhibitor, it might be able to cross the blood–brain barrier to provide effect therapeutic concentrations in cerebrospinal fluid. In mice with established brain metastases, treatment with lapatinib significantly suppressed the growth of brain metastases (Gril et al., 2008). In clinical trials, lapatinib monotherapy showed modest antitumor activity against brain metastases, and additional responses were observed for a combination of lapatinib and capecitabine (Lin et al., 2009; Metro et al., 2010; Ro et al., 2010). These data suggest that lapatinib is an effective therapeutic for brain metastases from breast cancer.

2.3.2 Erlotinib

Erlotinib is a highly potent reversible inhibitor of HER1/EGFR tyrosine kinase. It is activated by the extracellular binding of EGF, and is potentiated by the dimerization of activated receptors. Erlotinib has been shown to inhibit tumor cell growth in several human cancers (Moyer et al., 1997; Pollack et al., 1999). In clinical trials, erlotinib showed antitumor effects in patients with NSCLC, squamous cell carcinoma of the head and neck, and hepatocellular carcinoma (Pérez-Soler et al., 2004; Soulieres et al., 2004; Thomas et al., 2007); however, erlotinib monotherapy had minimal activity in patients with breast cancer (Dickler et al., 2009). In HER2-positive breast cancer models, the concurrent inhibition of HER2 and EGFR led to improved anticancer activity compared with the inhibition of HER2 alone. In breast cancer cell lines, trastuzumab and erlotinib demonstrated synergistic activity over a range of clinically relevant concentrations (Finn et al., 2003) and, in xenograft models, anti-EGFR plus VEGF therapy showed increased activity compared with either agent alone (Jung et al., 2002). These results provided a rationale for combining trastuzumab or bevacizumab with erlotinib in clinical studies. The combination of erlotinib and trastuzumab has been found to be well tolerated, with four PRs achieved in 12 patients, and a time to progression (TTP) of 9.03 months (Britten et al., 2009). The combination of erlotinib and bevacizumab was examined in 38 patients with MBC, one of whom achieved a PR, 15 had stable disease at first evaluation (at 9 weeks), and four of these had stable disease (SD) beyond 26 weeks. Although this combination therapy was well tolerated, it showed limited activity in unselected patients with previously treated MBC (Dickler et al., 2008). Current clinical trials are investigating the use of combination therapy with erlotinib and oral mTOR protein kinase inhibitor (Everolimus) (ClinicalTrials.gov 2), hormone therapy (fulvestrant) (ClinicalTrials.gov 3), and chemotherapy (docetaxel) (ClinicalTrials.gov 4) for breast cancer.

2.3.3 Gefitinib

Gefitinib is a small-molecule anticancer agent. This selective EGFR tyrosine kinase inhibitor blocks the signal-transduction pathway implicated in the proliferation and survival of cancer cells (Albanell et al., 2002; Woodburn, 1999). Preclinical studies clearly established that gefitinib potently inhibits growth in various human cancer cells (Ciardiello et al., 2000; Sirotnak et al., 2000; Wakeling et al., 2002), and similar growth-inhibitory effects of gefitinib have been reported in breast cancer models (Campiglio et al., 2004; Lu et al., 2003; Moulder et al., 2001). A significant antitumor effect was observed in the Iressa Dose Evaluation in Advanced Lung Cancer (IDEAL) clinical trial, and gefitinib is now approved in several countries for the treatment of advanced NSCLC (Bell et al., 2005; Fukuoka, 2003). However, clinical trials showed that gefitinib monotherapy did not appear to be efficacious in the treatment of advanced MBC patients (von Minckwitz et al 2005). A phase II clinical trial found that gefitinib in combination with docetaxel was an active regimen for patients with MBC (Dennison et al., 2007). Phase II clinical trials of gefitinib in combination with either the non-steroidal aromatase inhibitor anastrozole or tamoxifen showed improved PFS (Cristofanilli et al., 2010; Osborne et al., 2011). Although combined treatment with drugs that target EGFR (gefitinib) and HER2 (trastuzumab) resulted in efficient inhibition of tumor growth in breast cancer cells that co-expressed both receptors (Normanno et al., 2002), a phase I/II study showed that gefitinib in combination with trastuzumab was unlikely to result in clinical benefit compared with trastuzumab alone (Arteaga et al., 2008). Further investigation is warranted to clarify the effect of gefitinib in breast cancer patients.

2.4 mTOR inhibitors

PTEN exhibits tumor suppressor activity in the PI3K/Akt/mTOR signaling pathway, and its loss is associated with trastuzumab resistance. Everolimus (RAD001) is a rapamycin ester analog that inhibits mTOR, and in combination with trastuzumab, it has been reported to inhibit breast cancer growth in vitro and in vivo (Lu et al., 2007). These results strongly suggested promising results of the concomitant use of trastuzumab with mTOR inhibitor for treating cases of trastuzumab resistance by PTEN loss. A randomized phase II study evaluated patients with MBC and reported that their response rate with daily everolimus monotherapy was 12% (Ellard et al., 2009). Everolimus has also been studied in combination with chemotherapy. Combination therapy of everolimus with paclitaxel and trastuzumab in patients with HER2-overexpressing MBC pretreated with trastuzumab has been reported. The ORR of this therapy was 44% and it was generally well tolerated. When combined with vinorelbine and trastuzumab, everolimus exhibited an ORR of 19.1%, with a disease control rate of 83.0% and a median PFS of 30.7 weeks (Jerusalem et al., 2011). These clinical data suggested that everolimus combined with chemotherapy and trastuzumab is generally well tolerated and exhibits promising antitumor activity in heavily pretreated patients with HER2-overexpressing MBC that progressed on trastuzumab therapy. A summary of EGFR family signaling and target therapies for breast cancer is presented in Fig. 1.

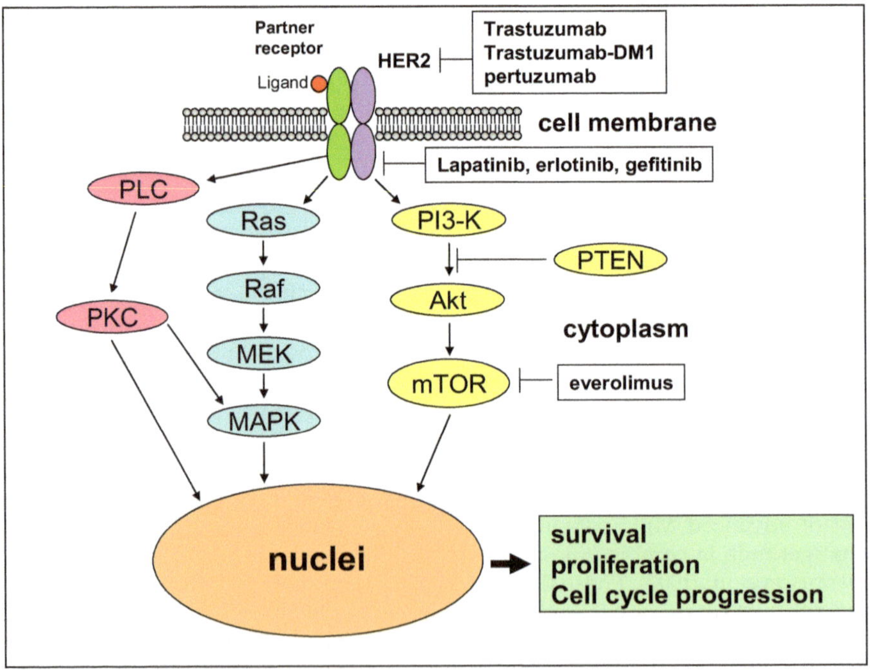

Fig. 1. EGFR family signaling and target therapies for breast cancer

2.5 Angiogenesis pathway

Angiogenesis is essential for tumor growth or metastasis. The primary factor controlling vessel formation is hypoxia, which triggers the secretion of pro-angiogenic factors, particularly VEGF, and stimulates new vessel formation to supply oxygen to the tumor. VEGF therefore plays a key role in tumor angiogenesis (Ferrara et al., 2003; Jain, 2003; Yancopoulos et al., 2000). It is a 34–46 KDa homodimeric glycoprotein that acts as a ligand for Flt-1 (VEGF receptor-1 or VEGFR-1) and KDR or Flt-2 (VEGFR-2). Under hypoxic conditions, the transcription factors hypoxia-inducible factor-1 alpha (HIF-1 alpha) and HIF-2 alpha are stabilized in cancer cells, then transported to the nucleus where they interact with HIF-beta. This complex binds to a specific sequence on the *VEGF* gene called the hypoxia response element (HRE), which stimulates *VEGF* gene transcription; VEGF protein is produced and then secreted from cancer cells (Fox et al., 2007; Shibuya, 2001). VEGF binds to VEGFR-2, which is expressed on the endothelial cell membrane, and homodimerization of the latter occurs. The effects of VEGF are mediated by the activation of various intracellular signaling transduction pathways, such as receptor tyrosine kinase activity or autophosphorylation of VEGFR-2, and the receptor mediates the biological action via the phospholipase C (PLC)–protein kinase C (PKC)–MAPK pathway. In other words, PLC directly binds to the autophosphorylated VEGFR-2, is tyrosine-phosphorylated then activated; this stimulates the activation of PKC and the Raf-1–MAPK cascade (Shibuya, 2001; Takahashi et al., 1999). Several preclinical studies showed that a VEGF-specific monoclonal antibody suppressed neovascularization and inhibited tumor growth arising from human cancer cell lines injected into nude mice (Fox et al., 2002; Kim et al., 1993). These results strongly suggest that VEGF inhibition blocks angiogenesis and tumor growth. The mechanism of the antitumor effect achieved through targeting VEGF might involve the stimulation of apoptosis of the tumor vasculature, the inhibition of metastasis, or the initiation of antitumor immune responses. VEGF inhibition might prevent its protective effect against apoptosis in tumor blood vessel-associated endothelial cells, leading to disruption of the tumor blood supply. In view of this antitumor activity, drugs targeting the VEGF system are currently in development. Mechanism of VEGF signaling is illustrated in figure 2.

2.5.1 Bevacizumab

The most promising approaches are offered by monoclonal antibodies directed against VEGF. Among the drugs in this class, bevacizumab, which consists of 93% human and 7% murine components, is currently at the most advanced stage of development. Bevacizumab is highly specific to VEGF-A and prevents angiogenesis by inhibiting the VEGF ligand thereby inhibiting VEGF signaling. Bevacizumab potently reduced the growth rate of several malignant tumors using xenograft models (Lee et al., 2008; Segerström et al., 2006) but, in a phase I/II trial, the clinical effects of bevacizumab monotherapy for breast cancer were unclear (Cobleigh et al., 2003); these might, however, be enhanced by using a combination of conventional chemotherapy and bevacizumab. The randomized phase III Eastern Cooperative Oncology Group 2100 (ECOG-E2100) trial compared paclitaxel with or without bevacizumab as first-line therapy for HER2-negative MBC; the addition of bevacizumab significantly increased the ORR (36.9% vs 21.2%; $p<0.001$) and the PFS (11.8 vs 5.9 months; $p<0.001$), but not the OS (26.7 vs 25.2 months; $p=0.16$) (Miller et al., 2007). Nevertheless, first-line anti-angiogenic therapy using bevacizumab clearly improved the response for earlier stage MBC. The Avastin and Docetaxel (AVADO) trial compared

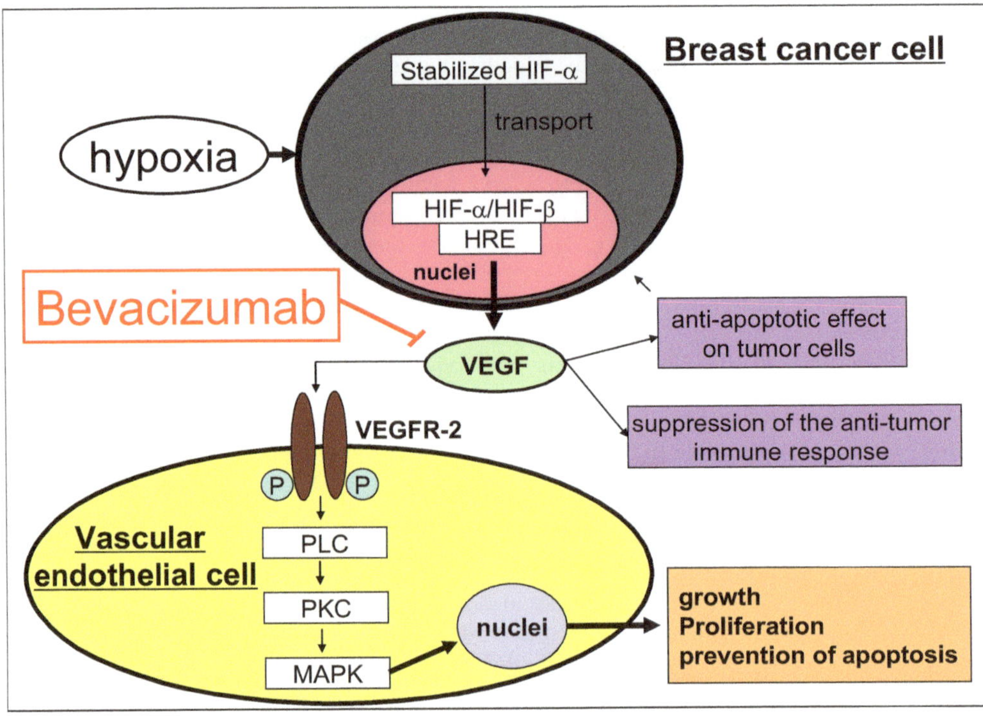

Fig. 2. Mechanisum of VEGF signaling

docetaxel with or without bevacizumab (at 7.5 mg/kg or 15 mg/kg) as first-line therapy for HER2-negative MBC (Miles et al., 2009). The combination therapy significantly increased the PFS (8.2 months for docetaxel plus placebo, 9.0 months for docetaxel plus bevacizumab at 7.5 mg/kg, and 10.1 months for docetaxel plus bevacizumab at 15 mg/kg), overall RR (46%, 55%, and 64%, respectively) and 1-year survival rates (76%, 81%, and 84%, respectively). As described above, a stronger antitumor effect is expected when prescribing bevacizumab to patients at an earlier stage of MBC. Several first or second-line clinical trials using bevacizumab are currently ongoing. The Regimens in Bevacizumab for Breast Oncology (RiBBON 1) trial is a phase III study that aims to establish standard first-line chemotherapy regimens and is comparing paclitaxel with or without bevacizumab for 722 HER2-negative MBC patients, while the RiBBON 2 trial is investigating second-line therapy. In addition, chemotherapy (an anthracycline-based regimen, taxane, or capecitabine) plus bevacizumab is being compared with chemotherapy plus placebo; the estimated enrollment for this study is 1,200 patients, and the primary endpoint is PFS (O'Shaughnessy & Brufsky, 2008). A first-line clinical trial using bevacizumab for triple-negative breast cancer is also ongoing. Triple-negative breast cancer does not react to hormone therapy or trastuzumab, so the prognosis is poor (Sørlie et al., 2001). Chemotherapy is the only suitable current treatment, but a combination of chemotherapy and bevacizumab is expected to be effective. Phase II trials of bevacizumab in combination with other regimens are currently underway for triple-negative MBC, these include an association with doxorubicin and carboplatin, an estimated enrollment of 50 patients and PFS as the primary endpoint (ClinicalTrials.gov 5), and an association with paclitaxel and carboplatin, an estimated enrollment of 46, and overall RR as the primary endpoint (ClinicalTrials.gov 6). If a stronger antitumor effect is shown by these clinical trials, it will suggest that bevacizumab is a good treatment strategy for triple-negative breast cancer. A first-line clinical trial of bevacizumab combined with other molecular targeting therapy is also ongoing. HER2 plays a specific role in the regulation of VEGF expression. A preclinical study showed a strong association between HER2 and VEGF (Klos et al., 2006; Konecny et al., 2004), while animal models showed superior efficacy when bevacizumab was combined with trastuzumab (Scheuer et al., 2006). Based on these results, a phase II trial of combined therapy targeting HER2-amplified MBC or local relapse, and surgically-unresectable breast cancer, was carried out using trastuzumab and bevacizumab as first-line treatment. A clinical response was documented in 13 of 28 patients (46%), all of whom showed a PR (Pegram 2006). These data support the clinical use of combination therapy with bevacizumab and trastuzumab, and suggest that it is an effective first-line therapy for HER2-overexpressing MBC.

The novel targeted agents that are currently being clinically evaluated for use in breast cancer are expected to show promising results. We are also continuing to investigate other molecules that might be useful for treatment of breast cancer. Our goal is to establish the potential of such agents to be translated into novel and useful approaches to breast cancer therapy, and to move promising lead compounds rapidly from the bench to the bedside. The preclinical molecular-targeting strategies that we are using against breast cancer focus on Cap43 and YB-1, as discussed below.

3. Cap43

Cap43 is a 43-kD protein identical to N-myc downstream-regulated gene 1 (NDRG1) and differentiation-related gene-1 (Drg-1). Cap43 expression is markedly influenced by several stimuli, including oxidative stress, metal ions, hypoxia, phorbol esters, vitamins A and D, and steroids, the oncogenes N-myc and C-myc, and the tumor-suppressor genes p53 and Von Hippel-Lindau (VHL). Although many studies have elucidated the characteristics of Cap43, its exact function remains unclear. Cap43 is expressed in various organs, including the prostate, ovary, colon, and kidney, and its expression changes dynamically during postnatal development in the kidney, brain, liver, and nerves (Lachat et al., 2002; Okuda et al., 1999; Shimono et al., 1999; Wakisaka et al., 2003). These observations suggested that Cap43 may be involved in normal organ maturation and differentiation. Cap43 expression has been reported to be higher than that in normal tissue in many types of human tumors, including colon, breast, prostate, kidney, liver, and brain cancers (Cangul et al., 2002). On the other hand, Cap43 expression is upregulated in normal cells and highly differentiated cancer cells, but downregulated in poorly differentiated cancer cells present in colon and prostate tumors (Bandyopadhyay et al., 2003; Guan et al., 2000). Although the exact function of Cap43 in malignant cells also remains unknown, a variety of studies has recently reported. In prostate cancer, Cap43 could be a novel marker for malignant progression and poor prognosis and is closely associated with the downregulation of E-cadherin expression (Song et al., 2010). In gastric cancer, Cap43 plays a significant role in carcinogenesis and in preventing metastasis and invasion (Jiang et al., 2010; Liu et al., 2010). Further, Cap43 enhanced portal vein invasion and intrahepatic metastasis in human hepatocellular carcinoma and the Cap 43 expression was thought to accelerate tumor invasion and metastasis (Akiba et al., 2008). In breast cancer, overexpression of the Cap43 gene inhibited cell growth and metastasis, and low Cap43 expression in breast cancer cells is closely correlated with poor clinical outcomes (Bandyopadhyay et al., 2004). These results indicate that one of the roles of Cap43 is suppression of metastasis; further, the Cap43 expression levels could serve as a good predictor of survival in breast cancer. Furthermore, Fotovati et al. (2011) reported that the endogenous Cap43 expression level was closely correlated with the differentiation status of breast cancer cell lines and that Cap43 overexpression expanded the differentiated areas in the xenograft model of breast cancer. Immunohistochemical analysis of human breast cancer specimens showed a close relationship between Cap43 and beta-casein or milk fat protein, which is a differentiation marker of breast tissue. Therefore, Cap43 is closely associated with the differentiation and/or malignant states of breast cancers. As reported in previous studies, the Cap43 gene could play a key role in breast cancer. Therefore, in order to assess the potential of Cap43 as a molecular target for the effects of anti-estrogenic agents in breast cancer, we investigated Cap43 gene expression during therapeutic treatment with anti-estrogenic drugs. Of the 8 breast cancer cell lines we examined, 4 expressed high levels of Cap43 and very low levels of estrogen receptor alpha□(ER alpha) and the remaining 4 expressed low levels of Cap43 and high ER alpha levels. Estradiol (E_2) treatment reduced Cap43 expression in a dose-dependent fashion in ER alpha-positive cell lines, but did not affect the expression in ER alpha-negative lines. Administration of the 2 anti-estrogenic agents tamoxifen and ICI 182780 inhibited the E_2-induced downregulation of Cap43. Overexpression of ER alpha in the ER alpha-negative cell lines SKBR-3 and MDA-MB-231 resulted in the downregulation of Cap43. Immunostaining revealed that Cap43 expression was inversely correlated with the expression of ER alpha. The E_2-induced downregulation of Cap43 appears to be mediated through ER alpha-dependent pathways in breast cancer cells, both in culture and in patients (Fotovati et al., 2006). Since Cap43 expression was very sensitive to E_2 and/or anti-estrogens in ER alpha-positive breast cancer cells, it is a potential molecular marker for determining the therapeutic efficacy of anti-estrogenic agents in breast cancer. In breast cancer therapy, when ER alpha(+) Cap43(-) patients are treated with tamoxifen, resulting in upregulation of Cap43, tamoxifen appears to be effective and the treatment should be continued. However, if Cap43 is not upregulated following tamoxifen administration in ER alpha(+) Cap43(-) patients, tamoxifen can be deemed ineffective, and the treatment should be changed. The postoperative blood Cap43 level can be easily measured; however, Cap43 is not a secreted protein. This poses clinical problems; to overcome these, we are currently exploring proteins that might be associated with Cap43. If the protein associated with Cap43 is identified, the Cap43 levels can be indirectly obtained by measuring the levels of this protein. Further studies are required in order to use Cap43 in clinical trials.

4. YB-1

YB-1 belongs to the cold shock domain protein family, members of which are found in both the cytoplasm and nucleus of human cells. It has pleiotropic functions in the regulation of gene transcription and translation, DNA repair, drug resistance, and cellular responses to environmental stimuli (Izumi et al., 2001; Kohno et al., 2003; Kuwano et al., 2003). YB-1 is normally present in the cytoplasm, although it is translocated to the nucleus when cells are exposed to anticancer drugs or ultraviolet (UV) light (Koike et al., 1997; Uchiumi et al., 1993). Nuclear localization of YB-1 is required for its transcriptional control of multidrug resistance (MDR)-related genes and for the control of repair of DNA damage caused by anticancer agents or radiation in cancer cells, resulting in the acquisition of global drug resistance to a wide range of anticancer agents (Kohno et al., 2003; Kuwano et al., 2004). Nuclear translocation of YB-1 is controlled by PKC and related proteins, protein tyrosine phosphatase, JAK1, and Akt (Basaki et al., 2007; Dooley et al., 2006; Koike et al., 1997; Sorokin et al., 2005; Stenina et al., 2000; Sutherland et al., 2005). Immunohistochemical labeling experiments have revealed that nuclear YB-1 expression was correlated with the expression of a representative MDR-related ATP-binding cassette superfamily protein, P-glycoprotein, which is encoded by the MDR1/ABCB1 gene; moreover, other drug resistance-related molecules have been reported in tumor specimens from a variety of cancers other than breast cancer (Bargou et al., 1997; Giménez-Bonafé et al., 2004; Janz et al., 2002; Kamura et al., 1999; Oda et al., 1998; Saji et al., 2003). In contrast, nuclear expression of YB-1 is often associated with a poor prognosis in various human malignancies, including breast cancer (Bargou et al., 1997; Dahl et al., 2009; Janz et al., 2002), ovarian cancer (Kamura et al., 1999), synovial sarcoma (Oda et al., 2003), and lung cancer (Shibahara et al., 2001). These findings strongly suggested that the nuclear expression of YB-1 can be used as a predictor in some human malignancies. Furthermore, the YB-1 gene was able to induce breast cancer in experimental animal models, suggesting its role as an oncogene that promotes the breast cancer progression (Bergmann et al., 2005). Additionally, YB-1 overexpression in human mammary epithelial cells can induce an EGF-independent growth phenotype through activation of the EGFR pathway (Berquin et al., 2005). Knockdown of YB-1 inhibited breast cancer cell growth and it is thought to be involved in the induction of apoptosis via the mTOR/STAT3 intracellular signaling pathway (Fujii et al. 2009, Lee et al., 2008). These studies all suggest a close linkage between YB-1 expression and the growth or proliferation potential of cancer cells via intracellular signaling, and indicate its association with poor prognosis of patients with breast cancer. Since YB-1 might play its key role not only by controlling the expression of drug resistance-related genes but also the expression of cell growth-related genes, we investigated the association of YB-1 localization to the nucleus with the expression of EGFR family proteins, hormone receptors, and other molecules whose expressions are probably associated with poor prognosis in patients with breast cancer. Knockdown of YB-1 with siRNA significantly reduced the expression levels of EGFR, HER2, and ER alpha in ER alpha-positive but not ER alpha-negative breast cancer cell lines. Nuclear YB-1 expression was positively correlated with HER2 ($P = 0.0153$) and negatively correlated with ER alpha ($P = 0.0122$) and chemokine (C-X-C motif) receptor 4 (CXCR4: which is known to play a critical role in the growth and metastasis of human breast cancers(Müller A et al., 2001, Liang, Z et al., 2004)) ($P = 0.0166$) in human breast cancer clinical specimens; however, it was not correlated with EGFR expression. Nuclear YB-1 expression was an independent prognostic factor for the overall ($P = 0.0139$) and progression-free ($P = 0.0280$) survival in these patients. These data strongly suggested that nuclear YB-1 localization could be a molecular target of intrinsic importance in not only the acquisition of multidrug resistance but also tumor growth dependent on HER2 and other growth factor receptors in breast cancer (Fujii et al., 2008). Intracellular signaling via Cap43 and YB-1 is illustrated in Fig. 3.

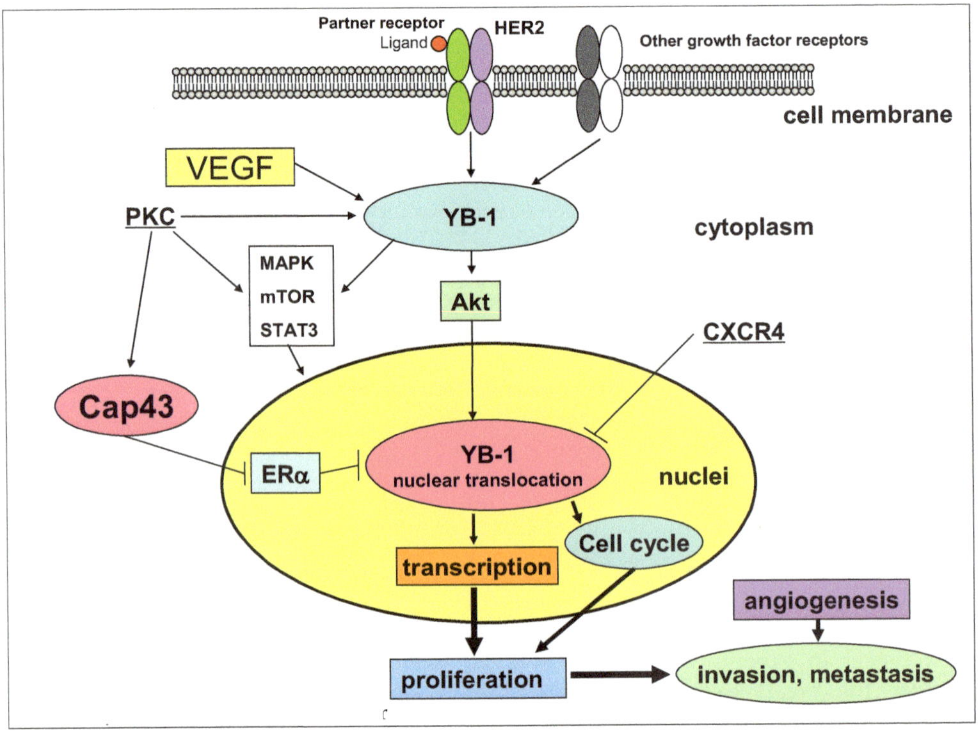

Fig. 3. Intracellular signaling via Cap43 and YB-1 in breast cancer

5. Conclusion

The development of effective adjuvant therapy, based on the post-operative administration of chemotherapy, hormone therapy, or trastuzumab, has significantly improved survival among breast cancer patients. However, therapy for adjuvant-resistant or metastatic disease is still palliative, and the possibility of inducing complete remission or a definitive cure for breast cancer remains remote. The research effort so far has identified key selective changes in molecules such as Cap43 and YB-1 that sustain breast cancer growth and progression. This provides the potential to develop specific, targeted therapies as the next generation of anticancer therapeutics.

6. References

Adams, CW., Allison, DE., Flagella, K., Presta, L., Clarke, J., Dybdal, N., McKeever, K. & Sliwkowski, MX. (2006) Humanization of a recombinant monoclonal antibody to produce a therapeutic HER dimerization inhibitor, pertuzumab. *Cancer Immunol Immunother,* Vol.55, No.6, pp. 717-727.

Akiba, J., Ogasawara, S., Kawahara, A., Nishida, N., Sanada, S., Moriya, F., Kuwano, M., Nakashima, O. & Yano H. (2008) N-myc downstream regulated gene 1

(NDRG1)/Cap43 enhances portal vein invasion and intrahepatic metastasis in human hepatocellular carcinoma. *Oncol Rep*, Vol.20, No.6, pp.1329-1335.

Albanell, J., Rojo, F., Averbuch, S., Feyereislova, A., Mascaro, JM., Herbst, R., LoRusso, P., Rischin, D., Sauleda, S., Gee, J., Nicholson, RI. & Baselga, J. (2002) Pharmacodynamic studies of the epidermal growth factor receptor inhibitor ZD1839 in skin from cancer patients: histopathologic and molecular consequences of receptor inhibition. *J Clin Oncol*, Vol.20, No.1, pp. 110-124.

Atalay, G., Cardoso, F., Awada, A. & Piccart, MJ. (2003) Novel therapeutic strategies targeting the epidermal growth factor receptor (EGFR) family and its downstream effectors in breast cancer. *Ann Oncol*, Vol.14, No.9, pp. 1346-1363.

Arteaga, CL., O'Neill, A., Moulder, SL., Pins, M., Sparano, JA., Sledge, GW. & Davidson NE. (2008) A phase I-II study of combined blockade of the ErbB receptor network with trastuzumab and gefitinib in patients with HER2 (ErbB2)-overexpressing metastatic breast cancer. *Clin Cancer Res*, Vol.14, No.19, pp. 6277-6283.

Bandyopadhyay, S., Pai, SK., Gross, SC., Hirota, S., Hosobe, S., Miura, K., Saito, K., Commes, T., Hayashi, S., Watabe, M. & Watabe, K. (2003) The Drg-1 gene suppresses tumor metastasis in prostate cancer. *Cancer Res*, Vol.63, No.8, pp.1731-1736.

Bandyopadhyay, S., Pai, SK., Hirota, S., Hosobe, S., Takano, Y., Saito, K., Piquemal, D., Commes, T., Watabe, M., Gross, SC., Wang, Y., Ran, S. & Watabe, K. (2004) Role of the putative tumor metastasis suppressor gene Drg-1 in breast cancer progression. *Oncogene*, Vol.23, No.33, pp.5675-5681.

Bargou, RC., Jürchott, K., Wagener, C., Bergmann, S., Metzner, S., Bommert, K., Mapara, M.Y., Winzer, KJ., Dietel, M., Dörken, B. & Royer, HD. (1997) Nuclear localization and increased levels of transcription factor YB-1 in primary human breast cancers are associated with intrinsic MDR1 gene expression. *Nat Med*, Vol.3, No.4, pp.447-450.

Basaki, Y., Hosoi, F., Oda, Y., Fotovati, A., Maruyama, Y., Oie, S., Ono, M., Izumi, H., Kohno. K., Sakai, K., Shimoyama, T., Nishio, K. & Kuwano, M. (2007) Akt-dependent nuclear localization of Y-box-binding protein 1 in acquisition of malignant characteristics by human ovarian cancer cells. *Oncogene*, Vol.26, No.19, pp.2736-2746.

Baselga, J., Gelmon, KA., Verma, S., Wardley, A., Conte, P., Miles, D., Bianchi, G., Cortes, J., McNally, VA., Ross, GA., Fumoleau, P. & Gianni, L. (2010a) Phase II trial of pertuzumab and trastuzumab in patients with human epidermal growth factor receptor 2-positive metastatic breast cancer that progressed during prior trastuzumab therapy. *J Clin Oncol*, Vol.28, No.7, pp. 1138-1144.

Baselga, J., Bradbury, I., Eidtmann, H., Di Cosimo, S., Aura, C., Azambuja, E., Gomez, H., Dinh, P., Fauria, K., Van Dooren, V., Paoletti, P., Goldhirsch, A., Chang, T-W., Lang, I., Untch, M., Gelber, RD. & Piccart-Gebhart M. (2010b) First results of the NeoALTTO trial (BIG 01-06/EGF 106903): A phase III, randomized, open label, neoadjuvant study of lapatinib, trastuzumab, and their combination plus paclitaxel in woman with HER2-positive primary breast cancer. *Cancer Res*, Vol.70, No.24, pp. 82s. (abstract S3-3).

Bell, DW., Lynch, TJ., Haserlat, SM., Harris, PL., Okimoto, RA., Brannigan, BW., Sgroi, DC., Muir, B., Riemenschneider, MJ., Iacona, RB., Krebs, AD., Johnson, DH., Giaccone, G., Herbst, RS., Manegold, C., Fukuoka, M., Kris, MG., Baselga, J., Ochs, JS. &

Haber, DA. (2005) Epidermal growth factor receptor mutations and gene amplification in non-small-cell lung cancer: molecular analysis of the IDEAL/INTACT gefitinib trials. *J Clin Oncol*, Vol.23, No.31, pp.8081-8092.

Bergmann, S., Royer-Pokora, B., Fietze, E., Jürchott, K., Hildebrandt, B., Trost, D., Leenders, F., Claude, J.C., Theuring, F., Bargou, R., Dietel, M. & Royer, H.D. (2005) YB-1 provokes breast cancer through the induction of chromosomal instability that emerges from mitotic failure and centrosome amplification. Cancer Res, Vol.65, No.10, pp.4078-4087.

Berquin, IM., Pang, B., Dziubinski, ML., Scott, LM., Chen. YQ., Nolan, GP. & Ethier, SP. (2005) Y-box-binding protein 1 confers EGF independence to human mammary epithelial cells. *Oncogene*, Vol.24, No.19, pp.3177-3186.

Blackwell, KL., Burstein, HJ., Storniolo, AM., Rugo, H., Sledge, G., Koehler, M., Ellis, C., Casey, M., Vukelja, S., Bischoff, J., Baselga, J. & O'Shaughnessy, J. (2010) Randomized study of Lapatinib alone or in combination with trastuzumab in women with ErbB2-positive, trastuzumab-refractory metastatic breast cancer. *J Clin Oncol*, Vol.28, No.7, pp. 1124-1130.

Britten, CD., Finn, RS., Bosserman, LD., Wong, SG., Press, MF., Malik, M., Lum, BL. & Slamon DJ. (2009) A phase I/II trial of trastuzumab plus erlotinib in metastatic HER2-positive breast cancer: a dual ErbB targeted approach. *Clin Breast Cancer*, Vol.9, No.1, 16-22.

Burris, HA 3rd., Rugo, HS., Vukelja, SJ., Vogel, CL., Borson, RA., Limentani, S., Tan-Chiu, E., Krop, IE., Michaelson, RA., Girish, S., Amler, L., Zheng, M., Chu, YW., Klencke, B. & O'Shaughnessy JA. (2011) Phase II study of the antibody drug conjugate trastuzumab-DM1 for the treatment of human epidermal growth factor receptor 2 (HER2)-positive breast cancer after prior HER2-directed therapy. *J Clin Oncol*, Vol.29, No.4, pp. 398-405.

Campiglio, M., Locatelli, A., Olgiati, C., Normanno, N., Somenzi, G., Viganò, L., Fumagalli, M., Ménard, S. & Gianni, L. J. (2004) Inhibition of proliferation and induction of apoptosis in breast cancer cells by the epidermal growth factor receptor (EGFR) tyrosine kinase inhibitor ZD1839 ('Iressa') is independent of EGFR expression level.*Cell Physiol.*, Vol.198, No.2, pp. 259-268.

Cangul, H.; Salnikow, K.; Yee, H.; Zagzag, D.; Commes, T.; Costa, M. Enhanced expression of a novel protein in human cancer cells: a potential aid to cancer diagnosis. *Cell Biol Toxicol*, Vol.18, No.2, pp.87-96.

Ciardiello, F., Caputo, R., Bianco, R., Damiano, V., Pomatico, G., De Placido, S., Bianco, A.R. & Tortora, G. (2000) Antitumor effect and potentiation of cytotoxic drugs activity in human cancer cells by ZD-1839 (Iressa), an epidermal growth factor receptor-selective tyrosine kinase inhibitor. *Clin Cancer Res*, Vol.6, No.5, 2053-2063.

ClinicalTrials.gov 1. A study of a combination of trastuzumab and capecitabine with or without pertuzumab in patients with HER2-positive metastatic breast cancer (PHEREXA). Available from http://clinicaltrials.gov/ct2/show/NCT01026142?term=pertuzumab+breast+cancer&rank=7.

ClinicalTrials.gov 2. Erlotinib and Everolimus in treating patients with metastatic breast cancer. Available from http://clinicaltrials.gov/ct2/show/NCT00574366?term=erlotinib+breast+cancer&rank=3.

ClinicalTrials.gov 3. Randomized, double blind multicenter phase II study of time to progression on fulvestrant in combination with erlotinib or placebo in hormone receptor-positive metastatic breast cancer (MBC) subjects who progressed on first line hormonal therapy. Available from http://clinicaltrials.gov/ct2/show/NCT00570258?term=erlotinib+breast+cancer&rank=18.

ClinicalTrials.gov 4. Erlotinib plus docetaxel in treating patients with stage IV or recurrent breast cancer. Available from http://clinicaltrials.gov/ct2/show/NCT00054275?term=erlotinib+breast+cancer&rank=8.

Clinicaltrials.gov 5. Phase II trial of doxil, carboplatin, bevacizumab in triple negative untreated metastatic breast cancer. Available from http://clinicaltrials.gov/ct2/show/NCT00608972?term=bevacizumab+AND+metastatic+breast+cancer&rank=1.

Clinicaltrials.gov 6. Weekly paclitaxel/carboplatin/ bevacizumab as first line therapy for triple negative breast cancer. Available from http://clinicaltrials.gov/ct2/show/NCT00691379?term=bevacizumab+AND+metastatic+breast+cancer&rank=63.

Cobleigh, MA., Langmuir, VK., Sledge, GW., Miller, KD., Haney, L., Novotny, WF., Reimann, JD. & Vassel, A. (2003) A phase I/II dose-escalation trial of bevacizumab in previously treated metastatic breast cancer. *Semin Oncol*, Vol.30, (5 Suppl 16), pp.117-124.

Cortes, J., Baselga, J., Petrella, T., Gelmon, K., Fumoleau, P., Verma, S., Pivot, X., Ross, G., Szado, T. & Gianni L. (2009) Pertuzumab monotherapy following trastuzumab-based treatment: activity and tolerability in patients with advanced HER2 positive breast cancer. J Clin Oncol, Vol. pp.46s. (abstract 1022).

Cristofanilli, M., Valero, V., Mangalik, A., Royce, M., Rabinowitz, I., Arena, FP., Kroener, JF., Curcio, E., Watkins, C., Bacus, S., Cora, EM., Anderson, E. & Magill, PJ. (2010) Phase II, randomized trial to compare anastrozole combined with gefitinib or placebo in postmenopausal women with hormone receptor-positive metastatic breast cancer. *Clin Cancer Res*, Vol.16, No.6, pp. 1904-1914.

Dahl, E., En-Nia, A., Wiesmann, F., Krings, R., Djudjaj, S., Breuer, E., Fuchs, T., Wild, PJ., Hartmann, A., Dunn, SE. & Mertens, PR. (2009) Nuclear detection of Y-box protein-1 (YB-1) closely associates with progesterone receptor negativity and is a strong adverse survival factor in human breast cancer. *BMC Cancer*, Vol.9, pp.410.

Dennison, SK., Jacobs, SA., Wilson, JW., Seeger, J., Cescon, TP., Raymond, JM., Geyer, CE., Wolmark, N. & Swain, SM. (2007) A phase II clinical trial of ZD1839 (Iressa) in combination with docetaxel as first-line treatment in patients with advanced breast cancer. *Invest New Drugs*, Vol.25, No.6, pp. 545-551.

Dickler, MN., Rugo, HS., Eberle, CA., Brogi, E., Caravelli, JF., Panageas, KS., Boyd, J., Yeh, B., Lake, DE., Dang, CT., Gilewski, TA., Bromberg, JF., Seidman, AD., D'Andrea, GM., Moasser, MM., Melisko, M., Park, JW., Dancey, J., Norton, L. & Hudis CA. (2008) A phase II trial of erlotinib in combination with bevacizumab in patients with metastatic breast cancer. *Clin Cancer Res,* Vol.14, No.23, pp. 7878-7883.

Dickler, MN., Cobleigh, MA., Miller, KD., Klein, PM. & Winer, EP. (2009) Efficacy and safety of erlotinib in patients with locally advanced or metastatic breast cancer. *Breast Cancer Res Treat,* Vol.115, No.1, 115-121.

Di Leo, A., Gomez, HL., Aziz, Z., Zvirbule, Z., Bines, J., Arbushites, MC., Guerrera, SF., Koehler, M., Oliv, C., Stein, SH., Williams, LS., Dering, J., Finn, RS. & Press MF. (2008) Phase III, double-blind, randomized study comparing lapatinib plus paclitaxel with placebo plus paclitaxel as first-line treatment for metastatic breast cancer. *J Clin Oncol,* Vol.26, No.34, pp. 5544-5552.

Dooley, S., Said, HM., Gressner, AM., Floege, J., En-Nia, A. & Mertens, PR. (2006) Y-box protein-1 is the crucial mediator of antifibrotic interferon-gamma effects. *J Biol Chem,* Vol.281, No.3, pp.1784-1795.

Ellard, SL., Clemons, M., Gelmon, KA., Norris, B., Kennecke, H., Chia, S., Pritchard, K., Eisen, A., Vandenberg, T., Taylor, M., Sauerbrei, E., Mishaeli, M., Huntsman, D., Walsh, W., Olivo, M., McIntosh, L. & Seymour L. (2009) Randomized phase II study comparing two schedules of everolimus in patients with recurrent/metastatic breast cancer: NCIC Clinical Trials Group IND.163. *J Clin Oncol,* Vol.27, No.27, pp.4536-4541.

Ferrara, N., Gerber, HP. & LeCouter, J. (2003) The biology of VEGF and its receptors. *Nat Med,* Vol.9, No.6, pp.669-676.

Finn RS, Wilson CA, Sanders J et al. Targeting the epidermal growth factor receptor and HER-2 with OSI-774 and trastuzumab, respectively, in HER-2 overexpressing human breast cancer cell lines in a therapeutic advantage in vitro. Proc Am Soc Clin Oncol 2003; 22. 235 (Abstract 940)

Fotovati, A., Fujii, T., Yamaguchi, M., Kage, M., Shirouzu, K., Oie, S., Basaki, Y., Ono, M., Yamana, H. & Kuwano M. (2006) 17 β-estradiol induces down-regulation of Cap43/NDRG1/Drg-1, a putative differentiation-related and metastasis suppressor gene, in human breast cancer cells. *Clin Cancer Res,* Vol.12, No.10, pp.3010-3018.

Fotovati, A., Abu-Ali, S., Kage, M., Shirouzu, K., Yamana, H. & Kuwano M. (2011) N-myc Downstream-regulated Gene 1 (NDRG1) a Differentiation Marker of Human Breast Cancer. Pathol Oncol Res, (Epub ahead of print).

Fox, SB., Generali, DG. & Harris AL. (2007) Breast tumour angiogenesis. *Breast Cancer Res,* Vol.9, No.6, pp.216.

Fox, WD., Higgins, B., Maiese, KM., Drobnjak, M., Cordon-Cardo, C., Scher, HI. & Agus, DB. (2002) Antibody to vascular endothelial growth factor slows growth of an androgen-independent xenograft model of prostate cancer. *Clin Cancer Res,* Vol.8, No.10, pp.3226-3231.

Franklin, MC., Carey, KD., Vajdos, FF., Leahy, DJ., de Vos, AM. & Sliwkowski, MX. (2004) Insights into ErbB signaling from the structure of the ErbB2-pertuzumab complex. *Cancer Cell,* Vol.5, No.4, pp. 317-328.

Fujii, T., Kawahara, A., Basaki, Y., Hattori, S., Nakashima, K., Nakano, K., Shirouzu, K., Kohno, K., Yanagawa, T., Yamana, H., Nishio, K., Ono, M., Kuwano, M. & Kage, M. (2008) Expression of HER2 and estrogen receptor alpha depends upon nuclear localization of Y-box binding protein-1 in human breast cancers. Cancer Res, Vol.68, No.5, pp.1504-1512.

Fujii, T., Seki, N., Namoto-Matsubayashi, R., Takahashi, H., Inoue, Y., Toh, U., Kage, M. & Shirouzu, K. (2009) YB-1 prevents apoptosis via the mTOR/STAT3 pathway in HER-2-overexpressing breast cancer cells. *Future Oncol*, Vol.5, No.2, pp.153-156.

Fukuoka, M., Yano, S., Giaccone, G., Tamura, T., Nakagawa, K,., Douillard, JY., Nishiwaki, Y., Vansteenkiste, J., Kudoh, S., Rischin, D., Eek, R., Horai, T., Noda, K., Takata, I., Smit, E., Averbuch, S., Macleod, A., Feyereislova, A., Dong, RP. & Baselga, J. (2003) Multi-institutional randomized phase II trial of gefitinib for previously treated patients with advanced non-small-cell lung cancer (The IDEAL 1 Trial) *J Clin Oncol*, Vol.21, No.12, pp.2237-2246.

Geyer, CE., Forster, J., Lindquist, D., Chan, S., Romieu, CG., Pienkowski, T., Jagiello-Gruszfeld, A., Crown, J., Chan, A., Kaufman, B., Skarlos, D., Campone, M., Davidson, N., Berger, M., Oliva, C., Rubin, S.D., Stein, S. & Cameron, D. (2006) Lapatinib plus capecitabine for HER2-positive advanced breast cancer. *N Engl J Med*, 2006, Vol.355, No.26, pp. 2733-2743.

Gianni, L., Eiermann, W., Semiglazov, V., Manikhas, A., Lluch, A., Tjulandin, S., Zambetti, M., Vazquez, F., Byakhow, M., Lichinitser, M., Climent, MA., Ciruelos, E., Ojeda, B., Mansutti, M., Bozhok, A., Baronio, R., Feyereislova, A., Barton, C., Valagussa, P. & Baselga, J. (2010a) Neoadjuvant chemotherapy with trastuzumab followed by adjuvant trastuzumab versus neoadjuvant chemotherapy alone, in patients with HER2-positive locally advanced breast cancer (the NOAH trial): a randomised controlled superiority trial with a parallel HER2-negative cohort. *Lancet,* Vol.375, No.9712, pp. 377-384.

Gianni, L., Lladó, A., Bianchi, G., Cortes, J., Kellokumpu-Lehtinen, PL., Cameron, DA., Miles, D., Salvagni, S., Wardley, A., Goeminne, JC., Hersberger, V. & Baselga, J. (2010b) Open-label, phase II, multicenter, randomized study of the efficacy and safety of two dose levels of Pertuzumab, a human epidermal growth factor receptor 2 dimerization inhibitor, in patients with human epidermal growth factor receptor 2-negative metastatic breast cancer. *J Clin Oncol*, Vol.28, No.7, pp. 1131-1137.

Gianni, L., Pienkowski, T., Im, Y-H., Roman, L., Tseng, L-M., Liu, M-C., Lluch-Hernandez, A., Semiglazov, V., Szado, T. & Ross, G. (2010c) Neoadjuvant pertuzumab (P) and trastuzumab (T): Antitumor and safety analysis of a randomized phase II study ('NeoSphere'). *Cancer Res*, Vol.70, No.24, pp. 82s (abstract S3-2).

Giménez-Bonafé, P., Fedoruk, MN., Whitmore, TG., Akbari, M., Ralph, JL., Ettinger, S., Gleave, ME. & Nelson, CC. (2004) YB-1 is upregulated during prostate cancer tumor progression and increases P-glycoprotein activity. *Prostate*, Vol.59, No.3, pp.337-349.

Goldhirsch, A., Ingle, JN., Gelber, RD., Coates, AS., Thürlimann, B. & Senn, HJ; Panel members. (2009) Thresholds for therapies: highlights of the St Gallen International Expert Consensus on the primary therapy of early breast cancer 2009. *Ann Oncol*, Vol.20, No.8, pp. 1319-1329.

Gomez, HL., Doval, DC., Chavez, MA., Ang, PC., Aziz, Z., Nag, S., Ng, C., Franco, SX., Chow, LW., Arbushites, MC., Casey, MA., Berger, MS., Stein, SH. & Sledge, GW. (2008) Efficacy and safety of lapatinib as first-line therapy for ErbB2-amplified locally advanced or metastatic breast cancer. *J Clin Oncol*, Vol.26, No.18, pp. 2999-3005.

Gonzalez-Angulo, AM., Litton, JK., Broglio, KR., Meric-Bernstam, F., Rakkhit, R., Cardoso, F., Peintinger, F., Hanrahan, EO., Sahin, A., Guray, M., Larsimont, D., Feoli, F., Stranzl, H., Buchholz, TA., Valero, V., Theriault, R., Piccart-Gebhart, M., Ravdin, PM., Berry, DA. & Hortobagyi, GN. (2009) High risk of recurrence for patients with breast cancer who have human epidermal growth factor receptor 2-positive, node-negative tumors 1 cm or smaller. *J Clin Oncol,* Vol.27, No.34, pp. 5700-5706.

Gril, B., Palmieri, D., Bronder, JL., Herring, JM., Vega-Valle, E., Feigenbaum, L., Liewehr, DJ., Steinberg, SM., Merino, MJ., Rubin, SD. & Steeg PS. (2008) Effect of lapatinib on the outgrowth of metastatic breast cancer cells to the brain. *J Natl Cancer Inst,* Vol.100, No.15, 1092-1103.

Guan, RJ., Ford, HL., Fu, Y., Li, Y., Shaw, LM. & Pardee, AB. (2000) Drg-1 as a differentiation-related, putative metastatic suppressor gene in human colon cancer. *Cancer Res,* Vol.60, No.3, pp. 749-755.

Hubbard, SR. (2005) EGF receptor inhibition: attacks on multiple fronts. *Cancer Cell,* Vol.7, No.4, pp. 287-288.

Izumi, H., Imamura, T., Nagatani, G., Ise, T., Murakami, T., Uramoto, H., Torigoe, T., Ishiguchi, H., Yoshida, Y., Nomoto, M., Okamoto, T., Uchiumi, T., Kuwano, M., Funa, K. & Kohno. K. (2001) Y box-binding protein-1 binds preferentially to single-stranded nucleic acids and exhibits 3'-->5' exonuclease activity. *Nucleic Acids Res,* Vol.29, No.5, pp.1200-1207.

Jain, RK. (2003) Molecular regulation of vessel maturation. *Nat Med,* Vol.9, No.6, pp.685–693.

Janz, M., Harbeck, N., Dettmar, P., Berger, U., Schmidt, A., Jürchott, K., Schmitt, M. & Royer HD. (2002) Y-box factor YB-1 predicts drug resistance and patient outcome in breast cancer independent of clinically relevant tumor biologic factors HER2, uPA and PAI-1. *Int J Cancer,* Vol.97, No.3, pp.278-282.

Jerusalem, G., Fasolo, A., Dieras, V., Cardoso, F., Bergh, J., Vittori, L., Zhang, Y., Massacesi, C., Sahmoud, T. & Gianni L. (2011) Phase I trial of oral mTOR inhibitor everolimus in combination with trastuzumab and vinorelbine in pre-treated patients with HER2-overexpressing metastatic breast cancer. *Breast Cancer Res Treat,* Vol.125, No.2, pp.447-455.

Jiang, K., Shen, Z., Ye, Y., Yang, X. & Wang S. (2010) A novel molecular marker for early detection and evaluating prognosis of gastric cancer: N-myc downstream regulated gene-1 (NDRG1). *Scand J Gastroenterol.* Vol.45, No.7-8, pp.898-908.

Joensuu, H., Kellokumpu-Lehtinen, PL., Bono, P., Alanko, T., Kataja, V., Asola, R., Utriainen, T., Kokko, R., Hemminki, A., Tarkkanen, M., Turpeenniemi-Hujanen, T., Jyrkkiö, S., Flander, M., Helle, L., Ingalsuo, S., Johansson, K., Jääskeläinen, AS., Pajunen, M., Rauhala, M., Kaleva-Kerola, J., Salminen, T., Leinonen, M., Elomaa, I., Isola, J.; FinHer Study Investigators. (2006) Adjuvant docetaxel or vinorelbine with or without trastuzumab for breast cancer. *N Engl J Med,* Vol.354, No.8, pp. 809-820.

Jung, YD., Mansfield, PF., Akagi, M., Takeda, A., Liu, W., Bucana, CD., Hicklin, DJ. & Ellis, LM. (2002) Effects of combination anti-vascular endothelial growth factor receptor and anti-epidermal growth factor receptor therapies on the growth of gastric cancer in a nude mouse model. *Eur J Cancer,* Vol.38, No.8, pp. 1133-1140.

Kamura, T., Yahata, H., Amada, S., Ogawa, S., Sonoda, T., Kobayashi, H., Mitsumoto, M., Kohno, K., Kuwano, M. & Nakano, H. (1999) Is nuclear expression of Y box-binding protein-1 a new prognostic factor in ovarian serous adenocarcinoma? *Cancer,* Vol.85, No.11, pp.2450-2454.

Kim, KJ., Li, B., Winer, J., Armanini, M., Gillett, N., Phillips, HS. & Ferrara N. (1993) Inhibition of vascular endothelial growth factor-induced angiogenesis suppresses tumour growth in vivo. *Nature,* Vol.362, No.6423, pp.841–844.

Klos, KS., Wyszomierski, SL., Sun, M., Tan, M., Zhou, X., Li, P., Yang, W., Yin, G., Hittelman, WN. & Yu, D. (2006) ErbB2 increases vascular endothelial growth factor protein synthesis via activation of mammalian target of rapamycin/p70S6K leading to increased angiogenesis and spontaneous metastasis of human breast cancer cells. *Cancer Res,* Vol.66, No.4, pp.2028–2037.

Kohno, K., Izumi, H., Uchiumi, T., Ashizuka, M. & Kuwano. M. (2003) The pleiotropic functions of the Y-box-binding protein, YB-1. *Bioessays,* Vol.25, No.7, pp.691-698.

Koike, K., Uchiumi, T., Ohga, T., Toh, S., Wada, M., Kohno, K. & Kuwano, M. (1997) Nuclear translocation of the Y-box binding protein by ultraviolet irradiation. *FEBS Lett,* Vol. 417, No.3, pp.390-394.

Konecny, GE., Meng, YG., Untch, M., Wang, HJ., Bauerfeind, I., Epstein, M., Stieber, P., Vernes, JM., Gutierrez, J., Hong, K., Beryt, M., Hepp, H., Slamon, DJ. & Pegram, MD. (2004) Association between HER-2/neu and vascular endothelial growth factor expression predicts clinical outcome in primary breast cancer patients. *Clin Cancer Res,* Vol.10, No.5, pp.1706–1716.

Konecny, GE., Pegram, MD., Venkatesan, N., Finn, R., Yang, G., Rahmeh, M., Untch, M., Rusnak, DW., Spehar, G., Mullin, RJ., Keith, BR., Gilmer, TM., Berger, M., Podratz, KC. & Slamon, DJ. (2006) Activity of the dual kinase inhibitor lapatinib (GW572016) against HER-2-overexpressing and trastuzumab-treated breast cancer cells. *Cancer Res,* Vol.66, No.3, pp. 1630-1639.

Koutras, AK., Fountzilas, G., Kalogeras, KT., Starakis, I., Iconomou, G. & Kalofonos, HP. (2010) The upgraded role of HER3 and HER4 receptors in breast cancer. *Crit Rev Oncol Hematol,* Vol.74, No.2, pp. 73-78.

Kuwano, M., Uchiumi, T., Hayakawa, H., Ono, M., Wada, M., Izumi, H. & Kohno. K. (2003) The basic and clinical implications of ABC transporters, Y-box-binding protein-1 (YB-1) and angiogenesis-related factors in human malignancies. *Cancer Sci,* Vol.94, No.1, pp9-14.

Kuwano, M., Oda, Y., Izumi, H., Yang, SJ., Uchiumi, T., Iwamoto, Y., Toi, M., Fujii, T., Yamana, H., Kinoshita, H., Kamura, T., Tsuneyoshi, M., Yasumoto, K. & Kohno K. (2004) The role of nuclear Y-box binding protein 1 as a global marker in drug resistance. *Mol Cancer Ther,* Vol.3, No.11, pp.1485-1492.

Lachat, P., Shaw, P., Gebhard, S., van Belzen, N., Chaubert, P. & Bosman, FT. (2002) Expression of NDRG1, a differentiation-related gene, in human tissues. *Histochem Cell Biol,* Vol.118, No.5, pp.399-408.

Lackey, KE. (2006) Lessons from the drug discovery of lapatinib, a dual ErbB1/2 tyrosine kinase inhibitor. *Curr Top Med Chem,* Vol.6, No.5, pp. 435-460.

Lee, C., Dhillon, J., Wang, MY., Gao, Y., Hu, K., Park, E., Astanehe, A., Hung, MC., Eirew, P., Eaves, CJ. & Dunn SE. (2008) Targeting YB-1 in HER-2 overexpressing breast cancer cells induces apoptosis via the mTOR/STAT3 pathway and suppresses tumor growth in mice. *Cancer Res,* Vol.68, No.21, pp.8661-8666.

Lee, SY., Kim, DK., Cho, JH., Koh, JY. & Yoon YH. (2008) Inhibitory effect of bevacizumab on the angiogenesis and growth of retinoblastoma. Arch Ophthalmol, Vol.126, No.7, pp.953-958.

Liang, Z., Wu, T., Lou, H., Yu, X., Taichman, RS., Lau, SK., Nie, S., Umbreit, J., Shim, H. (2004) Inhibition of breast cancer metastasis by selective synthetic polypeptide against CXCR4. *Cancer Res*, Vol.64, No.12, 4302-4308.

Lin, NU. & Winer, EP. (2004) New targets for therapy in breast cancer: small molecule tyrosine kinase inhibitors. *Breast Cancer Res,* Vol.6, No.5, pp. 204-210.

Lin, NU., Diéras, V., Paul, D., Lossignol, D., Christodoulou, C., Stemmler, HJ., Roché, H., Liu, MC., Greil, R., Ciruelos, E., Loibl, S., Gori, S., Wardley, A., Yardley, D., Brufsky, A., Blum, JL., Rubin, SD., Dharan, B., Steplewski, K., Zembryki, D., Oliva, C., Roychowdhury, D., Paoletti, P. & Winer EP. (2009) Multicenter phase II study of lapatinib in patients with brain metastases from HER2-positive breast cancer. *Clin Cancer Res,* Vol.15, No.4, 1452-1459.

Liu, YL., Bai, WT., Luo, W., Zhang, DX., Yan, Y., Xu, ZK. & Zhang FL. (2011) Downregulation of NDRG1 promotes invasion of human gastric cancer AGS cells through MMP-2. *Tumour Biol,* Vol.32, No.1, pp.99-105.

Lu, C., Speers, C., Zhang, Y., Xu, X., Hill, J., Steinbis, E., Celestino, J., Shen, Q. Kim, H., Hilsenbeck, S., Mohsin, SK., Wakeling, A., Osborne, CK. & Brown, PH. (2003) Effect of epidermal growth factor receptor inhibitor on development of estrogen receptor-negative mammary tumors. *J Natl Cancer Inst,* Vol.95, No.24, pp. 1825-1833.

Lu, CH., Wyszomierski, SL., Tseng, LM., Sun, MH., Lan, KH., Neal, CL., Mills, GB., Hortobagyi, GN., Esteva, FJ. & Yu D. (2007) Preclinical testing of clinically applicable strategies for overcoming trastuzumab resistance caused by PTEN deficiency. *Clin Cancer Res,* Vol.13, No.19, pp.5883-5888.

McArthur, HL., Mahoney, K., Morris, PG., Patil, S., Jacks, LM., Howard, J., Norton, L. & Hudis, C. (2010) Use of adjuvant trastuzumab with chemotherapy in women with small, node-negative, HER2-positive breast cancers. *J Clin Oncol,* Vol.28, pp 95s. (abstract 615).

Metro, G., Foglietta, J., Stocchi, L., Russillo, M., Papaldo, P., Crino, L., Giannarelli, D., Cognetti, F., Fabi, A. & Gori, S. (2010) Outcome of patients(pts) with brain metasitases (BMs) from HER2-positive breast cancer (BC) treated with lapatinib plus capecitabine (LC). *J Clin Oncol,* Vol.28, pp.152s, (abstract 1155)

Miles D et al. (2009) Final overall survival (OS) results from the randomized, double-blind, phase III AVADO study of bevacizumab (BEV) plus docetaxel (DOC) compared with placebo plus DOC for the first-line treatment of locally recurrent or metastatic breast cancer. San Antonio Breast Cancer Symposium (abstract 41)

Miller, K., Wang, M., Gralow, J., Dickler, M., Cobleigh, M., Perez, EA., Shenkier, T., Cella, D. & Davidson NE. (2007) Paclitaxel plus bevacizumab versus paclitaxel alone for metastatic breast cancer. *N Engl J Med,* Vol.357, No.26, pp.2666–2676.

Miller, K., Gianni, L., Andre, F., Dieras, V., Mahtani, RL., Harbeck, N., Huang, JE., Shih, T., Choi, Y. & Burris, HA III. (2010) A phase Ib/II trial of trastuzumab-DM1 (T-DM1) with pertuzumab (P) for women with HER2-positive, locally advanced or metastatic breast cancer (BC) who were previously treated with trastuzumab (T). *J Clin Oncol,* Vol.28, No15S, pp. 117s. (abstract 1012).

Moulder, SL., Yakes, FM., Muthuswamy, SK., Bianco, R., Simpson, JF. & Arteaga, C.L. (2001) Epidermal growth factor receptor (HER1) tyrosine kinase inhibitor ZD1839 (Iressa) inhibits HER2/neu (erbB2)-overexpressing breast cancer cells in vitro and in vivo. *Cancer Res*, Vol. 61, No.24, pp. 8887-8895.

Moyer, JD., Barbacci, EG., Iwata, KK., Arnold, L., Boman, B., Cunningham, A., DiOrio, C., Doty, J., Morin, MJ., Moyer, MP., Neveu, M., Pollack, VA., Pustilnik, LR., Reynolds, MM., Sloan, D., Theleman, A.& Miller, P. (1997) Induction of apoptosis and cell cycle arrest by CP-358,774, an inhibitor of epidermal growth factor receptor tyrosine kinase. *Cancer Res*, Vol.57, No.21, pp. 4838-4848.

Müller, A., Homey, B., Soto, H., Ge, N., Catron, D., Buchanan, ME., McClanahan, T., Murphy, E., Yuan, W., Wagner, SN., Barrera, JL., Mohar, A., Verástegui, E., Zlotnik, A. (2001) Involvement of chemokine receptors in breast cancer metastasis. *Nature*, Vol.410, No.6824, pp. 50-56.

NCCN Clinical Practice Guidelines in Oncology™ Breast Cancer Version 1. 2011 available from http://www.nccn.com.

Normanno, N., Campiglio, M., De, LA., Somenzi, G., Maiello, M., Ciardiello, F., Gianni, L., Salomon, DS. & Menard, S. (2002) Cooperative inhibitory effect of ZD1839 (Iressa) in combination with trastuzumab (Herceptin) on human breast cancer cell growth. *Ann Oncol*, Vol.13, No.1, pp.65-72.

Oda, Y., Sakamoto, A., Shinohara, N., Ohga, T., Uchiumi, T., Kohno, K., Tsuneyoshi, M., Kuwano, M. & Iwamoto, Y. (1998) Nuclear expression of YB-1 protein correlates with P-glycoprotein expression in human osteosarcoma. *Clin Cancer Res*, Vol.4, No.9, pp.2273-2277.

Oda, Y., Ohishi, Y., Saito, T., Hinoshita, E., Uchiumi, T., Kinukawa, N., Iwamoto, Y., Kohno, K., Kuwano, M. & Tsuneyoshi, M. (2003) Nuclear expression of Y-box-binding protein-1 correlates with P-glycoprotein and topoisomerase II alpha expression, and with poor prognosis in synovial sarcoma. *J Pathol*, Vol.199, No.2, pp.251-258.

Okuda. H., Hirai, S., Takaki, Y., Kamada, M., Baba, M., Sakai, N., Kishida, T., Kaneko, S., Yao, M., Ohno, S. & Shuin, T. (1999) Direct interaction of the beta-domain of VHL tumor suppressor protein with the regulatory domain of atypical PKC isotypes. *Biochem Biophys Res Commun*, Vol.263, No.2, pp.491-497.

Osborne, CK., Neven, P., Dirix, LY., Mackey, JR., Robert, J., Underhill, C., Schiff, R., Gutierrez, C., Migliaccio, I., Anagnostou, VK., Rimm, DL., Magill, P. & Sellers M. (2011) Gefitinib or placebo in combination with tamoxifen in patients with hormone receptor-positive metastatic breast cancer: A randomized phase II study. *Clin Cancer Res*, Vol.17, No.5, 1147-1159.

O'Shaughnessy, JA. & Brufsky AM. (2008) RiBBON 1 and RiBBON 2: phase III trials of bevacizumab with standard chemotherapy for metastatic breast cancer. *Clin Breast Cancer*, Vol.8, No.4, pp.370-373.

Pegram, M., Chan, D., Dichmann, RA., et al. (2006) Phase II combined biological therapy targeting the HER2 proto-oncogene and the vascular endothelial growth factor using trastuzumab (T) and bevacizumab (B) as first line treatment of HER2-amplified breast cancer. *Breast Cancer Res Treat*. Vol.100, S28, (Abstract 301).

Perez, EA., Romond, EH., Suman, VJ., Jeong, J., Davidson, NE., Geyer, CE., Martino, S., Mamounas, EP., Kauffman, PA., & Wolmark, N. (2007) Updated results of the combined analysis of NCCTG N9831 and NSABP B-31 adjuvant chemotherapy with/without trastuzumab in patients with HER2-positive breast cancer. *J Clin Oncol,* Vol.25, pp. 6s. (abstract 512).

Pérez-Soler, R., Chachoua, A., Hammond, LA., Rowinsky, EK., Huberman, M., Karp, D., Rigas, J., Clark, GM., Santabárbara, P. & Bonomi, P. (2004) Determinants of tumor response and survival with erlotinib in patients with non--small-cell lung cancer. J Clin Oncol, Vol.22, No.16, pp. 3238-3247.

Pollack, VA., Savage, DM., Baker, DA., Tsaparikos, KE., Sloan, DE., Moyer, JD., Barbacci, E.G., Pustilnik, LR., Smolarek, TA., Davis, JA., Vaidya, MP., Arnold, LD., Doty, JL., Iwata, KK. & Morin, MJ. (1999) Inhibition of epidermal growth factor receptor-associated tyrosine phosphorylation in human carcinomas with CP-358,774: dynamics of receptor inhibition in situ and antitumor effects in athymic mice. *J Pharmacol Exp Ther,* Vol.291, No.2, 739-748.

Ro, J., Park, S., Kim, T-Y., Im, Y-H., Rha, SY., Chung, JS., Moon, H. & Santillana S. (2010) Clinical outcomes of brain metastasis by lapatinib (L) and capecitabine (C) in an open-label expanded access study among Korean patients with HER2 positive metastatic breast cancer. Cancer Res, Vol.70, No.24, (abstract P1-14-04).

Rosen, LS., Ashurst, HL. & Chap, L. (2010) Targeting signal transduction pathways in metastatic breast cancer: a comprehensive review. *Oncologist,* Vol.15, No.3, pp. 216-235.

Russo, SM. & Ove, R. (2003) Molecular targets as therapeutic strategies in the management of breast cancer. *Expert Opin Ther Targets,* Vol.7, No.4, pp. 543-557.

Saji, H., Toi, M., Saji, S., Koike, M., Kohno, K. & Kuwano, M. (2003) Nuclear expression of YB-1 protein correlates with P-glycoprotein expression in human breast carcinoma. *Cancer Lett,* Vol.190, No.2, pp.191-197.

Segerström, L., Fuchs, D., Bäckman, U., Holmquist, K., Christofferson, R. & Azarbayjani F. (2006) The anti-VEGF antibody bevacizumab potently reduces the growth rate of high-risk neuroblastoma xenografts. Pediatr Res, Vol.60, No.5, pp.576-581.

Scheuer, W., Friess, T. & Hasmann, M. (2006) Enhanced antitumour effect by combination of HER2-targeting antibodies with bevacizumab in a human breast cancer xenograft model. *Eur J Cancer,* Suppl4, pp.66 (Abstract 213).

Scheuer, W., Friess, T., Burtscher, H., Bossenmaier, B., Endl, J. & Hasmann, M. (2009) Strongly enhanced antitumor activity of trastuzumab and pertuzumab combination treatment on HER2-positive human xenograft tumor models. *Cancer Res,* Vol.69, No.24, pp. 9330-9336.

Schlotter, CM., Vogt, U., Allgayer, H. & Brandt, B. (2008) Molecular targeted therapies for breast cancer treatment. *Breast Cancer Res,* Vol.10, No.4, pp.211.

Shibahara, K., Sugio, K., Osaki, T., Uchiumi, T., Maehara, Y., Kohno, K., Yasumoto, K., Sugimachi, K. & Kuwano, M. (2001) Nuclear expression of the Y-box binding protein, YB-1, as a novel marker of disease progression in non-small cell lung cancer. *Clin Cancer Res,* Vol. 7, No.10, pp.3151-3155.

Shibuya M. (2001) Structure and function of VEGF/VEGF-receptor system involved in angiogenesis. *Cell Struct Funct,* Vol.26, No.1, pp.25-35.

Shimono, A., Okuda, T. & Kondoh, H. (1999) N-myc-dependent repression of ndr1, a gene identified by direct subtraction of whole mouse embryo cDNAs between wild type and N-myc mutant. *Mech Dev,* Vol.83, No.1-2, pp.39-52.

Sirotnak, FM., Zakowski, MF., Miller, VA., Scher, HI. & Kris, MG. (2000) Efficacy of cytotoxic agents against human tumor xenografts is markedly enhanced by coadministration of ZD1839 (Iressa), an inhibitor of EGFR tyrosine kinase. Clin Cancer Res, Vol.6, No.12, 4885-4892.

Slamon, DJ., Leyland-Jones, B., Shak, S., Fuchs, H., Paton, V., Bajamonde, A., Fleming, T., Eiermann, W., Wolter, J., Pegram, M., Baselga, J. & Norton L. (2001) Use of chemotherapy plus a monoclonal antibody against HER2 for metastatic breast cancer that overexpresses HER2. N Engl J Med, Vol.344, No.11, pp. 783-792.

Slamon D, Eiermann W, Robert N, et al. (2006) BCIRG 006: 2nd interim analysis phase III randomized trial comparing doxorubicin and cyclophosphamide followed by docetaxel (AC->T) with doxorubicin and cyclophosphamide followed by docetaxel and trastuzumab (AC->TH) with docetaxel, carboplatin and trastuzumab (TCH) in Her2neu positive early breast cancer patients. Breast Cancer Res Treat 100(Suppl 1)(abstract 52).

Smith, I., Procter, M., Gelber, RD., Guillaume, S., Feyereislova, A., Dowsett, M., Goldhirsch, A., Untch, M., Mariani, G., Baselga, J., Kaufmann, M., Cameron, D., Bell, R., Bergh, J., Coleman, R., Wardley, A., Harbeck, N., Lopez, RI., Mallmann, P., Gelmon, K., Wilcken, N., Wist, E., Sánchez Rovira, P. & Piccart-Gebhart, MJ.; HERA study team. (2007) 2-year follow-up of trastuzumab after adjuvant chemotherapy in HER2-positive breast cancer: a randomised controlled trial. *Lancet*, Vol.369, No.9555, pp. 29-36.

Song, Y., Oda, Y., Hori, M., Kuroiwa, K., Ono, M., Hosoi, F., Basaki, Y., Tokunaga, S., Kuwano, M., Naito, S. & Tsuneyoshi M. (2010) N-myc downstream regulated gene-1/Cap43 may play an important role in malignant progression of prostate cancer, in its close association with E-cadherin. *Hum Pathol*, Vol.41, No.2, pp.214-222.

Sørlie T, Perou CM, Tibshirani R, Aas T, Geisler S, Johnsen H, Hastie T, Eisen MB, van de Rijn M, Jeffrey SS, Thorsen T, Quist H, Matese JC, Brown PO, Botstein D, Eystein Lønning P, Børresen-Dale AL. (2001) Gene expression patterns of breast carcinomas distinguish tumor subclasses with clinical implications. Proc Natl Acad Sci U S A, Vol.98, No.19, pp.10869-10874.

Sorokin, AV., Selyutina, AA., Skabkin, MA., Guryanov, SG., Nazimov, IV., Richard, C., Th'ng, J., Yau, J., Sorensen, PH., Ovchinnikov, LP. & Evdokimova, V. (2005) Proteasome-mediated cleavage of the Y-box-binding protein 1 is linked to DNA-damage stress response. *EMBO J*, Vol.24, No.20, pp.3602-3612.

Soulieres, D., Senzer, NN., Vokes, EE., Hidalgo, M., Agarwala, SS. & Siu, LL. (2004) Multicenter phase II study of erlotinib, an oral epidermal growth factor receptor tyrosine kinase inhibitor, in patients with recurrent or metastatic squamous cell cancer of the head and neck. *J Clin Oncol*, Vol.22, No.1, pp. 77-85.

Stenina, OI., Poptic, EJ. & DiCorleto, PE. (2000) Thrombin activates a Y box-binding protein (DNA-binding protein B) in endothelial cells. *J Clin Invest*, Vol.106, No.4, pp.579-587.

Sutherland, BW., Kucab, J., Wu, J., Lee, C., Cheang, MC., Yorida, E., Turbin, D., Dedhar, S., Nelson, C., Pollak, M., Leighton Grimes, H., Miller, K., Badve, S., Huntsman, D. Blake-Gilks, C., Chen, M., Pallen, CJ. & Dunn, SE. (2005) Akt phosphorylates the Y-box binding protein 1 at Ser102 located in the cold shock domain and affects the anchorage-independent growth of breast cancer cells. *Oncogene,* Vo.24, No.26, pp.4281-4292.

Takahashi, T., Ueno, H. & Shibuya, M. (1999) VEGF activates protein kinase C-dependent, but Ras-independent Raf-MEK-MAP kinase pathway for DNA synthesis in primary endothelial cells. *Oncogene,* Vol.18, No.13, pp.2221-2230.

Thomas, MB., Chadha, R., Glover, K., Wang, X., Morris, J., Brown, T., Rashid, A., Dancey, J. & Abbruzzese, JL. (2007) Phase 2 study of erlotinib in patients with unresectable hepatocellular carcinoma. *Cancer,* Vol.110, No.5, pp. 1059-1067.

Uchiumi, T.; Kohno, K.; Tanimura, H.; Matsuo, K.; Sato, S.; Uchida, Y.; Kuwano. M. (1993) Enhanced expression of the human multidrug resistance 1 gene in response to UV light irradiation. *Cell Growth Differ,* Vol.4, No.3, pp147-157.

Vogel, CL., Cobleigh, MA., Tripathy, D., Gutheil, JC., Harris, LN., Fehrenbacher, L., Slamon, DJ., Murphy, M., Novotny, WF., Burchmore, M., Shak, S., Stewart, SJ. & Press, M. (2002) Efficacy and safety of trastuzumab as a single agent in first-line treatment of HER2-overexpressing metastatic breast cancer. *J Clin Oncol,* Vol.20, No.3, pp. 719-726.

Vogel, C., Chan, A., Gril, B., Kim, SB., Kurebayashi, J., Liu, L., Lu, YS. & Moon, H. (2010) Management of ErbB2-positive breast cancer: insights from preclinical and clinical studies with lapatinib. *Jpn J Clin Oncol,* Vol.40, No.11, pp. 999-1013.

von Minckwitz, G., Jonat, W., Fasching, P., du Bois, A., Kleeberg, U., Lück, H.J., Kettner, E., Hilfrich, J., Eiermann, W., Torode, J. & Schneeweiss, A. (2005) A multicentre phase II study on gefitinib in taxane- and anthracycline-pretreated metastatic breast cancer. *Breast Cancer Res Treat,* Vol.89, No.2, pp. 165-172.

Wakeling, AE., Guy, SP., Woodburn, JR., Ashton, SE., Curry, BJ., Barker, AJ. & Gibson, KH. (2002) ZD1839 (Iressa): an orally active inhibitor of epidermal growth factor signaling with potential for cancer therapy. Cancer Res, Vol.62, No.20, pp. 5749-5754.

Wakisaka, Y., Furuta, A., Masuda, K., Morikawa, W., Kuwano, M. & Iwaki, T. (2003) Cellular distribution of NDRG1 protein in the rat kidney and brain during normal postnatal development. *J Histochem Cytochem,* Vol.51, No.11, pp.1515-1525.

Witton, CJ., Reeves, JR., Going, JJ., Cooke, TG. & Bartlett, JM. (2003) Expression of the HER1-4 family of receptor tyrosine kinases in breast cancer. *J Pathol,* Vol.200, No.3, pp. 290-297.

Woodburn, J.R. (1999) The epidermal growth factor receptor and its inhibition in cancer therapy. *Pharmacol Ther,* Vol.82,No.2-3, pp. 241-250.

Xia, W., Mullin, RJ., Keith, BR., Liu, LH., Ma, H., Rusnak, DW., Owens, G., Alligood, KJ. & Spector, NL. (2002) Anti-tumor activity of GW572016: a dual tyrosine kinase inhibitor blocks EGF activation of EGFR/erbB2 and downstream Erk1/2 and AKT pathways. *Oncogene,* Vol.21, No.41, pp. 6255-6263.

Xia, W., Gerard, CM., Liu, L., Baudson, NM., Ory, TL. & Spector, NL. (2005) Combining lapatinib (GW572016), a small molecule inhibitor of ErbB1 and ErbB2 tyrosine kinases, with therapeutic anti-ErbB2 antibodies enhances apoptosis of ErbB2-overexpressing breast cancer cells.*Oncogene,* Vol.24, No.41, pp. 6213-6221.

Yancopoulos, GD., Davis, S., Gale, NW., Rudge, JS., Wiegand, SJ. & Holash, J. (2000) Vascular-specific growth factors and blood vessel formation. Nature, Vol.407, No.6801, pp.242–248.

20

Validation of Growth Differentiation Factor (GDF-15) as a Radiation Response Gene and Radiosensitizing Target in Mammary Adenocarcinoma Model

Hargita Hegyesi[1], James R. Lambert[2], Nikolett Sándor[1],
Boglárka Schilling-Tóth[1] and Géza Sáfrány[1]
[1]Frédéric Joliot-Curie National Research Institute for Radiobiology and Radiohygiene,
[2]Department of Pathology, University of Colorado,
Anschutz Medical Campus, Aurora, CO,
[1]Hungary
[2]USA

1. Introduction

In this chapter we summarize the role of cytokines in the radiation response, focusing in particular on growth differentiation factor-15 (GDF-15), and give a brief overview of our ongoing experiments in a mouse mammary carcinoma model.

The principal function, receptor, and signaling pathway of GDF-15 remain uncertain, although several of its biological activities have already been described; the exact role of GDF-15 in cancer progression also remains poorly understood. Increased GDF-15 expression is a common feature of many cancers. Several studies have observed upregulation of GDF-15 mRNA and protein in tumor biopsy. Serum GDF-15 levels are often markedly elevated in cases of metastatic cancer, and appear to occur in parallel with the stages and extent of disease, particularly in cases of prostate and melanoma [Senapati et al., 2010, Boyle et al., 2009]. Indeed, a number of studies have described an antitumorigenic function for GDF-15, by which it induces apoptosis and may negatively affect tumor growth [Cekanova et al., 2009, Jutooru et al., 2009].

Prevention by eliminating tumor promoters, early diagnosis and new target treatment are keys to reduce the numbers of deaths caused by breast cancer. In our present study, we propose that GDF-15 increases radioresistance. We demonstrate that down regulated mouse GDF-15 by RNA interference improves the radiosensitivity of the tumor in an LM2 mouse breast cancer model. In this regard, GDF-15 overexpression in breast cancer cell has been shown to supply important cytoprotective roles and resistance to radiation treatments. The paradoxical role of GDF-15 in breast cancer could be related to its pleiotropic effect on different signal pathway.

Recent research has focused on molecular targets for radiation sensitization of cancer cells. It is of particular interest that several potential target proteins involved in radiation sensitization, which have been identified in growth related cellular signaling pathways.

2. Radiation response genes in breast cancer cells

Radiation causes DNA damage, which activates ATM (ataxia telangiectasia mutated/ATR (ATM and Rad3-related) protein that in turn promotes activation of receptors/ intracellular signaling pathways and stimulates cell cycle checkpoints, p53 (tumor protein 53) activity, and DNA repair pathways. Radiation generates ionizing events in water in the cytosol that are amplified, thought to be mediated by mitochondria, which generate large amounts of reactive oxygen species (ROS) and reactive nitrogen species (RNS) that inhibit protein tyrosine phosphatase (PTPase) activities. In addition, radiation activates acidic sphingomyelinase and increases the production of ceramide. Inhibition of PTPases leads to a general derepression (activation) of receptor and nonreceptor tyrosine kinases and the activation of downstream signal transduction pathways. Radiation-induced ceramide has been shown to promote membrane-associated receptor activation by facilitating the clustering of receptors within lipid rafts [Balaban et al., 1996, Goldkorn et al., 1997].

The inducible alteration in gene expression is a fundamental molecular event of mammalian cells in response to ionizing radiation, and the fate of cells will at least partially depend upon the inducible changes in expression of some genes involved in these complex regulatory pathways resulting in cell cycle delays, cell killing or apoptosis and DNA repair [Chaudhry et al., 2003, Cucinotta et al., 2002 Vallat et al., 2003]. The cDNA microarray technology, allowing a large-scale expression profiling analysis, can provide tremendous information for elucidating the complex cellular response to radiation. Until now, a great number of radiation-inducible target genes have already been identified. Some of the inducible genes were identified in cells exposed to high and even supra-lethal doses of ionizing radiation (IR) [Roy et al., 2001]; low doses or low dose rates [Ding et al., 2005, Amundson et al., 2003, Mercier et al., 2004]. These reports provide very valuable information for understanding the precise mechanisms of the diverse effects of IR. A simultaneously comparative analysis of gene responses to radiation from low, medium to high doses should be more informative for identifying the inducible genes with a dose-dependent expression.

It is well known that the p53 tumor suppressor plays a key role in mediating apoptosis and the cell cycle checkpoint by various intracellular and extracellular signals including IR. A number of proteins have been identified to be involved in the p53 pathway, including Proliferating cell nuclear antigen (PCNA), Cyclin-dependent kinase inhibitor 1A (CDKN1A/p21), Murine double minute 2 (MDM2), GDF-15, Tumor necrosis factor receptor superfamily member 10B (TNFRSF10B/TRAIL-R2), Tumor protein p53 inducible protein 3 (TP53I3/PIG3) and Growth arrest and DNA damage (GADD45) [Polyak et al., 1997, Contente et al., 2002]. In a microarray investigation showed that, only five genes were significantly induced by the radiotherapy in breast cancer tissue. The genes are DNA damage-binding protein 2 (DDB2), CDKN1A, GDF-15, Glutathione peroxidase 1 (GPX1) and Polo-like kinase 3 (PLK3) [Helland et al., 2006]. Additional studies demonstrated that the levels of mRNA and protein expression of PCNA, c-fos, c-Jun N-terminal kinase 2 (JNK2) and Fos-related antigen 1 (Fra-1) were increased in the mammary epithelial cell line compared to the levels in non-tumorigenic control cells. The transforming factor Rho A was significantly increased only in the tumor cell line. Furthermore, the levels of mRNA and protein expression of Human epidermal growth factor receptor 2 (ErbB2) were significantly increased in the transformed cell line and in tumor cells derived from the transformed cells after injecting them into nude mice [Yun et al., 2010]. A decrease in RbA/p48 protein expression and mRNA levels was observed in cells treated with double doses of alpha particle radiation in the presence of estrogen, regardless of tumorigenicity. Furthermore, radiation increased c-myc, c-jun and c-fos protein expression in the c-Ha-ras- relative to non-irradiated control cell line [Calaf & Hei, 2004].

The role that cytokines play in radiation toxicity was first discovered and described by Rubin and colleagues [Rubin et al, 1986]. Shortly thereafter, transforming growth factor β1 (TGF-β1) was identified in the circulation of breast cancer patients who developed pulmonary and hepatic complications from chemotherapy for bone marrow transplantation [Anscher et al, 1993]. Chen and colleagues found that subjects undergoing thoracic radiation who had elevated interleukine-1 (IL-1) or IL-6 before or during radiation all developed some degree of radiation changes (clinical or radiographic). Angiogenic factors have also been associated with late pulmonary toxicity. For example, Fibroblast growth factor 2 (FGF2) was markedly elevated in the circulation of most subjects with severe late radiation fibrovascular toxicity of the extremities [Chen et al, 2002].

Presently, we do not yet have adequate markers for the vast majority of clinical needs, and their discovery remains a very high priority in radiation research. The need for these markers has intensified due to the growing number of cancer survivors at risk for developing toxicity from radiation, chemotherapy, surgery, and combinations of all three.

2.1 GDF-15 expression in different normal and malignant cells

GDF-15 is expressed at high levels in placenta, macrophages, and epithelial cells. Its expression is very low in tumor cell lines originating from breast, cervix, and lung [Li et al., 2000], but elevated in some metastatic colon and gastric cancers [Buckhaults et al., 2001, Lee et al., 2003). GDF-15 expression is rapidly induced by a variety of cellular stresses in a p53-dependent and -independent manner, and it mediates cell cycle arrest and apoptosis in response to DNA damage, toxins, anoxia, liver injury, and other cellular stresses [Hsiao et al., 2000, Albertoni et al., 2002, Wilson et al., 2003]. GDF-15 induction may occur via Heat-shock protein 70-2 (Hsp70-2) depletion. In HeLa cells Hsp70-2 depletion resulted in increased p53 protein levels and activity as measured by a reporter gene assay [Rohde et al., 2005]. GDF-15 is a secreted protein that can inhibit tumor cell growth both in an autocrine and paracrine fashion [Tan et al., 2000]. Whereas the antiproliferative effect of GDF-15 depends on the intact TGF-β signaling pathway, receptor and mothers against 32 decapentaplegic homolog 4 (Smad4), endogenously expressed GDF-15 is highly cytotoxic also in Smad4-null breast cancer cells [Li et al., 2005, Tan et al., 2000). Thus, therapeutic strategies targeting GDF-15 are likely to affect also cancer cells with defective TGF-β signaling and additionally to induce a so-called bystander effect in GDF-15-responsive tumors.

GDF-15 has been reported to be regulated by many chemicals at the transcriptional level [Li et al., 2000, Baek et al., 2001, Baek et al., 2004, Baek et al., 2005] and some of which are dependent on de novo protein synthesis [Newman et al., 2003] Transcriptional regulation of GDF-15 is complex, and the promoter sequence has many different cis- and trans-acting promoter elements [Baek et al., 2001]. Induction of GDF-15 expression by doxorubicin, hypoxia and the hypoxia mimetic, cobalt chloride in LNCaP prostate tumor cells strictly was dependent on functional p53. LNCaP cells expressing dominant negative p53 failed to induce GDf-15 mRNA and protein under all of these experimental conditions. Similarly, p53 function was also required for induction of GDF-15 expression in response to high cell density [Kelly et al., 2009]. In addition, GDF-15 seems to be a potentially important downstream target of three tumor suppressor genes. GDF-15 expression is regulated by the tumor suppressor genes p53 and early growth response (EGR) gene-1 [Baek et al., 2004]. Recently, was identified GDF-15 as a novel negative downstream target of the phosphatidylinositol 3-kinase/protein kinase B (AKT)/glycogen synthase kinase (GSK)-3β pathway [Yamaguchi et al., 2004].

The role of GDF-15 has been implicated directly with cancer, in which both antiapoptotic and proapoptotic effects have been described in a variety of tumor cell types. GDF-15 induction by vitamin D via p53-dependent mechanism and inhibition of prostate cancer cell growth was reported previously [Lambert et al., 2006]. Experimental studies using human prostate LNCaP cells supported the role of GDF-15 in regulation of cell proliferation. Overexpression of GDF-15 by transfection in LNCaP-C33 cells induced aggressive cell growth, whereas knocking down GDF-15 in LNCaP-derived subclones (C81 and LNCaP-Ln3: LNCaP cells highly metastasis to lymph nodes) using antisense oligonucleotides inhibited cell growth and proliferation [Chen et al., 2007]. Also, GDF-15 overexpression in colon cancer cell lines reduced the growth of xenograft tumors [Baek et al., 2001), but serum GDF-15 levels were positively correlated with tumor stage and metastasis [Brown et al., 2003]. Despite ambiguous observations in various tumor cell types, data obtained from clinical studies has established that serum GDF-15 was the best diagnostic marker of bone metastasis in prostate cancer [Selander et al., 2007]. However in the tissue microenvironment various components individually and/or collectively cause tissue damage or injury, leading to inflammation. Inflammatory products, including GDF-15, could contribute to the tumor promotion environment. The tumorigenic function of GDF-15 could be modified by educating the macrophages. Or another possibility is that, thus GDF-15 is secreted from tumor cells together with vascular endothelial growth factor (VEGF) to promote vascular development mediated by serine/threonine-protein kinase B-Raf signaling as reported in malignant melanoma [Huh et al., 2010,].

Individual cancers have different levels of secreted GDF-15 protein because of differences in expression level and variation in the processing of mature GDF-15 [Bauskin et al., 2005]. Serum analyses of cancer patients showed a significant correlation between increased GDF-15 protein levels and the metastatic progression of colorectal, breast, and prostate cancers [Welsh et al., 2003, Koopmann et al., 2004, Baek et al., 2009]. The association of cancer progression with GDF-15 expression resembles that of TGF-β, which plays a role as a tumor suppressor during early stages of cancer and as a growth enhancer in later stages [Dumont & Artega 2003].

GDF-15 also induced the transactivation of HER2/neu (ErbB2 tyrosine kinase) in human breast and gastric cancer cells, and this activation stimulated Hypoxia-inducible factor 1-α (HIF-1α) protein accumulation and the expression of its target gene via the PI3K/Akt/mTOR and ERK-1/2 signaling pathways. These novel observations provide additional support for the notion that GDF-15 may operate as a positive regulator of tumor progression in certain ErbB2-overexpressing tumors, including breast and gastric cancers [Kim et al., 2008, Klos et al., 2006].

The increase of GDF-15 expression induced via environmental stimuli (irradiation, hypoxia, free radicals etc.) is indicated. Furthermore, several transcriptional factors have been shown to increase GDF-15 expression level in p53 –dependent or independent manner in cancer cells in vitro and in mice in vivo. Potentially GDF-15 is a downstream mediator of the radioprotection of LM2 tumor cells to DNA damage and oxidative stress. This suggests

GDF-15 has significant paracrine effects, which modulate the tumor environment; however what is clear, is that there is a strong evidence for GDF-15 measurement in blood and tissues to detect and monitor cancer progression.

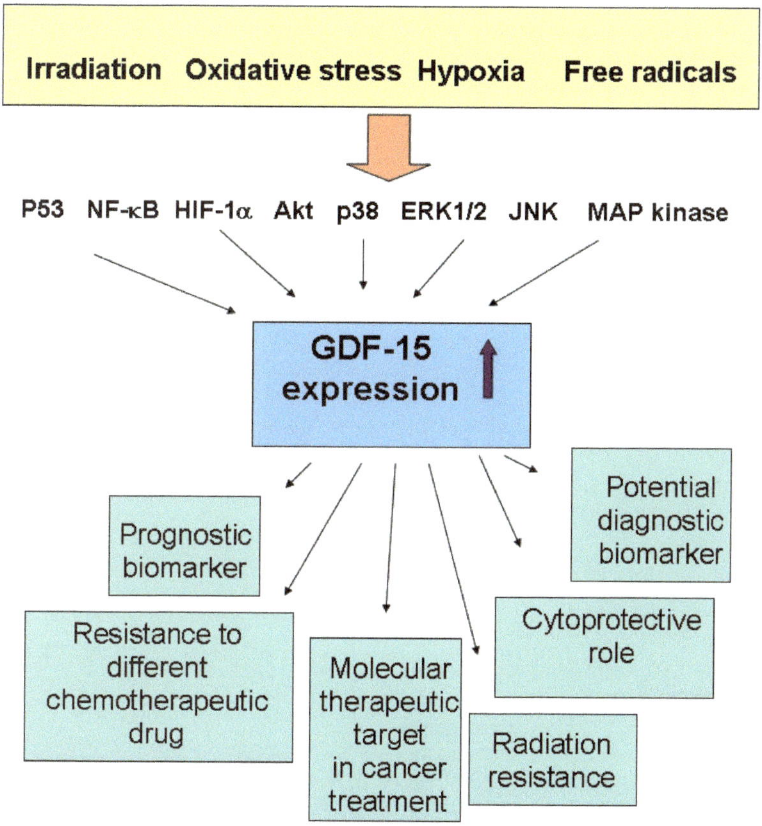

Fig. 1. Pleiotropic effect of GDF-15 overexpression.

3. Research result

3.1 Characteristics of LM2 cells as a model of breast cancer

Several years ago a mammary tumor cell line, LM2, derived from M2 mammary adenocarcinoma which spontaneously appeared in a Balb/c female mouse was described [Galli et al., 2000]. The LM2 cell line has been maintained in culture and grows as poorly differentiated elongated cells. Ultrastructural and immunocytochemistry analysis revealed characteristic features of adenocarcinoma. Cytogenetic studies showed that LM2 cells are fundamentally hypotetraploid. They express metalloproteinases (MMP) and show high levels of plasminogen activator type urokinase (uPA). They were sensitive to nitric oxide (NO)-mediated cytotoxicity when NO derived from an exogenous donor. In vivo, although LM2 cells were able to grow in the lungs, they could not metastasize to the same target organ from s.c. primary tumors. The LM2 mouse mammary adenocarcinoma cell line is a suitable model to examine different aspects of tumor biology [Hegyesi et al., 2007], in particular those related to the different pathways involved in the metastatic cascade and in the cytotoxicity mediated by NO. LM2 cells, kindly provided from the laboratory of Dr. Lucas Colombo (Research Area, Institute of Oncology Angel H. Roffo, C1417DTB, Buenos Aires, Argentina), were grown in DMEM medium supplied with 1% L-Glutamine and Penicillin/ Streptomycin and 10% FBS.

3.2 Radiation induced gene expression in LM2

It has been reported that GDF-15 is widely expressed, at low levels in different epithelial cells, but its expression is dramatically increased following inflammation, injury, or malignancy [Bauskin et al., 2006]. Our qRT-PCR data showed elevated transcriptional response of GDF-15 in LM2 cells, irradiated with 2 Gy and analyzed 2 hour later, but expression of TGF-β did not show the similar expression changes in these cells. It is likely that LM2 cells differently express TGF-β and the GDF-15.

The 2 Gy-induced changes in the transcript level of the GDF-15 and TGF-β gene were measured by qRT-PCR. The observed changes are shown in Figure 2. GDF-15 mRNA levels increased 2 hours after exposure with 2 Gy ($p<0.011$ with one-way ANOVA). Expression of TGF-β mRNA decreased 2 hours after exposure with 2 Gy ($p<0.039$ with one-way ANOVA). The dose-dependency of radiation-induced expression of GDF-15 at 2 hours with γ-ray exposure with doses 0.1 Gy, 2 Gy and 4 Gy was 196.9%± 17, 201.01%± 25 and 585.63%± 81, respectively in LM2 cells.

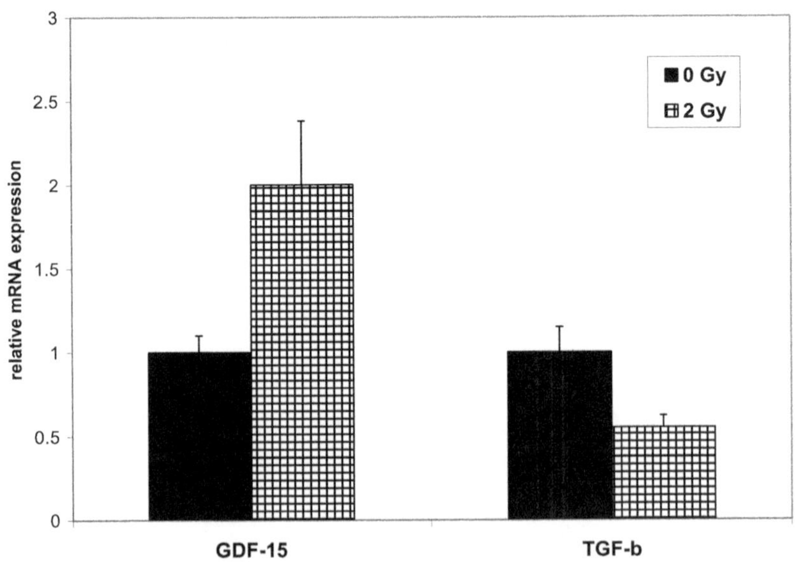

Fig. 2. 2 Gy induced expressional changes of GDF-15 and TGF-β measured by real time PCR. Real-time PCR was performed to test for radiation induced changes in GDF-15 and TGF-β mRNA expression. LM2 cells showed significant increased GDF-15 and decreased TGF-β mRNA expression after irradiation at 2h. The mRNA expression is normalized to the unirradiated controls. Error bars represent standard errors. Measurements were performed in duplicate, and experiments were repeated three times.

The identification of radiation-inducible genes, especially those exhibiting a dose-dependent response, not only expands our knowledge of the mechanisms underlying the diverse biological effects induced by ionizing radiation, but provides candidates for developing novel biomarkers of radiation injury.

3.3 Development of GDF-15 knocked down LM2 stable cell line

To establish a suitable cellular system to investigate a possible role of GDF-15 in breast cancer progression, we examined effect of GDF-15 silencing in LM2 cell lines.

To create GDF-15 expression silenced cell lines, we used plasmid vector construct kindly provided by Dr. Lambert (Anschutz Medical Campus, UCD-School of Medicine, Aurora, CO, USA). According to the manufacturer's protocol of OriGene shRNA (OriGene, Rockville, MD, USA) with different gene-specific shRNA expression pRS vectors (mouse GDF-15 shRNA) transfected into subconfluent LM2 cells for 48 hours. After transfection, puromycin (15 μg/ml) selection was commenced and maintained for two weeks to obtain the puromycin-resistant clones. Four clones were analyzed. The expectation was that a range of knockdown efficiencies will be achieved with at least 1 to 2 clones resulting in very high levels of knockdown. Expression of GDF-15 mRNA was measured by qRT-PCR. (We named the stable shGDF-15 expressing LM2 cells as "shGDF-15#1; #2; #3 or #4".) The puromycin-resistant stable transfected LM2 cells were propagated in the continual presence of puromycin (15 μg/ml).

Total RNA was isolated and used as a template to quantify the level of suppression of GDF-15 by qRT-PCR. GDF-15 expression data from several transfected clones is shown in Figure 3. Results showed that GDF-15 expression was indeed almost completely knocked down in

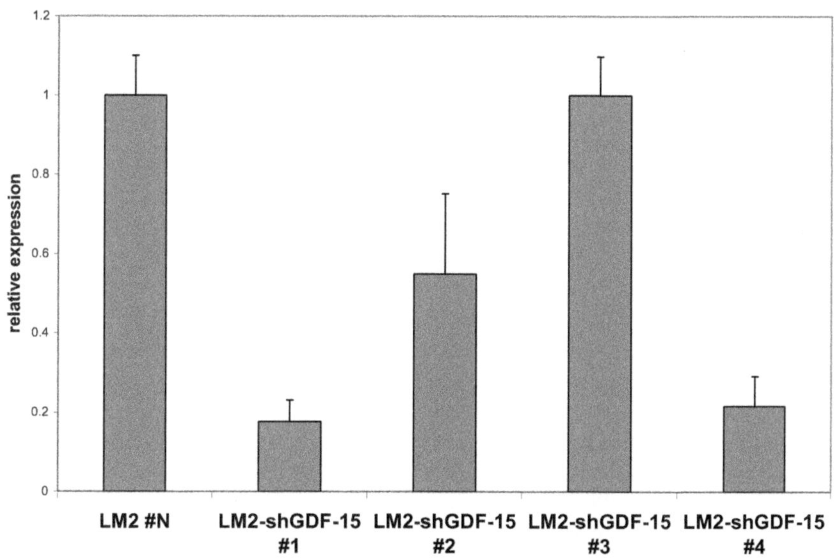

Fig. 3. The efficiency of down regulation of the GDF-15 gene was determined by qRT-PCR.

the transfected cells shGDF-15#1 and shGDF-15#4 at mRNA levels, whereas no effect was observed in scrambled shRNA-transfected control cells (LM2 #N). It can be seen that the expression of GDF-15 was most suppressed in the cell clone shGDF-15#1, which was generated from cells transfected with shRNA vector GDF-15#1. Therefore, the clone LM2-

shGDF-15#1 was used for further investigation of the involvement of GDF-15 in the cellular response to radiation.

The effect of 2 Gy exposure on expression of GDF-15 was almost completely abolished in GDF-15 silenced LM2 when compared with LM2#N + 2 Gy IR, as see on Figure 4 (2Gy induced elevation of GDF-15 in LM2#N: GDF-15 201%, LM2-shGDF-15#1: GDF-15 119,31%, was measured , respectively $p<0.05$).

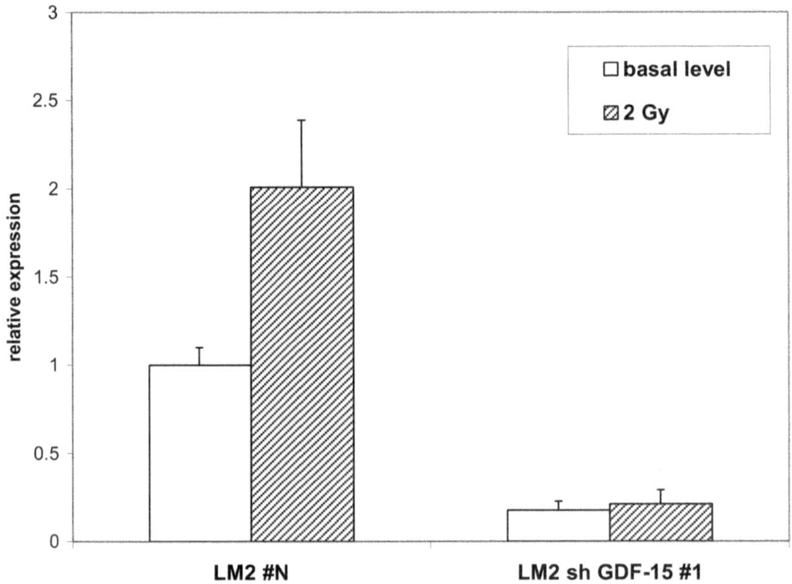

Fig. 4. 2 Gy induced expressional changes of GDF-15 measured by real time qRT-PCR.

3.4 Effect of GDF-15 silencing on survival of LM2 cells

In human colorectal HCT-116 cells, knockdown of GDF-15 impairs cell growth and survival [Baek et al, 2001]. Overexpression of GDF-15 in sense GDF-15 cells enhanced basal and indomethacin stimulated apoptosis, whereas the antisense GDF-15 exhibited an attenuated response to indomethacin treatment. Knockdown of GDF-15 in nasopharyngeal NPC cells resulted in growth delay and a reduction of clonogenic survival in response to radiation [Chang et al, 2007].

To gain a better understanding of how GDF-15 is involved in radiation response in mammary carcinoma cells, we determined the effects of stable knockdown of GDF-15 on radioresistance through expression of shRNA targeting GDF-15. In our study clonogenic survival assays further demonstrated that suppression of GDF-15 increased the sensitivity of LM2 shGDF-15#1 cells to radiation doses of up to 2 Gy (Figure 5). Our results suggest that cells with reduced GDF-15 expression were sensitive to radiation-induced cell death (Figure 5, $p<0.05$, LM2#N vs. LM2-shGDF-15#1). For statistical analysis Pearson's t test were used. Differences were accepted as statistically significant if $p<0.05$. These results further validate the specific role of GDF-15 pathway in regulation of radioresistance, and suggest that high level of expression of GDF-15 may be required for radioresistance of breast cancer cells.

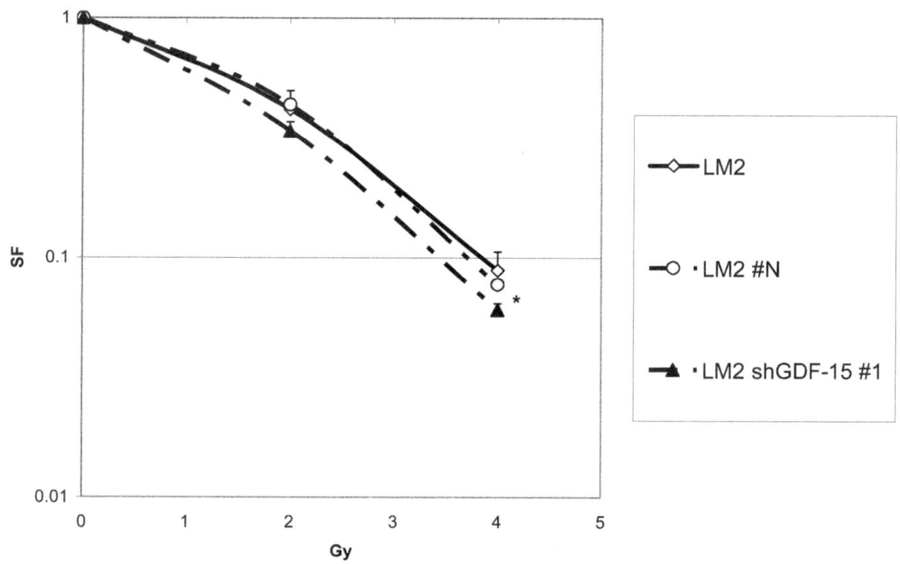

Fig. 5. Clonogenic survivals of irradiated LM2 cells after stable shGDF-15#1 transfection. Clonogenic survival was measured after stable transfection with GDF-15-specific shRNA (shGDF-15#1) in combination with irradiation at 2 Gy and 4 Gy. To examine the additional effects of irradiation all values of clonogenic survival at 0 Gy were set arbitrarily at 1. GDF-15 depleted cells showed significant increased radiosensitivity, after irradiation with 2 Gy or 4 Gy, respectively. Data represent the average values (± SE) of at least three independent experiments. (* $p < 0.05$).

3.5 Effect of GDF-15 silencing on in vivo tumor growth

The LM2 mammary adenocarcinoma and Balb/c mice was used for tumor growth delay assay. The mice were all female and 10 weeks old at the start of treatment. Exponentially growing cells cultured in DMeM medium supplemented with 10% fetal bovine serum were washed in PBS buffer and inoculated subcutaneously into the right flank. The growth delay assay was performed when the LM2 tumor reached 2 mm in average diameter, (6 days after inoculation).

In order to investigate the relevance of GDF-15 expression in tumor development, we examined whether GDF-15 silencing by shGDF-15 affects tumor growth in vivo. We used stable transfected LM2 shGDF-15#1 cell line or empty vector control LM2#N cells. The proliferation rate of LM2#N, and LM2-shGDF-15#1 cells, in vitro, was not affected significantly by GDF-15 expression and was comparable to the proliferation rate of the parental control cell line (Figure 6a).

We then analyzed whether GDF-15 silencing could affect the tumor growth capacity of these cells in vivo. The GDF-15 silencing clones LM2-shGDF-15#1 and the control LM2#N were injected subcutaneously into the flanks of the Balb/C mice. Tumor growth was observed and measured over a time period of 4 weeks (Figure 6b). Growth was delayed in GDF-15 knockdown cells, while the cells of the control pool retained high proliferative properties. Since the proliferation rate of GDF-15 silencing cells in vitro was almost similar to the proliferation rate of the control cells, inhibition of tumorigenicity by silencing of GDF-15 observed in vivo might involve in part a paracrine effect of GDF-15 on the host cells.

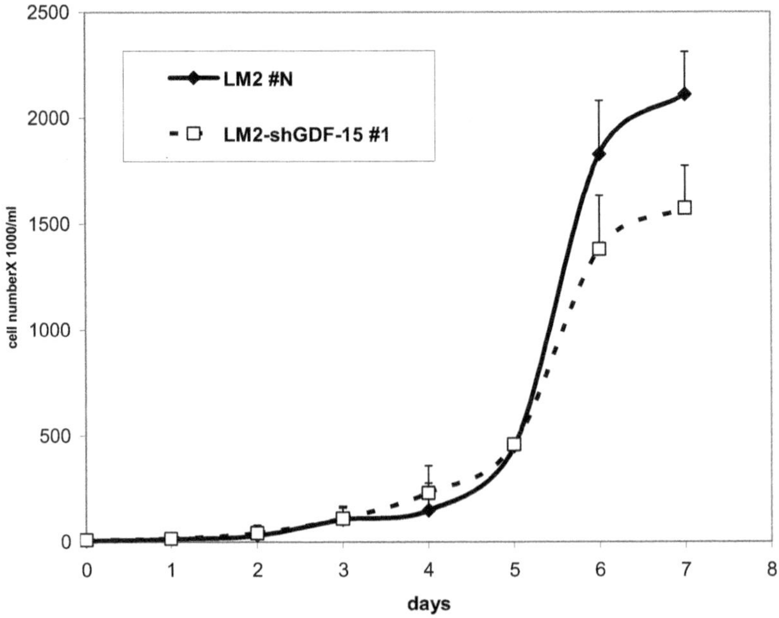

Fig. 6. a Effect of GDF-15 expression on cell growth in vitro.

Cells numbers were determined by manual counting using hemocytometer. Data are expressed as a mean± SE measured from three independent experiments but the difference on growing rate was not statistically significant.

In agreement with our result, Boyle et al. reported that melanoma cell lines and metastatic melanomas expressed larger amounts of GDF-15 than melanocytes, nevi, and primary lesions of melanoma. Knockdown of GDF-15 expression in three melanoma cell strains tested resulted in a significant decrease in tumorigenicity but did not affect anchorage-independent growth of the cells. The authors demonstrated that, in melanoma cells, expression of GDF-15 was at least partially dependent on the mitogen-activated protein kinase (MAPK) pathway and that stem cell factor–mediated c-Kit activation enhanced the level of GDF-15 [Boyle et al., 2009]. The decrease in GDF-15 levels by shRNA constructs reduced melanoma tumorigenesis, but did not alter cultured cell growth, suggesting a unique function other than growth control. GDF-15 may positively affect tumor progression via the Src-dependent transactivation of ErbB family receptors. Any activation of ErbB family tyrosine kinases by GDF-15 was likely to promote the ability of tumor cells to activate oncogenic signaling, most notably signaling of Akt and MAPKs in SK-BR-3 human breast cancer cells [Park et al., 2010].

In contrast, Baek and co- workers described an anti-tumorigenic function of GDF-15 ectopically expressed in the colon carcinoma cell line HCT-116 [Baek et al., 2001]. Ectopic expression of GDF-15 in the glioblastoma cell line LN-Z308, which are insensitive to GDF-15 mediated growth suppression in vitro, completely abolished tumorigenicity in vivo [Albertoni et al., 2002]. Additionally, GDF-15 expression in MCF-7 cells could directly inhibit tumor growth in an orthotopic tumor model using MCF-7 cells that overexpress GDF-15 [Martinez et al., 2006].

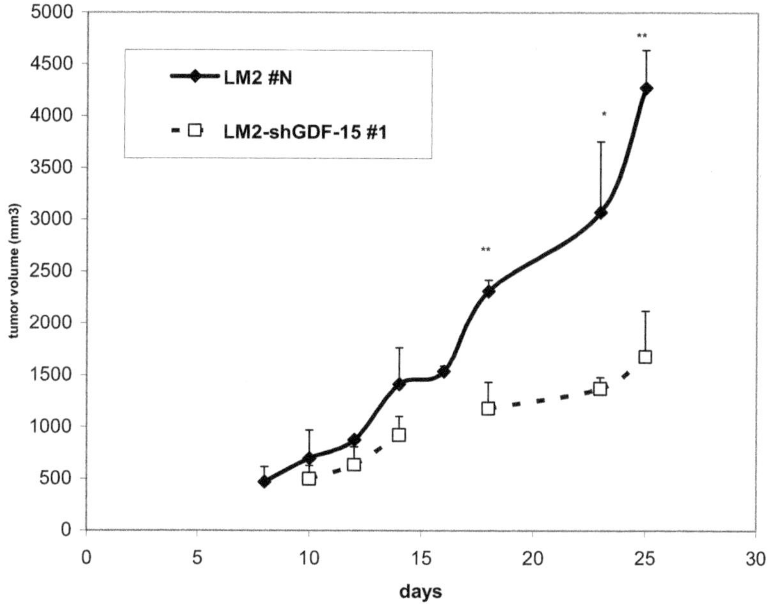

Fig. 6. b Effect of GDF-15 expression on tumor growth in vivo.

For statistical analysis Pearson's t test were used. Differences were accepted as statistically significant if $^*p<0.05$ and $^{**}p<0,001$

We speculated that the inhibitory or tumor promoter effect of GDF-15 on different tumor cell growth might be due to a defect in the TGF-β/Smad signaling pathway or the presence of the wild type p53 mediated cascade.

3.6 Therapeutic efficiency of combined radiotherapy with stable overexpression of shGDF-15 in preclinical mouse mammary tumor model

Irradiation was carried out using a cobalt-60 source at a dose rate of 0.45 Gy/min-, the total given dose was 4 Gy. For the growth delay assay, mice were given local irradiation. The two dimensions of each tumor were measured every second day with digital calipers, and the tumor volume was estimated using the formula $\Pi/6 \times w1 \times w2^2$ product of the longest (w1) and shortest (w2) dimensions.

To assess the long-term consequences of GDF-15 depletion in LM2 shGDF-15#1 cells on radiosensitivity, 4 Gy local exposure was applied, followed by implantation into Balb/c mice, to monitor the tumor growth. Cells depleted of GDF-15 showed no difference in tumor-forming capacity compared with LM2#N control cells (Figure 7), consistently with the modest in vitro effect. However, significant radiation-delayed tumor growth was observed compared with unirradiated LM2-shGDF-15#1 cells. The cytotoxic effect of 4 Gy exposure was significantly enhanced in GDF-15 depleted LM2 cells ($p<0.05$ in one-way ANOVA).

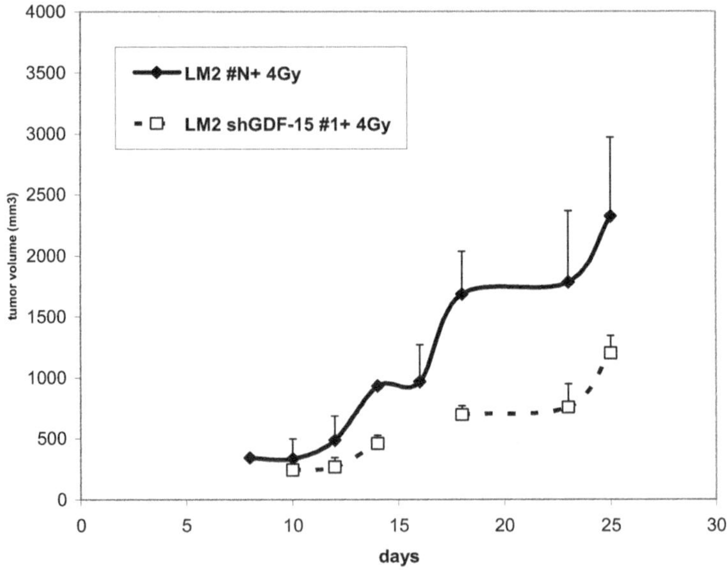

Fig. 7. Enhanced cytotoxicity and antitumor activity of a combination of GDF-15 silencing and ionizing radiation.

LM2 #N or LM2-shGDF-15#1 syngrafts grown in Balb/c mice were treated with ionizing radiation and tumor growth was monitored. A week after LM2 (5x105cell/50□l) cell injection, animals were give radiation treatment (4 Gy).

4. Conclusion

In order to investigate the role of GDF-15 in the cellular response to ionizing radiation, a cell line in which GDF-15 expression was silenced by shRNA interference was generated. In summary, in the present study we were able to demonstrate that GDF-15 silencing combined with irradiation has additive effects on clonogenic survival in-vitro, and the tumor growth delay in vivo. Furthermore, we showed that silencing of GDF-15 with shRNA causes radiosensitization of LM2 cells. This suggests that GDF-15 is an attractive target to improve the efficacy of radiotherapy. Additional radiobiological studies are necessary to investigate the role of GDF-15 and its association with radiosensitivity of other tumor cell lines.

Based on careful dissection of the complicated series of signaling changes within multiple pathways, it may in the future be possible to rationally combine multiple inhibitors of these processes to block cell survival, including inhibition of DNA damage sensing, receptor activation, paracrine ligand evolution, and intracellular signaling pathway, to achieve a better therapeutic response to radiotherapy.

5. Acknowledgment

This work was supported by the following grants: the European Union NOTE project (FP6-036465/2006), Hungarian OTKA K77766 and ETT 827-1/2009. The authors appreciate the expert technical assistance of Ms. Mária Frigyesi and Ms. Rita Lőkös.

6. References

Albertoni, M., Shaw, P.H., Nozaki, M., Godard, S., Tenan, M., Hamou, M.F., Fairlie, D.W., Breit, S.N., Paralkar, V.M., de Tribolet, N., van Meir, E.G., & Hegi, M.E. (2002). Anoxia induces macrophage inhibitory cytokine-1 (MIC-1) in glioblastoma cells independently of p53 and HIF-1. Oncogene, Vol. 21, No. 27, 4212–4219.

Amundson, S.A., Lee, R.A., Koch-Paiz, C.A., Bittner, M.L., Meltzer, P., Trent, J.M. and Fornace, A.J. Jr. (2003). Differential responses of stress genes to low dose-rate γ irradiation. Mol Cancer Res, Vol. 1, No. 6, 445-452.

Anscher, M.S., Peters, W.P., Reisenbichler, H., Petros, W.P., & Jirtle, R.L. (1993). Transforming growth factor beta as a predictor of liver and lung fibrosis after autologous bone marrow transplantation for advanced breast cancer. N Engl J Med, Vol. 328, No. 22, 1592–1598.

Balaban, N., Moni, J., Shannon, M., Dang, L., Murphy, E., & Goldkorn, T. (1996). The effect of ionizing radiation on signal transduction: antibodies to EGF receptor sensitize A431 cells to radiation. Biochimica et Biophysica Acta-Molecular Cell Research, Vol. 1314, No. 1-2, 147–156.

Baek, S.J., Horowitz, J.M. & Eling, T.E. (2001). Molecular cloning and characterization of human nonsteroidal anti-inflammatory drug-activated gene promoter. Basal transcription is mediated by Sp1 and Sp3. J Biol Chem, Vol. 276, No. 36, (Jul. 2001), 33384-33392.

Baek, S.J., Kim, J.S., Jackson, F.R., Eling, T.E., McEntee, M.F., & Lee, S.H. (2004). Epicatechin gallate-induced expression of NAG-1 is associated with growth inhibition and apoptosis in colon cancer cells. Carcinogenesis, Vol. 25, No. 12, (Aug. 2004), 2425-2432.

Baek, S.J., Kim, J.S., Moore, S.M., Lee, S.H., Martinez, J., & Eling, T.E. (2005). Cyclooxygenase inhibitors induce the expression of the tumor suppressor gene EGR-1, which results in the up-regulation of NAG-1, an antitumorigenic protein. Mol Pharmacol, Vol. 67, No. 2, (Oct. 2004), 356-364.

Baek, K.E., Yoon, S.R., Kim, J.T., Kim, K.S., Kang, S.H., Yang, Y., Lim, J.S., Choi, I., Nam, M.S., Yoon, M., Lee, H.G. (2009). Upregulation and secretion of macrophage inhibitory cytokine-1 (MIC-1) in gastric cancers. Clin Chim Acta, Vol. 401, No. 1-2, (Dec. 2008), 128–133.

Bauskin, A.R., Brown, D.A., Junankar, S., Rasiah, K.K., Eggleton, S., Hunter, M., Liu, T., Smith, D., Kuffner, T., Pankhurst, G.J., Johnen, H., Russell, P.J., Barret, W., Stricker, P.D., Grygiel, J.J., Kench, J.G., Henshall, S.M., Sutherland, R.L., & Breit, S.N. (2005). The propeptide mediates formation of stromal stores of PROMIC-1: role in determining prostate cancer outcome. Cancer Res, Vol. 65, No. 6, 2330–2336.

Bauskin, A.R., Brown, D.A., Kuffner, T., Johnen, H., Luo, X.W., Hunter, M., & Breit, S.N. (2006). Role of macrophage inhibitory cytokine-1 in tumorigenesis and diagnosis of cancer. Cancer Res, Vol. 66, No. 10, 4983–4986.

Boyle, G.M., Pedley, J., Martyn, A. C., Banducci, K.J., Strutton, G.M., Brown, D.A., Breit, S.N., & Parsons, P.G. (2009). Macrophage inhibitory cytokine-1 is overexpressed in malignant melanoma and is associated with tumorigenicity. Journ Invest Dermatol, Vol. 129, No. 2, (Aug. 2008), 383-391.

Brown, D.A., Ward, R.L., Buckhaults, P., Liu, T., Romans, K.E., Hawkins, N.J., Bauskin, A.R., Kinzler, K.W., Vogelstein, B., & Breit, S.N. (2003). MIC-1 serum level and genotype: associations with progress and prognosis of colorectal carcinoma. Clin Cancer Res, Vol. 9, No. 7, 2642–2650.

Buckhaults, P., Rago, C., St Croix, B., Romans, K.E., Saha, S., Zhang, L., Vogelstein, B., & Kinzler, K.W. (2001). Secreted and cell surface genes expressed in benign and malignant colorectal tumors. Cancer Res, Vol. 61, No. 19, 6996–7001.

Calaf, G.M., & Hei, T.K. (2004). Ionizing radiation induces alterations in cellular proliferation and c-myc, c-jun and c-fos protein expression in breast epithelial cells. Int J Oncol, Vol. 25, No. 6, 1859-1866.

Cekanova, M., Lee, S.H., Donnell, R.L., Sukhthankar, M., Eling, T.E., Fischer, S.M., & Baek, S.J. (2009). Nonsteroidal anti-inflammatory drug-activated gene-1 expression inhibits urethane-induced pulmonary tumorigenesis in transgenic mice. Cancer Prev Res, Vo. 2, No. 5, (Apr. 2009), 450-458.

Chaudhry, M.A., Chodosh, L.A., McKenna, W.G., & Muschel, R.J. (2003). Gene expression profile of human cells irradiated in G1 and G2 phases of cell cycle. Cancer Lett, Vol. 195, No. 2, 221-233.

Chen, S.J., Karan, D., Johansson, S.L., Lin, F.F., Zeckser, J., Singh, A.P., Batra, S.K., & Lin, M.F. (2007). Prostate-derived factor as a paracrine and autocrine factor for the proliferation of androgen receptor-positive human prostate cancer cells. Prostate, Vol. 67, No. 5, 557–571.

Chen, Y., Williams, J., Ding, I., Hernady, E., Liu, W., Smudzin, T., Finkelstein, J.N., Rubin P., & Okunieff, P. (2002). Radiation pneumonitis and early circulatory cytokine markers. Semin Radiat Oncol, Vol. 12, No. 1, 26–33.

Contente, A., Dittmer, A., Koch, M.C., Roth, J., & Dobbelstein, M. (2002). A polymorphic microsatellite that mediates induction of PIG3 by p53. Nat Genet, Vol. 30, No. 3, (feb. 2002), 315-320.

Cucinotta, F.A., Dicello, J.F., Nikjoo, H., & Cherubini, R. (2002). Computational model of the modulation of gene expression following DNA damage. Radiat Prot Dosimetry, Vol. 99, No. 1-4, 85-90.

Ding, L.H., Shingyoji, M., Chen, F., Hwang, J.J., Burma, S., Lee, C., Cheng, J.F., & Chen, D.J. (2005). Gene expression profiles of normal human fibroblasts after exposure to ionizing radiation: a comparative study of low and high doses. Radiat Res, Vol. 164, No. 1, 17-26.

Dumont, N., & Arteaga, C.L. (2003). Targeting the TGF beta signaling network in human neoplasia. Cancer cell, Vol. 3, No. 6, 531–536.

Galli, S., Colombo, L., Vanzuli, S., Daroqui, M.C., del Carmen Vidal, M., Jasnis, M.A., Sacerdote de Lustig, E., & Eijan, A.M. (2000). Characterization of a fibroblastoid mammary carcinoma cell line (LM2) originated from a mouse adenocarcinoma. Int J Oncol, Vol. 17, No. 6, 1259-1265.

Goldkorn, T., Balaban, N., Shannon, M., & Matsukuma, K. (1997). EGF receptor phosphorylation is affected by ionizing radiation. Biochimica et Biophysica Acta-Molecular Cell Research, Vol. 1358, No. 3, 289–99.

Hegyesi, H., Colombo, L., Pállinger, E., Tóth, S., Boer, K., Molnár, V., Falus, A. (2007). Impact of systemic histamine deficiency on the crosstalk between mammary adenocarcinoma and T cells. J Pharmacol Sci, Vol. 105, No. 1, 66-73.

Helland, A., Johnsen, H., Frøyland, C., Landmark, H.B., Saetersdal, A.B., Holmen, M.M., Gjertsen, T., Nesland, J.M., Ottestad, W., Jeffrey, S.S., Ottestad, L.O., Rodningen, O.K., Sherlock, G., & Børresen-Dale, A.L. (2006). Radiation-induced effects on gene expression: an in vivo study on breast cancer. Radiother Oncol, Vol. 80, No. 2, (Aug. 2006), 230–235.

Hsiao, E.C., Koniaris, L.G., Zimmers-Koniaris, T., Sebald, S.M., Huynh, T.V., & Lee, S.J. (2000). Characterization of growth-differentiation factor 15, a transforming growth factor beta superfamily member induced following liver injury. Mol. Cell Biol, Vol. 20, No. 10, 3742–3751.

Huh, S.J., Chung, C.Y., Sharma, A., & Robertson, G.P. (2010). Macrophage inhibitory cytokine-1 regulates melanoma vascular development. Am J Pathol, Vol. 176, No. 6, (Apr. 2010), 2948-2957.

Jutooru, I., Chadalapaka, G., Chintharlapalli, S., Papineni, S., & Safe, S. (2009). Induction of apoptosis and nonsteroidal anti-inflammatory drug-activated gene 1 in pancreatic cancer cells by a glycyrrhetinic acid derivative. Mol Carcinog, Vol. 48, No. 8, 692-702.

Kim, K.K., Lee, J.J., Yang, Y., You, K.H., & Lee, J.H. (2008). Macrophage inhibitory cytokine-1 activates AKT and ERK-1/2 via the transactivation of ErbB2 in human breast and gastric cancer cells. (2008). Carcinogenesis, Vol. 29, No. 4, (Feb. 2008), 704-712.

Kelly, J.A., Lucia M.S., & Lambert J.R. (2009). p53 controls prostate-derived factor/macrophage inhibitory cytokine/NSAID-activated gene expression in response to cell density, DNA damage and hypoxia through diverse mechanisms. Cancer Lett, Vol. 277, No. 1, (Dec. 2009), 38-47.

Klos, K.S., Wyszomierski, S.L., Sun, M., Tan, M., Zhou, X., Li, P., Yang, W., Yin, G., Hittelman, W.N., & Yu, D. (2006). ErbB2 increases vascular endothelial growth factor protein synthesis via activation of mammalian target of rapamycin/p70S6K leading to increased angiogenesis and spontaneous metastasis of human breast cancer cells. Cancer Res, Vol. 66, No. 4, 2028-2037.

Koopmann, J., Buckhaults, P., Brown, D.A., Zahurak, M.L., Sato, N., Fukushima, N., Sokoll, L.J., Chan, D.W., Yeo, C.J., Hruban, R.H., Breit, S.N., Kinzler, K.W., Vogelstein, B., & Goggins, M. (2004). Serum macrophage inhibitory cytokine1 as a marker of pancreatic and other periampullary cancers. Clin Cancer Res, Vol. 10, No. 7, 2386–2392.

Lambert, J.R., Kelly, J.A., Shim, M., Huffer, W.E., Nordeen, S.K., Baek, S.J., Eling, T.E., Lucia, M.S. (2006). Prostate derived factor in human prostate cancer cells: gene induction by vitamin D via a p53-dependent mechanism and inhibition of prostate cancer cell growth. J Cell Physiol, Vol. 208, No. 3, (sep 2006) 566-74.

Lee, D.H., Yang, Y., Lee, S.J., Kim, K.Y., Koo, T.H., Shin, S.M., Song, K.S., Lee, Y.H., Kim, Y.J., Lee, J.J., Choi, I., & Lee, J.H. (2003). Macrophage inhibitory cytokine-1 induces the invasiveness of gastric cancer cells by up-regulating the urokinase-type plasminogen activator system. Cancer Res, Vol. 63, No. 15, 4648–4655.

Li, P.X., Wong, J., Ayed, A., Ngo, D., Brade, A.M., Arrowsmith, C., Austin, R.C., & Klamut, H.J. (2000). Placental transforming growth factor-beta is a downstream mediator of the growth arrest and apoptotic response of tumor cells to DNA damage and p53 overexpression. J Biol Chem, Vol. 275, No. 26, 20127–20135.

Li, Y.M., Zhou, B.P., Deng, J., Pan, Y., Hay, N., & Hung, M.C. (2005). A hypoxia-independent hypoxia-inducible factor-1 activation pathway induced by phosphatidylinositol-3 kinase/Akt in HER2 overexpressing cells. Cancer Res, Vol. 65, No. 8, 3257-3263.

Liu, T., Bauskin, A.R., Zaunders, J., Brown, D.A., Pankhurst, S., Russell, P.J., & Breit, S.N. (2003). Macrophage inhibitory cytokine 1 reduces cell adhesion and induces apoptosis in prostate cancer cells. Cancer Res, Vol. 63, No. 16, 5034–5040.

Martinez, J.M., Sali, T., Okazaki, R., Anna, C., Hollingshead, M., Hose, C., Monks, A., Walker, N.J., Baek, S.J., & Eling, T.E. (2006). Drug-induced expression of nonsteroidal anti-inflammatory drug-activated gene/macrophage inhibitory cytokine-1/ prostate-derived factor, a putative tumor suppressor, inhibits tumor growth. J Pharmacol Exp Ther, Vol. 318, No. 2, (May. 2006), 899–906.

Mercier, G., Berthault, N., Mary, J., Peyre, J., Antoniadis, A., Comet, J.-P., Cornuejols, A., Froidevaux, C., & Dutreix, M. (2004). Biological detection of low radiation doses by combining results of two microarray analysis methods. Nucleic Acids Res, Vol. 32, No. 1, e12.

Newman, D., Sakaue, M., Koo, J.S., Kim, K.S., Baek, S.J., Eling, T., & Jetten, A.M. (2003). Differential regulation of nonsteroidal anti-inflammatory drug-activated gene in normal human tracheobronchial epithelial and lung carcinoma cells by retinoids. Mol Pharmacol, Vol. 63, No. 3, 557-564.

Polyak, K., Xia, Y., Zweier, J.L., Kinzler, K.W., & Vogelstein, B. (1997). A model for p53-induced apoptosis. Nature, Vol. 389, No. 6648, 300-305.

Rohde, M., Daugaard, M., Jensen, M.H., Helin K., Nylandsted J., & Jäättelä M. (2005). Members of the heat-shock protein 70 family promote cancer cell growth by distinct mechanisms. Genes Dev, Vol. 19, No. 5, 570-582.

Roy, D., Calaf, G. & Hei, T.K. (2001). Profiling of differentially expressed genes induced by high linear energy transfer radiation in breast epithelial cells. Mol Carcinog, Vol. 31, No. 4, 192-203.

Rubin, P., Finkelstein, J.N., Siemann, D.W., Shapiro, D.L., van Houtte, P., & Penney, D.P. (1986). Predictive biochemical assays for late radiation effects. Int J Radiat Oncol Biol Phys, Vol. 12, No. 4, 469–476.

Senapati, S., Rachagani, S., Chaudhary, K., Johansson, S.L., Singh, R.K., & Batra, S.K. (2010). Overexpression of macrophage inhibitory cytokine-1 induces metastasis of human prostate cancer cells through the FAK-RhoA signaling pathway. Oncogene, Vol. 29, No. 9, (Nov. 2009), 1293-1302.

Selander, K.S., Brown, D.A., Sequeiros, G.B., Hunter, M., Desmond, R., Parpala, T., Risteli, J., Breit, S.N., Jukkola-Vuorinen, A. (2007), Serum macrophage inhibitory cytokine-1 concentrations correlate with the presence of prostate cancer bone metastases. Cancer Epidemiol Biomarkers Prev, Vol. 16, No.3, 532-537.

Tan, M., Wang, Y., Guan, K., & Sun, Y. (2000). PTGF-beta, a type beta transforming growth factor (TGF-beta) superfamily member, is a p53 target gene that inhibits tumor cell growth via TGF-beta signaling pathway. Proc Natl Acad Sci USA, Vol. 97, No. 1, 109–114.

Vallat, L., Magdelénat, H., Merle-Béral, H., Masdehors, P., de Montalk, G.P., Davi, F., Kruhoffer, M., Sabatier, L., Orntoft, T.F., & Delic, J. (2003). The resistance of B-CLL cells to DNA damage induced apoptosis defined by DNA microarrays. Blood, Vol. 101, No. 11, (Feb. 2003), 4598-4606.

Welsh, J.B., Sapinoso, L.M., Kern, S.G., Brown, D.A., Liu, T., Bauskin, A.R., Ward, R.L., Hawkins, N.J., Quinn, D.I., Russell, P.J., Sutherland, R.L., Breit, S.N., Moskaluk, C.A., Frierson, H.F. Jr., & Hampton, G.M. (2003). Large-scale delineation of secreted protein biomarkers overexpressed in cancer tissue and serum. Proc Natl Acad Sci USA, Vol. 100, No. 6, (Mar. 2003), 3410–3415.

Wilson, L.C., Baek, S.J., Call, A., & Eling, T.E. (2003). Nonsteroidal anti-inflammatory drug-activated gene (NAG-1) is induced by genistein through the expression of p53 in colorectal cancer cells. Intl. J. Cancer, Vol. 105, No. 6, 747–753.

Yamaguchi, K., Lee, S. H., Eling, T. E., & Baek, S.J. (2006). A novel peroxisome roliferator-activated receptor gamma ligand, MCC-555, induces apoptosis via posttranscriptional regulation of NAG-1 in colorectal cancer cells. Mol Cancer Ther, Vol. 5, No. 5, 1352-1361.

Yun Jung Park, Y.J., Lee H., & Lee, H.-J. (2010). Macrophage inhibitory cytokine-1 transactivates ErbB family receptors via the activation of Src in SK-BR-3 human breast cancer cells. BMB Rep, Vol. 43, No. 2, 91-96.

21

Sentinel Lymph Node Biopsy: Actual Topics

L.G. Porto Pinheiro[1], P.H.D. Vasques[1],
M. Maia[2], J.I.X. Rocha[3] and D.S. Cruz[3]
[1]*Department of Surgery, Faculty of Medicine, UFC, Fortaleza - Ceará,*
[2]*Biochemistry, Laboratory for experimental surgery*
Saul Goldenberg MD, Fortaleza - Ceará,
[3]*Faculty of Medicine, UFC, Fortaleza - Ceará,*
Brazil

1. Introduction

The incidence of female breast cancer has increased 0.5% since the year 2000, as reported by the International Agency Research on Cancer. This number is greater in developing countries due to the increase in life expectancy and change in behavior resulting in increased exposure to risk factors.

Lymph node staging is an early event carried out during initial patient evaluation in developed countries. Some 20% to 30% of all cases are diagnosed quite early (in situ lesions) DCIS; 79% of the patients diagnosed at stage I and II has negative axillary nodes; (Holland et al., 2001). These values are somewhat different in developing countries where more than 50% of the cases are diagnosed at advanced stages of the disease.

Increased survival rates have been reported lately. According to Parkin (Parkin et al., 2001), the overall survival rate is 91% after the first year and 65% after five years in Europe. These values increase to 96.8% after the first year in the United States. As primary prevention of breast cancer is not available as yet, early detection and treatment in the initial phase of the disease are, therefore, the most important measures for its control (INCA, 2009). Available diagnostic methods include mammography, breast ultrasonography and fine-needle aspiration biopsy among others (Moore et al., 1996; Morton et al., 1998).

Until 1990, the assessment of axillary status of a patient with breast cancer depended on the histopathologic examination of lymph nodes from complete axillary dissection. With the definition of the sentinel lymph node as the first one which receives the drainage of the tumoral area (Cabanas, 1977), it was possible to ensure means for the proper staging of the illness and the therapeutic approach establishing less invasive surgery techniques.

Currently, it is admitted that the presence of metastatic lymph nodes is the main predictor factor for prognosis of the breast malignant neoplasia course and subsequent therapeutic program. Lymph nodes are also valuable for staging breast cancer. In the recent past dissection of the axillary lymph nodes was required for this matter, resulting in a series of additional complications (Veronesi et al., 1999).

2. Sentinel lymph node biopsy on breast cancer surgery

The status of the axillary lymph nodes is one of the most important prognostic factors in women with early stage breast cancer. Histologic examination of lymph nodes is the most accurate method for assessing spread of disease to these nodes.

Axillary lymph node dissection (ALND) has traditionally been a routine component of the management of early breast cancer. The benefits of ALND include its impact on disease control (ie, axillary recurrence and survival), its prognostic value, and its role in treatment selection. However, the anatomic disruption caused by ALND may result in lymphedema, nerve injury, and shoulder dysfunction, which compromise functionality and quality of life.

ALND remains the standard approach for women who have clinically palpable axillary nodes or positive nodes confirmed by methods such as ultrasound guided fine needle aspiration. For patients who have clinically negative axillary lymph nodes, sentinel lymph node biopsy (SLNB) is a less morbid method of staging the axilla than ALND.

Indications for and outcomes of SLNB will be reviewed here.

The sentinel lymph node (SLN) technique is based upon the observation that tumor cells migrating from a primary tumor metastasize to one or a few lymph nodes (LNs) before involving other LNs. Injection of vital blue dye and/or radiolabeled colloid around the area of the tumor permits identification of a SLN in the majority of patients, and its status accurately predicts the status of the remaining regional LNs.

In patients with clinically node negative breast cancer, SLNB identifies patients without axillary node involvement, thereby obviating the need for more extensive surgery. Several studies have shown that the risk of arm morbidity, particularly lymphedema, sensory loss, and shoulder abduction deficits, is significantly less for SLNB than with standard axillary dissection. As an example, the risk of lymphedema after 12 months was reported as 2 percent after SLNB alone as compared with 13 percent after SLNB with axillary lymph node dissection (ALND) in the American College of Surgeons Oncology Group (ACOSOG) Z-0011 trial.

Most surgeons and major cancer centers have adopted SLNB as a standard means of axillary nodal assessment. In a study of over 490,000 women with early breast cancer from the National Cancer Database, use of SLNB increased from 27 to 66 percent between 1998 and 2005 in the United States. Similar trends have been reported from Canada and the United Kingdom. SLNB is endorsed as an alternative to ALND for the diagnosis of axillary metastases in patients with clinically node-negative early breast cancer in guidelines from the American Society of Clinical Oncology (ASCO), the International Expert Consensus Panel on the Primary Therapy of Early Breast Cancer, and others.

Despite variability in selection criteria and technique, a SLN is consistently identified in approximately 96 percent of cases, and predicts the status of the remaining axillary LNs in ≥95 percent of cases in most series. The false negative rate of SLNB was originally reported as 5 to 10 percent (sensitivity 90 to 95 percent), but lower rates are attainable by experienced surgeons.

The greatest concern with SLNB is the potential of a false negative result, which could increase the potential for axillary recurrence. However, despite the approximately 5 to 10 percent false negative rate with SLNB found in studies in which completion ALND has been done, several series suggest that axillary recurrence rates are low after a negative SLNB alone in early stage breast cancer (range 0 to 4.5 percent). The details of key trials validating the SLNB are described below:

A landmark multicenter study of 443 patients with early breast cancer demonstrated that the SLNB technique could be learned and successfully applied by a diverse group of surgeons spanning private and academic practice. All patients underwent SLNB using radiolabeled colloid followed by completion ALND. At least one SLN was identified in 98 percent of cases and the predictive value of a negative SLN was 96 percent, with a false negative rate of 11 percent (sensitivity 88 percent). More intensive pathologic evaluation of the nodes in false negative cases with deeper sectioning of the sentinel node and immunohistochemical staining increased the yield of occult metastases in 18 percent of cases.

A systematic review, performed by the ASCO expert guidelines panel, included 69 eligible trials of SLNB in early stage breast cancer, representing 8059 patients. The SLN was identified using radiocolloid, blue dye, or both. SLN identification was successful in 95 percent of patients. The false negative rate was 7.3 percent (range 0 to 29 percent). The combination of radiocolloid and blue dye resulted in a significantly higher success rate in SLN mapping with a lower false negative rate as compared to blue dye alone.

The NSABP B-32 trial, published after the systematic review, enrolled 5611 patients with clinically negative nodes and compared SLNB followed by ALND versus SLNB followed by ALND only if the SLN was positive. Lymphatic mapping was successful in 97 percent, and the false-negative rate was 9.8 percent. No significant differences were observed in regional control, overall survival, or disease free survival between the groups at a median follow-up of almost eight years.

SLNB should be performed in most women with clinically node negative invasive or microinvasive breast cancer. SLNB can be omitted if the nodal information will not affect adjuvant treatment decisions. As an example, women ≥70 years of age who have a small (<2 cm) estrogen receptor-positive tumor and a clinically uninvolved axilla may be treated without a SLNB. Although older patients do not appear to be at increased risk of complications following axillary clearance, retrospective analyses and one randomised trial have questioned its value in older women with breast cancer (IBCSG, 1996). In a randomised trial, 473 women aged 60 or over. Interestingly in the ALMANAC trial (comparing sentinel node biopsy and standard axillary treatment), which used validated measures of patient reported quality of life and arm morbidity, older women (65 years and over) irrespective of axillary management had better quality of life outcomes at all stages of the 18-month follow-up than younger women (Fleissig et al, 2006).

SLNB should be performed in women with extensive ductal carcinoma in situ (DCIS), who are undergoing mastectomy. A SLNB will not be possible after mastectomy if invasive disease is found on final pathology, necessitating an axillary dissection for staging purposes. (See 'Ductal carcinoma in situ' below.)

When a SLNB is not successful or when clinically suspicious nodes are present in the axilla after all sentinel lymph nodes have been removed, the surgeon should perform an axillary dissection for staging purposes and to ensure locoregional control.

For women with clinically suspicious lymph nodes, preoperative axillary ultrasound (US) with fine needle aspiration (FNA) or core biopsy of suspicious areas provides a means to identify patients who have positive nodes, and thus need axillary lymph node dissection (ALND) rather than a SLNB. As an example, in a series of 653 consecutive patients, the preoperative diagnosis rate of axillary disease was 23 percent using axillary US and FNA, thereby avoiding the need for a second operation in 150 women. The efficacy of this approach is somewhat variable between centers because the accuracy of US examination is operator dependent.

Approximately 40 percent of patients with a positive sentinel lymph node (SLN) will be found to have residual disease in the axilla SLN metastases are categorized as isolated tumor cells, micrometastases or macrometastases, depending on the size of the largest tumor deposit in the SN. Treatment options will depend on the clinical situation and include completion axillary lymph node dissection (ALND) or axillary radiation therapy (RT).

Isolated tumor cells — The seventh edition of the American Joint Committee on Cancer (AJCC) tumor node metastasis (TNM) staging system for breast cancer includes a stringent classification for lymph node findings of isolated tumor cell clusters and single cells. Small clusters of cells not greater than 0.2 mm, or nonconfluent or nearly confluent clusters of cells not exceeding 200 cells in a single histologic lymph node cross section are classified as isolated tumor cells and are considered node negative. Malignant cells in regional lymph node(s) no greater than 0.2 mm (detected by H&E or IHC including ITC) are designated as pN0(i+). Isolated tumor cells are not considered an indication for further axillary surgery, radiation treatment or adjuvant systemic therapy.

SLNB allows the pathologist to perform a more detailed study of one or a few LNs that are most likely to contain metastases, compared to the 15 to 25 LNs obtained with ALND. This has the potential to improve staging accuracy, but has led to an increase in the identification of micrometastatic nodal involvement. For this reason, there is a separate designation of pN1mi (>0.2 mm and no greater than 2.0 mm) to indicate micrometastases alone.

Although it seems intuitive that the finding of axillary micrometastases should worsen prognosis, most studies show no reduction in patient survival compared to those without micrometastases. However, some analyses do suggest a negative impact of micrometastases on breast cancer outcomes.

There is debate about the prognostic value of the size of the SLN micrometastases (≤0.2 mm versus larger) in predicting the likelihood of involvement of axillary non-SLNs. Guidelines from ASCO and NCCN recommend that routine completion ALND be carried out for micrometastases detected on SLNB with standard hematoxylin and eosin (H&E) examination. However, the indications for a completion ALND for micrometastases are the subject of controversy.

The 2005 American Society of Clinical Oncology (ASCO) guidelines and 2010 National Comprehensive Cancer Network (NCCN) guidelines recommend that routine completion ALND be carried out for patients with SLNB macrometastases (≥2 mm). However, the indications for a completion ALND in patients with <3 positive sentinel nodes is the subject of controversy.

Role of IHC and RT-PCR in sentinel node evaluation — Occult micrometastases refers to nodal metastases that are not seen on hematoxylin and eosin (H&E) examination but are detected only by immunohistochemistry (IHC) or reverse transcriptase polymerase chain reaction (RT-PCR). The significance of occult micrometastases in terms of surgical management and patient outcome appears to be negligible.

Preliminary results from the American College of Surgeons Oncology Group (ACOSOG) study Z0010, a prospective multicenter study of 5210 patients with almost eight year follow up, confirm that IHC-detected metastases have no significant impact on overall survival. Thus, routine IHC or PCR is not recommended for the evaluation of SLNs in guidelines published by ASCO, NCCN, and others. Histologically negative nodes that are IHC or RT-PCR-positive are classified as pN0 disease in the TNM staging system for breast cancer.

Role of IHC in invasive lobular carcinoma – Although routine IHC staining with cytokeratin is not indicated for most breast cancers, it can be helpful for examination of the sentinel nodes in patients with invasive lobular carcinoma since the morphology of lobular cancer can be difficult to detect on H&E of axillary lymph nodes. In general, IHC should be used to definitively diagnose an area that is suspicious for, but not diagnostic of, lymph node metastases on H&E rather than as a routine method of evaluating nodes in cases of invasive lobular cancer.

When should completion axillary dissection be performed? The need for completion axillary lymph node dissection (ALND) is dependent upon the SLNB findings. There are some clear indications and some settings in which optimal surgical approach is controversial.

There is general acceptance for the following approaches:

For patients with a negative sentinel lymph node biopsy (SLNB), completion ALND is not indicated.

Patients with SLNB showing isolated tumor cells only are considered node negative and completion ALND is not indicated.

For patients with a positive SLNB showing micrometastases or macrometastases in three or more nodes, detected with standard hematoxylin and eosin (H&E) examination, completion ALND is recommended for staging purposes and to ensure local control. The timing of the procedure (ie, immediate [one operation] versus delayed [two separate operations]) does not seem to impact the total lymph node yield or the rate of long-term complications (particularly lymphedema).

In contrast, the need for a completion ALND is controversial in patients with a positive SLNB showing micrometastases or macrometastases in less than three nodes, detected with standard hematoxylin and eosin (H&E) examination. The SLN is the sole tumor-bearing node in up to 60 percent of cases overall, and in almost 90 percent of patients who harbor only micrometastatic disease. These observations have led to speculation that completion ALND may not be necessary in selected patients with a positive SLNB in less than three nodes because the need for systemic therapy is established and the risk of an axillary recurrence appears to be low.

The ACOSOG Z-0011 trial was designed to address the need for completion ALND for patients with T1 or T2 tumors that were clinically node negative and had less than three positive sentinel nodes; all patients were treated with radiation to the breast. Target accrual was 1900 patients. The study closed prematurely because of low accrual and low event rate after enrolling 425 patients in the SLNB alone arm and 388 in the SLNB plus ALND. The majority of patients had estrogen receptor positive tumors. At a median follow-up of 6.3 years, there were no significant differences between the SLNB plus ALND group versus the SLNB alone group in the locoregional recurrence rate (in breast recurrence 3.7 versus 2.1 percent; nodal recurrence 0.6 versus 1.3 percent), overall survival (91.9 versus 92.5 percent) or disease free survival (82.2 versus 83.8 percent). Estrogen receptor status and adjuvant systemic therapy were independent predictors of survival.

Based upon the apparent lack of benefit and low risk of events in this trial, some have suggested that completion ALND is not necessary for women with T1 or T2 tumors that are clinically node negative with less than three positive SLNs who will be treated with whole breast radiation, particularly in women with estrogen receptor positive tumors. Others prefer to wait for results from two ongoing randomized trials studying the benefit of ALND for clinically node negative women with positive SLNs: the EORTC 10981-22023 AMAROS trial; and Trial 23-01 of the International Breast Cancer Study Group (IBCSG).

Until more data are available, the need for completion ALND in clinically node negative women with less than three positive SLNs who will be treated with radiation to the breast is best resolved on a case-by-case basis, taking into account the patient's other risk factors and comorbidities and patient preference. When completion ALND is omitted in patients with a positive SLNB, radiotherapy is recommended.

Predictive nomograms — SLNB followed by a completion ALND results in significantly greater arm morbidity than SLNB alone. Because the majority of patients with a SLNB metastases will not have additional positive nodes on completion ALND, several predictive nomograms for estimating the risk of additional positive nodes have been developed in an effort to spare women from unnecessary and potentially morbid surgery. These nomograms include both clinical and pathologic features, such as the size and/or number of the SLN metastases, extranodal extension, and the size and/or presence of lymphovascular invasion in the primary tumor. A retrospective analysis of 319 patients with a positive SLNB who underwent completion axillary dissection compared the performance of four different nomograms. None of the nomograms was sufficiently reliable for clinical use.

Sentinel lymph node biopsy (SLNB) remains controversial in selected clinical settings.

Male breast cancer — The vast majority of published studies of SLNB for breast cancer are in women. Data are limited in men with breast cancer (MBC), because it is uncommon. A retrospective study of 30 men with breast cancer reported a 100 percent SLNB identification rate and a false negative rate of 0 percent. Prospective studies establishing the sensitivity and specificity of SLNB in MBC have not been carried out. However, the principles guiding SLNB in women appear to apply to men.

Due to the limited amount of data, the 2005 American Society of Clinical Oncology (ASCO) guidelines on SLNB did not make a specific recommendation about the use of SLNB in MBC, although it was deemed "acceptable".

Most studies have restricted SLNB to T1 or T2 breast cancers <5 cm in size, since larger tumors have a higher likelihood of positive axillary nodes. However, some studies have shown that SLNB is accurate in patients with T3 tumors and clinically negative axillae. Thus, many clinicians do not recognize large breast tumors as a contraindication to SLN dissection, as long as the axilla is clinically negative.

However, patients with T4 tumors (locally advanced) or inflammatory breast cancer are not considered candidates for SLNB. The false negative rate is high in patients with inflammatory breast cancer, presumably because of the presence of partially obstructed, functionally abnormal subdermal lymphatics.

The 2005 ASCO guidelines on SLNB did not recommend the routine use of SLNB in patients with locally advanced or inflammatory breast cancer for whom ALND was recommended to ensure locoregional control. Consensus recommendations from an International Expert Panel published in 2010 considered inflammatory breast cancer to be the one of the few absolute contraindications to SLNB. In addition, SLNB was not recommended for T4 tumors.

Many women with large primary breast tumors are offered neoadjuvant chemotherapy prior to definitive locoregional therapy. The optimal timing for sentinel lymph node biopsy (SLNB) in patients receiving neoadjuvant therapy has been debated, because some have reported a higher false negative rate for SLNB performed after induction therapy. Other uncontrolled studies support the accuracy of SLNB in such patients.

The 2005 ASCO guidelines concluded that there was insufficient information to guide the appropriate timing for SLNB in patients receiving preoperative systemic therapy. However, if prognostic information gained from examination of the axillary nodes is deemed valuable for planning locoregional treatment, SLNB can be considered before the institution of systemic therapy. Completion axillary dissection, if indicated, can be performed following chemotherapy at the time of definitive surgery. The ACOSOG trial Z1071, which is still accruing patients, is designed to answer the question of SLNB accuracy after neoadjuvant chemotherapy.

Studies that evaluated the functional anatomy of lymphatic drainage support the theory that all quadrants of the breast drain into the same lymph node(s). Thus, subareolar and intradermal (rather than peritumoral) injection of radiolabeled colloid or blue dye render SLNB feasible for patients with multicentric disease.

The success of SLNB for multicentric disease has been demonstrated in several studies. In a study of 142 women with multicentric breast cancer, SLNB was successful in 91 percent, with a false negative rate of 4 percent. However, the number of patients requiring completion ALND because of a positive SLN is higher in multicentric compared with unicentric disease. The likelihood of finding additional disease at the time of completion ALND is also higher with multicentric disease. The ASCO guidelines recommend SLNB as appropriate for patients with multicentric disease.

Most women with ductal carcinoma in situ (DCIS) do not require assessment of the axillary nodes, particularly if they are undergoing breast conserving therapy. However, women with DCIS may be candidates for SLN mapping if they are undergoing mastectomy, because the performance of SLNB will be impossible at a later time if invasive disease is found. An intact breast with its lymphatic plexus is necessary for injection of both the blue dye and the radioisotope tracers.

Some recommend that SLNB be considered in patients who are undergoing breast conserving therapy or mastectomy for DCIS only if the risk of node metastases is increased, as with extensive high-grade DCIS, a strong suspicion of invasive disease based upon ancillary imaging, or documented microinvasive disease in the core biopsy. However, if a lumpectomy is performed and invasive disease is identified, a SLNB can be done as a separate operation. This approach can minimize unnecessary morbidity, since SLNB can be associated with complications. SLNB is generally performed if microinvasion is found in the breast biopsy or if mastectomy is required for extensive or multifocal DCIS, where the risk of an occult invasive component is increased.

The finding of isolated tumor cell clusters (ie, pN0(i+)) in SLNs from patients with DCIS changes the clinical disease stage to stage IB in the seventh edition of the TNM staging system.

The safety and test performance of SLNB during pregnancy has not been fully evaluated. Supravital dyes such as isosulfan blue dye should not be administered to pregnant women. Available data suggests that the dose of radiation to the fetus is minimal using radiocolloid during SLNB. Nonetheless, 2005 guidelines from ASCO recommend against the use of SLNB in pregnant women with early stage breast cancer.

The feasibility of SLNB in women who have undergone other non-oncologic types of breast surgery such as reduction mammoplasty or augmentation with breast implants is unclear. The expert panel convened by ASCO did not make a recommendation for or against SLNB in women who have had breast reduction or augmentation because of insufficient data. They suggested that if SLNB were considered in this setting that it might best be performed with preoperative lymphoscintigraphy.

SLNB after axillary surgery has not been widely studied. In one retrospective series, a SLN could not be identified in 25 percent of 32 cases in which SLNB was attempted in women who had undergone prior axillary surgery. Guidelines from ASCO recommend against SLNB in women who have undergone prior axillary surgery. However, there are accumulating reports of successful second SLNB in patients with a local breast cancer recurrence following a previous SLNB and/or axillary dissection. This practice is becoming more frequently employed and further study is indicated, including the optimal interval before repeat sentinel node biopsy should be attempted. Lymphoscintigraphy should be performed if repeat sentinel node biopsy is planned, given that these patients often have alternate drainage patterns.

SLN techniques can identify non-axillary metastases in up to 43 percent of cases, depending upon the volume and type of colloid injected, injection technique, and primary tumor location and size. Whether or not this is useful remains controversial, since the majority of the data regarding treatment decisions and outcomes comes from evaluation of only axillary nodes.

Positive IM nodes are most common with medial tumors over 2 cm in size. The clinical relevance of finding and treating IM nodal disease in breast cancer is highly controversial.

Patients with multiple positive axillary nodes usually have the IM node chain included in the radiation field, if it can be safely undertaken without a significant dose to the heart. However, it remains unclear whether inclusion of the IM nodes in the treatment field is responsible for the survival benefit seen with chest wall radiation. Definitive demonstration of benefit for the treatment of IM nodes in the radiation field requires a clinical trial in which women are randomly assigned to IM-directed RT fields or not. Two such trials have completed accrual, and results are forthcoming: one sponsored by the EORTC (protocol 22922) and the other by the National Cancer Institute of Canada (protocol MA 20).

Patients with axillary node-negative disease will be found to have regional metastases to the IM nodes in 8 to 10 percent of cases. The diagnosis of positive IM nodes might benefit those patients who would otherwise not be candidates for adjuvant systemic therapy. Some have suggested that patients with primary IM nodal drainage on lymphoscintigraphy receive radiation treatment targeting the IM chain. However, many surgeons do not employ radiotracer injection and use only an intraoperative injection of blue dye to identify the sentinel nodes. Additional noninvasive methods for IM node assessment may be helpful, including MRI or PET scanning, although these imaging modalities are unable to definitively identify positive nodes.

There are also limitations to the SLN technique for identification of IM nodes. SLNB does not reliably identify involved IM LNs because of interference from radioactivity at the primary tumor site. There is a high rate of technical failure (20 to 39 percent) in patients with parasternal hot spots on lymphoscintigraphy. In addition, not all hot spots in the IM region represent tumor involvement.

In addition, the IM nodes are difficult to sample surgically if a positive hot spot is identified in this area. Although IM biopsy can be accomplished at the time of mastectomy by splitting the fibers of the pectoralis major, an IM node biopsy in a patient undergoing breast conserving surgery usually requires a second incision, which is cosmetically visible in many types of clothing. The procedure can be complicated by pneumothorax, pleural effusion or bleeding.

Not surprisingly, there is disagreement among major groups on the issue of surgical management of the IM nodes. There is no consensus on the need for IM nodal dissection in women with detection of an IM SLN. Internal mammary nodes are not routinely dissected in patients undergoing breast conserving therapy or mastectomy with axillary lymph node dissection. Thus, in the absence of definitive data, dissection of the IM nodes with sentinel lymph node biopsy should still be considered investigational.

Numerous case reports document identification of intramammary lymph nodes on SLNB, although few have explored the clinical significance of this finding. Intramammary LNs are present in 1 to 28 percent of women with breast cancer. Most series report a high likelihood of additional axillary nodal metastases when the intramammary nodes contain cancer.

If intramammary nodes contain tumor, they have the same prognostic significance as a positive axillary LN with respect to staging. ALND should be considered for women with a positive intramammary LN on SLNB, even if the axilla is clinically negative, because of the high rate of axillary LN involvement in these women.

Many studies have sought to determine the optimal technique for SLNB. Using a combination of isotope and blue dye for sentinel node localisation drastically reduces the rates of failed and false-negative procedures. In the ALMANAC study, in most patients both dye and isotope found the sentinel nodes, however, in approximately 10% of patients only one of the agents located the sentinel node. More importantly, in approximately 4% of patients the positive SLN was found by dye alone and in 3% by isotope alone; these would have been missed by relying on a single technique of localisation.

They have shown previously that replacement of the SLN by tumor significantly reduces the radioisotope uptake and may adversely affect intra-operative SLN identification. However, SLN identification using blue dye is not compromised by increased SLN tumor burden. The afferent lymphatic leading to the blocked node may be patent. The surgeon can identify the tumor-replaced node by following the blue lymphatic leading to the node. This result further suggests that a combination of blue dye and radioisotope should be used to optimise the localisation rate.

The ALMANAC study found that patient age, BMI, sentinel node visualisation on pre-operative lymphoscintiscan, tumor location, tumor size, tumor histology and presence of multifocality did not alter the false-negative rate. They have shown that high BMI adversely influences the successful mapping of SLNs. Patient age did not alter SLN localisation, though it has been reported in several other studies which have shown that accurate identification of the SLN decreases with increasing age as well as weight. The specific causes for mapping failure in overweight patients are unclear. Sentinel node identification may be difficult in obese women because of the higher content of subcutaneous and axillary adipose tissue. Furthermore, the increased fatty tissue may impede the flow of the tracer through the lymphatics in the breasts of these patients. Or the lymph nodes in obese patients may have undergone fatty degeneration reducing their capacity to concentrate the tracer. These findings, however, do not contraindicate SLNB in obese individuals as the rate of successful localisation remains high and unsuccessful mapping does not adversely affect their prognosis or treatment.

Arguments have been made in favour of pre-operative lymphoscintigraphy as a road map for surgeons. The ALMANAC results indicate that SLN visualisation on preoperative lymphoscintigraphy significantly improves the intra-operative SLN identification rate ($p<0.001$). If an SLN takes up enough radiocolloid to image with a camera, it should be easily detected with the intraoperative probe. Similar findings were reported by Birdwell et al.

They also found that tumors located in the upper outer quadrant had a higher SLN identification rate compared to other tumor locations. The simplest explanation relates to the transit distance for the blue dye or radioisotope from the peritumoral injection site to the axilla.

High false-negative rates may have a direct adverse impact on patient care including accurate staging, treatment decision making and long-term outcomes including survival. Clearly, the potential for both local as well as systemic under-treatment of patients increases as the false-negative rate increases. The ALMANAC study demonstrates a reduction in the predictive value of a negative SLNB in grade 3 tumors. Grade 3 tumors have a higher incidence of nodal metastases, thereby have an increased risk of lymphatic obstruction and re-routing of tracer leading to a false-negative result. Therefore, caution is required when applying the SLNB procedure in patients at considerably increased risk for lymph node positive disease.

The data from this study suggest that surgeons should not stop after finding just one SLN but should search thoroughly to be certain there are not more. This is important as the false-negative rate in patients who had multiple sentinel nodes (3 or more) removed was 1.1% compared with 10.1% in those with 1 sentinel node removed.

Then, sentinel node biopsy is a safe and accurate alternative to routine axillary dissection for patients with early stage breast cancer with clinically negative axillary nodes. The success and accuracy of sentinel node mapping in breast cancer is optimised by the combined use of blue dye and isotope. Body mass index >30, tumor location other than upper outer quadrant and non-visualisation of SLN on pre-operative lymphoscintiscan adversely affect the SLN identification rate. SLNB may not be appropriate for patients who have grade 3 tumors, and the decision to perform the procedure should be determined on the basis of the clinical judgement of the treating surgeon.

3. Hypersensitivity reactions and blue dye

Hypersensitivity reactions to anesthetics and associated agents used during the perioperative period have been reported with increasing frequency in most developed countries. Their estimated incidence ranges between 1 in 5000 to 1 in 13,000 anesthetics (Mertes et al., 2002). Although neuromuscular blocking agents, latex, and antibiotics are the leading causative agents, every substance used during the perioperative period can be responsible for an immediate hypersensitivity reaction. (Mertes et al., 2003)

The combination of isotope and blue dye is the current recommended technique for sentinel node localization in breast cancer in many countries with localization rates of over 99%. However, blue dye is associated with a range of allergic reactions. There have been a number of case reports and single case series of anaphylactic reactions following administration of patent blue V. Its allergic potential is also reflected in reports to the Committee of Safety of Medicines and to the manufacturer. No mortality has been reported but two cardio-respiratory arrests have been attributed to patent blue V (Mansel et el ., 2006; Montgomery et al., 2002).

Since the 1960s, blue dyes have been used in a variety of clinical situations, ranging from cardiac output determination (Al-Fadly et al., 1956) and lymphangiography (Biran et al., 1973) to intraoperative lymphatic mapping and sentinel lymphadenectomy in various types of neoplasms (Bilchik et al., 1998). They have long been considered a rare cause of anaphylaxis. This might in part be due to misleading nomenclature (Scherer et al., 2006). Patent BlueV (also called E131,Acid Blue 3, and disulfine blue) and isosulfan blue (also called Patent Blue violet or Lymphazurin),which belong to the group of triarylmethane dyes and share the same formula, are the most commonly used . A recent literature review that includes various names of these dyes reveals an impressive number of case reports of hypersensitivity reactions (Cimmino et al., 2001), and it has been suggested that sensitization occurs with everyday products containing blue dyes (Kalimo et al., 1981). In view of the increasing use of blue dyes for lymphatic mapping for sentinel lymph node biopsy, the incidence of anaphylaxis to these drugs can be expected to increase. Based on several retrospective and prospective studies, the estimated incidence of reactions of all grades of severity varies between 1% and 2%, with severe reactions being observed in 0.2% to 1.1% of cases (Cox et al., 2000; Montgomery et al., 2002; King et al., 2004; Albo et al., 2003; Blessinget al., 2002). In a series of 1013 patients, preoperative prophylaxis with glucocorticoids, diphenhydramine, and famotidine was found to reduce the severity but not the overall incidence of adverse reactions to dye (King et al., 2004). Similarly, a nonsignificant trend toward fewer allergic reactions with smaller volumes of blue dye has been reported (Raut et al., 2006).

The clinical diagnosis of an immediate hypersensitivity reaction during anesthesia is generally considered difficult. Many signs can be misinterpreted as an interaction between the clinical status of the patient and the drugs administered a dose-related side effect of the drugs, or excessively light anesthesia. Vigilance is essential because reactions might be well established before they are detected. Therefore information concerning the various clinical features encountered is essential, particularly when reactions caused by injected dye are considered. Indeed, the clinical diagnosis of anaphylaxis is, in fact, presumptive based on a close temporal relation with the administration of the implicated substance. This is clearly not the case for hypersensitivity reactions elicited by dyes. In general, the clinical reactions respond to the definition of an "immediate" reaction occurring within less than 1 hour after exposure, they significantly differ from those caused by neuromuscular blocking agents or antibiotics, which usually occur less than 10 minutes after intravenous administration in a sensitized patient (Mertes et al., 2003).

We recall that allergic reactions are classified into four grades (Montgomery et al, 2002):

- grade I corresponds to the cutaneous signs generalized erythema, urticaria with or without edema angioedema;
- grade II is a multi-organ damage moderate with cutaneous signs, hypotension but greater than 70 mm Hg and tachycardia unusual bronchial hyperreactivity (cough, difficulty breathing);
- grade III corresponds to a multiple organ damage severe threat ¸ ant life and requiring special treatment; collapse, tachycardia or bradycardia, heartbeat, bronchospasm. Cutaneous signs may be absent or appear after the Remon-Wu blood pressure;
- grade IV corresponds to circulatory arrest and / or respiratory.

The mechanism underlying the allergic reaction to blue dyes remains unclear. Both direct mast cell activation, basophil activation, or both and cross-linking of specific IgE antibodies are possible causative factors (Woltsche-Kahr et al., 2000).

In conclusion, the use of Patent Blue V for localization of sentinel lymph nodes is associated with a significant number of hypersensitivity reactions. Many groups around the world are doing protocols to identify a patient that will be affected with hypersensitivity reaction after the use of blue dyes (Mansel et al., 2003). Maybe, with the development of new markers with less risk, we`ll find a solution for this.

4. Sentinel lymph node biopsy: What's new?

Cancer is known to develop via a multistep carcinogenesis process. Cancer treatments are performed on the basis of clinical and pathologic staging that is determined using morphologic diagnostic tools, such as conventional radiological and histopathological examinations (Pinheiro et al., 2000). Sentinel node localization is one the most important parameters considered in cancer diagnosis and therapy. The concept of the sentinel lymph node has earned widespread importance with the advent of the sentinel lymph node biopsy technique. This technique has been explored in staging of various types of cancers to determine their spread. Recent advances in molecular, biological, and genetic diagnostic techniques have led to a considerable exploration of the sentinel lymph node diagnostic agents and modalities and their implication for the involvement of Sentinel node in development and progression of cancer.

In the last decade, methods for the precise localization of sentinel lymph node (SLN) have drawn tremendous attention by cancer surgeons and researchers in the field of medical diagnosis. The accurate identification and characterization of lymph nodes by imaging has important therapeutic and prognostic significance in patients with newly diagnosed cancers. Amongst the various exploited methods for SLN diagnosis, nanocarriers have received increasing attention as lymph node delivery agents. The present review will focus on various such particulate carriers namely radiolabeled sulfur colloids, liposomes, quantum dots, dendrimers and magnetic nanoparticles, which are most extensively studied and have been attributed with the most desirable characteristics for SLN imaging (Ratnesh et al., 2009).

Nanotechnology, one of the recent leaps in technology progress, has provided a big boost to sentinel lymph node imaging. The most important advantage of nanocarriers in this regards is their ability to enable the targeted delivery of imaging agents for specific sentinel lymph node imaging. Accurate and quick identification of Sentinel node has now been rendered as an achievable target due to the advances in nanotechnology. For example, the use of Quantum dots (Chan et al., 2002), potentially allows rapid and accurate sentinel lymph node localization. sentinel lymph node imaging using several types of nanocarriers has been investigated and systematic investigation of these carriers is a need of the hour. Quantum dots have been used as fluorescent imaging agents for the in vivo imaging of sentinel lymph node. Conjugation of Quantum dots with biomolecules, including peptides and antibodies, has been used to target tumors in vivo. Quantum dots have also been employed to identify metastatic cancer cells, quantitatively measure the level of specific molecular targets and guide targeted cancer therapy by providing biodynamicmarkers for target inhibition.

Amongst the other nanocarriers explored, dendrimers have displayed long circulating positive contrast enhancement by MRI/ NIR imaging in various animal models (Bellin et al., 1998). These investigations suggest the possibility of utilizing a labeled MRI/NIR optical hybrid contrast agent containing nanocarrier for sentinel lymph node imaging. Recent animal studies with targeted nanobubbles (Dayton et al., 2001) for lymph node imaging and therapy have exhibited a significantly improved therapeutic efficacy of these carriers when compared with the nontargeted nanoparticles. This nanocarrier formulation offers the advantage of providing real-time reports of the treatment by means of ultrasound imaging since the nanocarrier contains both the imaging as well as the therapeutic agent.

The development of multifunctional nanoparticles may contribute significantly to the localization of sentinel lymph node in multiple types of cancer. Ideally, for constructing multifunctional nanoparticles, an appropriate combination of agents (imaging agent and targeting moiety) will have to be chosen, based on accurate biological information within the tumor and lymph node with imaging material attached on the nanoparticle surface (Forsberg et al., 2001). Nanoparticles may eventually be capable of detecting sentinel lymph node, pinpointing and visualizing their location in the body (real-time in vivo imaging). This advancement may eventually lead to complete elimination of cancerous cells identified by accurate sentinel lymph node localization. Several types of nanocarriers have been evaluated to identify their potential for sentinel lymph node imaging.

Despite all the new initiatives in the sentinel lymph node biopsy, it was never published a novel marker derived from blood for replacing the blue dye (Pinheiro et al., 2009), a member of the current gold standard with the technetium.

During the management of two patients submitted to breast biopsy in our service, we observed their skin mapped as the lymphatic ducts draining to axillary lymph nodes (Photo 1).

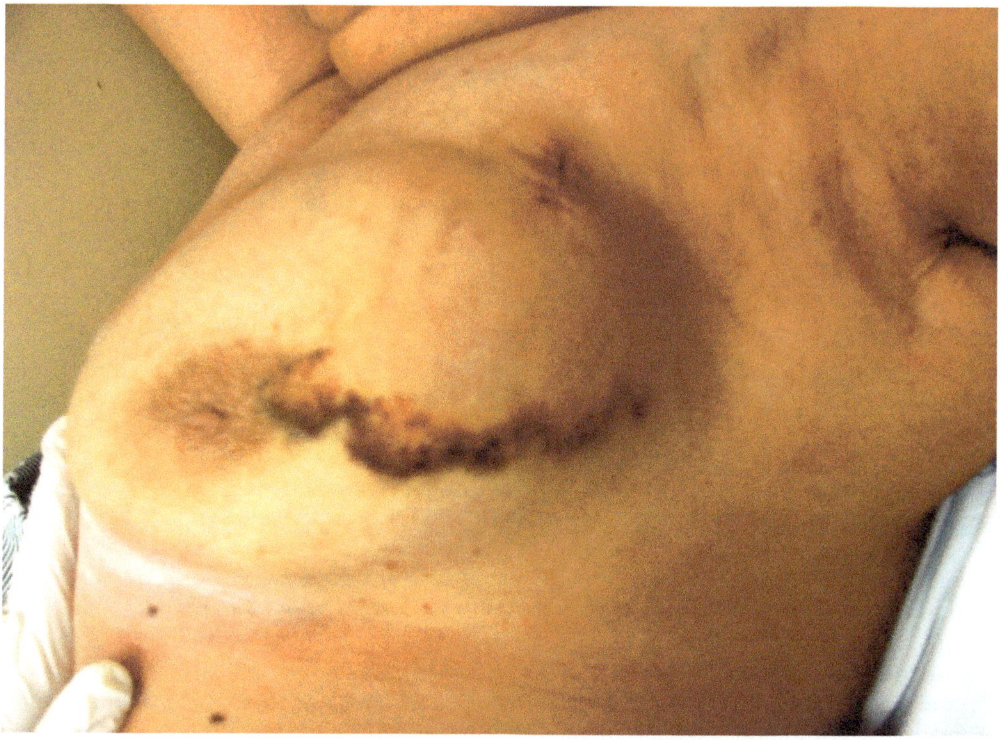

Photo 1. Skin mapped as a lymphatic duct in direction to the axilla

This observation stimulated us to try an animal model which was described for our group. Our theory was that some blood derivate (hemosiderin) was captured by macrophages and accessed the lymphatic duct in direction to the axilla.
In bid to replicate what was seen in patients, we developed an experimental protocol for obtaining a marker derived from blood and tested in a model of experimental surgery in dogs (Photo 2).

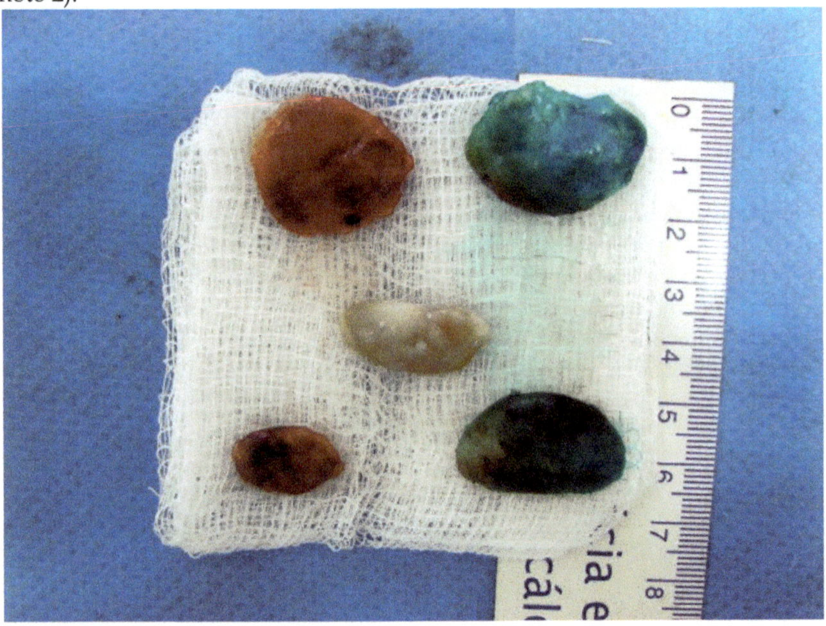

Photo 2. Sentinel lymph nodes marked with hemosiderin at left and with patent blue at right. Non-sentinel lymph node in the middle.

We found statistically significant and consistent data when comparing the group that underwent patent blue / technetium versus the group undergoing autologous blood-derived marker / technetium (Pinheiro et al., 2010).
The results of our experimental work showed that the blood derivate (hemosiderin) was capable of being used along with the radiomarker (technetium 99m) and coloring wonderfully the sentinel lymph node of female dogs.
The use of the blood derivate (hemosiderin) with the radiomarker also showed equal results comparing the use of the patent blue with the radiomarker in identifying the mammary sentinel lymph nodes of the female dog because they were always found in both axillas.
The hemosiderin, a blood-derived marker, theoretically does not cause side effects as allergic reactions. Besides, it may decrease personal and healthcare spendings, reduce the morbidity of the procedure and the emotional suffering, along with other indirect vantages.

4.1 Lipossomes

Liposomes have been used as delivery vehicles since the 1960s and their use for the delivery of imaging agents, for all imaging modalities, has a long history. Liposomes are defined as vesicles in which an aqueous volume is entirely surrounded by a phospholipid membrane.

They can vary in size from 30 nm to several micrometers, and can be uni- or multilamellar. Their properties have been extensively investigated and can vary substantially with respect to their size, lipid composition, surface charge, and method of preparation.

Currently, liposomes are one of the most widely explored nanocarriers for delivering imaging agents to the SLNs. Many imaging agents can be covalently or non-covalently incorporated into the different compartments of these nanocarriers. Also, they can be designed to encapsulate a wide range of hydrophilic agents (dyes, drugs etc) within their aqueous interior. They also serve as promising lymphoscintigraphic agents since their surface can easily be modified by attaching or coating with specific receptors or other molecules such as polyethylene glycol (PEG) for selective targeting. The relative efficiency of entrapment of imaging materials into these nanocarriers has been established. Liposomes have also been used for cellular labeling of contrasting agents such as iron oxide nanoparticles to facilitate enhanced imaging. Literature also reports loading of liposomes with gamma-emitters and other radionuclides as well as specific receptor targeting ligands for application in various imaging modalities to facilitate diagnostic imaging of liver, spleen, brain, cardio-vascular system, tumors, inflammation and infection.

Liposomal carriers for lymph node drug delivery were first investigated by Segal et al., where an intratesticular injection of liposomes, encapsulating the anticancer drug actinomycin D, was carried out. Lymph node imaging using 99mTc-labeled liposomes was first performed by Obsorne et al. Although several clinical studies were performed soon after these initial attempts and reported promising results, the use of 99mTc-liposomes for lymphoscintigraphy was questioned in an article by Patel et al. in 1984. In this report the stability of the 99mTc-liposome complex as well as the integrity of the liposomes with in the lymph nodes was put under surveillance.

The early liposome involving imaging studies employed stannous chloride as a reducing agent to associate reduced 99mTc with the liposomal surface. This labeling method was subsequently shown to be unstable in vivo and lead to the development of more effective liposome labeling methods. Another major drawback which hampered the successful liposome targeting to the SLN was the lack of effective preoperative staining of regional lymph nodes to improve their intraoperative identification and thus the selectivity of 'sentinel node' lymphadenectomy. Unfortunately the most commonly used staining agent, blue dye, used in these early trials failed to provide the requisite intensity and duration of contrast, for enhanced imaging.

Since then several attempts have been made by researchers all over the world towards the development stable and effective liposome/99mTc-liposome based SLN imaging agents to tackle the afore-mentioned problems. One of these early development trials by Hirnle et al. utilized blue dye-encapsulated liposomes to localize the SLNs during surgery.

With this technique, it was studied that following the injection of the blue liposomes into the lymphatic vessels, the lymph nodes were stained blue. Most notably, retroperitoneal lymph nodes in rabbits remained dark blue up to 28 days after the hind limb endolymphatic instillation of liposomal blue dye. Promising results of these studies further paved a way to human trials, in which blue liposomes were injected directly into the lymphatic vessels of the foot of a patient prior to retroperitoneal staging-lymphadenectomy. Twenty four hours after the intralymphatic injection of the blue liposomes, when a surgery was performed, the lymph nodes were well stained with the blue dye and were readily visualized.

These investigations proved the potential of liposomes as promising carriers for SLN imaging. However, the relatively low retention of liposomes in lymph nodes led to further investigations to improve this limitation.

4.2 Dendrimers

Dendrimers are perfectly cascade-branched, highly defined macromolecules, characterized by a combination of high end group functionality and compact molecular structures. The two major strategies of dendrimer synthesis in laboratories were initiated back in the year 1979.

The first method process included outward branching of an initiator core by a sequence of iterative reactions resulting in a three-dimensional organization of terminal groups. Fréchet et al. established the second process, known as the convergent growth process, which progressed inward from what would seem as a dendronmolecular surface to a reactive focal point at the root. The reaction of several, resulting reactive dendrons with a multifunctional core resulted in the formation of a dendrimer structure. The first dendrimer family, which was synthesized by structuring concentric shells of dendritic β-alanine units around a central initiator core, was the PAMAM (polyamidoamine) dendrimers.

These core–shell dendrimers grew linearly in diameter as additional shells/generations were added to their architecture. At the same time, at each generation, the surface groups underwent exponential amplification based on the dendritic-branching mathematics. Progression of this process over a few generations resulted in the formation of 'geometrically closed' nanostructure with guest–host container characteristics. Research over the years has resulted in the production and characterization of fifty such other dendrimer families, possessing interiors of varying compositions such as carbon, nitrogen, silicon, sulfur, phosphorus or metals. The architectural diversity of these nanostructures resulted in their application in biomedical functions including diagnostic imaging. Distinctive sizes, well defined structural design and the abundance of reactive and accessible peripheral functional groups were some of the features of this family of diagnostic vehicles which captured the interest of imaging experts. Other noteworthy features desirable for these applications included: structural control over size and shape of imaging-agent cargo space; biocompatibility; non-toxicity of the polymer/pendant functionality employed; nanoscale-vehicles and/or scaffolding properties with high imaging-agent capacity; lack of immunogenicity; appropriate cellular adhesion; endocytosis and intracellular trafficking to allow imaging in the cytoplasm or nucleus; acceptable bioelimination or biodegradation; minimal nonspecific cellular and blood-protein binding properties; ease of consistent, reproducible, clinical grade synthesis.

In view of these valuable traits, several research groups have been actively engaged in designing dendrimers for diagnostic applications.

Dendrimers bearing GdIII complexes are being used as imaging agents in magnetic resonance imaging. Pioneering work in this area has been carried out byWeiner et al. This research group has reported dendrimer-based GdIII chelates consisting of polyamidoamine (PAMAM) dendrimers of generations 2 (G2) and 6 (G6), and possessing 12 and 192 reactive terminal amines, respectively, conjugated to the chelating ligand 2-(4-isothiocyanatobenzyl)-6-methyldiethylenetria minepentaacetic acid (DTPA), through a thiourea linkage.

In vivo experiments on rabbits have revealed that intravenous injections of larger dendrimer conjugates provides enhanced circulation times of these structures of greater than 100min thus resulting in excellent MRI images of the blood vessels. Another interesting area of research included the construction of DNA dendrimers which were synthesized by sequential hybridizations of partially complementary heteroduplexes (DNA monomers). After each generation, the structure was fixed by a crosslinking step. These DNA dendrimers were employed for high sensitivity detection of oligonucleotides since numerous radioactive or fluorescent labels could be tagged subsequent to the modification of the terminal polynucleotide strands. Such DNA dendrimers with capacity of selective recognition of specific RNA strands have been employed as selective markers of the Epstein–Barr virus in post transplant patients. Polynucleotide dendrimers labeled with fluorescent tags have also been proved as promising tools in DNA microarray technology for signal amplification in high-throughput functional genomic analysis.

Rapid diagnosis of genetic and pathogenetic diseases has been made possible by dendrimer-based biosensors for DNA hybridization. The single-stranded oligonucleotides immobilized on these structures specifically hybridize with their complementary target sequence. Also PAMAM dendrimers loaded with 111 In or 153 Gd complexes have been used as the anchoring vehicles for highly specific, radiolabeled monoclonal antibodies. In yet another study, the dendrimer arms were tagged with dye molecules which upon hybridization with a complementary fluorescently labeled DNA strand, generated energy transfer to provide enhanced imaging.

The first dual purpose dendrimers loaded with MRI-fluorescent imaging agents were described by Talanov et al. where PAMAM dendrimers were covalently attached to GdIII-DTPA chelates and units of the NIR fluorescent dye, Cy 5.5. In these systems, the bifunctional DTPA derivative, 2-(4-isothiocyanatobenzyl)-6-methyldiethylenetriaminepentaacetic acid (1B4M-DTPA) was chosen as the sequestering agent for GdIII , whereas the cyanine dye, Cy 5.5, was included to facilitate NIR imaging. These systems resulted in clear magnetic resonance and fluorescence images of the SLN(s). These dendrimers resulted in enhanced optical imaging, despite their powerful enhancement in the NIR, thus allowing the node localization through the skin. The blurred imaging by OI was taken care of by MRI which enabled the visualization of the node as well as its associated lymphatic channel. The superficial location of the node, in this study, resulted in the visualization of both the afferent and efferent lymphatic channels in the fluorescent image of the surgically exposed tissues. The research clearly demonstrates the immense potential of dendrimers as a platform for the development of efficient imaging agents for both magnetic resonance and optical imaging modalities.

Parallel work on the development of such dual mode dendrimers has also been reported by Koyama et al. where they have described the successful synthesis and utilization of dual labeled MRI/NIR optical hybrid contrast dendrimers for reoperative and intraoperative localization of SLNs. Yet another application of dendrimers in diagnostics is their application in dynamic MR lymphangiography. Gd-labeled dendrimer-based imaging agents have been used in mice models to detect the location of the SLN as well as to diagnose the presence or absence of metastatic cancer. Waldmann et al. have shown PAMAM-G6 dendrimers to be one of the best MRI imaging agents since they provide high concentrations of GdIII within the node, even in the presence of lymph node metastases.

These dendrimers exhibited most rapid and intense enhancement as compared to the other lymphatic agents tested. This utility of G6 dendrimers for lymphatic draining tumors opens up yet another avenue of their application for regional lymph nodes. However the widespread use of G6 dendrimers is limited due to certain drawbacks.

For instance their application may be restricted in overt lymphatic metastases, where the metastases can obstruct lymphatic flow, leading to collateral lymphatic circulation, and thus prevent the dendrimers from entering into the SLN.

Another limitation is that since the GdIII concentrations within the lymph nodes are estimated based on both phantom studies and T1 measurements, it could not be accurately calculated based on relaxivity in the lymph node tissue. Since the tissue in the lymph node is not as homogenous as serum phantoms, this non-homogeneity was found to change the relaxivity of G6 and affect the T1 signal intensity due to susceptibility artifacts. However, since the values obtained with two different methods were nearly consistent, these MRI methods were deemed to provide a close estimation to the actual concentrations of GdIII within the lymph nodes, although the validation of this estimationwas found to be difficult in case of the lymph node specimens, which were too small to be resected and accurately weighed. The study thus revealed that the PAMAM-G6 Gd dendrimer not only provided excellent opacification of SLNs but also acted as potential carriers for targeted SLN therapy.

Intensive research in the area of dendrimers as a potential tool for SLN imaging has thus revealed that certain pervasive biological patterns and biomimicry have played a distinctive role in the development of many biomedical applications for dendrimers. Research in this area has gained a huge momentum and around 3000 papers and patents about dendrimers as biomedical tools have been published in just last 5 years. The structural preciseness and control, reproducible and convenient size scale and comparable physico-chemical properties as that of globular proteins, antibodies and enzymes support the potential application of these tools in diagnostic imaging, particularly SLN imaging. This gamut of unique diagnostic properties offered by the dendrimers, along with their possible application in proteomics, clearly indicates their huge potential in the development of new biomedical devices and approaches for the detection and treatment of human diseases.

4.3 Quantun dots

Quantum dots (QDs) are nearly spherical semiconductor particles with diameters between 2-8 nm and containing roughly 200-10,000 atoms. They are generally composed of atoms from group II and VI elements (e.g. CdSe and CdTe) or group III and V elements (e.g. InP and InAs) of the periodic table. The semiconducting nature and the size-dependent fluorescence of these nanocrystals have rendered them an extremely attractive approach for use in optoelectronic devices, biological detection, and also as fundamental prototypes for the study of colloids and the size-dependent properties of nanomaterials.

QDs provide a new class of biomarkers that could overcome the limitations of conventional diagnostics. Thus their application as luminescent imaging probes has significantly increased in the recent times.

When compared to the currently employed diagnostic techniques, QD based detection is rapid, easy and cost effective. The unique properties which make them ideal for use in diagnostics, include intense and stable fluorescence for a longer time; resistance to photobleaching, large molar extinction coefficients and highly sensitive detection due to their ability to absorb and emit light very efficiently. Due to their large surface area-to-volume ratio, a single QD can be conjugated to various molecules, thus making QDs appealing for employment in the fabrication of more complex and multifunctional nanostructures.

QDs have been covalently linked to a variety of biomolecules such as antibodies, peptides, nucleic acids and other ligands for fluorescence probing applications. Some of the applications of QDs in biology along with their tremendous potential for in vivo molecular imaging have already been explored. One of the greatest advantages which makes them suitable for imaging in living tissues is that their emission wavelengths can be tuned throughout the near-infrared spectrum by adjusting their composition and size, resulting in photostable fluorophores that are stable in biological buffers.

One of the first in vivo applications of quantum dots included mapping of the reticuloendothelial system (RES) and localization of SLNs. Fluorescence imaging provided a simple optical readout, a higher resolution as well as a wider dynamic range than dye absorption or scientigraphy techniques. For exposed tissues, the localization capability and sensitivity by QDs were found to be potentially better than those obtained by either visible dyes or radioactives, especially when using near-infrared emission. This could be attributed to the good tissue penetration and lowered background in the infrared offered by QDs.

Near-infrared (NIR) fluorescent QDs have been used for SLN mapping and resection. NIR light, otherwise invisible to the human eye, provides extremely high signal-to-background ratios without changing the look of the surgical field. A thorough discussion of the use of NIR light in biomedical imaging has been published previously.

With a suitable intraoperative imaging system, the NIR QDs provided several advantages for SLN mapping which included high sensitivity, real-time and simultaneous visualization of both surgical anatomy and lymphatic flow and non-radioactive detection. Kim et al. explored the possibility of employing NIR QDs emitting at 850 nm for SLN mapping. In this investigation, QDs injected intradermally into live mice were followed in real-time even up to 1 cm below the skin in the SLN. A series of 3D MR lymphangiograms recorded at 24 min after injecting G6 nano-size contrast agents. Possible accumulation of high concentrations of Gd(III) within the nodes as indicated by the phantom having 400 and 800 ppm of Gd(III) of the G6 agent.

In yet another study in pigs, the quantum dots were introduced into the lungs as a method of finding the SLN draining from lung cancer. The lymph node draining from the lung was rapidly identified. This rapid SLN identification using a non-radioactive method was thought to attribute a significant advantage to the method.

Various studies have been carried out for exploring the application of different materials that could be used in the fabrication of either the QD surface or core. Quantum dots with a core/shell/shell structure consisting of an alloyed core of InAsxP1-x, an intermediate shell of InP, and an outer shell of ZnSewere developed by Kimet al. Here, the cores contained a zinc blend structure for all compositions and exhibited a tunable emission in the NIR region. The first shell of InP was instrumental for bringing about a red-shift and subsequent increase in quantum yield, while the final shell of ZnSe stabilized the system for applications in aqueous environments, including NIR biomedical fluorescence imaging. This NIR-emitting core/shell/shell In AsxP1-x/InP/ZnSe was successfully used in SLN mapping experiments in various animal models.

In a recent study, PEG-coated quantum dots with terminal carboxyl, amino, or methoxyl groups have been used for SLN imaging. After injection, these quantum dots were shown to rapidly migrate to SLNs. At least two nodes could usually be defined when their passage from the tumor through lymphatics to adjacent nodes was visualized dynamically through the skin. Also, imaging studies performed during necropsy confirmed the confinement of quantum dots to the lymphatic system and thus proved them to be effective markers of SLN pathology.

Several studies have been carried out to determine the in vivo fate of QDs. In one such investigation, within minutes of intradermal injection into female SKH-1 hairless mice, the highly UV fluorescent QDs could be observed moving from the injection sites, through the lymphatic duct system to the regional lymph nodes. These results indicated the potential of sentinel organs as effective locations for monitoring the transdermal penetration of these systems.

All these investigations have led to the emergence of QDs as technological conjectures with characteristics that could greatly improve SLN imaging and detection. However future concerted efforts are required in this promising area of research. Some of the important considerations which could be focused in future studies include: 1. Overcoming the possibility of toxicity from the heavy metal, particularly cadmium, which forms a major component of these systems. Toxicology investigations including their distribution, excretion, metabolism, pharmacokinetics, and pharmacodynamics would be imperative for the development of novel and more effective QDs for application in SLN imaging and beyond. 2. Combining quantum dot fluorescence imaging with other noninvasive techniques (e.g., scientigraphy, MRI, or PET) would allow mapping of deep nodes and more detailed information about SLN. 3. Quantum dots conjugated to appropriate ligands and fluorescing at different wavelengths could be explored to localize metastases in SLNs. 4. Development of biocompatible QDs with specificity may be explored to avoid their nonspecific organ uptake and RES scavenging. They could thus provide a better clinical option for effective imaging of SLN. 5. Optimizing the size, shape, and surface chemistry of QDs may lead to the development of novel QDs with enhanced and specific applications.

4.4 Nanoparticles

Nanoparticles have now been developed as widely used diagnostic agents in medicine. They possess unique features that can be exploited to suit the various imaging modalities. Many types of nanoparticles exhibit significant retention, sometimes as high as 40%, in the first lymph node that they encounter during their movement from the injection site. This makes them ideal system for enhanced identification and localization of SLNs. Various studies had been reported for SLN imaging using different types of nanoparticles.

4.4.1 Radiopharmaceutical colloidal nanoparticles

Radiopharmaceutical colloidal preparations were developed soon after World War II. In 1955, Hultborn et al. reported the preoperative use of interstitial colloidal gold injections in breast cancer patients. With future investigations, 99mTc was introduced as a replacement for radioactive gold since it is readily available, inexpensive and has ideal imaging and dosimetry characteristics when compared to the latter. The standard radiopharmaceutical nanoparticles range in size from 10 nm to 1000 nm and are clinically approved for use as imaging agents.

However, numerous other radiopharmaceuticals have also been reported for this purpose which include 99mTc-labeled dextran, 99mTc hydroxy ethyl starch, 99mTc human serum albumin (HSA) and several labeled colloids, including gold-198-colloid, 99mTc stannous phytate, 99mTc antimony trisulfide colloid, 99mTc rhenium colloid and 99mTc colloidal albumin. However, none of these entirely fulfill the desired criteria of an ideal imaging agent. The search for an optimal nanoparticulate radiopharmaceutical is still in progress. The most essential requirement for SLN detection is that, the developed colloids should

move to the SLN with minimal further migration. However most of these nanoparticulate systems are not ideal agents for the detection of the SLN, due to the retention of the majority of the injected dose at the peritumoral site of injection.
Studies in animals have demonstrated a very low clearance with less than 5% of the injected dose being cleared from the site of injection within the first 60 min and less than 2% of the injected dose accumulated in the SLN at 60 min. The resulting low intensity of the 99mTc activity frequently makes the SLN localization difficult, either by imaging or with a handheld detector probe used in surgery. Filtered particles have been used for greatermovement although there is still a debate as to whether filtered particles are better than standard particles due to the possible loss of imaging agents during filtration.
The retention of nanoparticles in the first lymph node is mainly due to phagocytosis of the nanoparticles by macrophages. The total retention in the sentinel node is higher than the retention in the subsequent draining lymph nodes, since only a very small fraction of nanoparticles encountered in various studies led to the introduction of radioactive technetium-99m-sulfur colloid particles (99mTc-SC) particles as yet another method to localize the SLN in addition to the blue dye being conventionally used by the surgeons. The use of 99mTc-SC, in addition to blue dye resulted in a significant improvement in the quality of image over, that obtained by the use of blue dye alone. The blue dye was not well retained in the SLN and moved very rapidly, thus creating a difficulty for the surgeons to distinguish the sentinel node from the secondary lymph nodes. This problem was solved by the additional use of 99mTc-SC which proved to be a better marker of the sentinel node. Although the blue dye provided the desired visual guide for the surgeon, the inclusion of 99mTc-SC provided the desired verification that the correct lymph node was biopsied. As the imaging could be performed in the operating room prior to and during the surgery, it frequently led to a smaller operative incision and decreased the time span required for locating the sentinel node. The use of radiolabeled nanocolloids along with the blue dye thus proved to be complementary imaging agents which performed the best when used simultaneously.

4.4.2 Magnetic nanoparticles

The application of magnetic nanoparticles in combination with the other imaging modalities is gaining a major momentum in diverse areas of biology and medicine. Unlike many of the newer probes used in the field molecular imaging, the magnetic nanoparticles are chemically similar to a large number ofmaterials with a long history of clinical use.
Magnetic nanoparticles consist of a core of superparamagnetic iron oxide (usuallymagnetite, $Fe3O4$, ormaghemite, γ-$Fe2O3$) and are coated with a biocompatible polymer, and to this basic design, biomolecules are attached. Polymer-coated iron oxides have been used in the treatment of iron anemias since the 1960s.
Magnetic nanoparticles can be broadly categorized into two basic types namely the polymer coated and the molecularly targeted. Polymer-coated magnetic nanoparticles are those that are not designed to be recognized by a specific biomolecule (e.g. receptor, antigen). "Molecularly targeted" magnetic nanoparticles are those that are designed to bind to a specific target, typically by the attachment of a biomolecule (antibody, peptide, polysaccharide). Dextran-coated magnetic nanoparticles (SPIOs) were first introduced for hepatic imaging. Following the intravenous injection, these particles have been reported to be rapidly taken up by the liver Kupffer cells and appear hypointense or black on the MR

images. Subsequently ultra-small magnetic nanoparticles (often referred as USPIOs) were developed, that displayed a longer blood half-life, and were taken up by the macrophages including those in lymph nodes.

Superparamagnetic particles (USPIOs) find preferential application in SLN imaging, due to the fact that they behave non-magnetically when they are not under the influence of an external magnetic field, thus preventing undesired magnetic agglomeration. To further assist in preventing agglomerations, to optimize bio-interactions with the host environment and to maximize biocompatibility, the choice of appropriate surface chemistries and functionalizations is also important. Different surface modifications have been reported to accommodate these characteristics in to the magnetic nanoparticles. These include tuning the particle size in the size range 3–30 nm with the particles displaying an ellipsoidal shape. A comprehensive characterization of such particles has been reported by Jolivet et al.

USPIO enhanced magnetic resonance imaging (MRI) is now being used as a potential biomarker for the diagnosis of lymph node metastases. USPIOs are transported into the interstitial space and reach the SLN via the lymphatic circulation, acting as 'negative imaging' agents due to T2- and T2-weighted sequences, which can potentially identify the metastases independent of the lymph node size. However, reports also indicate that this predominant effect of USPIOs on the T2 relaxation time does not prevent the use of their properties for the T1 relaxation time when appropriate imaging sequences are chosen [150–154]. USPIO nanoparticles are disseminated to the lymph nodes by two discrete pathways: a) USPIOs move into the medullary sinuses of the lymph node through venules via direct transcapillary passage, followed by phagocytosis by macrophages, b) USPIOs move into the interstitial space in the body through endothelial transcytosis, followed by uptake of the nanoparticles by draining lymphatic vessels and transport to the lymph nodes via afferent lymphatic channels. USPIOs with minor macrophage uptake and prolonged blood half-life have been shown to be useful for metastatic lymph node imaging.

Various studies have shown that USPIO particles taken up by the macrophages are transported to the interstitial spaces and subsequently to the lymph node via the lymph vessels. Thus healthy lymph node tissues produce a dark signal with a T2/T2 sequence since they are rich in macrophages which phagocytose the USPIOs. However, no such contrast modification is observed in the metastatic lymph node tissue which lacks the presence of macrophages, thus facilitating the effective imaging of this tissue. Additionally, the prolonged blood half-life of USPIOs allows their progressive access to the lymph nodes thus helping in further enhancement of the quality of image which can be procured.

Nodal disease is a self-determining adverse prognostic aspect in many types of cancers. By and far, measurement of the node size by means of imaging is the only widely established method for assessing this nodal involvement. In this regards, the superparamagnetic agents have raised immense attention because normal nodes posses high affinity towards these agents following intravenous or subcutaneous injection. The first agent, and also the most explored one is ferumoxtran-10. Numerous studies on ferumoxtran-10 have demonstrated its efficacy in metastatic lymph node imaging in various types of cancer with significant results being reported especially in case of breast cancer.

Early results with ferumoxtran-10 MRI in breast cancer showed a sensitivity of 78%, a specificity of 96% and a negative predictive value of 97%. The SLN procedure in breast cancer has a 3%–10% false negative rate; furthermore, positive internal mammary lymph nodes are missed in 17%. Finally, the SLN is the only positive node in 61% lymph node positive patients. These patients all undergo axillary dissection, with subsequent high rate of clinically significant lymph edema. The high negative predictive value in patients with a negative ferumoxtran-10 MRI thus exhibits a possibility that axillary dissection may potentially be avoided [163]. Further studies are required to confirm the potential use of these nanoparticles in SLN localization.

Apart from the above discussed nanoparticulate systems, a variety of studies have been reported for SLN localization with various other types of magnetic nanoparticles. In one of the studies, SLN mapping of the stomach cancer has been reported using fluorescent magnetic nanoparticles (FMNP). Here the use of these nanoparticles was found to overcome problems such as unpredictable lymphatic drainage patterns and skipmetastases which are of common occurrences in these cancers and which limit the available imaging techniques for their precise diagnosis. Biocompatible silica-overcoated magnetic nanoparticles containing rhodamine B isothiocyanate (RITC) within a silica shell of controllable thickness of about 60 nm have also been used in some of the studies.

In another study, Surguladze et al. have reported novel magnetic nanoparticles, UNIMAG, for SLN imaging. UNIMAG represents a magnet-sensitive stable suspension of magnetite nanoparticles (magnetic fluid). After the peritumoral injection of UNIMAG, the magnetite nanoparticles have been proposed to be absorbed by the macrophages,which deliver themthrough the lymphatic capillaries to regional lymph nodes. This mechanism of magnetite nanoparticle transport is responsible for the SLN detection. As compared to the other dyestuff agents used in this direction, magnetite nanoparticles were found to actively fill the lymphatic nodes and colored them in bold black. This significantly facilitated the atraumatic separation of the lymph nodes during lymphadenectomy. Besides the intraoperative indication of lymphatic nodes, UNIMAG also provided the possibility of X-ray and ultrasound imaging of SLNs and the possibility of performing their biopsy in the preoperative period. Despite these promising results, there are several problems associated with the use of magnetic nanoparticles. These limitations include (i) the possibility of embolization of the blood vessels in the target region due to accumulation of the magnetic carriers, (ii) difficulties in scaling up from animal models due to the larger distances between the target site and the magnet, and (iii) toxic responses to the magnetic carriers. However, recent pre-clinical and experimental results indicate that there is still a possibility of overcoming these limitations and use the magnetic nanoparticles to provide enhanced imaging simultaneously handling the safety issues.

4.5 Ultrasound nanobubbles

Particulate agents are important for the regional lymph node contrast enhancement following their subcutaneous administration.

These agents appear to traverse the endothelium of the peripheral lymphatics with subsequent localization in regional draining lymph nodes. Like other particulate nanocarriers, nanobubbles have been attempted for the ultrasound contrast enhancement of the regional lymph nodes. Nanobubble is a novel nanocarrier currently being widely investigated for the localization of the sentinel lymph node.

Nanobubbles combine properties of polymeric drug carriers, ultrasound imaging imaging agents, and enhancers of ultrasound mediated drug delivery. In biological fluids and tissues, nanobubbles are efficient reflectors of sound. Ultrasound is the most common biomedical imaging modality and ultrasound imaging agents are used to increase the reflectivity or backscatter of blood and tissues.

Nanobubbles either comprise perfluorocarbon nanodroplets stabilized by walls made of biodegradable block copolymers or bilayered shell of albumin and an inner layer of a biodegradable polymer known as polycaprolactone. This shell encapsulates a gas such as nitrogen. Following their subcutaneous injection, these nanobubbles are tracked using ultrasound imaging.

In a study carried out in dogs for comparing the activity of microbubbles with that of sub-micron nanobubbles, the nanobubbles were found to bemore effective in detecting the sentinel nodes. In this study these nanobubbles were injected subcutaneously into normal dogs to target the cervical and popliteal lymph nodes. First-order (sentinel) lymph nodes and second-order sublumbar nodes were imaged intermittently from 0 h to at least 2 h following the contrast injection using continuous power Doppler mode. To confirm the lymphatic drainage patterns and sentinel lymph nodes of nanobubbles, lymphoscintigraphy studies were performed in dogs. Approximately 94% (30 of the 32) sentinel nodes were detected during this study.

This nanobubble technology could serve as an alternative method for detecting the sentinel lymph node. This approach is also unique in that the use of ultrasound to detect the bubbles also causes the bubbles to break apart and formsmaller bubbles. It has been proposed that jets released from these nanobubbles following exposure to high-frequency ultrasound could be used to nanoinject drugs into cells. As these nanobubbles can also carry drugs, they could be used to deliver high levels of drugs to lymph nodes which could be rapidly released following insonation. However, concerns have been expressed that the energy released during this procedure lead to thermal tissue damage and thus harmful bioeffects and further investigations to verify these possible problems, are required in order to facilitate the introduction of a safe imaging modality.

5. References

Pinheiro, L.G.P. ; Oliveira Filho, R.S. ; Vasques, P.H.D. ; Filgueira, P.H.O. ; Aragão, D.H.P.; Barbosa, P. M. E. ; Beserra, H.E.O. ; Cavalcante, R.V. Hemosiderin: a new marker for sentinel lymph node identification. Acta Cirurgica Brasileira (Impresso), v. 24, p. 432/06, 2009.

Holland JF, Frei E, Kufe DW, Bast RC. Principles of Medical Oncology 6th ed. Philadelphia: Saunders, 2001.

Parkin DM, Bray FI, Devesa SS. Cancer burden in the year 2000. The global picture. Eur J Cancer. 2001; 37:64-66.

Instituto Nacional do Câncer. Estimativas da incidência e mortalidade por câncer no Brasil em 2008. [cited 2009 April 12]. Available from: URL: http://www.inca.gov.br/estimativa/2008/index.asp

Moore MP, Kinne DW. Is axillary lymph node dissection necessary in the routine management of breast cancer? Yes. Important Adv Oncol. 1996; 12:245-50.

Morton DL, Ollila DW. Critical review of the sentinel node hypothesis. Surgery. 1999; 126:815-9.

Cabanas RM. An approach for the treatment of penile carcinoma. Cancer. 1977; 39(2):456-66.

Veronesi U, Paganelli G, Niale G, Galimberti V, Luini A, Zurrida S, et al. Sentinel lymph node biopsy and axillary dissection in breast cancer: results in a large series. J Natl Cancer Inst. 1999; 91:368-73.

Morton DL, Wen DR, Wong JH, Economou JS, Cagle LA, Storm FK, et al. Technical details of intraoperative lymphatic mapping for early stage melanoma. Arch Surg. 1992; 127:392-9.

Giuliano AE, Kirgan DM, Guenther JM, Morton DL. Lymphatic mapping and sentinel lymphadenectomy for breast cancer. Ann Surg. 1994; 220:391-401.

Krag DN, Weaver DL, Alex JC, Fairbank JT. Surgical resection and radiolocalization of the sentinel lymph node in breast cancer using a gamma probe. Surg Oncol. 1993; 2:335-9.

Pinheiro LGP, Moraes MO, Soares AH, Lopes AJT, Naguére MASP, Gondim FAL, et al. Estudo Experimental de Linfonodo sentinela na mama da cadela com azul patente e tecnécio 99. Acta Cirurgica Brasileira. 2003; 18(6):545-552.

Mertes PM, Malinovsky JM, Mouton-Faivre C, Bonnet-Boyer MC, Benhaijoub A, Lavaud F, et al. Anaphylaxis to dyes during the perioperative period: reports of 14 clinical cases. J Allergy Clin Immunol. 2008; 122:348-52.

Salhab M, Al Sarakbi W, Mokbel K. Skin and fat necrosis of the breast following methylene blue dye injection for sentinel node biopsy in a patient with breast cancer. Int Semin Surg Oncol. 2005; 2:26.

Sleth JC. Un accident anaphylactoïde imputé au bleu patenté. Faut-il changer de colorant? Ann Fr Anesth Reanim. 2008; 27:515.

Mulan MH, Deacock SJ, Quiney NF, Kissin MW. Anaphylaxis to patent blue dye during sentinel lymph node biopsy for breast cancer. Eur J Surg Oncol. 2001; 27: 218-9.

Scherer K, Studer W, Figueiredo V, Bircher AJ. Anaphylaxis to isosulfan blue and cross-reactivity to patent blue V: case report and review of the nomenclature of vital blue dyes. Ann Allergy Asthma Immunol. 2006; 96: 497–500.

Wohrl S, Focke M, Hinterhuber G, Stingl G, Binder M. Near-Fatal Anaphylaxis to Patent Blue V. Br J Dermatol. 2004; 150:1037-8.

M. Hamoudeh, M.A. Kamleh, R. Diab, H. Fessi, Radionuclides delivery systems for nuclear imaging and radiotherapy of cancer, Adv. Drug Deliv. Rev. 60 (2008) 1329–1346.

A.D. Bangham, M.M. Standish, J.C. Watkins, Diffusion of univalent ions across the lamellae of swollen phospholipids, J. Mol. Biol. 13 (1965) 238–252.

H.E.Wang,H.M. Yu, Y.C. Lu,N.N.Heish, Y.L. Tseng, K.L.Huang, K.T. Chuang, C.H. Chen, J.J. Hwang,W.J. Lin, S.J.Wang, G. Ting, P.J. Whang,W.P. Deng, Internal radiotherapy and dosimetric study for 111In/177Lu-pegylated liposomes conjugates in tumor bearing mice, Nucl. Instrum. Methods, A 569 (2) (2006) 533–537.

W.T. Phillips, R. Klipper, B. Goins, Use of (99m)Tc-labeled liposomes encapsulating blue dye for identification of the sentinel lymph node, Nucl. Med. 42 (2001) 446–451.

T.A. Elbayoumi, V.P. Torchilin, Enhanced accumulation of long-circulating liposomes modified with the nucleosome-specific monoclonal antibody 2C5 in various tumours in mice: gamma-imaging studies, Eur. J. Nucl.Med.Mol. Imaging 33 (2006) 1196–1205.

S. Dagar, A. Krishnadasa, I. Rubinstein,M.J. Blend, H. Önyüksel, VIP grafted sterically stabilized liposomes for targeted imaging of breast cancer: in vivo studies, J. Control. Release 91 (2003) 123–133.

V.P. Torchilin, Surface-modified liposomes in γ and MR imaging, Adv. Drug Deliv. Rev. 24 (1997) 301–313.

A.W. Segal, G. Gregoriadis, C.D. Black, Liposomes as vehicles for the local release of drugs, Clin. Sci. Mol. Med. 49 (1975) 99–106.

M.P. Osborne, V.J. Richardson, K. Jeyasingh, B.E. Ryman, Radionuclide-labelled liposomes—a newlymphnode imaging agent, Int. J.Nucl.Med.Biol. 6 (1979) 75–83.

H.M. Patel, K.M. Boodle, R. Vaughan-Jones, Assessment of the potential uses of liposomes for lymphoscintigraphy and lymphatic drug delivery. Failure of 99m- technetiumto represent intact liposomes in lymph nodes, Biochim. Biophys. Acta 801 (1984) 76–86.

G.M. Barratt, N.S. Tuzel, B.E. Ryman, The labeling of liposomal membranes with radioactive technetium, in: G. Gregoriadis (Ed.), Liposome Technology, vol. 2, CRC Press, Boca Raton, FL, 1984, pp. 94–105.

P. Laverman, E. Dams,W. Oyen, G. Storm, E. Koenders, R. Prevost, J. van derMeer, F. Corstens, O. Boerman, A novel method to label liposomes with 99mTc by the hydrazino nicotinyl derivative, J. Nucl. Med. 40 (1999) 192–197.

C. Tilcock, Q.F. Ahkong, D. Fisher, 99mTc-labeling of lipid vesicles containing the lipophilic chelator PE-DTPA: effect of tin-to chelate ratio, chelate content and surface polymer on labeling efficiency and biodistribution behavior, Nucl. Med. Biol. 21 (1994) 89–96.

P. Hirnle, R. Harzmann, J.K. Wright, Patent blue V encapsulation in liposomes: potential applicability to endolympatic therapy and preoperative chromolym phography, Lymphology 21 (1988) 187–189.

B. Pump, P. Hirnle, Preoperative lymph-node staining with liposomes containing patent blue violet. A clinical case report, J. Pharm. Pharmacol. 48 (1996) 699–701.

W.T. Phillips, R. Klipper, B. Goins, Novel method of greatly enhanced delivery of liposomes to lymph nodes, Pharmacol. Exp. Ther. 295 (2000) 309–313.

L.A.Medina, S.M. Calixto, R. Klipper,W.T. Phillips, B. Goins, Avidin/biotinliposome system injected in the pleural space for drug delivery to mediastinal lymph nodes, J. Pharm. Sci. 93 (2004) 2595–2608.

L.A. Medina, R. Klipper,W.T. Phillips, B. Goins, Pharmacokinetics and biodistribution of [111ln]-avidin and [99mTc]-biotin-liposomes injected in the pleural space for the targeting of mediastinal nodes, Nucl. Med. Biol. 31 (2004) 41–51.

E.M. Plut, G.H. Hinkle, W. Guo, R.J. Lee, Kit formulation for the preparation of radioactive blue liposomes for sentinel node lymphoscintigraphy, J. Pharm. Sci. 91 (2002) 1717–1732.

M. Dieter, R. Schubert, P. Hirnle, Blue liposomes for identification of the sentinel lymph nodes in pigs, Lymphology 36 (2003) 39–47.

V.P. Torchilin, Recent advances with liposomes as pharmaceutical carriers, Nat. Rev., Drug Discov. 4 (2005) 145–160.

S. Stiriba, H. Frey, R. Haag, Dendritic polymers in biomedical applications: from potential to clinical use in diagnostics and therapy, Angew. Chem., Int. Ed. Engl. 41 (2002) 1329–1334.

D.A. Tomalia, H. Baker, J.R. Dewald,M. Hall, G. Kallos, S.Martin, J. Roeck, J. Ryder, P. Smith, A new class of polymers: starburst-dendritic macromolecules, Polym. J. 17 (1985) 117–132.

V.J. Venditto, C.S. Regino, M.W. Brechbiel, PAMAM dendrimer based macro molecules as improved contrast agents, Mol. Pharmaceutics 2 (2005) 302–311.

J.M. Fréchet, M. Henni, I. Gitsov, S. Aoshima, M.R. Leduc, R.B. Grubbs, Self-condensing vinyl polymerization: an approach to dendritic materials, Science 269 (1995) 1080–1083.

R. Esfand, D.A. Tomalia, Poly (amidoamine) (PAMAM) dendrimers: from biome 1351 micry to drug delivery and biomedical applications, Drug Discov. Today 6 (2001) 1352 427–436.

V.S. Talanov, C.A. Regino, H. Kobayashi, M. Bernardo, P.L. Choyke, M.W. Brechbiel, Dendrimer-based nanoprobe for dual modality magnetic resonance and fluorescence imaging, Nano Lett. 6 (2006) 1459–1463.

E.C.Wiener,M.W. Brechbiel, H. Brothers, R.L.Magin, O.A. Gansow, D.A. Tomalia, P.C. Lauterbur, Dendrimer-based metal chelates: a new class of magnetic resonance imaging contrast agents, Magn. Reson. Med. 31 (1994) 1–8.

R.H.E. Hudson, M. Damha, Nucleic acid dendrimers: novel biopolymer structures, J. Am. Chem. Soc. 115 (1993) 2119–2124.

Y. Koyama, V.S. Talanov, M. Bernardo, Y. Hama, C.A.S. Regino, M.W. Brechbiel, P.L. Choyke, H. Kobayashi, A dendrimer-based nanosized contrast agent dual-labeled for magnetic resonance and optical fluorescence imaging to localize the sentinel lymph node in mice, J. Magn. Reson. Imaging 25 (2007) 866–871.

H. Kobayashi, S. Kawamoto, Y. Sakai, P.L. Choyke, R.A. Star,M.W. Brechbiel, N. Sato, Y. Tagaya, J.C. Morris, T.A. Waldmann, Lymphatic drainage imaging of breast cancer in mice by micro-magnetic resonance lymphangiography using a nano size paramagnetic contrast agent, J. Natl. Cancer Inst. 96 (2004) 703–708.

H. Kobayashi, S. Kawamoto, P.L. Choyke, N. Sato, M.V. Knopp, R.A. Star, T.A. Waldmann, Y. Tagaya, M.W. Brechbiel, Comparison of dendrimer-based macromolecular contrast agents for dynamic micromagnetic resonance lymphangiography, Magn. Reson. Med. 50 (2003) 758–766.

A.P. Alivisatos, Semiconductor clusters, nanocrystals, and quantum dots, Science 271 (1996) 933–937.

M. Bruchez, M. Moronne, P. Gin, S. Weiss, A.P. Alivisatos, Semiconductor nanocrystals as fluorescent biological labs, Science 281 (1998) 2013–2016.

S. Liu, C.M. Lee, S. Wang, D.R. Lu, A new bioimaging carrier for quantum dot nanocrystals – phospholipid nanoemulsion mimicking natural lipoprotein core, Drug Deliv. 13 (2006) 159–164.

B. Dubertret, P. Skourides, D.J. Norris, V. Noireaux, A.H. Brivanlou, A. Libchaber, In vivo imaging of quantum dots encapsulated in phospholipid micelles, Science 298 (2002) 1759–1762.

X. Gao,Y. Cui, R.M. Levenson, L.W. Chung, S.Nie, Invivo cancer targeting and imaging with semiconductor quantum dots, Nat. Biotechnol. 22 (2004) 969–976.

W.C.W. Chan, S. Nie, Quantum dot bioconjugates for ultrasensitive nonisotopic detection, Science 281 (1998) 2016–2018.

W.C.W. Chan, D.J.Maxwell, X. Gao, R.E. Bailey,M. Han, S. Nie, Luminescent QDs for multiplexed biological detection and imaging, Curr. Opin. Biotechnol. 13 (2002) 40–46.

M. Han, X. Gao, J.Z. Su, S. Nie, Quantum dot-tagged microbeads for multiplexed optical coding of biomolecules, Nat. Biotechnol. 19 (2001) 631–635.

C.M. Niemeyer, Nanoparticles, proteins, and nucleic acids: biotechnology meets materials science, Angew. Chem., Int. Ed. Engl. 40 (2001) 4128–4158.

C.A. Leatherdale, W.K. Woo, F.V. Mikulec, M.G. Bawendi, On the absorption cross section of CdSe nanocrystal quantum dots, J. Phys. Chem. Biol. 106 (2002) 7619–7622.

B. Ballou, Quantumdot surfaces for use in vivo and in vitro, Curr. Top. Dev. Biol. 70 (2005) 103–120.

B. Ballou, B.C. Lagerholm, L.A. Ernst, M.P. Bruchez, A.S. Waggoner, Noninvasive imaging of quantum dots in mice, Bioconjug. Chem. 15 (2004) 79–86.

S. Kim, Y.T. Lim, E.G. Soltesz, A.M. De Grand, J. Lee, A. Nakayama, J.A. Parker, T. Mihaljevic, R.G. Laurence, D.M. Dor, L.H. Cohn,M.G. Bawendi, J.V. Frangioni, Near infrared fluorescent type II quantum dots for sentinel lymph node mapping, Nat. Biotechnol. 22 (2004) 93–97.

B. Ballou, L.A. Ernst, A.S.Waggoner, Fluorescence imaging of tumors in vivo, Curr. Med. Chem. 12 (2005) 795–805.

J.V. Frangioni, In vivo near-infrared fluorescence imaging, Curr. Opin. Chem. Biol. 7 (2003) 626–634.

Y.T. Lim, S. Kim, A. Nakayama,N.E. Stott,M.G. Bawendi, J.V. Frangioni, Selection of QD wavelengths for biomedical assays and imaging, Mol. Imaging 2 (2003) 50–64.

A. Nakayama, F. Del Monte, R.J. Hajjar, J.V. Frangioni, Functional near-infrared fluorescence imaging for cardiac surgery and targeted gene therapy,Mol. Imaging 1 (2002) 365–377.

A.M. De Grand, J.V. Frangioni, An operational near-infrared fluorescence imaging system prototype for large animal surgery, Technol. Cancer Res. Treat. 2 (2003) 553–562.

X.Michalet, F.F. Pinaud, L.A. Bentolila, J.M. Tsay, S. Doose, J.J. Li, G. Sundaresan, A.M. Wu, S.S. Gambhir, S. Weiss, Quantum dots for live cells, in vivo imaging, and diagnostics, Science 307 (2005) 538–544.

S. Kim, J.P. Zimmer, S. Ohnishi, J.B. Tracy, J.V. Frangioni,M.G. Bawendi, Engineering InAsxP1-x/InP/ZnSe III-V alloyed core/shell quantum dots for the near-infrared, J. Am. Chem. Soc. 127 (2005) 10526–10532.

B. Ballou, L.A. Ernst, S. Andreko, T. Harper, J.A.J. Fitzpatrick, A.S. Waggoner, M.P. Bruchez, Sentinel lymph node imaging using quantum dots in mouse tumor models, Bioconjug. Chem. 18 (2007) 389–396.

N.V. Gopee, D.W. Roberts, P.Webb, C.R. Cozart, P.H. Siitonen, A.R.Warbritton,W.W. Yu, V.L. Colvin, N.J. Walker, P.C. Howard, Migration of intradermally injected quantum dots to sentinel organs in mice, Toxicol. Sci. 98 (2007) 249–257.

A.M. Derfus, W.C.W. Chan, S.N. Bhatia, Probing the cytotoxicity of semiconductor quantum dots, Nano Lett. 4 (2004) 11-18.

R. Hardman, A toxicologic review of quantum dots: toxicity depends on physicochemical and environmental factors, Environ. Health Perspect. 114 (2006) 165–172.

A. Hoshino, K. Fujioka, T. Oku,M. Suga, Y.F. Sasaki, T. Ohta,M. Yasuhara, K. Suzuki, K. Yamamoto, Physicochemical properties and cellular toxicity of nanocrystal quantum dots depend on their surface modification, Nano Lett. 4 (2004) 2163–2169.

R. Jain et al. / Journal of Controlled Release 138 (2009) 90–102[120] C. Kirchner, T. Liedl, S. Kudera, T. Pellegrino, A. Munoz Javier, H.E. Gaub, S. Stolzle, N. Fertig, W.J. Parak, Cytotoxicity of colloidal CdSe and CdSe/ZnS nanoparticles, Nano Lett. 5 (2005) 331-338.

S.M. Moghimi, A.E. Hawley, N.M. Christy, T. Gray, L. Illum, S.S. Davis, Surface engineered nanospheres with enhanced drainage into lymphatics and uptake by macrophages of the regional lymph nodes, FEBS Lett. 344 (1994) 25–30.

K.A. Hultborn, L.G. Larsonn, I. Ragnhult, The lymph drainage from the breast to the axillary and parasternal lymph nodes studied with the aid of colloidal Au 198, Acta. Radiol. 43 (1955) 52–63.

J. Weinberg, E.M. Greaney, Identification of regional lymph nodes by means of vital staining dye during surgery of gastric cancer, Surg. Gynecol. Obstet. 90 (1950) 561–567.

D.L.Morton, D.R.Wen, J.H.Wong, J.S. Economou, L.A. Cagle, F.K. Storm, L.J. Foshag, A.J. Cochran, Technical details of intraoperative lymphatic mapping for early stage melanoma, Arch. Surg. 127 (1992) 392–399.

J.C. Alex, D.N. Krag, Gamma probe guided localization of lymph nodes, Surg. Oncol. 2 (1993) 137–143.

A.J. Wilhelm, G.S. Mijnhout, E.J. Franssen, Radiopharmaceuticals in sentinel lymph-node detection – an overview, Eur. J. Nucl. Med. 26 (1999) S36–42.

J.C. Hung, G.A. Wiseman, H.W. Wahner, B.P. Mullan, T.R. Taggart, W.L. Dunn, Filtered technetium-99m-sulfur colloid evaluated for lymphoscintigraphy, J. Nucl. Med. 36 (1995) 1895–1901.

R.C.Martin 2nd,M.J. Edwards, S.L.Wong, T.M. Tuttle, D.J. Carlson, C.M. Brown, R.D. Noyes, R.L. Glaser, D.J. Vennekotter, P.S. Turk, P.S. Tate, A. Sardi, P.B. Cerrito, K.M. McMasters, University of Louisville breast cancer sentinel lymph node study, practical guidelines for optimal gamma probe detection of sentinel lymph nodes in breast cancer: results of a multi-institutional study, Surgery 128 (2000) 139–144.

C. Oussoren, G. Storm, Role of macrophages in the localisation of liposomes in lymph nodes after subcutaneous administration, Int. J. Pharm. 183 (1999) 37–41.

S.L. Focht, Lymphatic mapping and sentinel lymph node biopsy, AORN J. 69 (1999) 802–809.

A. Gradilone, D. Ribuffo, I. Silvestri, E. Cigna, P. Gazzaniga, I. Nofroni, G. Zamolo, L. Frati, N. Scuderi, A.M. Agliano̖, Detection of melanoma cells in sentinel lymph nodes by reverse transcriptase-polymerase chain reaction: prognostic significance, Ann. Surg. Oncol. 11 (2004) 983–987.

J.H.Wong, L.A. Cagle, D.L.Morton, Lymphatic drainage of skin to a sentinel lymph node in a feline model, Ann. Surg. 214 (1991) 637–641.

H.S. Cody III, J. Fey, T. Akhurst, M. Fazzari, M. Mazumdar, H. Yeung, S.D.J. Yeh, P.I. Borgen, Complementarity of blue dye and isotope in sentinel node localization for breast cancer: univariate and multivariate analysis of 966 procedures, Ann. Surg. Oncol. 8 (2001) 13–19.

D.L. Burns, E.A. Mascioli, B.R. Bistrian, Parenteral iron dextran therapy: a review, Nutrition 11 (1995) 163–168.

S.T. Callender, Treatment of iron deficiency, Clin. Haematol. 11 (1982) 327–338.

L. Josephson, Magnetic nanoparticles for MR imaging, in: M. Ferrari (Ed.), BioMEMS and Biomedical Nanotechnology, vol. 1, Springer Science, New York, 2006, pp. 227–228.

A. Moore, R. Weissleder, A. Bogdanov Jr., Uptake of dextran-coated monocrystalline iron oxides in tumor cells and macrophages, J. Magn. Reson. Imaging 7 (6) (1997) 1140–1145.

D.D. Stark, R.Weissleder,G. Elizondo, P.F.Hahn, S. Saini, L.E. Todd, J.Wittenberg, J.T. Ferrucci, Superparamagnetic iron oxide: clinical application as a contrast agent for MR imaging of the liver, Radiology 168 (1988) 297–301.

R. Weissleder, G. Elizondo, J. Wittenberg, A.S. Lee, L. Josephson, T.J. Brady, Ultrasmall superparamagnetic iron oxide: an intravenous contrast agent for assessing lymph nodes with MR imaging, Radiology 175 (1990) 494–498.

M.G. Harisinghani, J. Barentsz, P.F. Hahn, W.M. Deserno, S. Tabatabaei, C.H. van de Kaa, J. de la Rosette, R.Weissleder, Noninvasive detection of clinically occult lymph node metastases in prostate cancer, N. Engl. J. Med. 348 (2003) 2491–2499.

R.E. Rosensweig, Magnetic fluids, Sci. Am. 247 (1982) 136–145.

H. Itoh, T. Sugimoto, Systematic control of size, shape, structure, and magnetic properties of uniform magnetite and maghemite particles, Colloid Interface Sci. 265 (2002) 283–295.

O. Bomati-Miguel, M.P. Morales, P. Tartaj, J. Ruiz-Cabello, P. Bonville,M. Santos, X.Q. Zhao, S. Veintemillas-Verdaguer, Fe-based nanoparticulate metallic alloys as contrast agents for magnetic resonance imaging, Biomaterials 26 (2005) 5695–5703.

R. Vijayakumar, Y. Koltypin, I. Felner, A. Gedanken, Sonochemical synthesis and characterization of pure nanometer-sized Fe304 particles, Mater. Sci. Eng., A 286 (2000) 101–105.

R.M. Cornell, U. Schwertmann, The Iron Oxides. Structure, Properties, Reactions, Occurrence and Uses, VCH, Weinheim, Germany, 1996, pp. 344–345.

E. Tronc, J.P. Jolivet, Surface effects on magnetically coupled gamma-Fe2O3 colloids, Hyperfine Interact. 28 (1986) 525–528.

E. Tronc, D. Fiorani, M. Nogues, A.M. Testa, F. Lucari, F. D'Orazio, J.M. Greneche,W. Wernsdorfer, N. Galvez, C. Chaneac, D. Mailly, J.P. Jolivet, Surface effects in noninteracting and interacting y-Fe2O3 nanoparticles, J. Magn. Magn. Mater. 262 (2003) 6–14.

E.D. Parker, V. Dupuis, F. Ladieu, J.P. Bouchaud, E. Dubois, R. Perzynski, E. Vincent, Spin-glass behavior in an interacting γ-Fe2O3 nanoparticle system, Phys. Rev., B 77 (2008) 104428.

J.L. Dormann, L. Dormann, L. Spinu, E. Tronc, J.P. Jolivet, F. Lucari, F. D'Orazio, D. Fiorani, Effect of interparticle interactions on the dynamical properties of y-Fe203 nanoparticles, J. Magn.Magn. Mater. 183 (1998) L255–L260.

S. Saini, D.D. Stark, P.F. Hahn, J. Wittenberg, T.J. Brady, J.T. Ferrucci Jr., Ferrite particles: a superparamagnetic MR contrast agent for the reticulo endothelial system, Radiology 162 (1987) 211–216.

A. Hemmingsson, J. Carlsten, A. Ericsson, J. Klaveness, G.O. Sperber, K.A. Thuomas, Relaxation enhancement of the dog liver and spleen by biodegradable superparamagnetic particles in proton magnetic resonance imaging, Acta. Radiol. 28 (1987) 703–705.

J.T. Ferrucci, D.D. Stark, Iron oxide-enhanced MR imaging of the liver and spleen: review of the first 5 years, AJR Am. J. Roentgenol. 155 (1990) 943–950.

A. Chachuat, B. Bonnemain, European clinical experience with Endorem. A new contrast agent for liver MRI in 1000 patients, Radiologe 35 (1995) S274–S276.

P. Reimer, B. Tombach, Hepatic MRI with SPIO: detection and characterization of focal liver lesions, Eur. Radiol. 8 (1998) 1198–1204.

C. Corot, P. Robert, J.M. Idee, M. Port, Recent advances in iron oxide nanocrystal technology for medical imaging, Adv. Drug Deliv. Rev. 58 (2006) 1471–1504.

M. Ferrari, Cancer nanotechnology: opportunities and challenges, Nat. Rev., Cancer 5 (2005) 161–171.

Q.A. Pankhurst, J. Connolly, S.K. Jones, J. Dobson, Applications of magnetic nanoparticles in biomedicine, J. Phys., D, Appl. Phys. 36 (2003) R167–R181.

J. Dobson, Magnetic nanoparticles for drug delivery, Drug Dev. Res. 67 (2006) 55–60.

M.G. Harisinghani, J. Barentsz, P.F. Hahn, W.M. Deserno, S. Tabatabaei, C. Hulsbergen van de Kaa, J. De la Rosette, R. Weissleder, Noninvasive detection of clinically occult lymph-node metastases in prostate cancer, N. Engl. J. Med. 348 (2003) 2491–2499.

J.M. Rogers, J. Lewis, L. Josephson, Visualization of superiormesenteric lymph nodes by the combined oral and intravenous administration of the ultra-small superparamagnetic iron oxide AMI-227, Magn. Reson. Imaging 12 (1994) 1161–1165.

Y. Anzai, S. McLachlan, M. Morris, R. Saxton, R.B. Lufkin, Dextran-coated superparamagnetic iron oxide an MR contrast agent for assessing lymph nodes in the head and neck, Am. J. Neuroradiol. 15 (1994) 87–94.

M.F. Bellin, C. Roy, K. Kinkel, D. Thoumas, S. Zaim, D. Vanel, C. Tuchmann, F. Richard, D. Jacqumin, A. Delcourt, E. Challier, T. Lebret, P. Cluzel, Lymph node metastases: safety and effectiveness of MR imaging with ultrasmall superparamagnetic iron oxide particles—initial clinical experience, Radiology 207 (1998) 799–808.

S.C.A.Michel, T.M. Keller, J.M. Fröhlich, D. Fink, R. Caduff, B. Seifert, B.Marincek, R. Kubik-Huch, Preoperative breast cancer staging: MR imaging of the axilla with ultrasmall superparamagnetic iron oxide enhancement, Radiology 225 (2002) 527–536.

J.S. Kim, T.J. Yoon, H.K. Kim, S.S. Kim, H.S. Chae,M.G. Choi, Y.J. Kim, G.C. Yi, Y.S. Cho, Sentinel lymph node mapping of the stomach using fluorescent magnetic nanoparticles in rabbits, Korean J. Gastroenterol. 51 (2008) 19–24.

G.B. Surguladze, R. Zhorzoliani, T. Tskitishvili, Novel method of sentinel lymph node detection in malignant tumors using preparation 'UNIMAG', Breast Cancer Res. 9 (2007) P15.

C. Chambon, O. Clément, A. Le Blanche, E. Schouman-Claeys, G. Frija, Superparamagnetic iron oxides as positive MR contrast agents: in vitro and in vivo evidence, Magn. Reson. Imaging 11 (1993) 509–519.

E. Canet, D. Revel, R. Forrat, C. Baldy-Porcher, M. de Lorgeril, L. Sebbag, J.P. Vallee, D. Didier, M. Amiel, Superparamagnetic iron oxide particles and positive enhancement for myocardial perfusion studies assessed by subsecond T1-weighted MRI, Magn. Reson. Imaging 11 (1993) 1139–1145.

F. Forsberg, W.T. Shi, Physics of contrast microbubbles, in: B.B. Goldberg, J.S. Raichlen, F. Forsberg, Martin Dunitz (Eds.), Ultrasound Contrast Agents: Basic Principles and Clinical Applications, 2001, pp. 15–24.

P.A. Dayton, J.E. Chomas, A.F. Lum, J.S. Allen, J.R. Lindner, S.I. Simon, K.W. Ferrara, Optical and acoustical dynamics of microbubble contrast agents inside neutrophils, Biophys. J. 80 (2001) 1547–1556.

E.C. Unger, T.O. Matsunaga, T. McCreery, P. Schumann, R. Sweitzer, R. Quigley, Therapeutic applications of microbubbles, Eur. J. Radiol. 42 (2002) 160–168.

F. Robert, M.D. Mattrey, M.D. Yuko Kono, K. Baker, T. Peterson, Sentinel lymph node imaging with microbubble ultrasound contrast material, Acad. Radiol. 9 (2002) S231–S235.

N. Rapoport, Z. Gao, A. Kennedy, Multifunctional nanoparticles for combining ultrasonic tumor imaging and targeted chemotherapy, J. Natl. Cancer Inst. 99 (2007) 1095–1106.

F. Yang, A. Gu, Z. Chen, N. Gu, M. Ji, Multiple emulsion microbubbles for ultrasound imaging, Mater. Lett. 62 (2008) 121–124.

Z. Gao, A.M. Kennedy, D.A. Christensen, N.Y. Rapoport, Drug-loaded nano/ microbubbles for combining ultrasonography and targeted chemotherapy, Ultrasonics 48 (2008) 260–270.

N. Rapoport, K.H. Nam, Z. Gao, D.A. Cristensen, A.M. Kennedy, Acoustic properties of multifunctional nanomicrobubbles used in ultrasonography and ultrasound-mediated chemotherapy, J. Acoust. Soc. Am. 123 (2008) 3217.

E.R. Wisner, K.W. Ferrara, R.E. Short, T.B. Ottoboni, J.D. Gabe, D. Patel, Sentinel node detection using contrast-enhanced power Doppler ultrasound lymphography, Invest. Radiol. 383 (2003) 58–65.

M. Postema, A.V.Wamel, C.T. Lancee, N.D. Jong, Ultrasound-induced encapsulated microbubble phenomena, Ultrasound Med. Biol. 30 (2004) 827–840.

P.A. Dijkmans, Microbubbles and ultrasound: from diagnosis to therapy, Eur. J. Echocardiog. 5 (2004) 245–256.

E. Stride, N. Saffari, The potential for thermal damage posed by microbubble ultrasound contrast agents, Ultrasonics 42 (2004) 907–913.

Hung WK, et al.: Randomized clinical trial comparing blue dye with combined dye and isotope for sentinel lymph node biopsy in breast cancer. Br J Surg 92: 1494–1497, 2005.

Goyal A, Douglas-Jones AG, Newcombe RG, Mansel RE: Effect of lymphatic tumor burden on sentinel lymph node biopsy in breast cancer. Breast J 11: 188–194, 2005.

Cox CE, et al.: Age and body mass index may increase the chance of failure in sentinel lymph node biopsy for women with breast cancer. Breast J 8: 88–91, 2002.

Derossis AM, Fey JV, Cody HS III, Borgen PI: Obesity influences outcome of sentinel lymph node biopsy in early-stage breast cancer. J Am Coll Surg 197: 896–901, 2003.

Birdwell RL, et al.: Breast cancer: variables affecting sentinel lymph node visualization at preoperative lymphoscintigraphy. Radiology 220: 47–53, 2001.

Goyal A, et al.: Sentinel lymph node biopsy in male breast cancer patients. Eur J Surg Oncol 30: 480–483, 2004.

Permissions

The contributors of this book come from diverse backgrounds, making this book a truly international effort. This book will bring forth new frontiers with its revolutionizing research information and detailed analysis of the nascent developments around the world.

We would like to thank Susan J. Done, for lending his expertise to make the book truly unique. He has played a crucial role in the development of this book. Without his invaluable contribution this book wouldn't have been possible. He has made vital efforts to compile up to date information on the varied aspects of this subject to make this book a valuable addition to the collection of many professionals and students.

This book was conceptualized with the vision of imparting up-to-date information and advanced data in this field. To ensure the same, a matchless editorial board was set up. Every individual on the board went through rigorous rounds of assessment to prove their worth. After which they invested a large part of their time researching and compiling the most relevant data for our readers. Conferences and sessions were held from time to time between the editorial board and the contributing authors to present the data in the most comprehensible form. The editorial team has worked tirelessly to provide valuable and valid information to help people across the globe.

Every chapter published in this book has been scrutinized by our experts. Their significance has been extensively debated. The topics covered herein carry significant findings which will fuel the growth of the discipline. They may even be implemented as practical applications or may be referred to as a beginning point for another development. Chapters in this book were first published by InTech; hereby published with permission under the Creative Commons Attribution License or equivalent.

The editorial board has been involved in producing this book since its inception. They have spent rigorous hours researching and exploring the diverse topics which have resulted in the successful publishing of this book. They have passed on their knowledge of decades through this book. To expedite this challenging task, the publisher supported the team at every step. A small team of assistant editors was also appointed to further simplify the editing procedure and attain best results for the readers.

Our editorial team has been hand-picked from every corner of the world. Their multi-ethnicity adds dynamic inputs to the discussions which result in innovative outcomes. These outcomes are then further discussed with the researchers and contributors who give their valuable feedback and opinion regarding the same. The feedback is then collaborated with the researches and they are edited in a comprehensive manner to aid the understanding of the subject.

Apart from the editorial board, the designing team has also invested a significant amount of their time in understanding the subject and creating the most relevant covers. They scrutinized every image to scout for the most suitable representation of the subject and create an appropriate cover for the book.

The publishing team has been involved in this book since its early stages. They were actively engaged in every process, be it collecting the data, connecting with the contributors or procuring relevant information. The team has been an ardent support to the editorial, designing and production team. Their endless efforts to recruit the best for this project, has resulted in the accomplishment of this book. They are a veteran in the field of academics and their pool of knowledge is as vast as their experience in printing. Their expertise and guidance has proved useful at every step. Their uncompromising quality standards have made this book an exceptional effort. Their encouragement from time to time has been an inspiration for everyone.

The publisher and the editorial board hope that this book will prove to be a valuable piece of knowledge for researchers, students, practitioners and scholars across the globe.

List of Contributors

Alfred O. Mueck, Harald Seeger and Hans Neubauer
University Women's Hospital, Tübingen, Germany

Zhor Bouizar
U676 INSERM, Hôpital Robert Debré AP-HP, Paris Université Paris Diderot, Paris, France

Jan Baumann, Christopher Karch, Antonis Kourtidis and Douglas S. Conklin
University at Albany, State University of New York, USA

Becuwe Philippe
Henri Poincaré's University-Nancy, France

Pengcheng Fan and Yu Wang
Department of Pharmacology and Pharmacy, The University of Hong Kong, Hong Kong SAR, China

Ming-Ta Hsu
Institute of Biochemistry and Molecular Biology, VGH-YM Genome Center, National Yang-Ming University, Taipei, Taiwan

Ching Cheng and Ming-Ta Hsu
Institute of Biochemistry and Molecular Biology, National Yang-Ming University, Taipei, Taiwan

Chian-Feng, Chen and Ming-Ta Hsu
VGH-YM Genome Center, National Yang-Ming University, Taipei, Taiwan

Chien-Yi Tung and Chi-Hung Lin
Institute of Microbiology and Immunology, National Yang-Ming University, Taipei, Taiwan

Yiin-Jeng Jong, Yann-Jang Chen, Sheng Wang-Wuu, Ling-Hui Li and Shih-Feng Tsai
Institute of Genome Sciences, National Yang-Ming University, Taipei, Taiwan

Mei-Hua Tsou, Skye H. Cheng, Chii-Ming Chen and Andrew T. Huang
Koo Foundation Sun Yat-Sen Cancer Center, Taipei, Taiwan

Nisha Kanwar and Susan Done
Department of Laboratory Medicine and Pathobiology, University of Toronto, Campbell Family Institute for Breast Cancer Research, University Health Network, Toronto, Canada

Hsiu-Chuan Chou
Department of Applied Science, National Hsinchu University of Education, Hsinchu, Taiwan

Hong-Lin Chan
Institute of Bioinformatics and Structural Biology and Department of Medical Science, National Tsing Hua University, Hsinchu, Taiwan

Chu Khoi, Zaiming Ye, Annie Z. Luo, Kimberly M. Boley, Moishia C. Wright, Erik M. Freiter and Fredika M. Robertson
The Department of Experimental Therapeutics, The University of Texas M.D. Anderson Cancer Center, Houston, TX, USA

Fredika M. Robertson
The Morgan Welch Inflammatory Breast Cancer Research Program, The University of Texas MD Anderson, Cancer Center, Houston, TX, USA
The University of Texas Graduate School of Biomedical Sciences, Houston, TX,USA

Rita Circo
Istituto Superiore di Sanità, Rome, Italy

Rita Circo, Julia Wulfkuhle, Emanuel F. Petricoin and Lance A. Liotta
The Center for Applied Proteomics and Molecular Medicine, George Mason University, Manassas, VA, USA

Savitri Krishnamurthy
The Department of Pathology, The University of Texas M.D. Anderson Cancer Center, Houston, TX, USA

Sanford H. Barsky
The Department of Pathology, The University of Nevada School of Medicine, Reno NV and The Nevada Cancer Institute, Las Vegas, NV, USA

Massimo Cristofanilli
The Department of Medical Oncology, Fox Chase Cancer Center, Philadelphia, PA, USA

Amal T. Qattan and Jasminka Godovac-Zimmermann
Molecular Cell Dynamics, Division of Medicine, University College London, UK

Michel Eisenblätter Thorsten Persigehl and Carsten Höltke
Dept. of Clinical Radiology, University Hospital Münster, Germany

Christoph Bremer
Dept. of Radiology, St. Franziskus Hospital Münster, Germany

Tadaharu Matsunaga
Nagumo Clinic, Japan

Fan-Lin Kong and David J. Yang
Department of Experimental Diagnostic Imaging, University of Texas MD Anderson Cancer Center, Houston, Texas, USA

Andrew B. Jackson, Lauren B. Retzloff, Prasant K. Nanda and C. Jeffrey Smith
University of Missouri Department of Radiology, Columbia, MO, United States of America

Pornchai Phukpattaranont, Somchai Limsiroratana, Kanita Kayasut and Pleumjit Boonyaphiphat
Prince of Songkla University, Thailand

Chenbo Zeng, Jinbin Xu and Robert H. Mach
Department of Radiology, USA

Robert H. Mach
Department of Cell Biology and Physiology, USA
Department of Biochemistry and Molecular Biophysics, Washington University School of Medicine, St. Louis, MO, USA

Arutselvan Natarajan
Department of Radiology, Stanford University, California, USA

Senthil Kumar Venugopal
Institute of Liver and Biliary Sciences, New Delhi, India

Teruhiko Fujii, Hiroki Takahashi and Yuka Inoue
Breast Care Center, Clinical Research Institute, National Hospital Organization Kyushu Medical Cancer, Japan

Teruhiko Fujii, Hiroki Takahashi and Kazuo Shirouzu
Department of Surgery, Kurume University, Japan

Teruhiko Fujii and Masayoshi Kage
Center for Innovative Cancer Therapy, Kurume University, Japan

Masayoshi Kage
Department of Pathology, Kurume University, Japan

Hideaki Yamana
Multidisciplinary Treatment Center, Kurume University, Japan

Hargita Hegyesi, Nikolett Sándor, Boglárka Schilling-Tóth and Géza Sáfrány
Frédéric Joliot-Curie National Research Institute for Radiobiology and Radiohygiene, Hungary

James R. Lambert
Department of Pathology, University of Colorado, Anschutz Medical Campus, Aurora, CO, USA

L.G. Porto Pinheiro and P.H.D. Vasques
Department of Surgery, Faculty of Medicine, UFC, Fortaleza - Ceará, Brazil

M. Maia
Biochemistry, Laboratory for experimental surgery, Saul Goldenberg MD, Fortaleza - Ceará, Brazil

J.I.X. Rocha and D.S. Cruz
Faculty of Medicine, UFC, Fortaleza - Ceará, Brazil